BIOPSY INTERPRETATION SERIES

BIOPSY INTERPRETATION OF THE SKIN

Primary Non-Lymphoid Cutaneous Neoplasia

BIOPSY INTERPRETATION SERIES

Series Editor: Jonathan I. Epstein, MD

Interpretation of Breast Biopsies, 4th Ed.
Darryl Carter, 2002

Prostate Biopsy Interpretation, 3rd Ed.
Jonathan I. Epstein and Ximing J. Yang, 2002

Bladder Biopsy Interpretation
Jonathan I. Epstein, Mahul B. Amin, and Victor E. Reuter, 2004

Biopsy Interpretation of the Gastrointestinal Tract Mucosa
Elizabeth A. Montgomery, 2005

Biopsy Interpretation of the Upper Aerodigestive Tract and Ear
Edward B. Stelow and Stacey E. Mills, 2007

Biopsy Interpretation of the Prostate, 4th Ed.
Jonathan I. Epstein and George Netto, 2007

Biopsy Interpretation of the Breast
Stuart J. Schnitt and Laura C. Collins, 2008

Biopsy Interpretation of the Liver, 2nd Ed.
Stephen A. Geller and Lydia M. Petrovic, 2009

Biopsy Interpretation of the Uterine Cervix and Corpus
Anais Malpica, Michael T. Deavers, and Elizabeth D. Euscher, 2009

Biopsy Interpretation: The Frozen Section
Jerome B. Taxy, Aliya N. Hussain, and Anthony G. Montag, 2009

Biopsy Interpretation of the Skin
A. Neil Crowson, Cynthia M. Magro, and Martin C. Mihm, 2009

Biopsy Interpretation of the Thyroid
Scott L. Boerner and Sylvia L. Asa, 2009

Biopsy Interpretation of the Soft Tissue Tumors
Cyril Fisher and Elizabeth A. Montgomery, 2010

Biopsy Interpretation of the Bladder, 2nd Ed.
Jonathan I. Epstein, Mahul B. Amin, and Victor E. Reuter, 2010

Biopsy Interpretation of the Lung
Saul Suster and Cesar Moran, 2011

Biopsy Interpretation of the Central Nervous System
Daniel J. Brat and Matthew J. Schniederjan, 2011

BIOPSY INTERPRETATION SERIES

BIOPSY INTERPRETATION OF THE SKIN

Primary Non-Lymphoid Cutaneous Neoplasia

A. Neil Crowson, MD

Clinical Professor
Departments of Dermatology, Pathology, and Surgery
University of Oklahoma

and

Chairman, Department of Pathology,
St John Medical Center
Tulsa, Oklahoma

Cynthia M. Magro, MD

Professor of Pathology
Division of Dermatopathology
Department of Pathology
Weill Medical College of Cornell University
New York, New York

Martin C. Mihm Jr, MD

Clinical Professor
Departments of Dermatology and Pathology
Harvard Medical School
Massachusetts General Hospital
Boston, Massachusetts

Wolters Kluwer Health | Lippincott Williams & Wilkins

Philadelphia • Baltimore • New York • London
Buenos Aires • Hong Kong • Sydney • Tokyo

Senior Executive Editor: Jonathan W. Pine, Jr
Senior Manufacturing Manager: Benjamin Rivera
Senior Marketing Manager: Angela Panetta
Creative Director: Doug Smock
Production Service: Aptaracorp

530 Walnut Street
Philadelphia, PA 19106 USA
LWW.com

Printed in the People's Republic of China

Library of Congress Cataloging-in-Publication Data
Crowson, A. Neil.
Biopsy interpretation of the skin : primary non-lymphoid cutaneous neoplasia / A. Neil Crowson, Cynthia M. Magro, Martin C. Mihm Jr.
p. ; cm. – (Biopsy interpretation series)
Includes bibliographical references and index.
ISBN 978-0-7817-7205-1 (alk. paper)
1. Skin–Cancer Diagnosis. 2. Skin–Biopsy. I. Magro, Cynthia M. II. Mihm, Martin C., 1934– III. Title. IV. Series: Biopsy interpretation series.
[DNLM: 1. Skin Neoplasms–diagnosis. 2. Biopsy–methods. 3. Skin Neoplasms–pathology. WR 500 C953b 2009]

RC280.S5C76 2009
616.99'477075–dc22

2009029430

To purchase additional copies of this book, call our customer service department at (800) 638-3030 or fax orders to (301) 223-2320. International customers should call (301) 223-2300.

Visit Lippincott Williams & Wilkins on the Internet: at LWW.com. Lippincott Williams & Wilkins customer service representatives are available from 8:30 am to 6 pm, EST.

10 9 8 7 6 5 4 3 2

RRS1003

CONTENTS

PREFACE

Dermatopathology has evolved as a subspecialty discipline of anatomic pathology and of dermatology in a fashion that has reflected certain peculiar dynamics of medical practice over the last century and a half. The first dynamic is rooted in the nascent observational medical science that spawned a plethora of clinical terms applied to inflammatory dermatoses. It has been suggested that there are over 9,000 discrete dermatological entities; the diagnostic terminology that applies to them derives from eponyms, from Latin, or more recently from the native tongue of the clinician who first described an "entity," which may have merely reflected one or another reaction pattern as opposed to a distinct pathophysiological condition. In consequence, these inflammatory dermatoses have mainly, until the last few decades, fallen under the rubric of "dermatologic conditions" and have largely been the realm of clinical dermatologists. Other physicians in different specialties have found the terminology perplexing and, in the frequent absence of a unifying pathophysiologic basis, obscure. Most anatomic pathologists without specific training or expertise in dermatopathology find these conditions intimidating.

By contrast, neoplastic pathology of the skin frequently falls under the purview of general anatomic pathology. Roughly one third of the surgical pathology specimens in any given community or academic hospital are biopsy or excision specimens of the skin. The nature of referral patterns for outpatient skin biopsy specimens has meant that many anatomic pathology programs have been starved of teaching material and in many cases, in part reflecting economic pressures, expertise in the discipline has moved away from the teaching hospital environs. For these reasons, a surgical pathologist will find himself or herself in practice facing cutaneous neoplasms with the sense of less than perfect diagnostic certainty that flows from relative inexperience. Thus, this book.

Its purpose is to address the primary non-lymphoid cutaneous neoplasia. Dermatologists, and to an increasingly greater extent, plastic surgeons, oculoplastic surgeons, and general surgeons, will require ever heightening specificity of diagnosis as a guide to management. It is no longer sufficient, for example, to render a diagnosis of "basal cell carcinoma" without an attempt at subclassification that may define aggressive versus indolent biologic behavior. It is hoped that this book will contribute to a more informed standard of surgical pathology practice in community and teaching hospitals where anatomic pathologists face lesions such as those described herein on a daily basis. It is hoped as well that this book will be of interest to practicing dermatologists who find classification schemes for more obscure neoplasms, such as those of the sweat glands, to be perplexing.

A. Neil Crowson
Cynthia M. Magro
Martin C. Mihm, Jr.

CONTRIBUTORS

Raymond L. Cornelison, MD
Professor and Carl Herzog Chair
Department of Dermatology
University of Oklahoma
Tulsa, Oklahoma

A. Neil Crowson, MD
Clinical Professor
Departments of Dermatology, Pathology and Surgery
University of Oklahoma;
Chairman of Pathology,
St John Medical Center and
President, Pathology Laboratory Services,
Tulsa, Oklahoma

Henry D. Haskell
Clinical Assistant Professor
Department of Dermatology
University of Oklahoma and
Regional Medical Laboratory,
Tulsa, Oklahoma

Cynthia M. Magro, MD
Professor of Pathology Laboratory
Director of Dermatopathology
Weill Medical College of Cornell University
New York, New York

Martin C. Mihm Jr, MD
Clinical Professor
Departments of Dermatology and Pathology
Harvard Medical School
Massachusetts General Hospital
Boston, Massachusetts

Carlos N. Prieto-Granada, MD
Research Fellow,
Department of Pathology
Tufts Medical Center,
Boston, Massachusetts

Phoebe Rich, MD
Adjunct Professor
Department of Dermatology
Oregon Health Sciences University
Portland, Oregon

1

HOW AND WHEN TO BIOPSY THE SKIN

The skin is a complex organ that has a number of appendageal structures as well as different types of epidermis and dermis that vary in thickness and conformation dependant upon anatomic site, aging factors, and the influence of actinic damage. Because of these differences in various regions of the body, the decision of which biopsy technique to use depends on the area of the skin being biopsied as well as the type of lesion to be biopsied. Dermatologists and other physicians who perform skin biopsies with regularity know that it is as critically more important to decide when to biopsy as it is to know how to biopsy. Biopsies help the clinician discern the type of skin disease and/or lesion with which they are dealing. The decision to biopsy the lesion on the skin should be made only if the biopsy would be helpful to the diagnosis and provide the information needed to the clinician.

There are multiple types of biopsies of the skin that will be discussed in the text below. It is impossible in the scope of this chapter to cover every nuance, but the major biopsy techniques will be discussed in detail.

PUNCH BIOPSY

The dermal punch is a valuable tool for biopsy. Dermal punches range in size from 1 to 6 mm in diameter. Generally, every biopsy of 3 mm or more will require a sutured closure for optimal cosmetic results. However, in certain places that are highly visible, such as the face, even a 2 mm biopsy may need to be sutured for optimal results. The dermal punch consists of a plastic or metal upper portion that narrows to a small piece of about 2 mm of steel with slight narrowing near the lower end of the dermal punch just above the actual cutting portion that limits the depth of the dermal punch since it creates a shelf that will limit the depth of the biopsy. This type of biopsy is usually relatively easy and safe, but caution will be needed if the lesion being biopsied overlies an important neurological or vascular structure. In areas of the skin such as the upper back where the dermis is quite thick, it will not provide a full-thickness portion of the dermis. A punch biopsy is particularly helpful when one does not need an extensive width of tissue, but is more interested in the vertical relationship of the epidermis, dermis, and in some cases, subcutaneous tissue. This allows optimal correlation between epidermal and dermal findings. The punch biopsy is not suitable for biopsies of the subcutaneous tissue.

SHAVE BIOPSY

A shave biopsy is usually done when the skin lesion is macular or slightly elevated. This is particularly helpful in lesions where a very thin piece of tissue is needed to give an accurate histologic diagnosis. An example would be a junctional melanocytic proliferation, which shows features clinically suspicious for a melanoma. It is possible with a shave biopsy to obtain the entire specimen to give optimal tissue for the dermatopathologist to examine. Shave biopsies are generally done with a razor blade usually broken in half and slowly and carefully entering the skin just below the depth of the clinical lesion. In addition to this modality, iris scissors may be used, particularly if the lesion is elevated, to allow the scissors to remove the lesion with minimal cosmetic consequences. Some clinicians use a no. 15 blade for biopsies, but the authors find this less helpful for controlling depth and width. This biopsy technique is not used when one wants to obtain the entire specimen, and the specimen is particularly large in diameter. If this is the case, other biopsy techniques discussed below will be more appropriate.

Consistent with the cosmetic result desired, it is best to biopsy the entire lesion if possible. This is particularly important in a pigmented lesion where melanoma is suspected. A complete shave excisional biopsy of the lesion provides the dermatopathologist with an opportunity to examine not only the cytologic details of the specimen but also the architecture. It is sometimes impossible to remove the entire lesion with a shave biopsy. In such cases, the area that is clinically most suspicious should be preferentially biopsied. An example of this would be a large suspect lentigo maligna on the face. Until the diagnosis is established, it is not prudent to excise the entire lesion with a significant cosmetic defect. In such cases, the clinician should determine the most suspicious area of the lesion and preferentially sample that.

EXCISIONAL BIOPSY

An excisional biopsy is generally done when a clinician feels that it is important to remove the entire lesion for examination. These biopsies are usually done with an elliptical technique with a range of 2½ to 3 × length versus width. Almost without exception, these biopsies are closed primarily with sutures. The excisional biopsy is particularly helpful if the clinician is almost certain that a pigmented lesion is malignant. It is best if one is going to remove a pigmented lesion for biopsy purposes to excise the lesion the first time it is biopsied. There is no evidence in literature that a biopsy of a melanoma or carcinoma leads to lymphatic or vascular spread. Excisional biopsies at times may be so large that they need to be closed with a tissue transfer technique.

CURETTAGE BIOPSIES

Curettage biopsies are fragmented biopsies or surgical margins that are only useful if one does not need to particularly see the architecture of the lesion. The most common example is a curettage biopsy of a basal cell carcinoma, which, at the same time, is then further curetted and removed in its entirety. Curettage biopsies are not appropriate for infiltrative growth, morpheaform or sclerosing basal cell carcinomas, and basosquamous carcinoma. They are also not appropriate for pigmented lesion biopsies.

WEDGE BIOPSIES

Wedge biopsies are generally done for subcutaneous or deep dermal processes. The wedge biopsy allows the dermatopathologist to examine a continuum from the adjacent normal skin in continuity with the pathologic process. The wedge biopsy is generally done to include all or most of the subcutaneous layer. It is particularly helpful in lesions that are deep dermal or subcutaneous in nature on the lower extremities. It is important for the dermatopathologist to be able to compare the adjacent skin, which may show, for example, stasis changes on the lower extremities within the lesion itself, as well as the normal tissue.

BIOPSIES OF THE SCALP

When a biopsy of the scalp is being done, particularly with respect to the investigation of alopecia states, a punch biopsy of 4 to 6 mm is often used. The specimen can be sectioned both vertically and horizontally to provide maximum information about the hair follicle complex, adjacent adnexal structures, and the surrounding dermis and epidermis. A shave biopsy or excisional biopsy may be done for other abnormalities that involve the scalp.

Nail Biopsy Indications and Methods

Prerequisites for a successful nail biopsy are (i) thorough knowledge of nail anatomy, (ii) adequate anesthesia and hemostasis, (iii) proper surgical technique, and (iv) an abnormal nail caused by a neoplastic or inflammatory process. Nail biopsy is a safe procedure provided the idiosyncrasies of the nail unit are understood and the logical principles of nail surgery are followed (Table 1.1).[1–6]

The clinical features of a nail disease are determined by the location of the pathology within the nail unit. For example, nail plate dystrophy and dyschromia result from pathologic processes in the nail matrix. Nail bed changes may be visible through the nail plate and may elevate or distort the nail plate by exerting pressure from below. Inflammatory nail disorders such as psoriasis or lichen planus may have pathologic processes in the nail bed, the nail matrix, and the proximal nail fold and hyponychium.

TABLE 1.1 Biopsies of Nail Matrix, Nail Bed, and Nail Fold

Nail matrix biopsy
1. Visualize the full matrix by reflection of proximal nail fold after releasing incisions are made in the nail fold. 2. Remove or cut through the nail plate to obtain the matrix tissue beneath the proximal nail plate. 3. Orient the nail matrix specimen on a paper template so that it will be processed and sectioned in the correct orientation, especially when longitudinal sectioning is helpful with architectural features of certain nail tumors.
Nail bed biopsy
1. If the nail lesion is clearly visible through the nail plate, a punch excision through the nail plate can be performed. 2. If the lesion is not visible, avulsion of the nail plate is preferable. In some situations, it is useful to mark the location of the nail bed lesion on the nail folds prior to removal because the lesion may disappear if not carefully mapped. 3. After the lesion is removed, the nail plate may be repositioned as a biologic dressing to protect the wound and facilitate healing.
Nail fold and hyponychium biopsies
1. Specimens are taken as from other cutaneous areas.

Adequate anesthesia is crucial for patient acceptance of nail surgery. Lidocaine or bupivacaine is injected into the nail fold for a wing block. The advantages of wing block over digital block (Fig. 1.1) include (i) onset of action is more rapid, (ii) less anesthesia is used, (iii) there is less risk of inadvertently injecting into a blood vessel, and (iv) injection itself is more comfortable. Recent reports have shown that epinephrine is safe in surgery on digits and its use reduces the need for a tourniquet for hemostasis.[3,4,5]

Basic nail surgical procedures include nail avulsion followed by matrix exploration, nail matrix punch or shave biopsy, lateral longitudinal biopsy, nail bed biopsy, and nail fold biopsy. Each of these procedures has specific indications and techniques.

Nail avulsion is the basic nail procedure, which involves loosening the nail plate from its attachment to the underlying nail bed. This procedure does not result in permanent nail dystrophy.

The nail folds are biopsied using the same techniques as elsewhere on the skin. It is often useful to protect the underlying matrix by inserting a freer elevator under the nail fold prior to the excision (e-figs. 1.1–1.3).

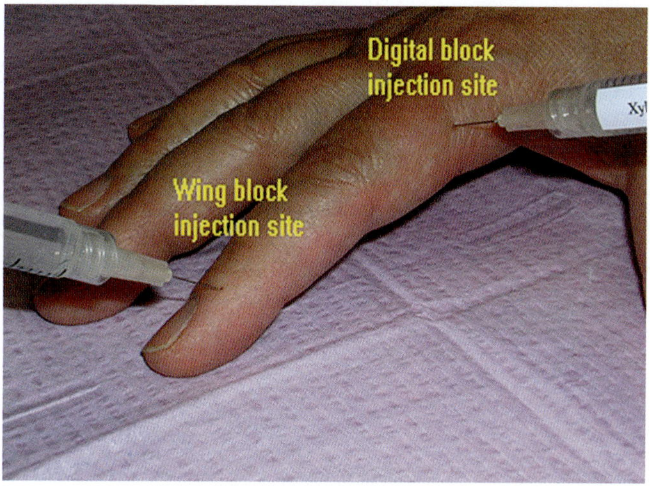

FIGURE 1.1 Location of injection of wing block.

Nail bed lesions such as glomus tumors may be removed through the nail plate with a punch biopsy or by opening a window in the nail plate, which can be replaced after the tumor is removed and will act as a biologic dressing as the new nail grows in (e-figs. 1.4–1.7).

When both the matrix and the nail bed are involved with a pathologic process, a full excision of the nail bed, nail fold, and nail matrix can be obtained. This specimen should be oriented and sectioned in a longitudinal plane so that the various structures of the nail unit are seen together in the same section.

Nail matrix biopsy may be performed after full or partial avulsion of the nail plate and exposure of the nail matrix by reflecting the proximal nail fold (e-figs. 1.8–1.11). Full-thickness excision of the matrix may result in permanent nail dystrophy unless sutures are used to approximate the nail matrix, whereas a shave biopsy of the matrix does not usually leave a defect and there is very little risk of transecting the tumor because the matrix is a thick epithelium. Nail specimens are often small fragile pieces of tissue and can be easily misoriented or cut tangentially. It is useful to place the fresh specimen on a paper template of a nail in the correct orientation prior to placing it in formalin. The specimen sticks to the paper template and can be placed in the cassette and sectioned while still attached to the paper in order to preserve the orientation (Fig. 1.2).

The only situation in which nail plate biopsy may be of some value is in the diagnosis of onychomycosis when the periodic acid–Schiff stain (PAS)-positive hyphae may be seen in the substance of the nail plate. However, onychomycosis is thought to originate in the nail bed and involve the nail plate secondarily; therefore, a nail bed specimen is more likely to yield a positive result and the nail plate is involved secondarily, so a better specimen for diagnosis is from the nail bed.

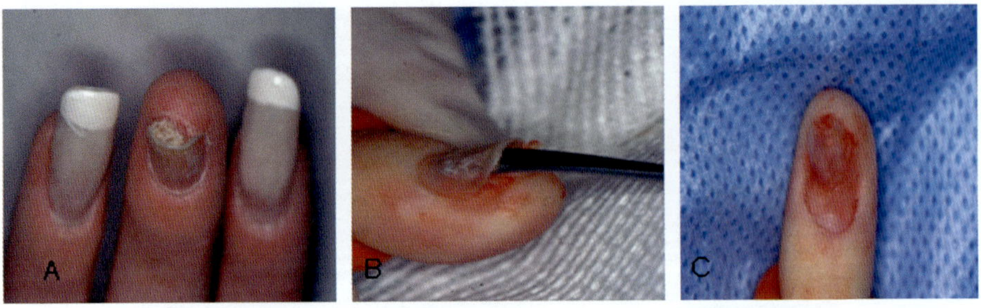

FIGURE 1.2 Nail avulsion for exostosis **(A)**. Freer elevator is inserted beneath the nail plate **(B)**. Nail plate avulsed and tumor visualized **(C)**.

REFERENCES

1. Rich P. Nail biopsy: Indication and methods. *Dermatol Surg* 2001;27:229–234.
2. Rich P. Nail surgery. In: Bolognia J, Jorrizzo J, Rapini R, et al., eds. *Dermatology*. 2nd Ed. New York: Mosby, 2008.
3. Thomson CJ, Lalonde DH, Denkler KA, Feicht AJ. A critical look at the evidence for and against elective epinephrine use in the finger. *Plast Reconstr Surg* 2007;119:260–266.
4. Lalonde D, Bell M, Benoit P, et al. A multicenter prospective study of 3,110 consecutive cases of elective epinephrine use in the fingers and hand: The Dalhousie Project clinical phase. *J Hand Surg (Am)* 2005;30:1061–1067.
5. Krunic AL, Wang LC, Soltani K, et al. Digital anesthesia with epinephrine: An old myth revisited. *J Am Acad Dermatol* 2004;51:755–759.
6. Collins S, Cordova K, Jellinek N. Alternatives to complete nail plate avulsion. *J Am Acad Dermatol* 2008;59:619–626.

2

BENIGN MELANOCYTIC PROLIFERATIONS AND PRECURSOR LESIONS TO MELANOMA

Melanocytic lesions are among the most diversified and difficult proliferations in the realm of cutaneous neoplasia. They encompass a broad range of lesions ranging from benign–typified by such lesions as the common acquired nevus, congenital nevus, and blue nevus and even those lesions that fall under the designation of dysplastic nevus–to overtly malignant, i.e., melanoma. Other lesions are a diagnostic conundrum for even the most experienced dermatopathologist but are encountered on a frequent basis in referral centers, namely, those lesions whose biological potential for metastasis cannot be predicted by light microscopic analysis alone. In this chapter, we describe a spectrum of melanocytic lesions that range from indisputably benign, through those dysplastic melanocytic lesions that are precancerous and lack metastatic capability, to the indeterminate melanocytic tumors in the context of those arising in the deep-penetrating nevus and the so called atypical Spitz tumor. Also considered are conventional Spitz nevi and atypical nevi of special sites such as those nevi from the genitalia, axilla, and acral sites.

NON-NEVUS BENIGN MELANOCYTIC LESIONS CONFINED TO THE EPIDERMIS

Freckles and lentigines are not precancerous melanocytic proliferations but are important as they can be mistaken for precancerous melanoses and, as in the context of lentiginosis syndromes, they may be a clue to a systemic disease process.

FRECKLES (EPHELIDES)

Freckles are light brown macules typically less than 2 mm in diameter seen in light-skinned individuals on sun-exposed areas that become more obvious after sun exposure and are inconspicuous in the winter.[1] They appear in childhood and persist into adulthood; some manifest an autosomal dominant pattern of inheritance.

Histopathology

Increased melanin production generates increased melanization of basal layer keratinocytes unaccompanied by elongated retia or increased numbers of melanocytes.

Differential Diagnosis

The differential diagnosis of the freckle encompasses the café au lait spot, the melanotic macule of Albright, and the lentigo simplex. While the café au lait spot can be distinguished by virtue of giant melanosomes, and the lentigo simplex by its elongated retia with variable melanocytic hyperplasia, the melanotic macule of Albright may be indistinguishable from the freckle.[2] An identical histology but with a different clinical appearance is seen with reticulate pigmentation of the neck,[3] reticulate pigmentary anomaly of the flexures (Dowling–Degos disease),[4] and reticulate acropigmentation of Kitamura[5] with which it overlaps.

LENTIGINES: LENTIGO SIMPLEX AND THE LENTIGINOSES

A lentigo is a pigmented macule less than 1 cm in diameter and classically 1 to 5 mm in diameter. There are clinical variants of lentigines, and several genodermatoses are associated with multiple lentigines, the so-called *lentiginosis* syndromes. Classically, lentigo simplex arises in childhood anywhere on the body with no relationship to sun exposure[6] and manifests tan, brown, or dark nonpalpable macules that do not exceed 4 mm in diameter. Some patients manifest disseminated lentigines with a lesional morphology similar to that of lentigo simplex, either as isolated cutaneous lesions[7] or associated with other systemic manifestations[6] such as **LAMB** syndrome that may have family members who only manifest skin lesions while others may manifest anomalies of the cardiac, musculoskeletal, neurologic, reproductive, gastrointestinal, auditory, and respiratory systems and have been categorized into different syndromes; the best characterized are Carney's syndrome and the **LEOPARD** syndrome. The latter is an acronym for **L**entigines, **E**CG abnormalities, **O**cular hypertelorism/obstructive cardiomyopathy, **P**ulmonary valve stenosis, **A**bnormalities of genitalia in males, **R**etardation of growth, and **D**eafness.[7] Carney complex comprises multiple neoplasms including myxomas at various sites, endocrine tumors, epithelioid blue nevus, melanotic schwannoma, and lentiginosis; in many of these syndromes, pattern of inheritance is autosomal dominant.[8]

Histopathology

There is panepidermal hyperpigmentation with elongated retia that is either thin or, at times, club shaped, with a variable, albeit usually slight, increase in melanocytes. Melanophages and a sparse chronic inflammatory infiltrate are typical. Some lesions show eosinophilic fibrosis around the tips of retia and fused retia mimicking with dysplastic nevi. On occasion, clustered melanocytes may be seen at the tips of retia and giant melanosomes may be observed (Figs. 2.1 and 2.2). There is some variation in the light microscopic findings in the setting of systemic disorders. In the LEOPARD syndrome, lesions mimic lentigo simplex but may also show melanocytes

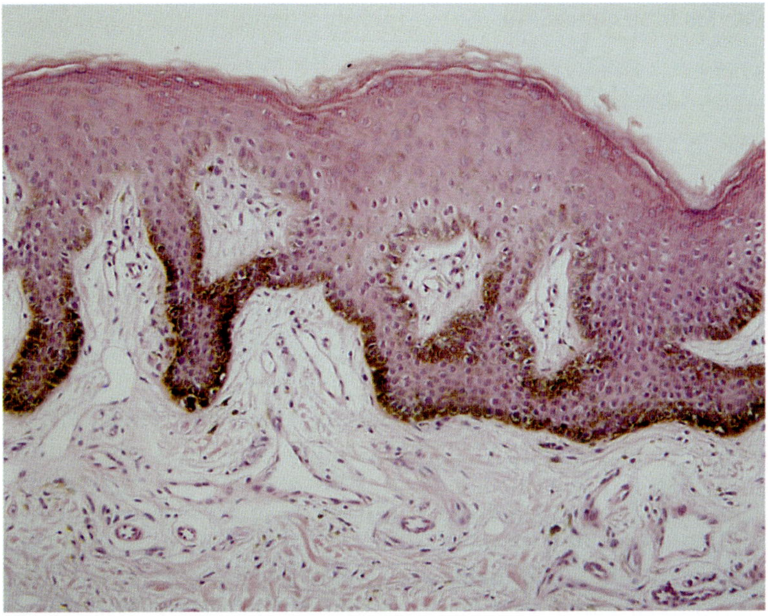

FIGURE 2.1 Classic features of a lentigo with elongated retia exhibiting hypermelanosis and a slight increase in melanocytes. The hypermelanosis is seen throughout the epidermis and cornified layer.

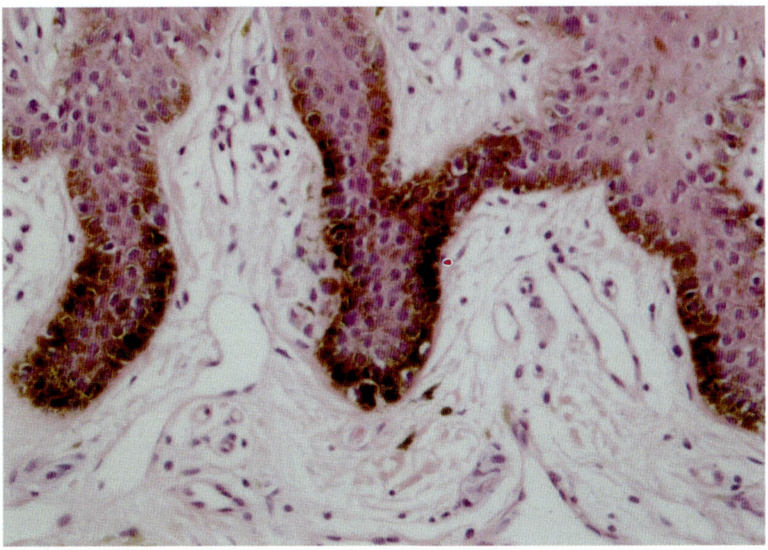

FIGURE 2.2 Classic features of a lentigo with elongated retia exhibiting hypermelanosis and a slight increase in melanocytes. The hypermelanosis is seen throughout the epidermis and cornified layer.

distributed in the upper epidermis as micronests; this histology is similar to that of Moynahan's syndrome. In Peutz–Jeghers's syndrome, there may be no accompanying increase in melanocytes, and large melanosomes may be seen within keratinocytes at all levels of the epidermis. In **LAMB** syndrome, melanocytes tend to assume an exaggerated dendritic morphology.

MUCOSAL LENTIGINES

Labial Melanotic Macule

Classically seen on the lower lip, labial melanotic macule can occur anywhere in the oropharynx[9] and is a benign lesion.[10] Epithelial hyperplasia is accompanied by parakeratosis, slightly increased numbers of melanocytes with an often dendritic morphology, basilar epithelial pigmentation, and subepithelial melanophages (Figs. 2.3 and 2.4).

Genital Lentigines

In men on the glans penis, corona, sulcus, and penile shaft or in women anywhere on genital mucosa, genital lentigines are tan to dark brown macules up to 15 mm in diameter. They may be exaggerated by pregnancy and in the postpartum period, at times localizing to episiotomy sites. Elongation of retia, basal layer hyperpigmentation, increased numbers of melanocytes with prominent dendritic processes, and subepithelial melanophages are characteristics of vulvar and penile lentigines (Fig. 2.5).

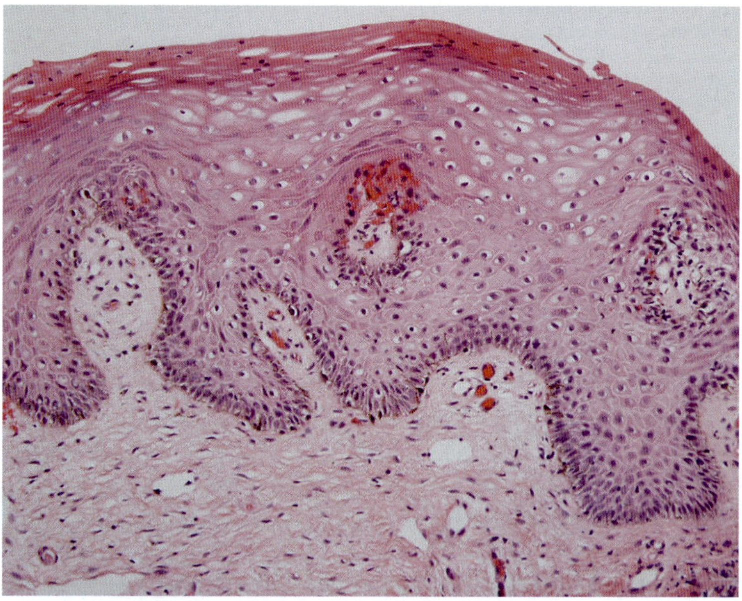

FIGURE 2.3 **In the Classic Lower Labial Melanotic Macule, There Is Epidermal Hyperplasia with Basilar Hypermelanosis.** A few of the melanocytes have a dendritic quality. There is no melanocytic atypia.

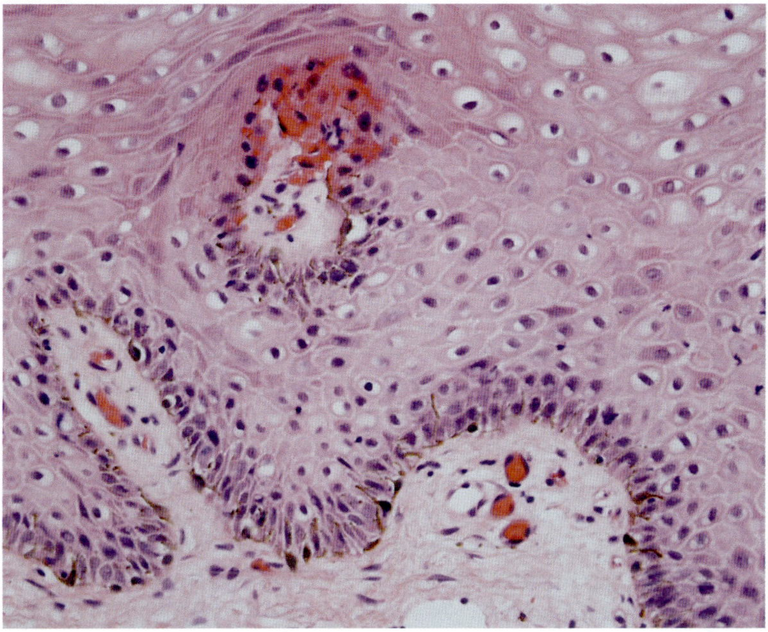

FIGURE 2.4 **In the Classic Lower Labial Melanotic Macule, There is Epidermal Hyperplasia with Basilar Hypermelanosis.** A few of the melanocytes have a dendritic quality. There is no melanocytic atypia.

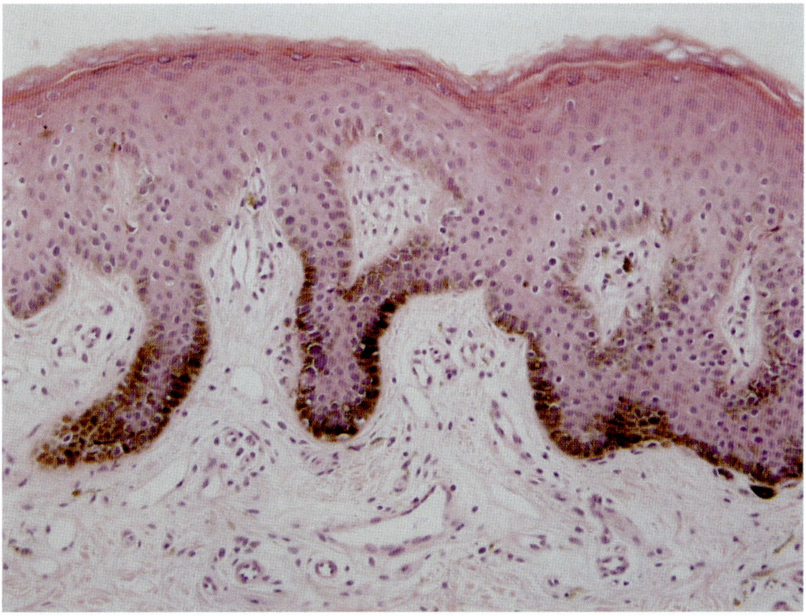

FIGURE 2.5 In the classic genital lentigo, the morphology closely resembles lentigo simplex with elongation of the retia, basal layer hyperpigmentation, and a mild increase in basal layer melanocytes. The melanocytes can have a dendritic appearance.

Vulvar and Penile Melanosis

Vulvar and penile melanosis manifests as solitary or multiple, intensely pigmented, irregular macules,[11–13] often several centimeters in diameter. If there are any irregularities in pigmentation, several biopsies may be warranted to exclude radial growth phase melanoma of mucosal lentiginous type. Pigmented Bowen's disease, pigmented Paget's disease, and patch-type bowenoid papulosis can mimic genital melanosis. The genital lentigines raise consideration to melanoma and, as they cannot usually be separated on clinical grounds, a biopsy is typically warranted.[14]

Vulvar melanosis histologically resembles vulvar lentigo but does not usually demonstrate elongation of the retia, and, thus, there is histologic overlap between vulvar lentiginosis and melanosis. Nested melanocytes are not observed. There is uniform hypermelanosis and, although there may be slight melanocytic hyperplasia, melanocytic atypia should not be observed; its presence indicates atypical genital melanocytic hyperplasia/atypical genital melanosis, a precursor to melanoma. A similar phenomenon on plantar surfaces has been termed *atypical melanosis* in those lesions showing only a slightly atypical lentiginous melanocytic hyperplasia and *premalignant plantar melanosis* in those lesions showing greater atypia (Fig. 2.6).

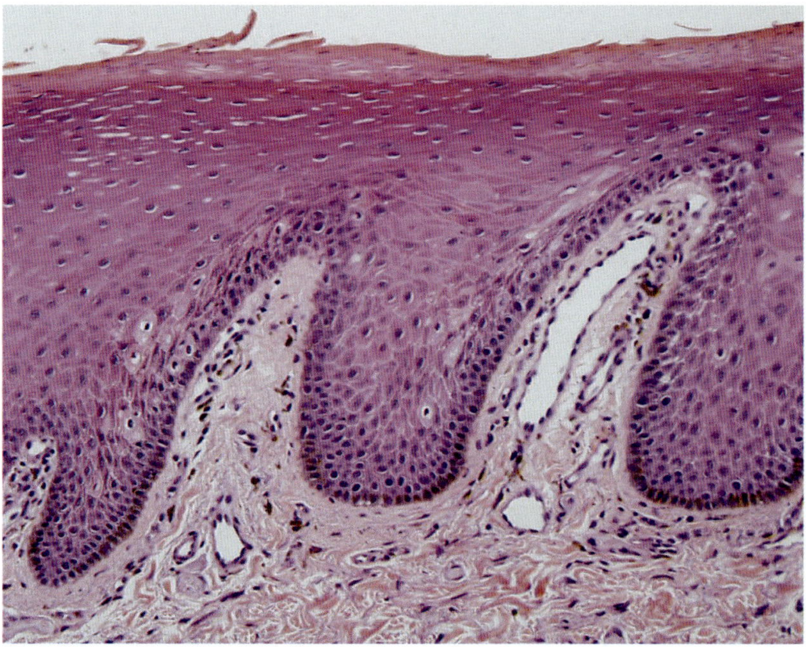

FIGURE 2.6 Vulvar melanosis histomorphologically resembles vulvar lentigo but does not usually demonstrate elongation of the retia, although acanthosis may be seen.

Acral Lentigines

Acral lentigines from palms and soles of persons of African extraction comprise 1- to 5-mm circumscribed pigmented macules[6] having elongated retia, hypermelanosis, and a single-cell proliferation of dendritic melanocytes lacking cytologic features of atypia and confined to the basal layer of the epidermis.

ACTINIC (SOLAR) LENTIGO

Actinic lentigines are tan to brown 1 to 10 mm macules on sun-damaged skin of the face, the dorsa of the hands, etc. that appear as early as the second decade of life and are nearly ubiquitous in elderly Caucasians. Occasional lesions form confluent, large patches. The histology depends on the age of lesion biopsied, initially manifesting a slight increase in basal layer melanocytes having features of photoactivation, namely, increased cell size, dendritic processes, and preserved nucleocytoplasmic ratios. Hypermelanosis extends from the basal layer into the midspinous layers. Progressively, the retia elongate and manifest angulation as the stroma becomes more elastotic (Fig. 2.7); retia become irregular with a foot-like form likened to the blade of a hockey stick wrapped in black tape. There may be some architectural disarray with keratinocytic atypia, raising consideration to a superficial pigmented actinic keratosis; however, the statum corneum is either orthokeratotic or hyperkeratotic rather than parakeratotic as in an actinic keratosis. The two processes may coexist. Evolution into a pigmented reticulated seborrheic keratosis or a benign lichenoid keratosis often eventuates. The differential diagnosis includes the large cell acanthoma, the "ink spot" lentigo, and lentigo maligna. The large cell acanthoma is a variant of actinic lentigo in which keratinocytes have expanded cytoplasms and large, aneuploid nuclei.[15,16] The "ink spot" lentigo is characterized clinically by a black reticulated lesion and histologically by prominent epidermal melanization with transepithelial elimination of pigment to the cornified layer[17] and densely pigmented retia.

Actinic lentigines with chronic photoactivation can manifest a proliferation of plump, somewhat atypical melanocytes with hyperchromatic nuclei, and so they can mimic lentigo maligna. The correct diagnosis hinges upon recognition that:

1. The dominant lesion is actinic lentigo.
2. There is no nesting or upward migration of melanocytes into the upper epidermis.
3. The melanocytic hyperplasia is of low to moderate density with no areas of confluent lentiginous growth.
4. Retia are usually hyperplastic in actinic lentigo; no areas of retiform effacement are seen. The exception to this rule is the incipient actinic lentigo, which shows minimal or no acanthosis and a retiform pattern that is usually cognate to that of normal skin. Conversely, there are cases of lentigo maligna where the epidermis may appear hyperplastic.

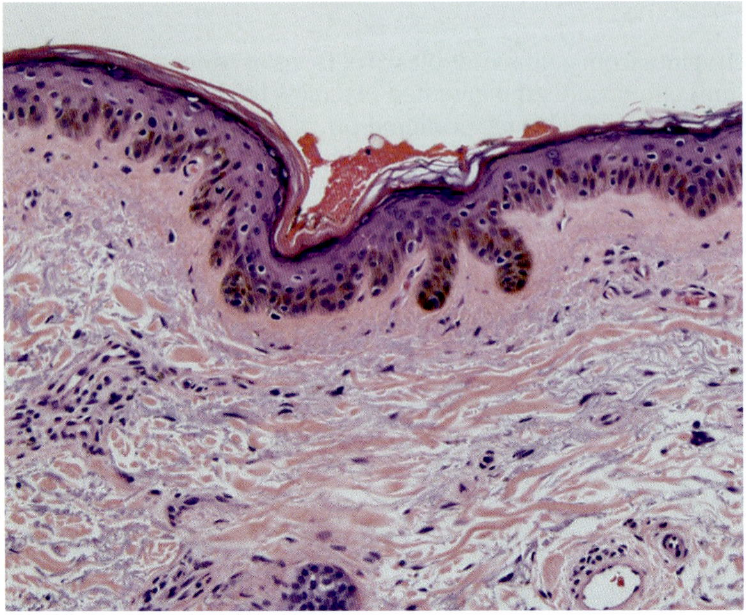

FIGURE 2.7 **In the Classic Solar Lentigo, There is Rete Ridge Elongation with Hypermelanosis, Solar Elastosis, and Mild Squamous Atypia.** The melanocytes are oftentimes increased in number reflecting chronic photoactivation of melanocytes rather than signifying a true melanocytic dysplasia; the cells nonetheless show nuclear hyperchromasia and angulation.

COMMON ACQUIRED NEVUS AND OTHER BENIGN ACQUIRED NEVI

Nevi are circumscribed anomalies of embryonic development that present at birth or later in life as collections of pigment-producing cells of melanocytic origin present in the epidermis and/or dermis. The constituent cell of the nevus is a pigment-synthesizing melanocyte that differs from its normal counterpart by virtue of a nondendritic morphology, by having the capability for division, and by virtue of representing, in at least some cases, a clonal proliferation.[18] One melanocyte provides melanin for approximately 5 to 20 keratinocytes. The prototypic banal nevi are classified by their onset (congenital or acquired), by their microscopic location in the skin (junctional when confined to the epidermis, compound when involving the epidermis and dermis, or dermal when confined to the dermis), and by architecture, i.e., Miescher's nevus, Unna's nevus, etc. Most common acquired nevi show a stereotypic evolutionary pattern and are initially flat, tan lesions 1 to 2 mm in diameter that slowly assume a dimension of up to 4 to 5 mm. As a nevus progresses, it becomes slightly raised, reflecting the acquisition of a dermal population derived from migration of nevus cells from the epidermis to the dermis.[19] Later, the nevus becomes a papule or nodule that may be dark blue, light tan, or flesh-colored. Common acquired nevi manifest cephalocaudal spread, and are thus most common in the head and neck area. The average white person will have from 20 to 100 benign acquired melanocytic nevi with the incidence climbing in proximity to the equator; there is a clear relationship to sun exposure.[20] The number of banal nevi is an independent risk factor for the development of melanoma; the average number of nondysplastic melanocytic nevi 2 mm or greater in diameter is 97 for melanoma patients and 36 for control subjects. Rarely, nevi may appear as a disseminated eruption resembling a lichenoid rash in apparently healthy young adults.[21]

Histology

Nevomelanocytes, derived from neural crest migrants to the skin, are classified as type A, type B, or type C cells.[22] The type A or epithelioid nevus cell has abundant coarsely melanized cytoplasm; these cells are found with the epidermis and superficial dermis. The type B or lymphocytelike nevus cell is a round to cuboidal, nonpigmented cell with a round hyperchromatic nucleus containing an inconspicuous nucleolus and with scant cytoplasm. They are slightly larger than mature resting small lymphocytes or mast cells, i.e., in the 8 to 10 μm range. The type C or neuroid nevus cell has a spindled morphology with fibrillary elongated cytoplasmic processes reminiscent of a Schwann cell.[19] Senescent change may be observed in the dermal component as multinucleation of melanocytes with close nuclear apposition and hyperchromasia along with complete loss of nuclear detail. Pleomorphism may be striking in different portions of the lesion, but in any one high-power field, there is uniformity. Balloon cell change is also thought to represent a senescent phenomenon due to degeneration of melanosomes. The prototypic common acquired nevi initiate as a lentiginous proliferation of single cells dispersed along the basal layer of epidermis, forming tan-colored or dark macules, sometimes with an irregular contour. These then manifest accumulations of cells as discrete junctional nests. Migration of nevus cells into the dermis then forms a compound nevus, the clinical concomitant being a palpable lesion. Complete nevus cell migration into the dermis forms a dermal nevus, manifested clinically as a palpable lesion with a tan or pale color. The junctional nevus demonstrates discrete intraepidermal nests of nevomelanocytes[19] localized to the tips of slightly hyperplastic rete ridges. Pagetoid spread of nevomelanocytes may occur, especially in children's nevi or in specific anatomic locations such as acral sites, but is not the dominant form of melanocytic growth and is usually orderly, emanating from basal nests and thus being accentuated, overlying the retia. This directed pagetoid migration yields discrete columns of melanin in the stratum corneum. The junctional nevus nests may be associated with a lentiginous proliferation of nevus cells arranged as single cells along the basal layer and not extending at lateral edges beyond the nested component; these are termed *lentiginous junctional nevi*. Mirror-image symmetry is the rule. An individual section may impart an apparent intradermal location to a junctional nest whose true epidermal residence is only demonstrable by serial sections (Fig. 2.8).[23]

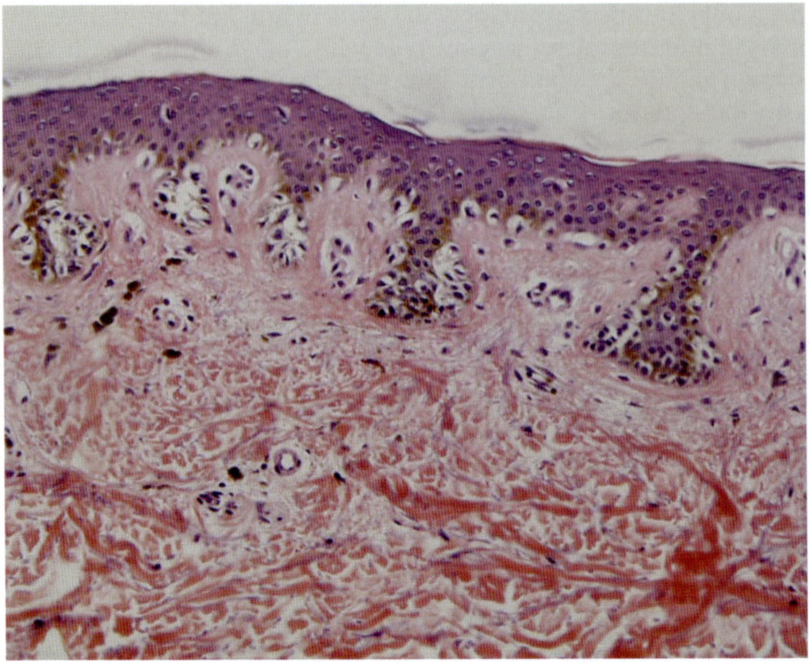

FIGURE 2.8 **Example of a Junctional Nevus.** Note the proliferation of melanocytes confined to the basal layer. The cells are disposed singly and in small nests primarily situated at the tips of rete ridges. The cells are bland appearing, manifesting a small round nucleus with an inconspicuous nucleolus.

The cells comprising the nests have nuclei that are round to oval, containing finely dispersed chromatin and small nucleoli; five or more such nevomelanocytes define a junctional thèque or nest.[22] The cells within the nests are monotonous in size and shape and have either a type A or a type B morphology. Mitoses are rare. Marked heterogeneity of melanization is mainly a feature of dysplastic melanocytic proliferations characterized by coarse, variably sized melanin granules with giant melanosomes. The stroma beneath the junctional nests may exhibit mild periretal fibroplasia but not the patterned lamellar or concentric eosinophilic fibrosis seen in dysplastic nevi, nor is there inflammation or increased vascularity. Halo junctional nevi, in contrast, manifest a brisk lymphohistiocytic inflammatory response that is symmetrical; as it subsides, a uniform pattern of delicate fibroplasia with neovascularization occurs. In compound nevi, melanocytes are found in both the epidermis and dermis; the intraepidermal component of the benign acquired nevus is usually delimited by the lateral boundaries of the subjacent dermal component, while any extension beyond the dermal domain exhibits bilateral mirror-image symmetry. The size of the dermal nests is usually similar to that of the intraepidermal nests. The nests are encased in a delicate stroma and may assume a coalescent

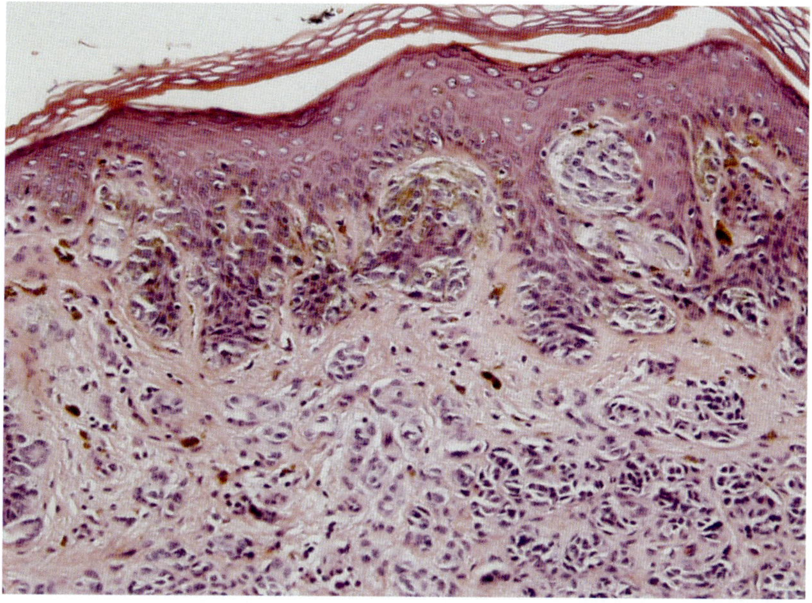

FIGURE 2.9 **In the Compound Nevus, There Is a Benign Proliferation of Melanocytes Both in the Epidermis and the Dermis.** The epidermal component does not extend beyond the intraepidermal component and vice versa. There is no true supervening cytologic melanocytic atypia. In the superficial dermis, the cells have a plump, rounded appearance while those cells in the deeper dermis appear smaller, almost lymphocyte-like, defining the concept of the type B nevus cell. Pigmentation can be observed amidst the melanocytes in the epidermis and superficial dermis.

bandlike disposition but are still discernible as separate nests as opposed to an expansile nodule. The dermal component typically stops at the papillary–reticular dermal junction, without extension into the reticular or adventitial dermis, and in adulthood, a stromal proliferation occurs at the base of the nevus and separates it from the papillary–reticular dermal junction. Mast cells are then often admixed and mucin may be observed (Fig. 2.9).

The intraepidermal cytology is identical to that described for the prototypic benign common acquired junctional nevus, but the dermal component shows progressive maturation of cell type toward the base of the lesion. The superficial component comprises type A cells, while type B cells are often situated at the base and may be admixed with type C, or neurotized, nevus cells. Infiltration by fat cells is a frequent concomitant of this involuting phase. The dermal nevus has, by definition, no intraepidermal component; in practice, we allow up to two junctional thèques. Senescent change as described above may be seen in the dermal component as may fibrous involution, the likely derivation of the fibrous papule, the angiofibroma, and the perifollicular fibroma. Formation of pseudovascular spaces may be seen, in part due to a fixation artifact, whereby stroma manifests a cleft caused by shrinking of the nevus cells. Mitoses are

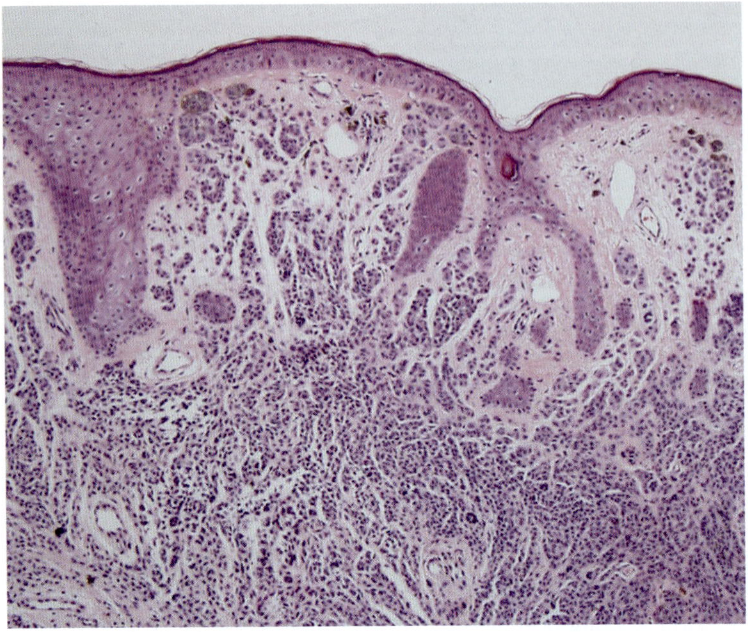

FIGURE 2.10 The last phase in the evolution of the common acquired nevus is the presence of a pure dermal component without an intraepidermal contribution. Nevertheless, in facial and auricular nevi, the intraepidermal melanocytic proliferation may be quite florid and may show pagetoid intraepidermal ascent.

rarely observed unless there has been an inciting factor such as trauma; the presence of more than three mitoses in one section should prompt the study of multiple levels to exclude nevoid melanoma. A conservative re-excision of such cases may be advised if they are not completely excised. Dermal nevi may be associated with an intraepidermal single-cell proliferation of plump melanocytes, most often disposed in a lentiginous array. This proliferation is focal, is most conspicuous centrally, and is held to represent a photoactivation effect in facial nevi in particular. We incorporate microscopic descriptions in reports of melanocytic neoplasms to describe such findings. The presence of senescent atypia does not herald a significant risk of malignant degeneration (Fig. 2.10).

OTHER ACQUIRED BENIGN NEVI

Balloon Cell Nevus

The balloon cell nevus clinically has an appearance similar to other common acquired nevi, manifesting as a dome-shaped, flesh-colored papule, typically less than 6 mm in diameter,[24,25] most often in patients under the age of 30 years and occurring mainly in the head and neck.

Histology

Diagnosis hinges on the recognition of balloon cell change involving more than 50% of dermal nevomelanocytes; balloon cells manifest abundant clear, finely vacuolated cytoplasm and small hyperchromatic nuclei with a scalloped contour. Multinucleation may be observed. The main differential diagnostic consideration is that of balloon cell melanoma. The distinction rests on the recognition of a malignant neoplastic cytology; in balloon cell melanoma, the majority of cells manifest pleomorphism, the nuclei appearing large with irregularly distributed chromatin, mitoses, and necrosis.

Nevus Spilus

We use the term nevus spilus to denote the entity of speckled lentiginous nevus characterized by a light brown macule on which darker macular or papular lesions are superimposed, most often seen on the trunk, sometimes with a dermatomal distribution. The lightly pigmented foci are consistent with a lentigo simplex, while the superimposed darker spots have features of a junctional or compound nevus of common acquired or dysplastic subtype and, rarely, a dermal Spitz nevus or a blue nevus[26,27]; the combined nevus of blue nevus and nevus spilus subtypes is also called Kawamura nevus. Reports of melanoma arising in lesions of nevus spilus have led to concerns regarding malignant potential.[28] By 1997, 17 patients had been reported in the literature; the most common type is a superficial spreading melanoma.[29] In some of these cases, features of a dysplastic nevus were present, but most of them had a banal junctional nevus morphology. Thus, our current recommendation is to completely excise the nevus spilus if it is of congenital onset. For large, atypical lesions, we propose periodic examination using baseline photography and selective excision of clinically atypical elements.

Histology

Those lesions with uniform pigmentation clinically have a histology indistinguishable from a lentigo simplex, with slight elongation of retia manifesting increased basilar keratinocyte pigment and an increase in bland melanocytes in a lentiginous distribution. Such lesions are difficult to distinguish from a café au lait spot, in which the density of melanocytes along the dermoepidermal junction is higher; giant melanosomes can be observed in both café au lait macules and nevi spilus.[30] Agminated blue and Spitz nevi with overlying lentigo simplex-like changes are reported.[31,32]

Effects of Exogenous or Endogenous Hormones on Melanocytic Nevi

Nevi become larger and darker during pregnancy, a phenomenon that correlates histologically to an increase in melanocyte proliferation, an increase in cell size, increased chromatin content, and conspicuous nucleolation, although the chromatin remains evenly distributed, the N/C ratios are maintained, and there is uniformity of nuclear shape and size. Significant atypia in melanocytic lesions excised from pregnant patients should not be discounted as a reactive estrogen effect; rather, it could reflect inherent melanocytic dysplasia unmasked by the altered hormonal milieu.[22] The lesion must be examined for standard cytologic and architectural features associated with dysplasia as described below. Prominent pagetoid growth and effacement of architecture may also indicate severe melanocytic dysplasia.

CONGENITAL NEVUS

Congenital pigmented lesions are identified in approximately 1% of newborn infants; though usually 3 to 4 mm in size, a rare lesion may be several centimeters in size. These are designated as giant congenital nevi or garment congenital nevi, the latter term used for lesions greater than 20 cm in diameter or lesions that cover the entire trunk or limb. Lesions are considered as intermediate when measuring 1.5 to 5 cm and small when less than 1.5 cm. The giant congenital nevus has a bimodal age peak of melanoma incidence, the first occurring in the first 5 years of life and the second occurring from puberty into adulthood. Small congenital nevi, on the other hand, are not reported to undergo malignant transformation during the first two decades of life, but the risk of malignancy appears during late adolescence and the incidence progressively rises in adult life. A series of 160 patients with large congenital nevi showed 3 patients who developed melanomas and did so in extracutaneous sites, namely, central nervous system and retroperitoneum; the 5-year cumulative risk for melanoma was 2.3%.[33] Lesions located in the head and neck may be associated with melanocytic proliferations of the meninges with extension into the cisterna magni causing secondary hydrocephalus; termed neurocutaneous melanosis, this may be associated with intracranial melanoma. Congenital nevi covering 4% or less of the body surface may not be at significant risk for malignant transformation.[34]

Irrespective of its size, the morphology of the congenital nevus changes with age, darkening in the first 5 to 6 years of life and then again at puberty. It is flat at birth and becomes palpable with age, gradually acquiring terminal hairs. As the patient ages, the lesions develop areas of hyperkeratosis, "doughy" alterations associated with mucinous degeneration, and the formation of neurofibromata. The appearance of firm nodules in congenital nevi is worrisome and any nodular proliferation should be excised to exclude malignant transformation. One diagnostic consideration in this setting is the development of proliferative nodules; up to 5 mm in diameter with smooth or sometimes ulcerated surfaces, these are held to reflect self-limited, slowly growing proliferations.[35]

Histology

We consider the following diagnostic of the congenital origin of a nevus:

1. Intramural or subendothelial nesting of nevus cells in small to medium size arteries, veins, and lymphatics.
2. Nevus cell nests in the papilla of the hair follicle.

3. Nevus cells scattered in single cell array throughout the lower reticular dermis and the subcutaneous fat.
4. Nevus cells in arrector pili muscles.
5. Nevus cells in tight perivascular array mimicking an inflammatory infiltrate throughout the reticular dermis (Figs. 2.11 and 2.12).[36]

Perineural infiltration and permeation of the adventitial dermis and adnexal epithelium are also seen in lesions of congenital nevi; however, such changes are only suggestive of potential congenital origin of lesions. Involvement of adnexal structures including the pilar erector muscle is seen in acquired nevi in the head and neck area, and hence cannot be used as a diagnostic criterion of congenital onset.

Treatment

Each patient is carefully followed and evaluated with gross inspection and palpation for subcutaneous nodules, changes in lesional consistency, and surface topography or coloration. Should any such change occur, an excision of this area with a margin of the nevus is recommended. We recommend complete excision or partial extensive excision of a giant congenital nevus in a patient in whom biopsy shows foci worrisome for evolution into melanoma or consistent with overt melanoma. Nevi up to 5 cm in size can be excised in a one-stage procedure, but larger lesions

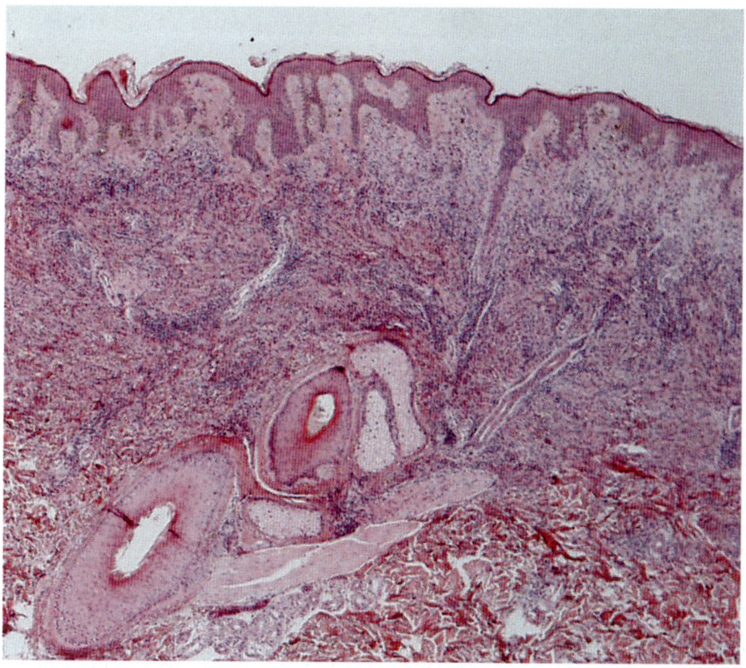

FIGURE 2.11 The congenital nevus is characteristically larger than the common acquired nevus and hence the lateral breadth of these lesions oftentimes exceeds 1 cm. Nevus cells track along adnexae into the deep reticular dermis.

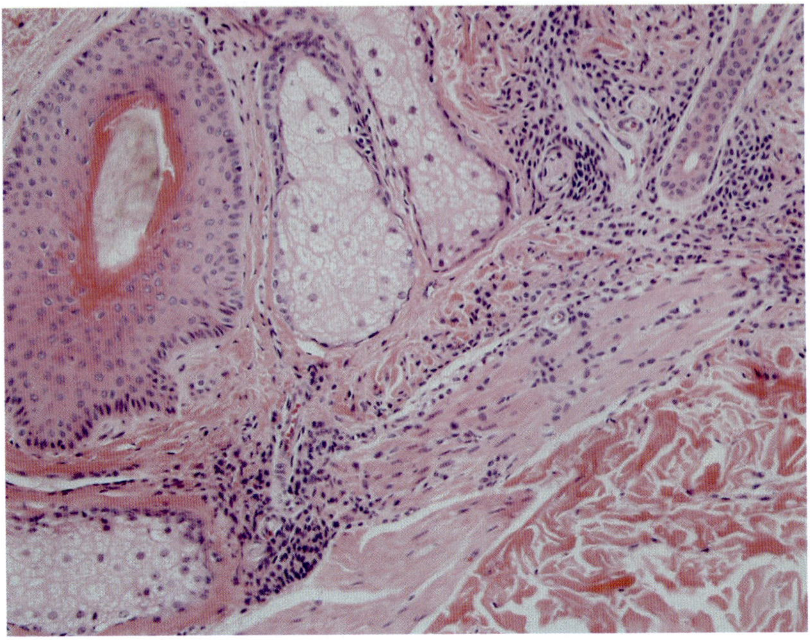

FIGURE 2.12 Additional clues to the diagnosis of the congenital nevus include infiltration of the pilar arrector muscle and protrusion of nevus cells into lymphatic channels. It should be emphasized that in the head and neck area, it is very common for common acquired nevi to show deep periadnexal extension into the pilar erector muscle and protrude into intralymphatic protrusion.

may mandate the use of a tissue expander, sometimes with staged therapy using full-thickness or intermediate-thickness grafts following superficial partial removal of the nevus, with the proviso that no histologic evidence of atypia is identified.

RECURRENT MELANOCYTIC NEVUS

Recurrence of a nevus manifests as repigmentation in the scar at the site of a previous incomplete excision, electrodessication, or dermabrasion of a melanocytic lesion. The pigmentation within or adjacent to the scar is irregular or stippled with a variegated color ranging from tan to dark brown or black.[37] Similar changes appear in nevi partly ablated through trauma of which the patient may be unaware. Repigmentation occurs within weeks to months of the original excision, unlike recurrent melanoma, where repigmentation occurs years later.[37,38]

Histology

The original lesion is usually a compound nevus, an intradermal nevus being seen in 32% of cases and a junctional nevus in 5% of cases. Less than 10% of recurrent nevi arise from prior dysplastic nevi. The recurrent nevus can be easily recognized at scanning magnification by virtue of an intraepidermal melanocytic growth over a dermal scar with a subjacent remnant of benign nevus. While the dominant localization of the recurrent nevus is within the epidermis, there can be recurrent nevus within the dermis. Other features help to differentiate it from two other common scenarios associated with dermal fibrosis and an atypical intraepidermal melanocytic growth, namely, regressed and/or recurrent melanoma.[39] The intraepidermal growth in recurrent nevi manifests sharp lateral circumscription, with lateral boundaries defined by the scar from the prior procedure[37]; if there is residual lesion peripheral to the main scar, the intraepidermal component is cytologically that of a nevus, be it of common acquired, dysplastic, or congenital subtypes. Over the scar, the melanocytes are enlarged with epithelioid cytology, round to oval nuclei, abundant pigment, variable sizes and shapes, nucleolation, and a single-cell and nested array with confluence of growth, nest variability of shape, location, and orientation, and dyshesion.[37] There may be upward pagetoid growth to the suprabasilar epidermis and spinous layer, sparing the granular cell layer (Figs. 2.13–2.16).

The epidermis is often flattened. Mitotic activity, seen in a minority of cases, is typically superficially confined. Melanocytes may grow along the basal layer of adnexal structures. The dermis demonstrates parallel arrangement of collagen with neovascularization and banal nevus cells. There may be patchy perivascular lymphocytic infiltrates but lichenoid inflammation is absent. Nucleolated nevomelanocytes similar to those in the epidermis

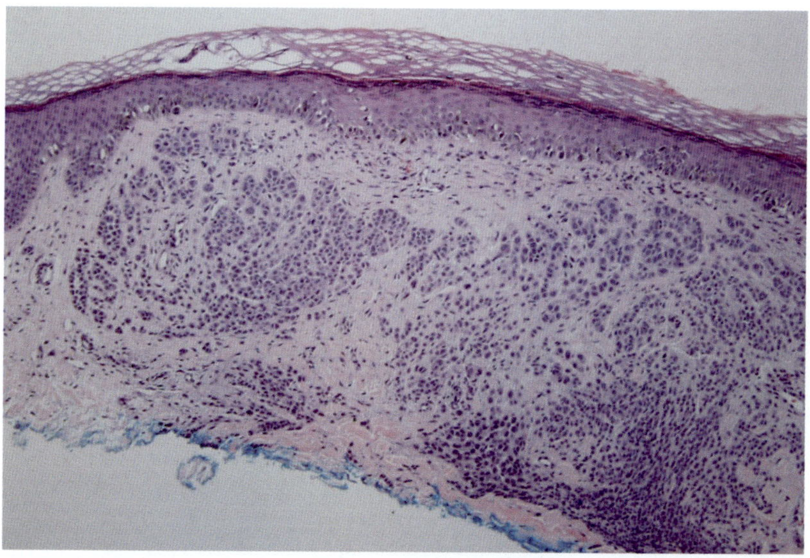

FIGURE 2.13 **Recurrent Nevus: There Is an Obvious Scar.** The scar is of recent onset as revealed by the delicate nature of the connective tissue fiber network. Overlying the scar there is a relatively high-density growth of melanocytes. The cells are disposed singly and in large irregular, somewhat dyshesive, nests. The epidermis is attenuated.

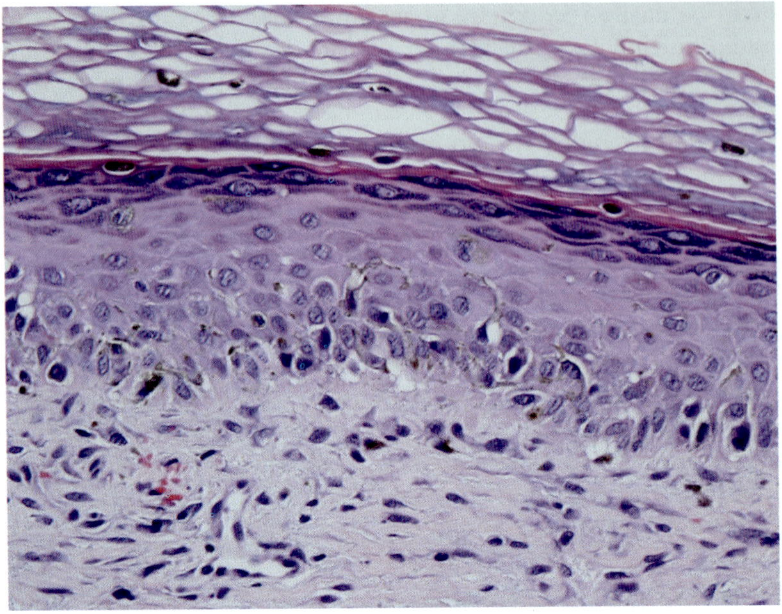

FIGURE 2.14 Higher-power magnification reveals significant epithelioid cell atypia. The cells are noticeably larger, with conspicuous nucleolation and irregular pigment disposition within the cytoplasms. The rete ridge pattern is effaced and there is Pagetoid ascent.

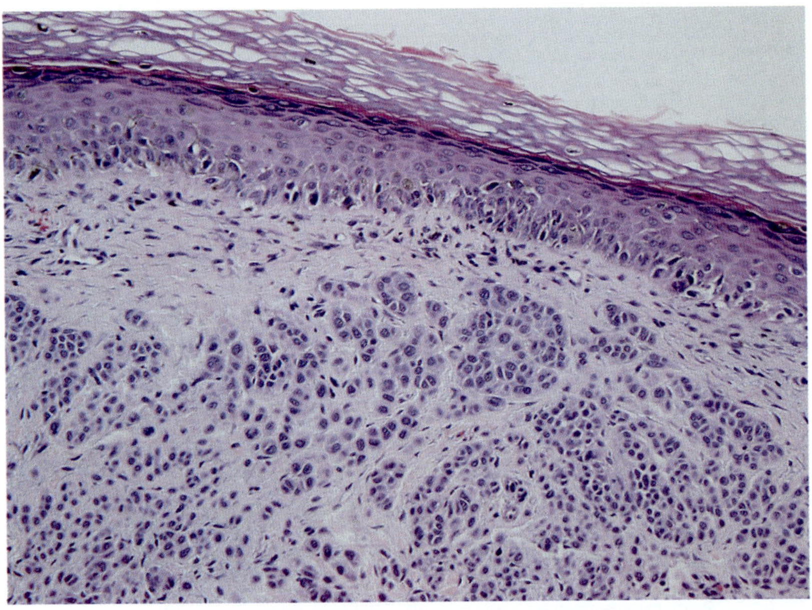

FIGURE 2.15 Although the dominant aspect of the recurrent nevus is in the context of intraepidermal melanocytic atypia, there may be superficial dermal recurrence as well. The cells in the zone of recurrent dermal nevus show moderate epithelioid cell atypia.

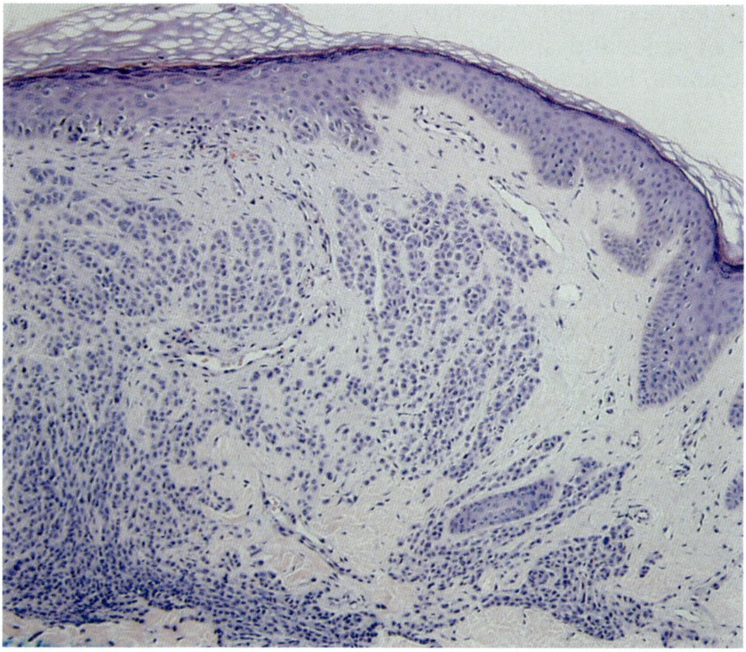

FIGURE 2.16 Despite the extent of atypia that can be observed within the region of recurrence, peripheral to the scar, the lesion may appear quite bland if the original lesion was a benign nevus. The recurrent atypia will be greatest in the recurrent dysplastic nevus; examination of the prior excision specimen is important for confirming the diagnosis of recurrent nevus over one of recurrent melanoma. An asymmetrical architectural shoulder past the confines of the scar indicates a recurrent dysplastic, as opposed to a recurrent banal, nevus.

may be seen within the scar in the superficial dermis. The cells are usually nested. The atypia can be significant and can closely mimic a high-grade melanocytic dysplasia. We do not grade atypia in recurrent nevi; it always looks worse than in the original biopsy and, especially in young children and adolescents, may be severe with upward epidermal migration of melanocytes. More valuable is the assessment of the original specimen and the melanocytes in the residual nevus peripheral to the scar. If it is a recurrence of a dysplastic nevus, we indicate the following tissue review.

The recurrent Spitz nevus is typically intradermal in location and may permeate the subcutis. Recurrent Spitz nevi resemble the desmoplastic Spitz nevus by virtue of dermal fibrosis.[40] There is a low incidence of recurrence in classic Spitz nevi; one study failed to show any recurrences in 49 such patients during a follow-up period of 5 years.[41] Recurrent dysplastic nevi manifest cytoplasmic retraction artifact as clear spaces and clefts around nests or individual nevus cells showing variable cytologic atypia indistinguishable from the recurrent common acquired nevus. In our own experience, the atypia in recurrent dysplastic nevus exceeds the one that is seen in the common acquired nevus; the key is to look past the scar where classic features of residual dysplastic nevus are identifiable and the diagnosis can often be made. Review of prior material is essential when available.

Differentiation from Melanoma with Regression and Recurrent Melanoma

Regressive fibrosis in melanoma is different from a scar, with a delicate pattern of thin collagen fibers in an edematous matrix containing scattered mononuclear cells with prominent ectatic venules oriented perpendicularly to the epidermis. A scar is often hypovascular with laminated thick bundles of collagen in a parallel disposition to the epidermis. When vessels are present, they are small and may be closely aggregated. In regressed melanoma, there is usually prominent inflammation that may be lichenoid with conspicuous melanophage accumulation (i.e. tumoral melanosis).

In regressed melanoma, there may be no discernible melanocytes. In recurrent nevi, the epidermis shows melanocytic hyperplasia and hypermelanosis. In regressed melanoma, a severely atypical intraepidermal or dermoepidermal melanocytic proliferation is found outside the areas of regressive stromal fibrosis, in contrast to recurrent nevi where the pattern and cytology of melanocytic growth is typically banal outside the scar. The residual dermal lesion in melanoma is usually severely atypical while the residual dermal lesion in a recurrent nevus is not.

DERMAL DENDRITIC MELANOCYTIC PROLIFERATIONS

The dermal melanocytoses are characterized by dendritic melanocytes within the dermis: the mongolian spot, the blue nevus and its variants, the nevus of Ota, the nevus of Ito, Sun's nevus, and the dermal melanocytic hamartoma. Thought to evolve from a dermal arrest in the migration of melanocytes from the neural crest to the epidermis, these lesions share a common constituent cell, the dendritic melanocyte, which exhibits dense melanosomes and is partly surrounded by basal lamina cognate to a Schwann cell. The subtype of melanocytosis rests on correlation of clinical and histologic findings.

COMMON BLUE NEVUS OF JADASSOHN–TIECHE

The common blue nevus is mainly a lesion of childhood, but can occur later in life on the dorsa of the hands and feet and less often on the buttock, head and neck, and trunk[42] or subunguum[43] and on mucosal surfaces[44] including the vagina,[45] lymph nodes,[46] meninges, internal organs, such as the prostate gland,[47] and cervix.[48] The lesions average 3 to 4 mm in size but can grow as large as 1 cm and have a blue to blue–black color; they are rarely multiple and/or familial with an autosomal dominant inheritance[49] and are then seen throughout the body surface or in a large agminated cluster, i.e., a plaque-type blue nevus[50] up to 24 cm in diameter.[51] Satellitosis and an irregular border have been described.[52]

Histology

The blue nevus manifests pigmented cells of melanocytic and histiocytic origin in the upper to midreticular dermis in close apposition to collagen (Fig. 2.18). In most cases, a grenz zone of uninvolved papillary dermis is present and there is no overlying intraepidermal melanocytic proliferation; a small minority exhibit a dendritic junctional component.[53] The dermal proliferation may be poorly defined or may have a circumscribed nodular pattern. The cytoplasm of the dendritic melanocyte has a symmetrical bipolar extension from a central nucleus and contains fine, evenly distributed pigment granules and a nucleus that is round to oval with a small nucleolus, a delicate nuclear rim, and even chromatin. Admixed are melanophages that form the dominant component in some cases and contain coarse, irregular melanin granules within rounded cytoplasmic contours. Mitoses are almost never seen. The center of the lesion may assume a hypocellular collagenized nodular appearance with dendritic melanocytes dispersed between collagen bundles; this lesion is termed the sclerosing or desmoplastic blue nevus (Figs. 2.17 and 2.18).

When blue nevi may manifest small hypercellular foci of lightly pigmented spindle cells in an otherwise classic background, we apply the term

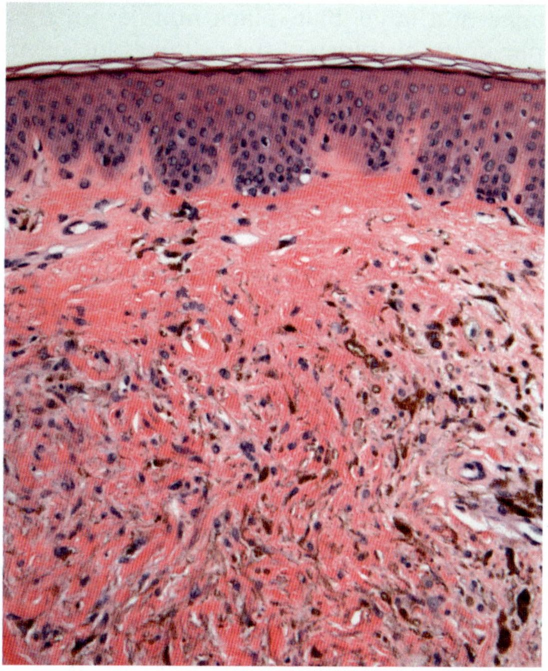

FIGURE 2.17 **Blue Nevus: There Is a Proliferation of Slender Dendritic Nevomelano-cytes Amidst a Sclerotic Hyalinized Appearing Dermis.** The cells are HMB-45 positive as opposed to those encountered in desmoplastic melanoma that are HMB-45 negative. In Figure 2.19, the blue nevus coexists with common acquired type A and type B melanocytes defining the concept of the combined nevus.

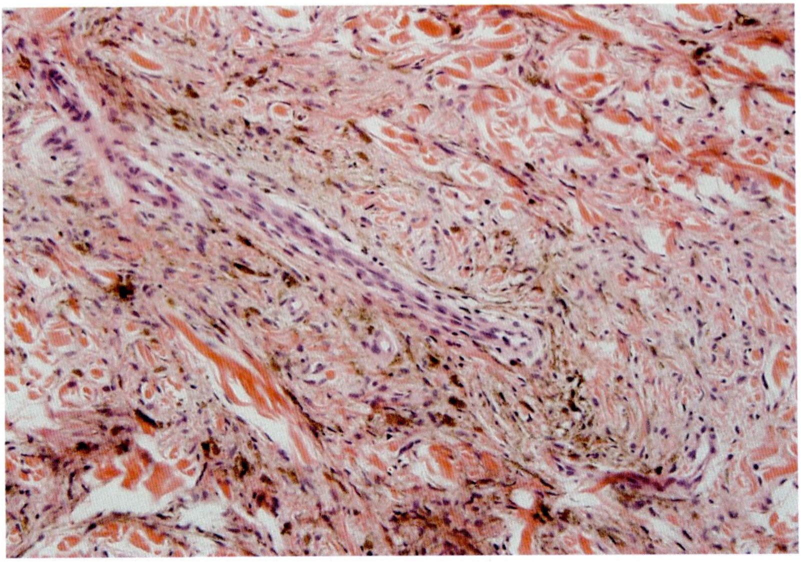

FIGURE 2.18 **Blue Nevus: There Is a Proliferation of Slender Dendritic Nevomelanocytes Amidst a Sclerotic Hyalinized Appearing Dermis.** The cells are HMB-45 positive as opposed to those encountered in desmoplastic melanoma that are HMB-45 negative. In Figure 2.19, the blue nevus coexists with common acquired type A and type B melanocytes defining the concept of the combined nevus.

blue nevi with hypercellularity (Fig. 2.19A–C); neither the clinical appearance of a large, blue–black nodule nor the striking expansile pandermal plexiform histology of the cellular blue nevus is observed.

A variant of blue nevus, designated as the hypopigmented common blue nevus, has minimal deposition of melanin and a clinical and histologic appearance that mimics a dermatofibroma.[54] We have encountered a case recently that resembled a pigmented epithelioid melanocytoma based on its large size, the extent of cellularity, and a nodular pattern of extension into the dermis. We designated the lesion as an unusual blue nevus with hypercellularity and sclerosis. The distinguishing feature from pigmented epithelioid melanocytoma was that the cells in the former include dendritic melanocytes admixed with heavily pigmented rounded cells that are melanophages; in the latter case the round cells are pigmented epithelioid melanocytes and/or melanophages. Illustrated is a classic pigmented epithelioid melanocytomal cell (Figs. 2.20 and 2.21). Incompletely excised blue nevi that persist or "recur" may, in the re-excision specimens, manifest greater cellularity but lack necrosis en masse, marked cytologic atypia, or abundant mitoses of a malignant blue nevus.[55]

Antibodies HMB-45 or Melan-A are of use in confirming that the lesion is of melanocytic derivation. Blue nevi, like melanomas, are diffusely positive throughout the lesion,[56] unlike desmoplastic melanoma where there is a sharp decline in HMB-45 or Melan-A expression in the lesional base or where some or most examples are entirely negative.

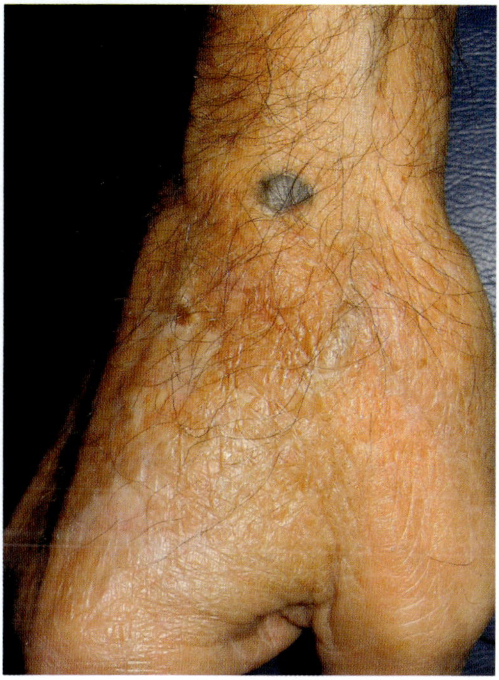

A

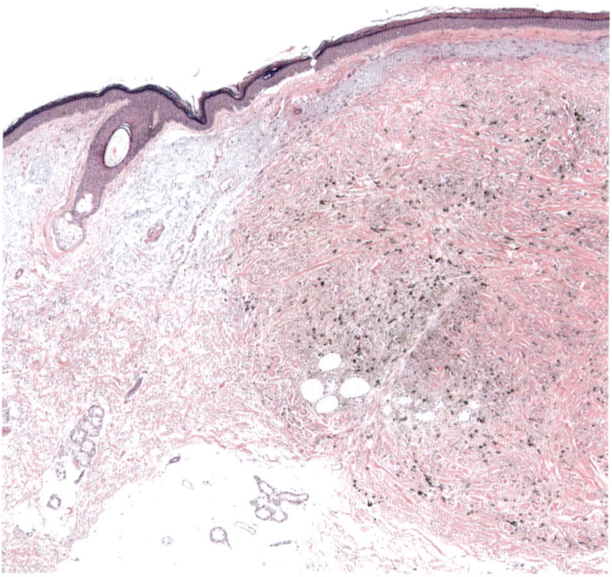

B

FIGURE 2.19 **Blue Nevus with Hypercellularity.** The clinical morphology in this case does not deviate from the conventional blue nevus **(A)**. The histomorphology differs by virtue of more cellular fascicles of the classic cell types, oftentimes with a more prominent epithelioid cell component **(B, C)**. (Case courtesy Dr George Monks, Tulsa, OK.)

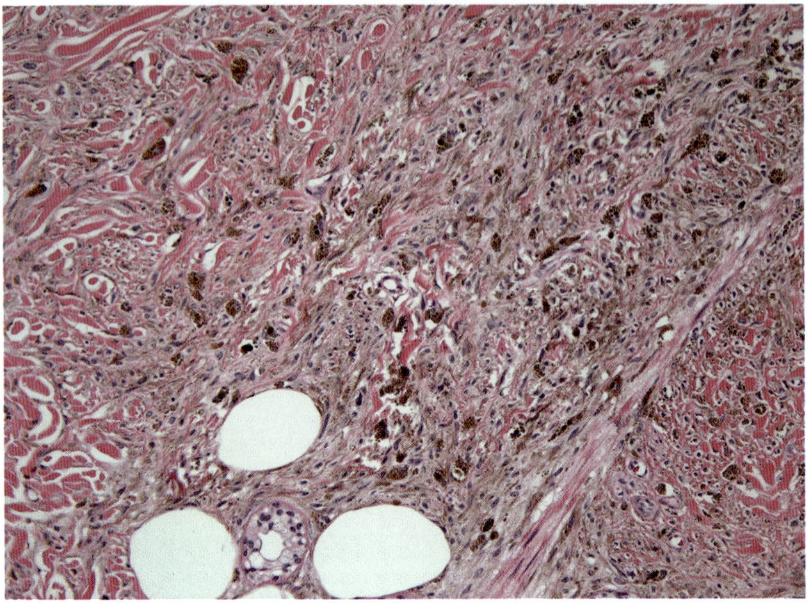

C

FIGURE 2.19 Cont'd.

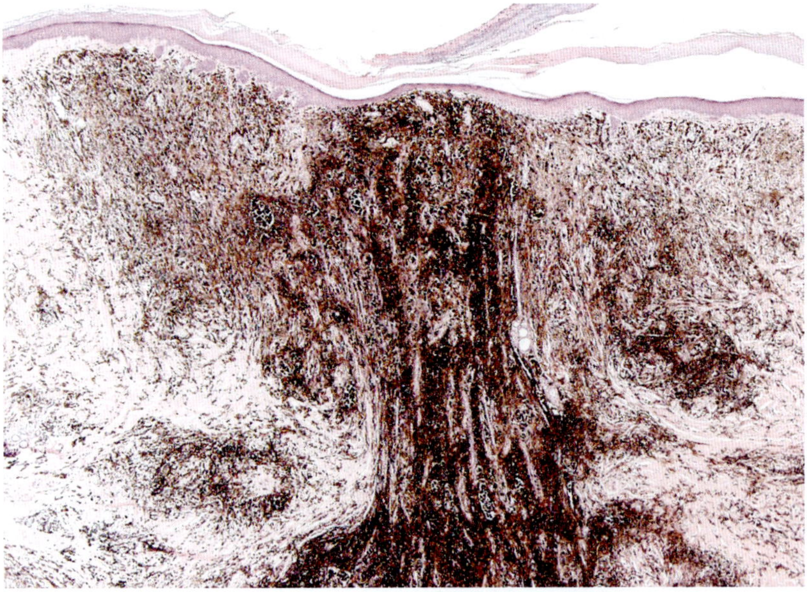

FIGURE 2.20 **Pigmented Epithelioid Melanocytoma: This Lesion Shows a Nodular Growth Pattern in the Deeper Dermis.** This particular architectural finding is usually a worrisome one. However, in this context, the cells appearing polygonal are melanocytes rather than representing melanophages. The cells in the classic pigmented epithelioid melanocytoma have a bland cytology.

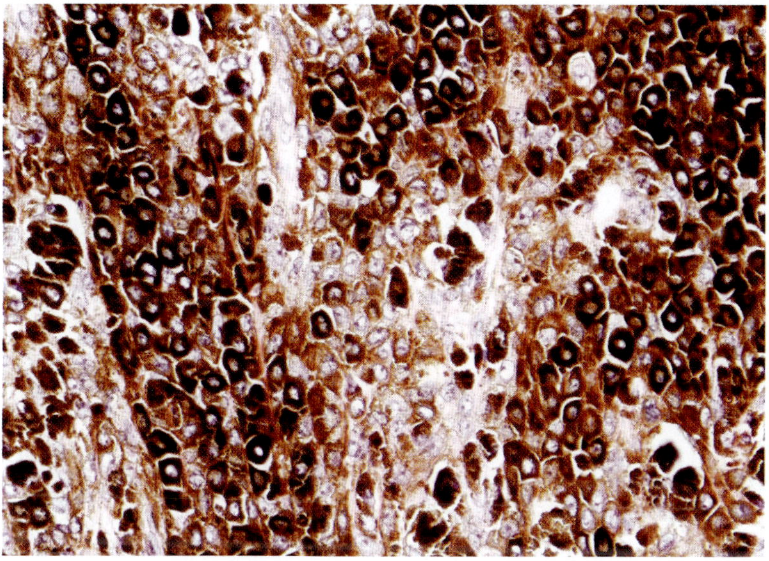

FIGURE 2.21 **Pigmented Epithelioid Melanocytoma: This Lesion Shows a Nodular Growth Pattern in the Deeper Dermis.** This particular architectural finding is usually a worrisome one. However, in this context, the cells appearing polygonal are melanocytes rather than representing melanophages as one would encounter in the classic pigmented epithelioid melanocytoma.

EPITHELIOID BLUE NEVUS

The epithelioid blue nevus is seen in 10% of patients with Carney complex, usually appears in childhood, is dome shaped, is under a centimeter in diameter, and has dark hues. Lesions tend to involve the trunk and extremities and, less frequently, the head and neck, do not recur, and, to our knowledge, do not undergo malignant degeneration. The epithelioid blue nevus may occur in a sporadic fashion.[57]

Histology

Epithelioid blue nevi have poorly defined or pushing margins or a combination and involve the subcutis in one-half of cases, comprising pigmented epithelioid cells admixed with a pigmented, spindled cell population as seen in typical blue nevi disposed between the collagen bundles singly and in small rows, clusters, and short fascicles imparting a checkerboard appearance. The epithelioid component has two morphologies, one being globular and heavily pigmented and the other being polygonal and lightly pigmented. When discernible, the nuclei of the former are small and spherical with an indistinct nucleolus. The polygonal cell nuclei have a single prominent nucleolus and do not mature.[57,58] The fusiform component is typical of a blue nevus. The lesion may be part of a combined nevus. Mitoses are rare and typical. Epithelioid blue nevi do not manifest sclerosis.[57,58] These lesions are held to be morphologically indistinguishable from the pigmented epithelioid melanocytoma.

CELLULAR BLUE NEVUS

The cellular blue nevus (CBN) classically occurs in children and young adults with a mean age of 33 years[59] but can present at any age as a large multinodular mass with a mean diameter of over 1 cm, sometimes showing progressive enlargement to a size of 10 cm or more. Lesions may ulcerate. Characteristic locations are the dorsa of the feet or the buttocks, but they occur anywhere on the body including the scalp, the conjunctiva, and spinal canal (termed "melanocytoma").[60] They are sometimes mistaken for melanoma when invasion of subjacent brain occurs.[61,62] Some CBNs are associated with palpable lymph nodes reflecting rests.

Histology

A low-power "dumbbell" configuration oriented perpendicularly to the epidermis with extension deep into the dermis and subcutis is classic, whereby alternating zones of hypercellularity and collagenous acellular pigmented foci are seen. The cellular component comprises nodules or fascicles of cuboidal, oval, or spindled cells; the former within the nodular foci and the latter in the fascicular zones (Figs. 2.22 and 2.23).

The cells have vacuolated, clear cytoplasms with coarse granular melanin and nuclei with delicate chromatin and small nucleoli. Draped around these cell balls are pigmented dendritic cells (Figs. 2.24 and 2.25).

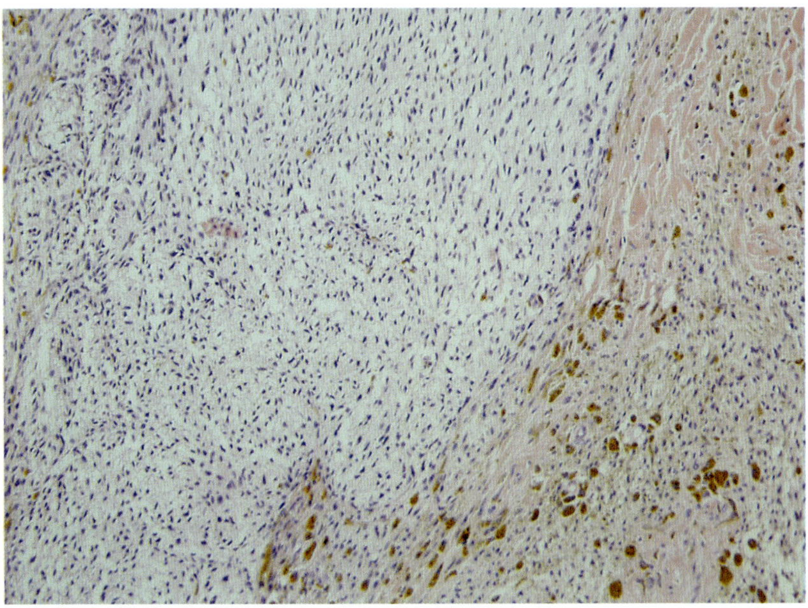

FIGURE 2.22 **Cellular Blue Nevus: Zones of Hypercellularity are Juxtaposed with Collagenous Acellular Pigmented Foci.** The lesion is extensive assuming a nodular configuration and may extend into fat. This particular architectural growth pattern may also be seen in melanoma.

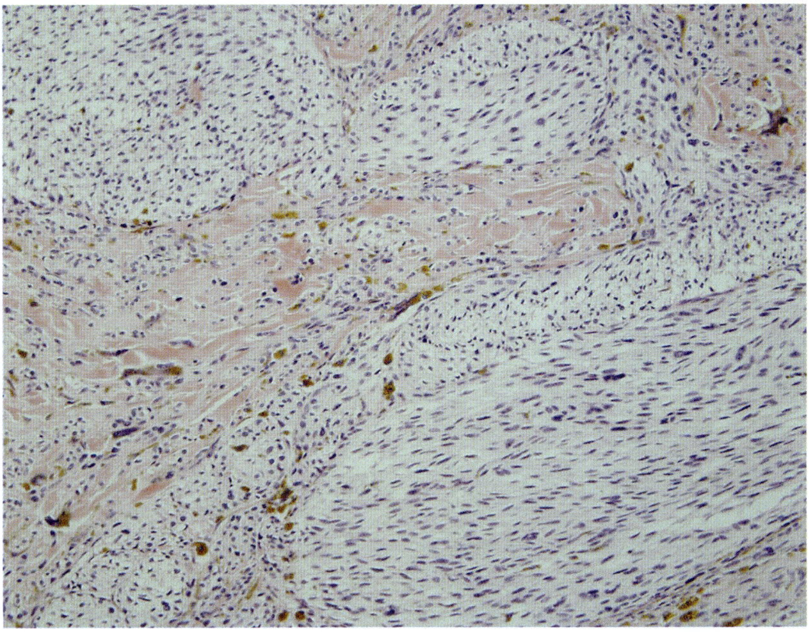

FIGURE 2.23 **Cellular Blue Nevus: Higher-power Magnification of the Cellular Foci Reveals that the Cells Are Oval to Spindled in Quality with Clear Cytoplasm.** The adjacent collagenized foci are more typical for the classic composition that defines a blue nevus.

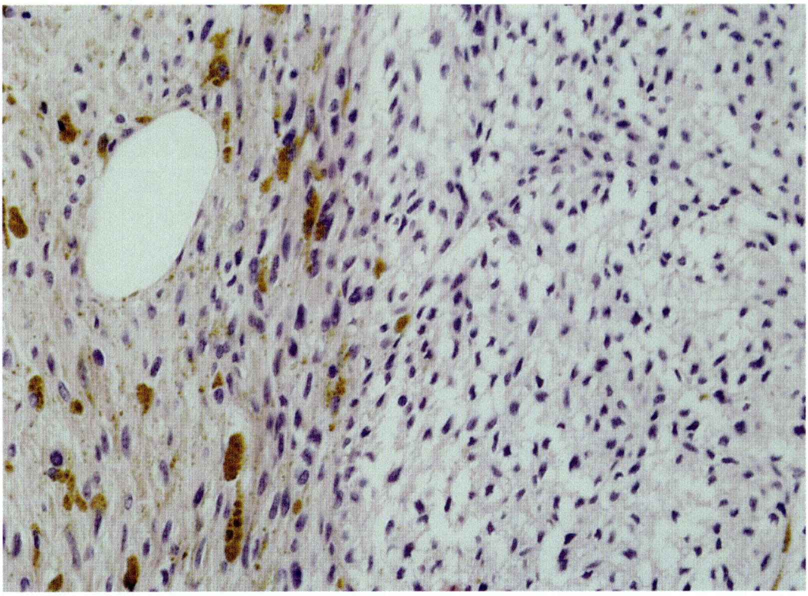

FIGURE 2.24 **Cellular Blue Nevus: Higher-power Magnification of the Cellular Foci Reveals that the Cells Are Oval to Spindled in Quality with Clear Cytoplasm.** The adjacent collagenized foci are more typical for the classic composition that defines a blue nevus.

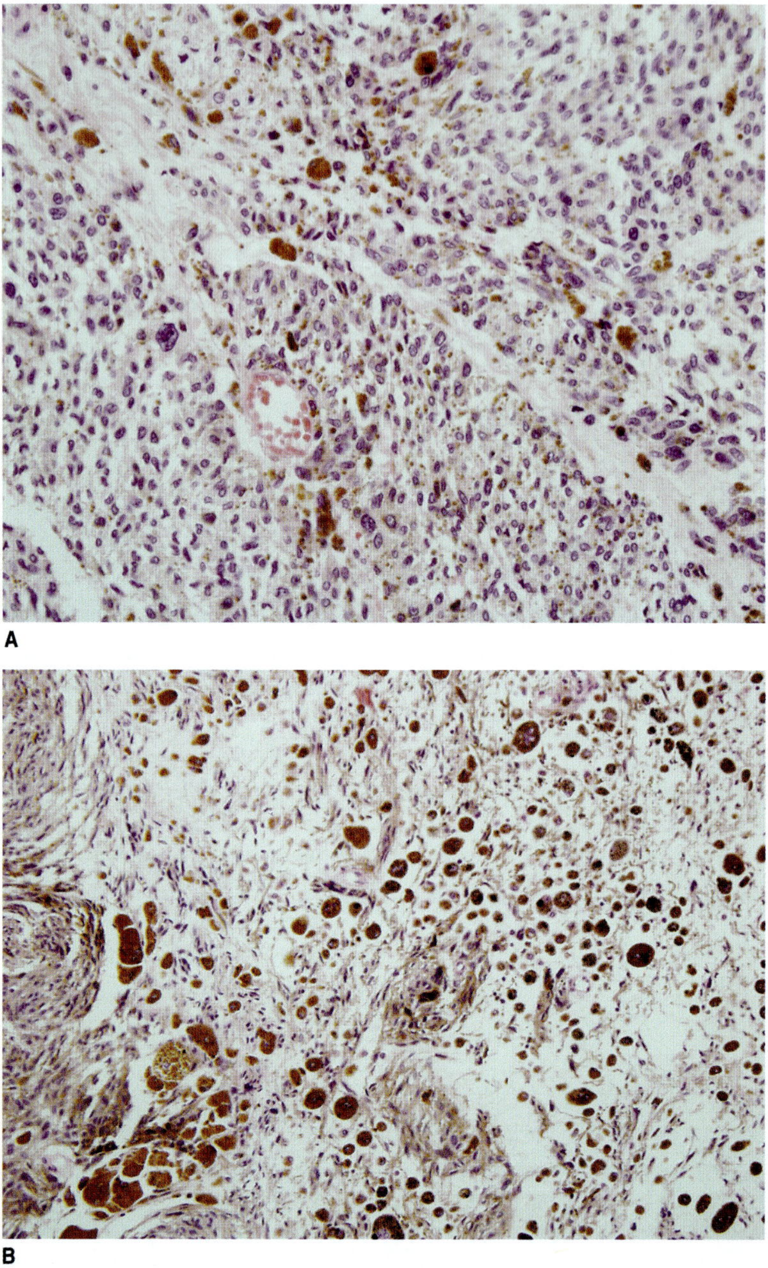

FIGURE 2.25 **Senescent Atypia may be Observed in the CBN and should not be Confused with Anaplasia.** Multinucleated giant cells may be seen and typical mitoses may be observed but are few in number (less than one per 40× high-power field) **(A)**. There is oftentimes cystification with adjacent melanophages as typified in **(B)** and **(C)**. **(D)** shows a malignant blue nevus. It is critical to make the distinction between the random senescent atypia of the CBN and the confluent high-grade atypia with mitoses and necrosis en masse that characterize the malignant blue nevus.

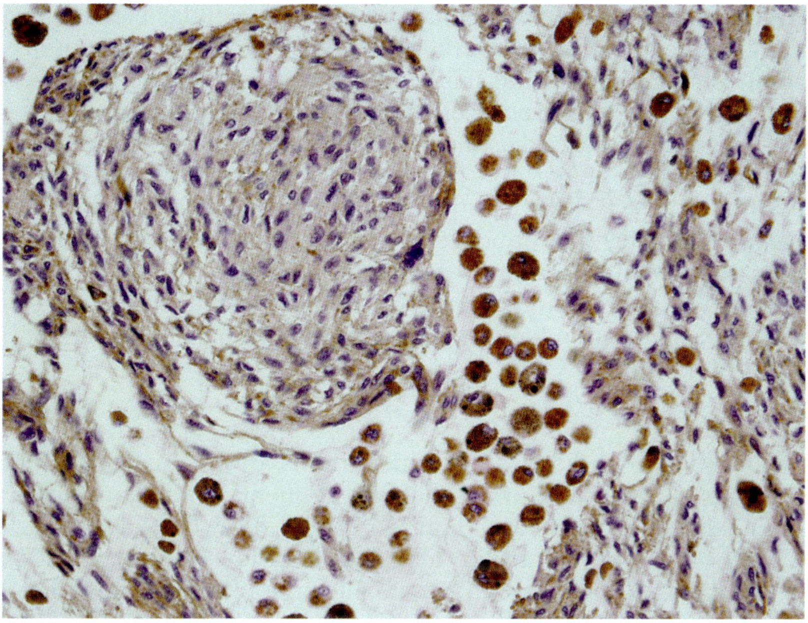

C

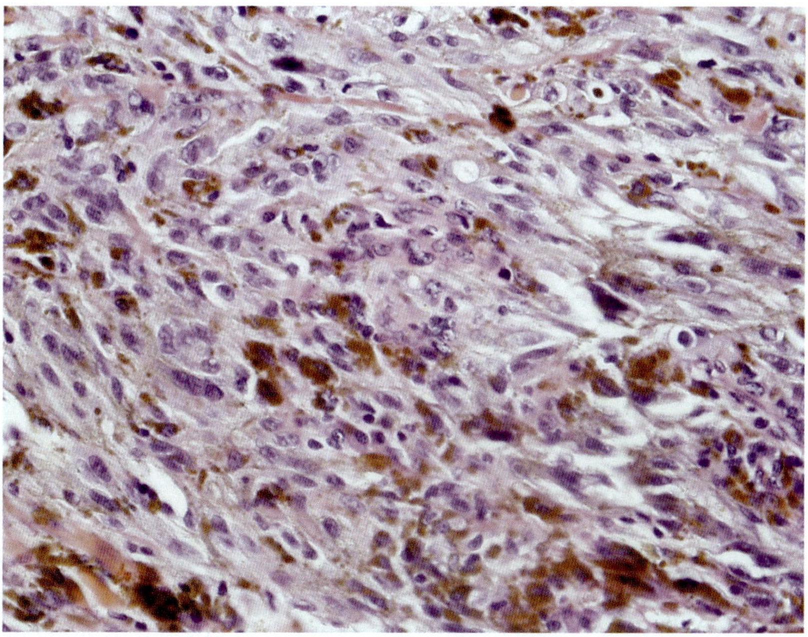

D

FIGURE 2.25 Cont'd.

Cystic degeneration may occur but the residual cellular elements within such foci appear viable and are embedded within an edematous and mucinous stroma, unlike the malignant blue nevus where cystic change reflects tumor necrosis. Senescent atypia may be observed in the CBN (Fig. 2.25); multinucleated giant cells may be seen and typical mitoses are few (less than one per 40× high-power field). A variant designated as the desmoplastic CBN has abundant desmoplastic stroma.[63] Balloon cell change is described.[64] The appellation *atypical blue nevus* has been applied to cases that manifest certain architectural and cytologic features that include an infiltrative margin, asymmetry, hypercellularity, pleomorphism, hyperchromasia, mitotic figures, and/or focal necrosis[65] superimposed on a background lesion of CBN.

Differential Diagnosis

The main differential diagnostic considerations are the malignant melanocytic neoplasms with prominent melanin pigment production, the first of which is the exceedingly rare "malignant blue nevus"[66] that occurs most often on the scalp of men in the fifth decade of life; an occurrence in the vulva with ovarian metastases 15 years after the initial diagnosis has been described.[67] The malignant blue nevus has atypical pigmented spindled cells showing marked variability of nuclear size and shape with overtly malignant cytology, numerous and atypical mitoses, and confluent necrosis. The biphasic elements of the CBN are absent and there is effacement of the dermal architecture.[66,68] Neurotropism may be observed in both. While the CBN may exhibit "aggressive" local growth with extension into the underlying tendons, the muscle, and even the brain, the histology remains typical. The second pigmented neoplasm entering into the differential diagnosis of the CBN is the melanoma with prominent pigment synthesis or "animal type" melanoma.[69]

NEVI OF OTA AND ITO

The nevus of Ota is a congenital lesion that occurs most often in Asians,[70] in African-Americans, and, less commonly, in Caucasians in a distribution that follows the first two (and sometimes the third) branches of the trigeminal nerve to involve conjunctiva, sclera, choroid, retina, and, rarely, the optic nerve, orbital fat, and periosteum (i.e., orbital melanocytosis)[71] with variable involvement of the eyelids, forehead, temple, nose, and the malar eminence of the cheek and rare involvement of the tympanum, hard palate, uvula, nasopalantine ganglion, and nasopharynx. Lesions are bilateral in 10% of cases[72,73] and are rarely first expressed in adult life with a 4:1 female preponderance. Rare malignant degeneration has been reported.[74] Some patients with ophthalmic involvement may develop melanoma of the choroid, retina, brain, or meninges; malignant lesions have a histology that resembles malignant blue nevi. The nevus of Ito is a unilateral pigmentary abnormality in the anterior or posterior upper shoulder area in the distribution of the acromioclavicular nerve[75]; typically, a subtle

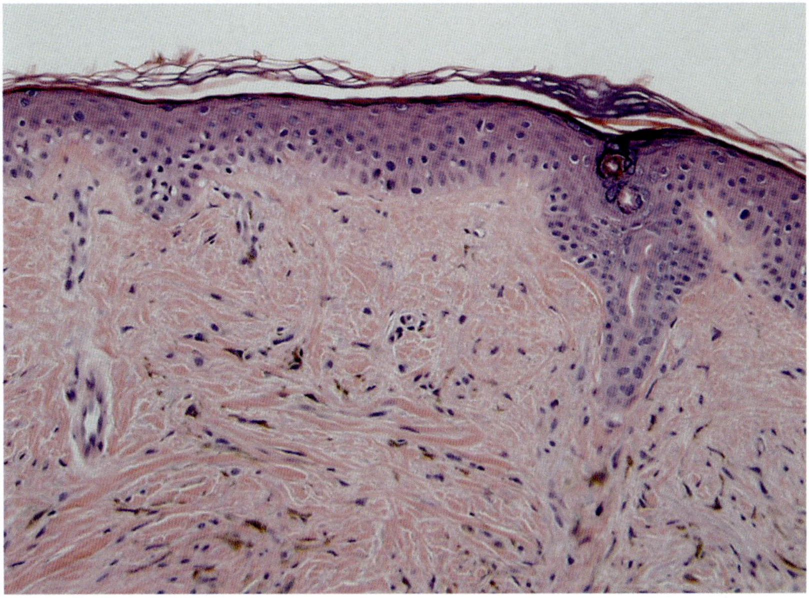

FIGURE 2.26 **Dermal Melanocytosis: There Is a Proliferation of Very Bland Appearing Dendritic Nevomelanocytes in the Superficial Reticular Dermis Compatible with a Nevus of Ito.** It is not possible to discriminate between nevus of Ito and Ota without the clinical history.

light gray macular pigmentation no more than 5.5 × 2.0 cm presents in the first or second decades of life but is likely to present at birth. Nevi of Ito and Ota may coexist.

Histology

The histology of the nevi of Ota and Ito is similar, namely, a subtle band-like disposition of dendritic melanocytes and melanophages in the upper third of the reticular dermis. Extension into the lower dermis or subcutaneous fat is uncommon (Figs. 2.26 and 2.27). Cellularity in scleral lesions may be greater than in those of skin.

MONGOLIAN SPOT

The mongolian spot is a gray area of macular pigmentation typically 3 to 5 cm in diameter in the lower lumbosacral area in 90% of Asian, African-American, and Native American newborns and 20% of Caucasians examined with a Wood lamp. Lesions are rarely multiple; the "ectopic" mongolian spot may appear anywhere on the body surface. We are not aware of malignant transformation in mongolian spots.

Histology

Dendritic melanocytes are scattered throughout the mid- and lower-reticular dermis and even into the subcutis, at a lower density than in the nevi of Ota, Ito, or Sun.

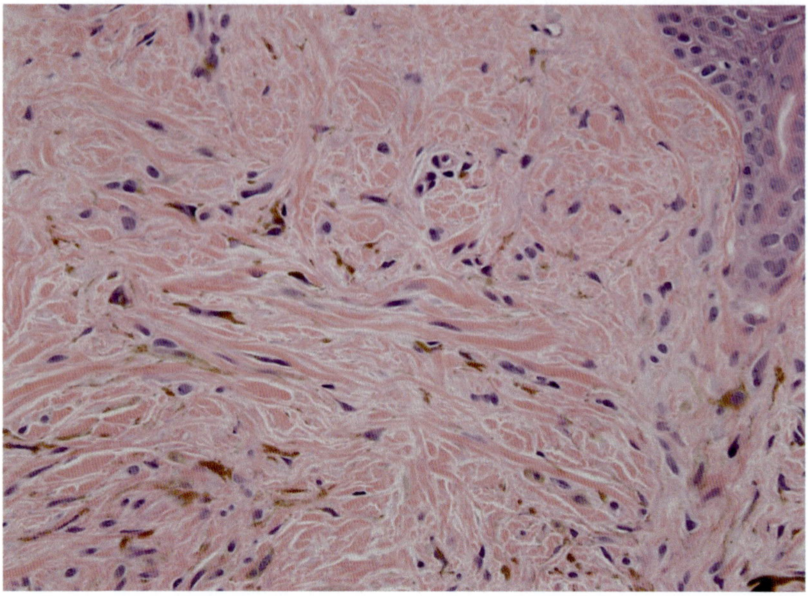

FIGURE 2.27 **Dermal Melanocytosis: There Is a Proliferation of Very Bland Appearing Dendritic Nevomelanocytes in the Superficial Reticular Dermis Compatible with a Nevus of Ito.** It is not possible to discriminate between nevus of Ito and Ota without the clinical history.

SUN'S NEVUS AND DERMAL MELANOCYTE HAMARTOMA

A speckled pattern of bilateral pigmentation in the zygoma occurs in the second decade of life or later in patients of Chinese extraction with a 6:1 female preponderance and with occasional familial clustering in the absence of ocular or mucosal pigmentary alteration.[76] Slender pigmented melanocytes are noted within the upper dermis in the absence of a fibrous response. This dermal melanocytosis is an extensive pigmentation of the buttocks with superimposed darker pigmented macules, often extending in a dermatomal distribution down one leg.[77] The histology is identical to that of the nevi of Ito and Ota.

NEVI OF SPECIAL ANATOMIC SITES

The main melanocytic lesions in the genital area include the mucosal lentigo, the common acquired nevus, the dysplastic nevus, melanoma, and a distinctive form of nevus termed "atypical melanocytic nevus of the genital type," the latter being clinically and histologically distinctive from the dysplastic nevus and frequently showing changes reflecting alterations in hormone levels such as during pregnancy. As identical lesions are seen throughout the anatomic milk line–the axillae, the breasts, the periumbilical region, the groins, and the genital areas of men and women[78]–we prefer the term "nevus of milk-line type, although nevi with a similar morphology may be seen on the ears or in fold areas of the skin." Typically located on either the mucosal surface or glabrous skin of the labia, clitoris, or mons pubis, the clinical morphology ranges from a polypoid evenly pigmented lesion to a flat one with variable pigmentation that ranges in size from 2 mm to 2 cm. More challenging is the occurrence of a nevus in the setting of vulvar lichen sclerosus, where flat pigmented lesions usually no greater than 5 to 6 mm but often only 2 to 3 mm in size contrast with a white-colored, depigmented background reflecting the lichen sclerosis component; the histologic and clinical concern is that of regressed melanoma.[79] Some designate these lesions as "atypical nevi of special sites." These lesions can show varying degrees of atypia; as with other atypical pigmented lesions, any such lesion with moderate or severe atypia should be completely excised if clinical circumstances permit.

Histology

The "atypical" melanocytic nevus of special sites, including the milk-line, manifests an intraepidermal component comprising epithelioid nevomelanocytes arranged in both a lentiginous and a dominantly nested fashion. An admixture of giant melanocytes and pigmented dendritic melanocytes is typical. The nuclei range in size from 8 to 12 μm and manifest open chromatin patterns distinct from those of adjacent nonlesional vulvar melanocytes, which are smaller with uniformly dense chromatin. The nested epithelioid cells assume an aberrant disposition along the sides of the rete ridges and in apposition to suprapapillary plates.[80] Some lesions show oval nests of spindled cell tracking obliquely along the junction of the epidermis and the retia. These nests may extend into the superficial dermis and are of variable size, sometimes showing dyshesion and retraction artifact. Melanin granules are typically large and coarse, unlike the dustlike melanin granules in the cytoplasms of intraepidermal melanoma cells. The junctional nests sometimes form a confluent plaquelike array with pagetoid spread of intact nests and/or single melanocytes in most cases; such cells have a nuclear morphology identical to those of the junctional nevomelanocytes. Lentiginous growth may extend on either side of the nested junctional proliferation. The epidermis often shows areas of hyperplasia and papillomatosis with areas of epidermal thinning centrally. The pagetoid growth pattern is invariably focal, never represents the dominant intraepidermal pattern, and is infrequently present at the lateral borders. There is typically sharp lateral circumscription, with termination as cohesive junctional and dermal nests, but these lesions can be asymmetrical. Cytologic atypia of either the epithelioid or the so-called lentiginous type is seen in the majority of cases (Figs. 2.28–2.31).

The fibrotic dermal reaction characteristic of milk-line/special site nevi comprises broad, amorphous collagen in the papillary and reticular dermis in which dermal nevus cells are embedded. The collagen does not resemble the organized periretal stromal response that typifies dysplastic nevi or the desmoplastic response seen with some invasive melanomas. The nevus cells are smaller than those cells found in the overlying epidermis and mature in the base.

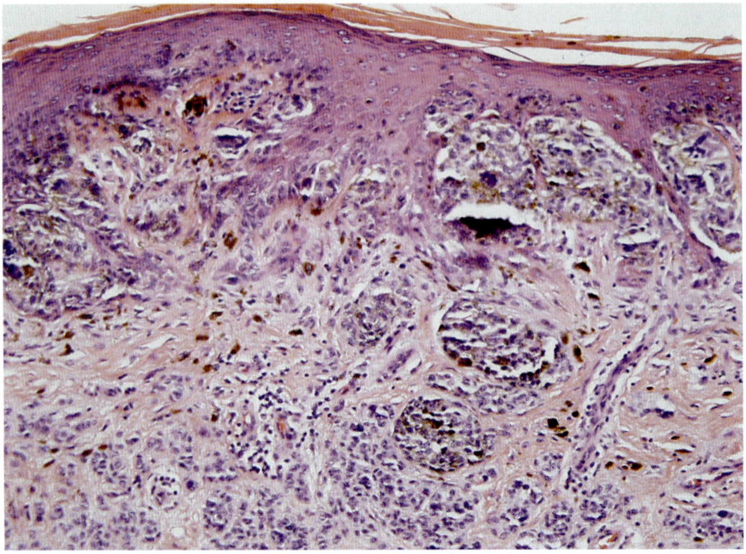

A

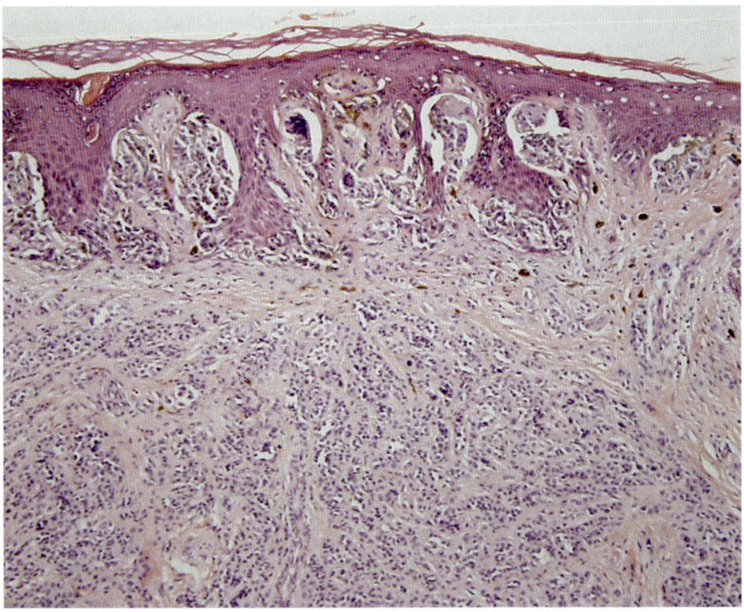

B

FIGURE 2.28 A–C: **Nevus of Special Anatomic Sites: This Biopsy Shows an Intraepidermal Proliferation of Epithelioid Appearing Nevomelanocytes Arranged in Both a Lentiginous and a Dominantly Nested Fashion.** There are scattered multinucleated nevus cells. Note that the nests are very dyshesive and irregular in regard to shape and location within the epidermis.

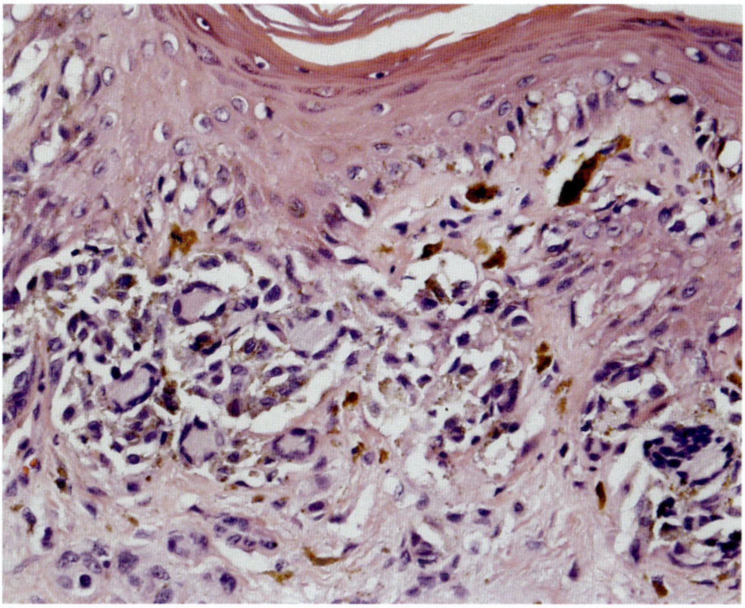

C

FIGURE 2.28 A–C: Cont'd.

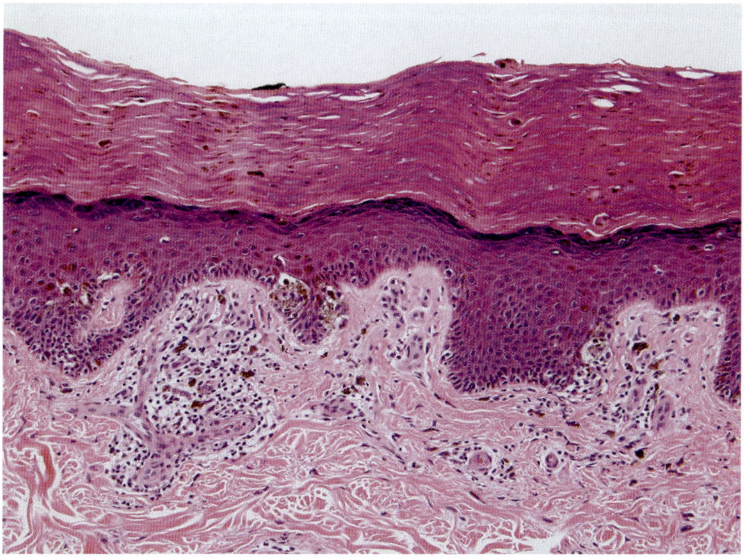

FIGURE 2.29 **Nevus of Special Anatomic Sites/Milk Line Nevus: Cytologically One Observes Atypia with Nuclear Size and Shape Variation and Irregular Melanization.** Scattered dendritic appearing and multinucleated melanocytes are observed.

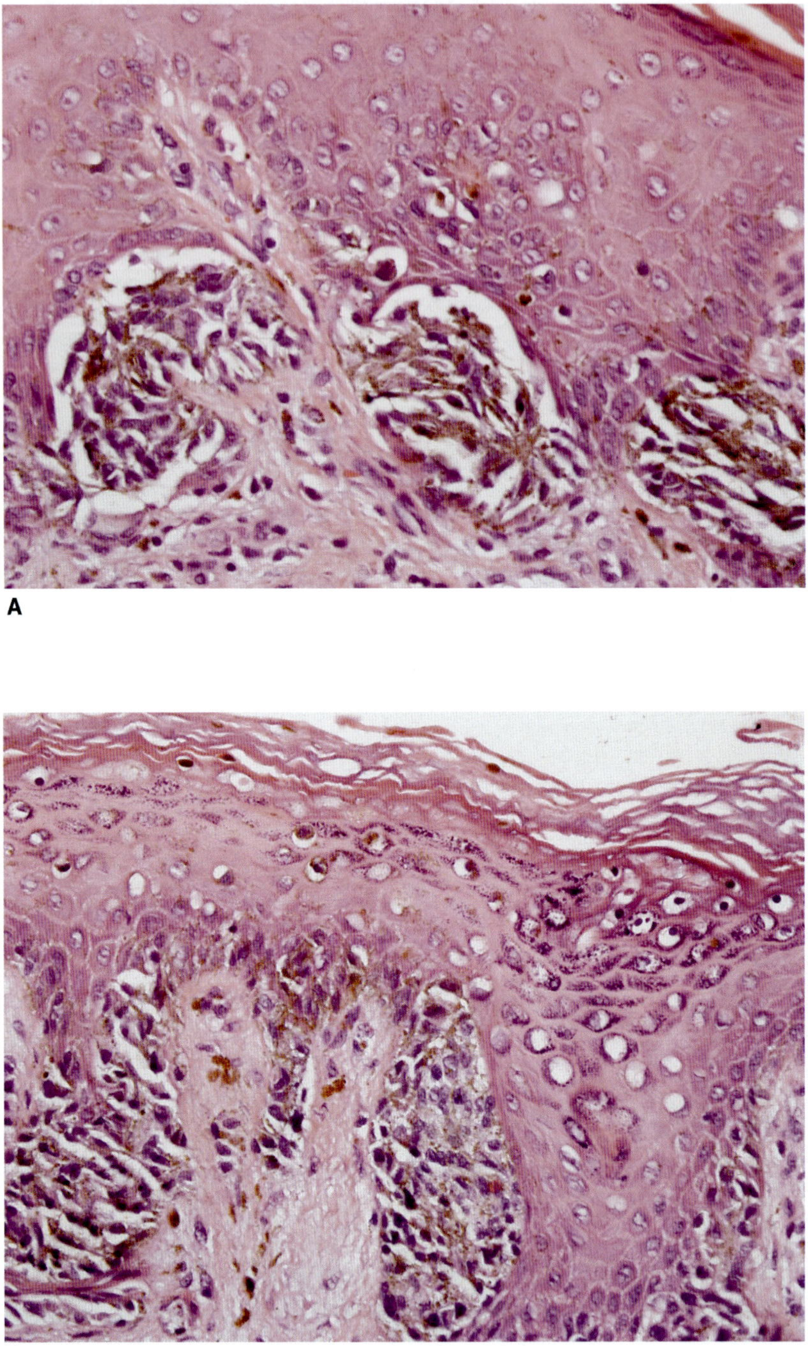

A

B

FIGURE 2.30 A, B: **Nevus of Special Anatomic Sites (Milk Line Nevus).** There may be focal pagetoid ascent; however, the dominant growth pattern within the epidermis is along the dermal epidermal junction.

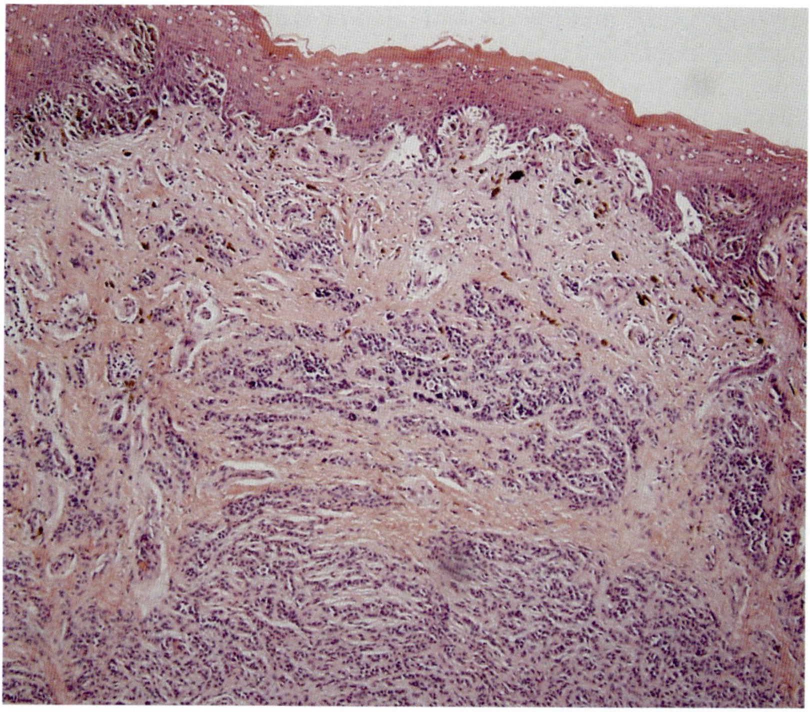

FIGURE 2.31 **Nevus of Special Anatomic Sites (Auricular Nevus).** Instead of the drape-like fibroplasias typical of the dysplastic nevus, these particular lesions show a common pattern of stromal fibroplasias whereby the stroma appears hyalinized and can be quite expansive oftentimes encasing the entire dermal component.

SPITZ NEVUS

Spitz nevi are seen most frequently in prepubertal children and are sometimes present at birth,[81] but 25% of lesions are biopsied or excised from patients older than 25 years of age and some patients present in the seventh decade. The classic Spitz nevus presents as a flesh-colored, dome-shaped, hairless papule on the trunk (39%), lower (25%) or upper (12%) extremity, or head and neck area (24%).[82]

Histology

Pigmented spindled cells predominated in the flat pigmented variants, whereas dome-shaped lesions usually comprised both spindled and epithelioid cells. The average size is 60 mm in diameter, with a range of 0.2 to 1.7 cm; less than 5% of lesions are greater than 1 cm in diameter. Occasionally, a compound Spitz nevus will present as a variegated plaque with mottled brown or tan pigmentation mimicking melanoma, i.e., the "plaque-type Spitz nevus." Rare clinical variants are the agminated Spitz nevus, comprising multiple pigmented or flesh-colored papules localized to a discrete area,[83] and the disseminated or eruptive variant.[84] Implicated etiologies of disseminated and agminated Spitz nevi include trauma, sunburn exposure,[85] pregnancy,[86] and radiotherapy.[87] Clinical differential diagnostic considerations include juvenile xanthogranuloma, mastocytoma, hemangioma, and, in the case of the sclerosing Spitz nevus, dermatofibroma.

Spitz nevi may be junctional, compound, or intradermal. Compound nevi account for two thirds and junctional Spitz nevi for 10% of lesions; purely dermal lesions are seen mainly in adults and represent the balance.[88] With respect to cytology, spindle cells predominate in 45% of cases and epithelioid cells in 20% of cases. An admixture of spindle and epithelioid cells is seen in the remainder.[82] Some authors suggest that certain histologic features are more common in childhood than in adult Spitz nevi, namely, papillomatosis, dermal edema and telangiectasia, and a dominant epithelioid cytomorphology.

The compound Spitz nevus manifests a sharply circumscribed dermal and epidermal proliferation that assumes the architecture of an inverted cone with its base oriented parallel to the dermoepidermal junction and its apex pointing toward the subcutis. Large thèques of nevomelanocytes at the dermoepidermal junction are separated by cleftlike spaces from the adjacent epidermis and are accompanied by acanthosis that may be pseudoepitheliomatous with overlying hyperkeratosis and hypergranulosis. The papillary dermis appears edematous, and there is vascular ectasia with junctional nests exhibiting a vertical orientation to the long axis of the epidermis (i.e., “Raining down” fascicles); cells in these arrays typically exhibit a spindle cell morphology. The nests are cohesive but show retraction from the epidermis. Eosinophilic globular structures in the epidermis, termed “Kamino bodies,” are hyalinelike bodies typically in the 30- to 40-μm size range seen in isolation or in association with a junctional nest in the majority of cases. These distinctive structures represent extracellular filaments with basement membrane components including types IV and VII collagen and laminin[89] and fibronectin[90] with components of the cytosolic shell. They are also present in melanomas and are hence not a specific criterion.

The cytology of the Spitz nevus is distinctive (Figs. 2.32–2.36). Cytoplasms are abundant with undulating rather than spherical cytoplasmic margins and are eosinophilic with variable deposition of melanin pigment; nuclear to cytoplasmic ratios are low. The melanocytes are two to three times the size of the small cuboidal nevomelanocytes that typify the common acquired nevus. The spindled component manifests banal nuclear characteristics, but with fusiform shapes and cytoplasms ranging from clear to heavily pigmented. Cell variability between cells of the same type is low.

Characteristic of Spitz nevi are the bizarre, “ganglionlike” mononuclear cells or bi- and multinucleated melanocytes disposed singly within the superficial dermis and/or along the dermal–epidermal junction in a single cell array. They may also be located in those junctional thèques composed of epithelioid cells. While epithelioid cells can demonstrate

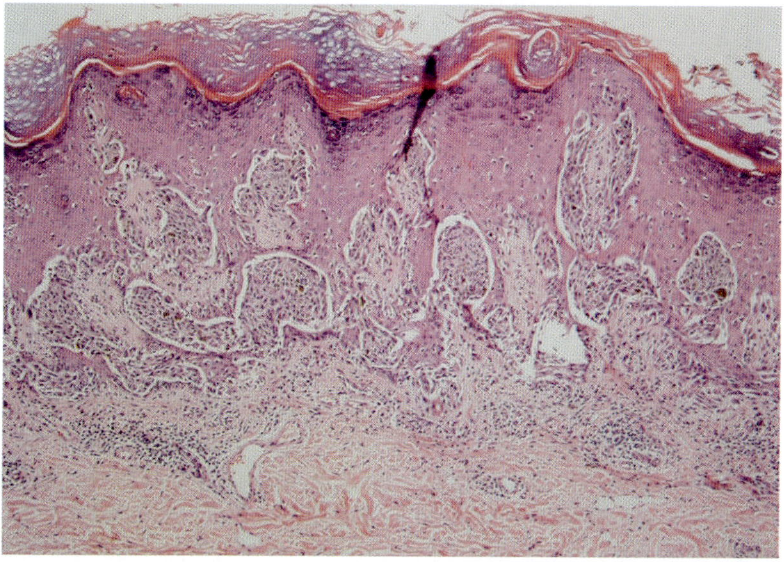

FIGURE 2.32 The intraepidermal component is predominantly in a nested array whereby the nests assume a vertical disposition to the long axis of the epidermis with retraction and epidermal hyperplasia.

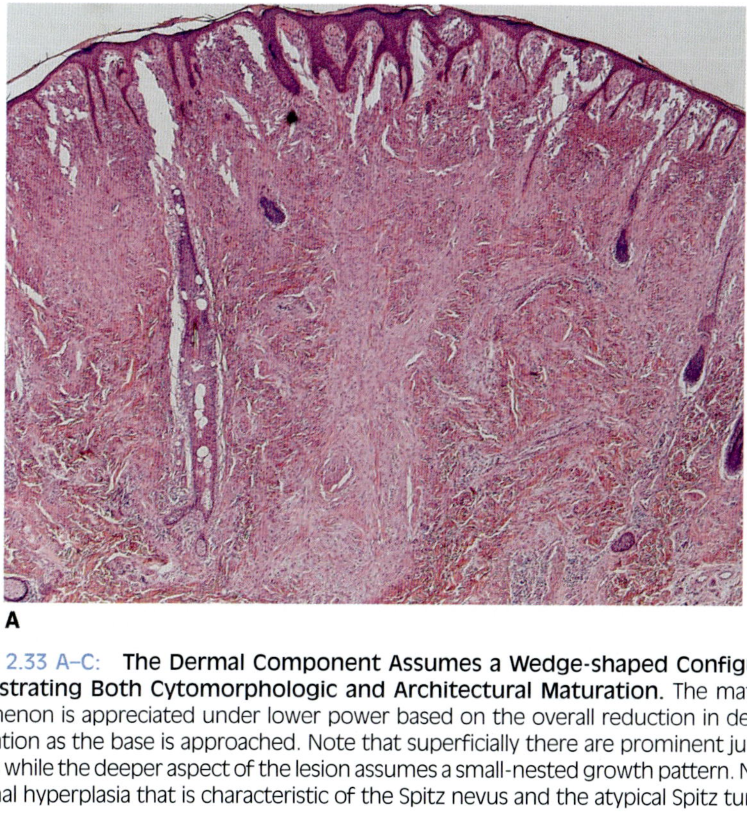

A

FIGURE 2.33 A–C: **The Dermal Component Assumes a Wedge-shaped Configuration Demonstrating Both Cytomorphologic and Architectural Maturation.** The maturation phenomenon is appreciated under lower power based on the overall reduction in density of proliferation as the base is approached. Note that superficially there are prominent junctional thèques while the deeper aspect of the lesion assumes a small-nested growth pattern. Note the epidermal hyperplasia that is characteristic of the Spitz nevus and the atypical Spitz tumors.

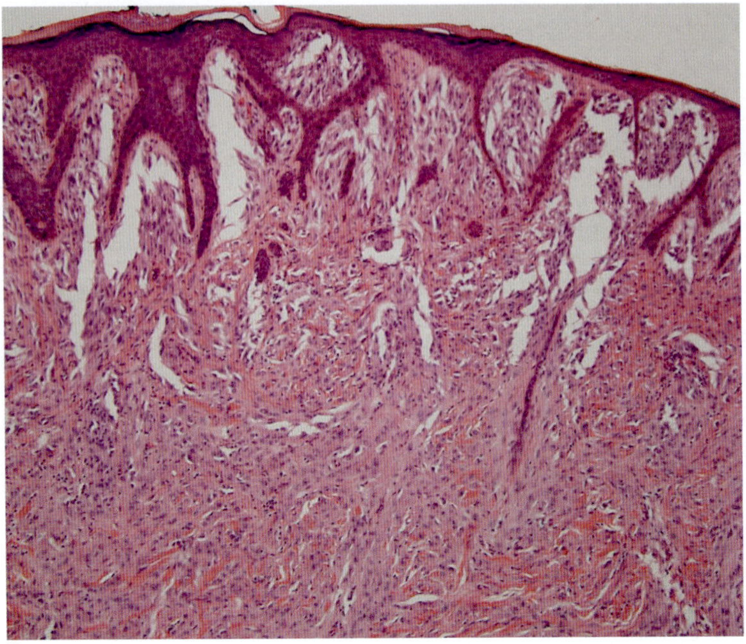

B

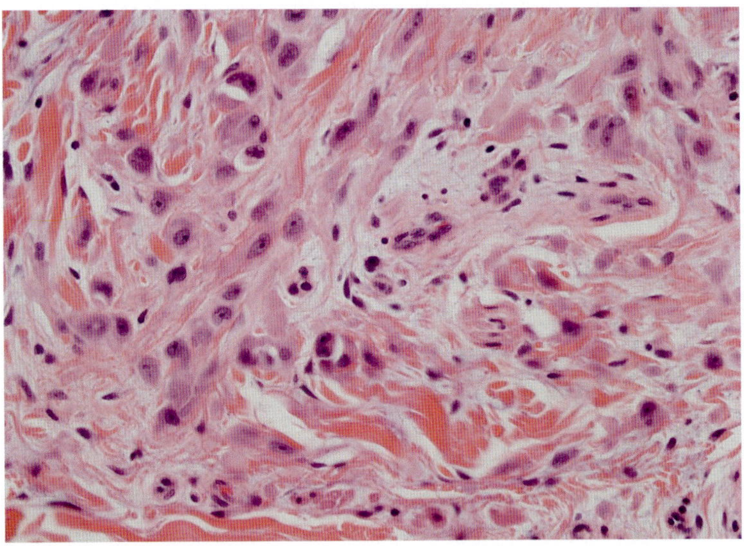

C

FIGURE 2.33 A–C: Cont'd.

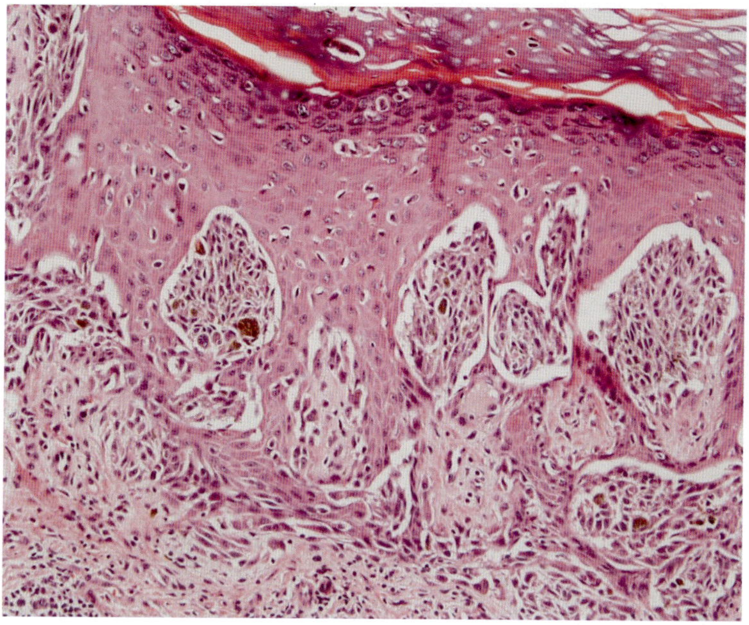

FIGURE 2.34 Pagetoid ascent is also present whereby there are foci of singly disposed and nests of nevomelanocytes ascending into the spinous layer of the epidermis.

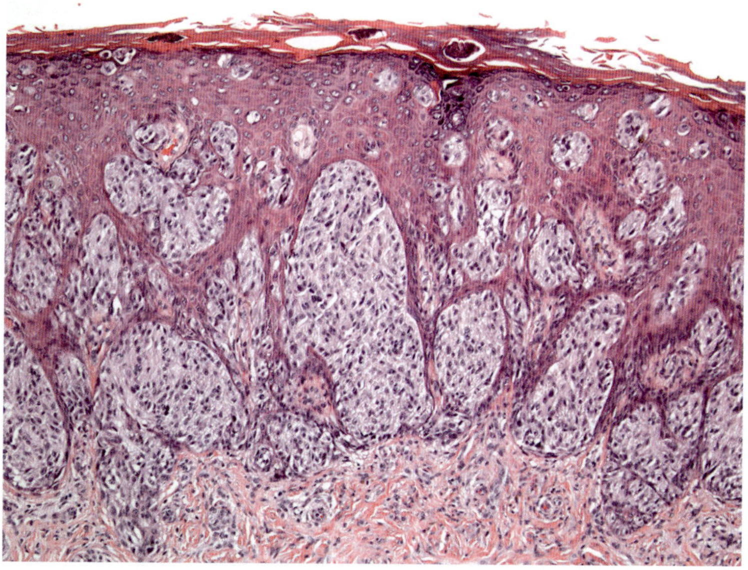

FIGURE 2.35 Epidermal hyperplasia is characteristic of Spitz nevus.

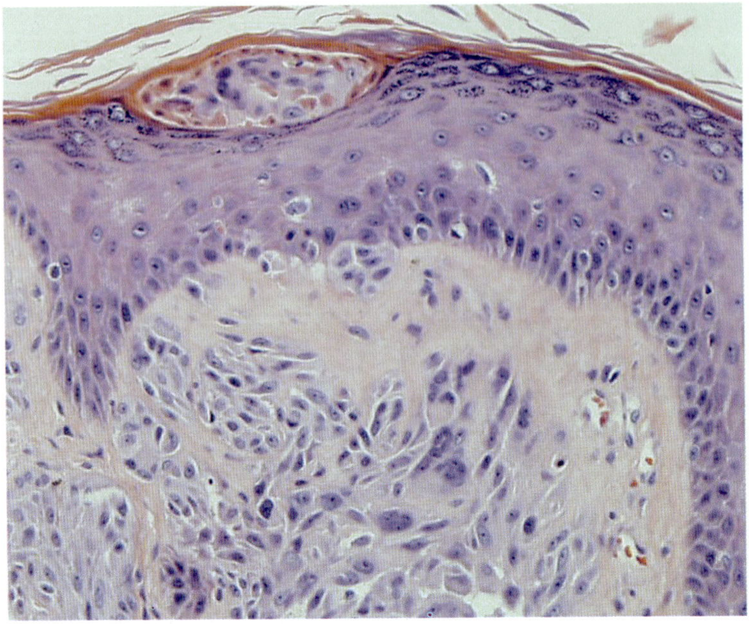

FIGURE 2.36 In the zones of nested growth, there is focal pagetoid ascent although in no areas does the pagetoid component dominate over areas of junctional nested activity.

pagetoid ascent, it is rare for the atypical multinucleated giant cell to permeate the spinous layer of the epidermis (Figs. 2.37–2.39). Pagetoid spread is seen in most Spitz nevi and is most obvious in childhood; it is characteristically maximal in the central portion of the lesion and is most conspicuous in the overlying junctional nests. It would be considered a disturbing finding to see zones of dominant pagetoid spread, especially at the lateral borders. Such lesions are better categorized as atypical Spitz tumors but may indicate melanoma. In acral Spitz nevi, the pagetoid spread is also confined to the area over the junctional nested component that tends to be broader; pagetoid spread is more extensive and may be confluent. A single-cell pattern of epidermal growth is common but it is reassuring when the pagetoid component is predominantly in a nested array. Invasion of eccrine ducts, hair follicles, and nerve twigs is routine and does not necessarily imply congenital onset. Intravascular nevus cells are identified in 14% of all Spitz nevi in children.[91] Mitoses are identified in roughly 20% of Spitz nevi,[88] mainly in the junctional and superficial dermal components. Any "marginal mitoses" defined as those seen within 0.25 mm of the lesional edge should prompt concern with respect to malignancy.[92,93] While it is held that features favoring a Spitz nevus include the intraepidermal eosinophilic bodies, relative superficial confinement, and architectural maturation, no specific criterion is decisive. Maintaining a uniform and benign cytologic character, the cells of a Spitz nevus diminish in size away

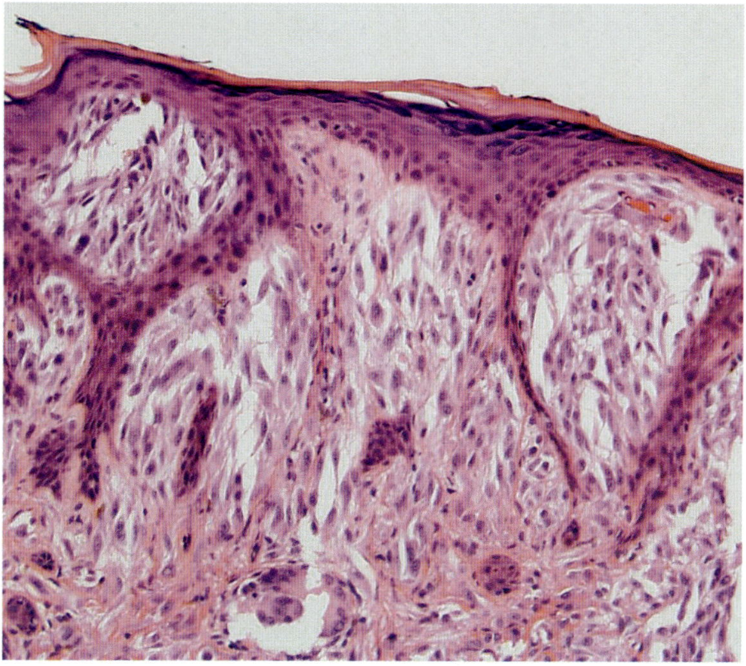

FIGURE 2.37 From a cytomorphologic perspective, the cells in the epidermis have an epithelioid appearance. They are round with abundant eosinophilic cytoplasm. The nuclei are round and nucleoli are conspicuous and have an eosinophilic quality.

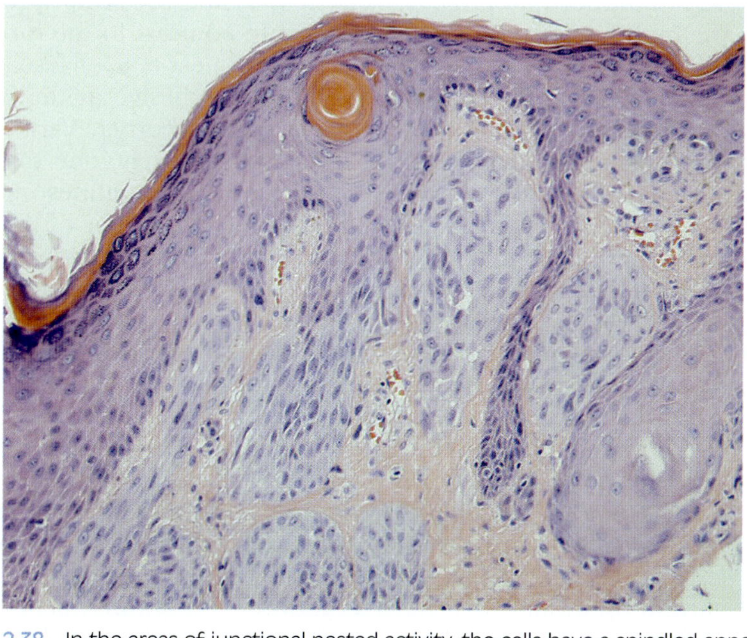

FIGURE 2.38 In the areas of junctional nested activity, the cells have a spindled appearance.

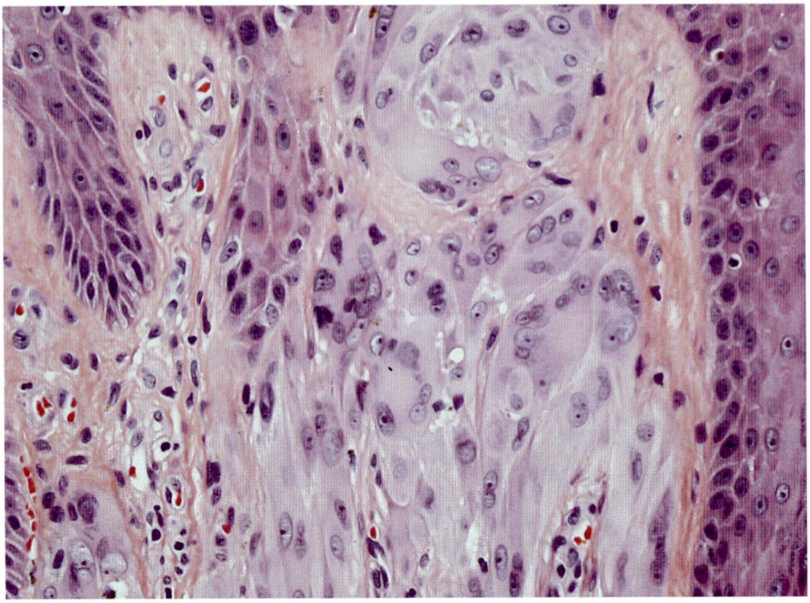

FIGURE 2.39 **The Minor Cell Component Is One Characterized By Pleomorphic Giant Cells.** These cells exhibit multinucleation and show considerable nuclear variability both in terms of nuclear shape and the quality of the chromatin pattern.

from the epidermal surface; the cells are superficially disposed in nests and fascicles that become progressively smaller and break up into single cells in the mid- and lower-reticular dermis. In contrast to the foregoing, atypical Spitz tumors do not show a decrease in nest and/or fascicle size or a single cell pattern of dispersal but remain cohesive at the lesional margin to produce a pushing, nodular, or expansile border. Variations in the low-power morphologic features of a lesion, namely, one that lacks the architecture of an inverted cone, fail to mature, or manifest marginal mitoses, or large fascicles or expansile nodules in the depths of the lesion should prompt concern that the lesion may represent an atypical Spitz tumor whose biological behavior is uncertain, versus a melanoma. When in doubt, consultation is advisable.

It has been suggested that 3% of dysplastic nevi have a Spitz nevus phenotype; we make this diagnosis when classic stromal and other features of dysplasia are superimposed.[94] In our experience, the most common cell type is a spindled nevomelanocyte defining an overlap between a dysplastic nevus and a pigmented spindle cell nevus of Reed. A lymphocytic host response may be observed in Spitz nevi; it is uniform throughout the lesion, imparts a symmetrical wedge-shaped morphology, and varies from a pandermal patchy perivascular infiltrate to a dense one obscuring the nevus.[95]

Regarding the dermal Spitz nevus of adulthood, scanning magnification reveals a symmetrical inverted triangular architecture while the epidermis shows hyperplasia with variable hypermelanosis. There is dissipation of cellularity in the depths of a lesion that terminates as small nests or as single cells dispersed between collagen bundles and along adnexal structures in the center. The dominant cell of the dermal Spitz nevus is usually epithelioid, but admixed spindle cells may be observed. The cells show mild hyperchromasia with irregular chromatin distribution; cytoplasms are usually devoid of pigment. Variable numbers of giant cells are present; some cases have none. A delicate reactive fibrosis surrounds individual nevus cells, but is not prominent as in the desmoplastic Spitz nevus and is in sharp contrast to the fibroplasia provoked by melanoma, where tumor cell invasion disrupts the pre-existing collagen network.

We recommend a conservative re-excision of all Spitz nevi that have not been completely excised or of those cases with atypical light microscopic features if narrowly excised. These recommendations derive from the fact that one must examine an entire lesion microscopically to arrive at a correct diagnosis. Atypical lesions may recur and in their recurrence, the histology may appear even more atypical; persistent recurrence of any pigmented lesion is always an ominous sign. Further excision at the outset will obviate these problems.

SCLEROSING OR DESMOPLASTIC SPITZ NEVUS

The sclerosing or desmoplastic Spitz nevus is a variant of the dermal Spitz nevus.[96] Stromal desmoplasia can accompany virtually any type of benign dermal melanocytic nevus.[97] Desmoplastic nevi are located preferentially on the extremities and trunk and spare the palms and soles.

Histology

The low-power architecture is that of a poorly circumscribed fibrotic plaque without sharp lateral or vertical margins. In contrast, desmoplastic melanoma has a diffuse pattern of growth. The epidermis shows hyperplasia as one sees overlying a dermatofibroma; small junctional nests may be present. Higher-power examination reveals an interpolation of bizarre cells between sclerotic collagen bundles in a low-density proliferation. Inflammation is minimal to absent. There is cell-to-cell variability with little cytoplasmic pigment deposition; the cells have a large polygonal ganglionlike morphology with multinucleated forms that may resemble a Touton giant cell, but lacking cytoplasmic lipid vacuoles. Nucleolation may be observed but mitoses are absent or rare (i.e., no more than 1 in 20 high-power fields). The cells are primarily singly disposed, although a few small clusters of cells may be observed. Maturation is observed in only a minority of cases. An "angiomatoid desmoplastic Spitz nevus" has a richly vascular stroma with plump endothelia[98] (Figs. 2.40 and 2.41).

The lesion must be distinguished from desmoplastic melanoma. Metastatic carcinoma of breast ductal primary derivation may enter into the differential diagnosis because of the pleomorphic epithelioid quality of

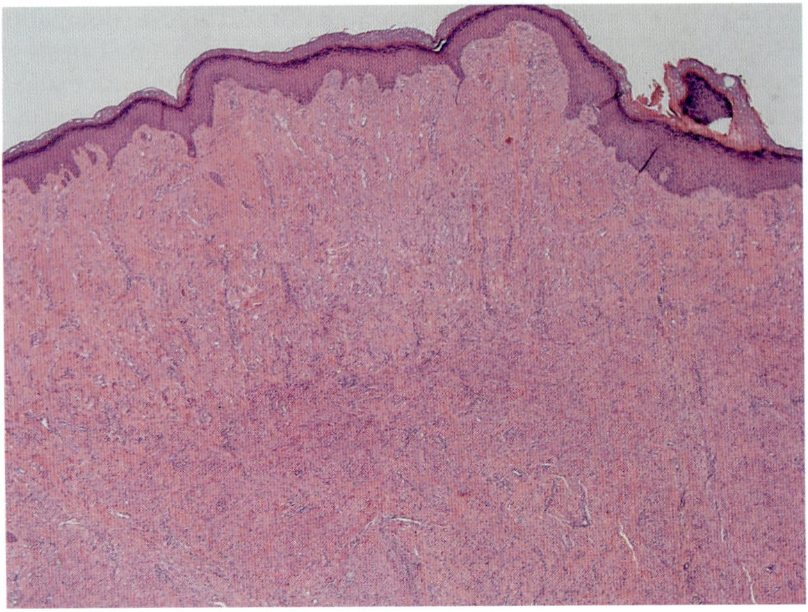

FIGURE 2.40 **Desmoplastic Spitz Nevus.** Amidst a sclerotic dermis, there are scattered bizarre appearing pleomorphic giant cells. At low power, this lesion could be mistaken for a cicatrix and/or a dermatofibroma.

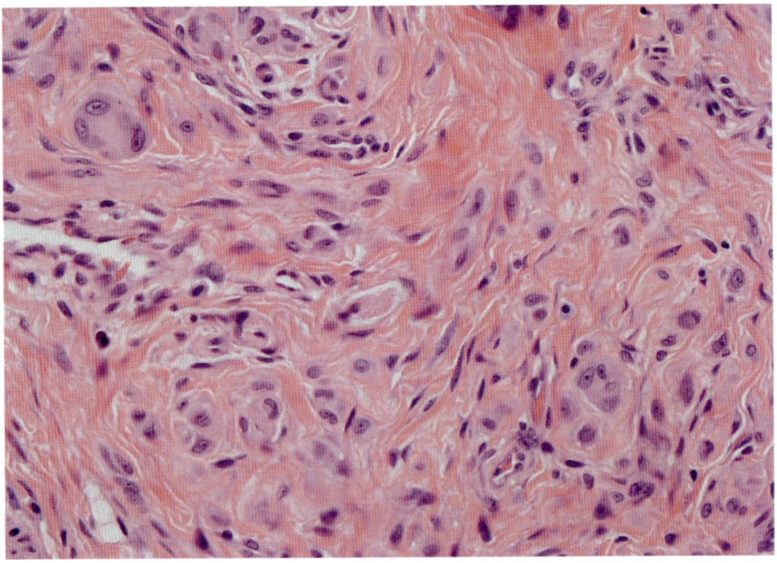

FIGURE 2.41 **Desmoplastic Spitz Nevus.** Amidst a sclerotic dermis, there are scattered bizarre appearing pleomorphic giant cells. At low power, this lesion could be mistaken for a cicatrix and/or a dermatofibroma.

the cells and the desmoplastic nature of the stroma. Immunohistochemistry should enable this distinction.

PAGETOID SPITZ NEVUS

This entity appears as a clinically innocuous, small pigmented macule in a young patient, typically less than 0.4 cm in diameter.[99]

Histology

The dominant pattern of growth is as single cells in a pagetoid array with variable nest formation and a symmetrical profile with sharp lateral circumscription. The cytology is typical of the epithelioid cell component of the common Spitz nevus; the nuclei are round or oval and do not exhibit the aberrant, folded or angulated contours encountered in high-grade melanocytic dysplasia. Cytoplasms are abundant with an eosinophilic or lightly pigmented staining quality and heterogeneity of melanization is not a feature.[100] Distinction of such lesions from high-grade de novo intraepidermal epithelioid melanocytic dysplasia/melanoma in situ is difficult; we advise re-excision. In our opinion, a certain subset of lesions designated as so-called pagetoid Spitz nevus represents de novo intraepidermal epithelioid melanocytic dysplasia, a distinctive form of melanocytic dysplasia seen in patients with the atypical mole phenotype (Fig. 2.42).

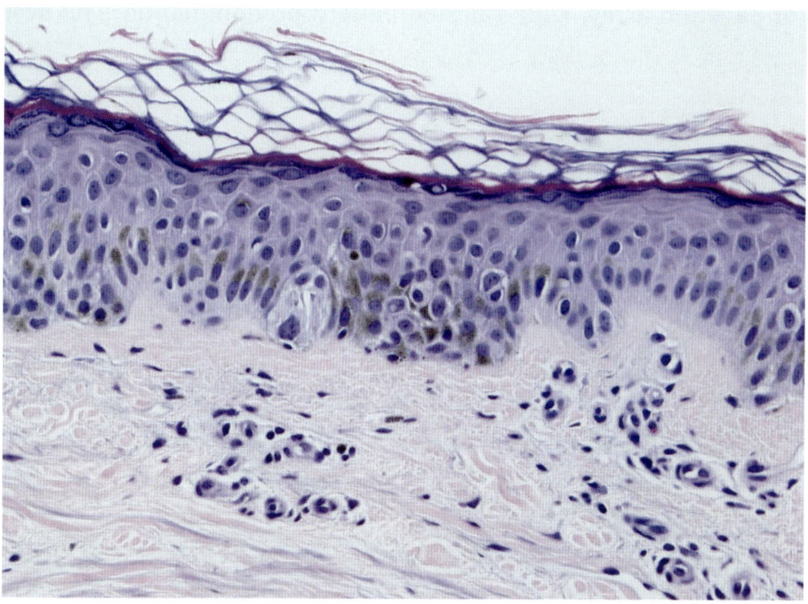

FIGURE 2.42 De novo intraepidermal epithelioid melanocytic dysplasia. There is a single cell Pagetoid growth pattern melanocytes. This is a precursor to melanoma in situ.

PIGMENTED SPINDLE CELL NEVUS OF REED

The pigmented spindle cell nevus presents as a black or dark brown dome-shaped lesion, 2 to 6 mm papule on the proximal extremities, back, or abdomen of a young woman.[101] A minority has an irregular border.[102]

Histology

This is a variant of the Spitz nevus dominated by spindle cells (Fig. 2.43) showing heavy melanization, accompanied by a variable admixture of epithelioid cells (Fig. 2.43). Such lesions are either purely intraepidermal or else have only a superficial dermal contribution. The lower border often abuts the papillary–reticular dermal interface as a broad horizontal shelf; the average thickness is 0.67 mm. Three-quarters of lesions showed sharp lateral circumscription, but 2% have an ill-defined edge and roughly one fourth show sharp lateral demarcation at one margin and gradual diminution of junctional activity at the opposite margin.[103] Some show a recent change such as rapid growth, peripheral erythema, or a halo effect after intense sun exposure. The epidermis is of variable thickness; pagetoid growth is seen in most cases, being maximal in the overlying areas of prominent nested junctional activity.[104] In our experience, a nested pattern of upward migration often predominates. The cytology resembles that of the spindle cell component of the classic Spitz nevus. There is often transepidermal elimination of melanin pigment to the cornified layer and melanophages in the superficial dermis.[104] The cells in the epidermis are disposed in a nested, lentiginous and/or pagetoid array, with a nested pattern predominating. The nests lie

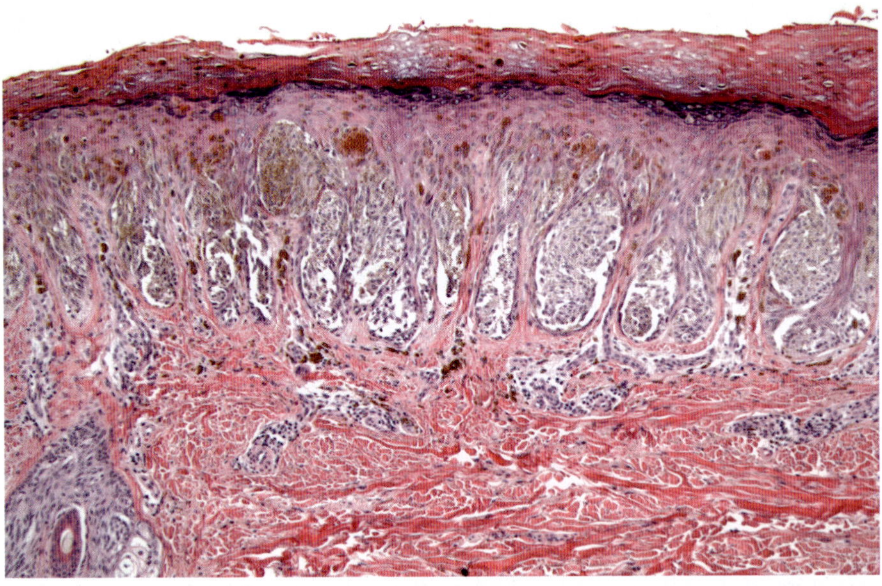

FIGURE 2.43 The biopsy shows a principally intraepidermal melanocytic proliferation of spindled melanocytes assuming a dominantly nested growth pattern along the dermal epidermal junction.

within elongated retia that may fuse; cells are often vertically oriented at the tips of retia or horizontally oriented when associated with fusion of retia. Careful attention to the banal cytology will prevent false-positive diagnoses when pagetoid spread is prominent; mitoses may be observed but are always typical. Vertical arrays of papillary dermal collagen may be seen, but lamellar fibroplasia is uncommon. Maturation is invariable. Perivascular dermal inflammation is frequent, although regressive stromal changes are uncommon. Kamino bodies are often seen.[105]

The pigmented epithelioid cell nevus manifests the same clinical features as the pigmented spindle cell nevus with an identical histology save that the constituent cell has a cytology typical of the epithelioid cell component of the Spitz nevus.[106]

HISTOLOGIC AND MOLECULAR ADJUNCTS TO THE DIAGNOSIS OF THE SPITZ NEVUS

Spitz nevi have a higher proliferation index relative to common acquired nevi; however, the Ki-67 staining pattern is a predictable one that is largely confined to the superficial dermis. This is contradistinction to the atypical Spitz tumor and to the melanoma in which Ki-67 expression is found at all depths of the lesion. There is enhanced apoptosis in Spitz nevi that may be the basis of the Kamino bodies; conversion of a cell into a senescent state ensures that DNA damage does not accumulate in aging cells, defining the concept of replicative senescence reflecting a gradual loss of short repeated sequences called telomeres. The loss of telomeres from the chromosome results in cell senescence; telomerases stabilize telomers and lead to immortalization. Telomerase activity is increased in melanomas[107] in a fashion that correlates with ulceration, angioinvasion, and increasing Breslow depth[108]; reduction of telomerase activity causes acquisition of a dendritic cell morphology and of tyrosinase function, characteristics of a mature melanocyte phenotype that would correlate with benignancy.[109] There are conflicting data on the detection of differences in telomerase activity between common acquired nevi and Spitz nevi. In lesions categorized as a Spitz nevus, there is also conflicting data regarding evidence of BRAF or N-RAS mutations, which are seen in sporadic melanomas[110]; some authors have reported a subset of Spitz nevi with atypical histology that have BRAF mutations.[110] Spitz nevi have a characteristic increase of chromosome 11p, the site of the H-RAS gene which, in 67% of all cases, is also mutated.[110] In short, there is at present no recourse but the astute use of the light microscope.

ATYPICAL SPITZ TUMOR INCLUDING THE SUPERFICIAL PLAQUE TYPE VARIANT

A subset of Spitzoid neoplasms has clinically and pathologically disturbing features.[111] Such lesions are likely indolent; although metastatic disease may occur, it tends to remain localized to the regional lymph nodes despite the identification of cytogenetic abnormalities similar to those reported in lymph node deposits of metastatic melanoma.[112,113] Unfortunately, lethal

Spitzlike melanomas are also described.[113] We feel that the atypical Spitz tumor has histologic features at variance with Spitzlike melanoma and that such lesions have a clinical appearance similar to the subtypes of Spitz nevi described above, but are often larger, reaching sizes of 2 cm or more, and may have a history of recent change. In addition, within this borderline group is a subset whereby the tumors are primarily confined to the superficial dermis, often with a pattern of stromal alteration reminiscent of regression. Because of their superficial nature and the platelike architecture with or without fibrosis, we have proposed the appellation plaque-type, superficial atypical Spitz tumor for this distinctive lesion.[114]

Histology

The atypical Spitz tumor manifests a failure of maturation; the cells do not diminish in size toward the base and may even appear larger than their superficial counterparts. Mitotic figures may be seen in this deep-seated component, as may one or more expansile dermal nodules. A grading system for risk stratification of atypical Spitz tumors in children and adolescents has been proposed in an attempt to identify lesions at greater risk for aggressive behavior. Among the parameters studied, only diagnosis at age greater than 10 years, lesional diameter greater than 10 mm, presence of ulceration, involvement of the subcutaneous fat, and mitotic activity of at least six per square millimeter carried a significant risk of metastasis.[115] Patient age, sharp demarcation, symmetry, maturation of melanocytes at the base, and epithelial hyperplasia were all signs of benignity.[115] Of particular significance as discussed above are marginal mitoses within 0.25 mm of the lesional edge.[116,117] In some cases, confident distinction of Spitz nevi from malignant melanoma cannot be made, another fact that prompts us to advise complete excision of all Spitz nevi and atypical Spitz tumors irrespective of histology or age. The atypical Spitz tumor, in our view, merits a more aggressive therapeutic strategy. In our recent study addressing the borderline melanocytic tumor, we examined 14 cases of the atypical Spitz tumor measuring 1 mm or more in thickness. All cases showed classic Spitzoid features including pseudoepitheliomatous change of the epidermis. Kamino body formation, prominent superficial vascular ectasia, and edema and a baseline cytology are reminiscent of a Spitz nevus. A mixed spindle and epithelioid cell morphology was seen in the majority of the cases while others had a dominance of epithelioid cells with a variable number of ganglionlike cells. The epithelioid cell-dominant cases had more pleomorphism than did those in which spindled cells were dominant. Maturation was observed; mitoses never exceeded two per ten high-power fields. At variance with the classic Spitz nevus were an architectural growth pattern resembling vertical growth phase melanoma and significant penetration into the reticular dermis, which in half was equal to or in excess of one millimeter. Five of fourteen patients had positive sentinel lymph nodes characterized by intraparenchymal deposits of tumor that in one case exceeded the atypia in the original biopsied lesion leading to recategorization as a Spitzoid melanoma. All of these patients had completion lymphadenectomy and apart from the one patient who was recategorized as spitzoid melanoma, further positive lymph nodes were not uncovered in any other instances (Figs. 2.44–2.48).

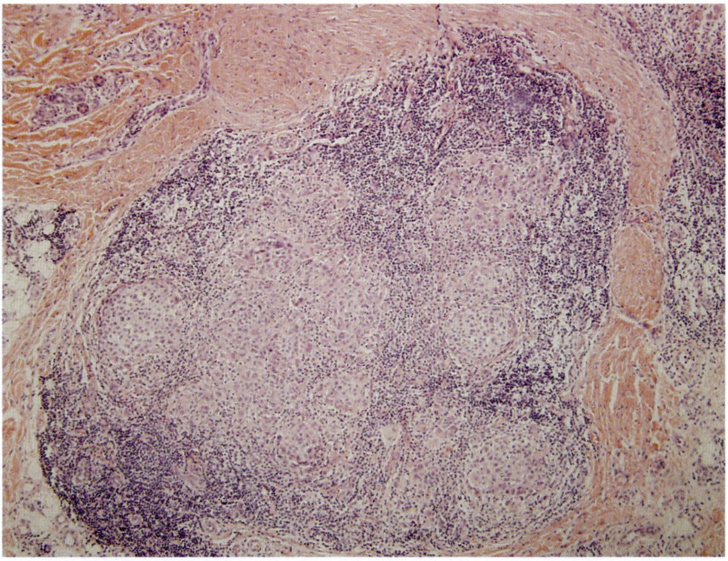

A

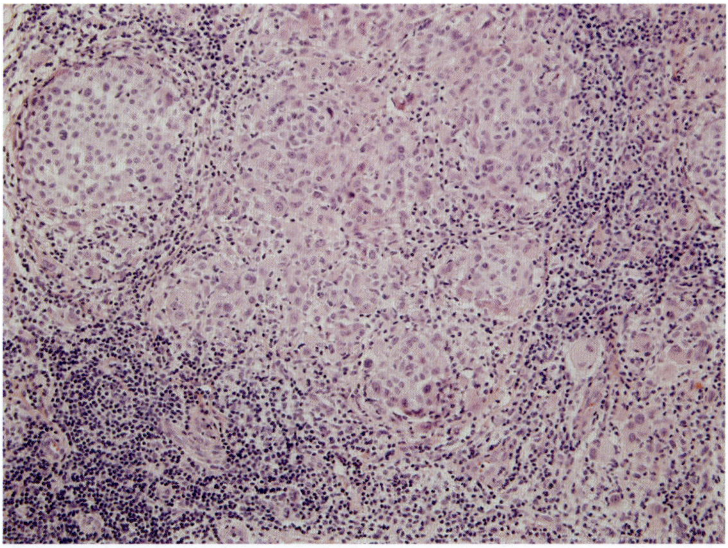

B

FIGURE 2.44 A, B: The atypical Spitz tumor may manifest a failure of maturation; the cells do not diminish in size toward the base and may even appear larger than their superficial counterparts. The deepest aspect of the dermal component may demonstrate a nodular configuration. This particular case represents a residual atypical Spitz tumor in the re-excision specimen from the ear of a 4 year old. Higher-power magnification reveals a monotonous population of moderate to severely atypical epithelioid cells; note the accompanying immunogenic host response.

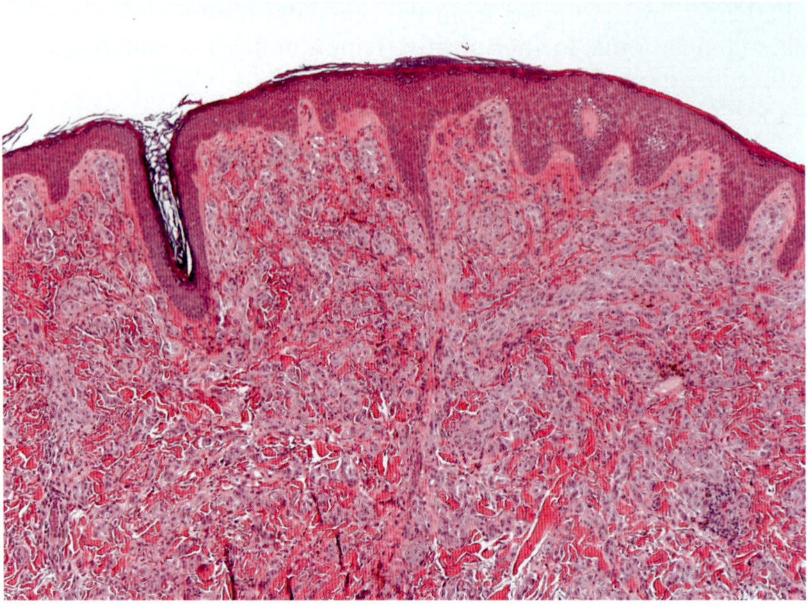

A

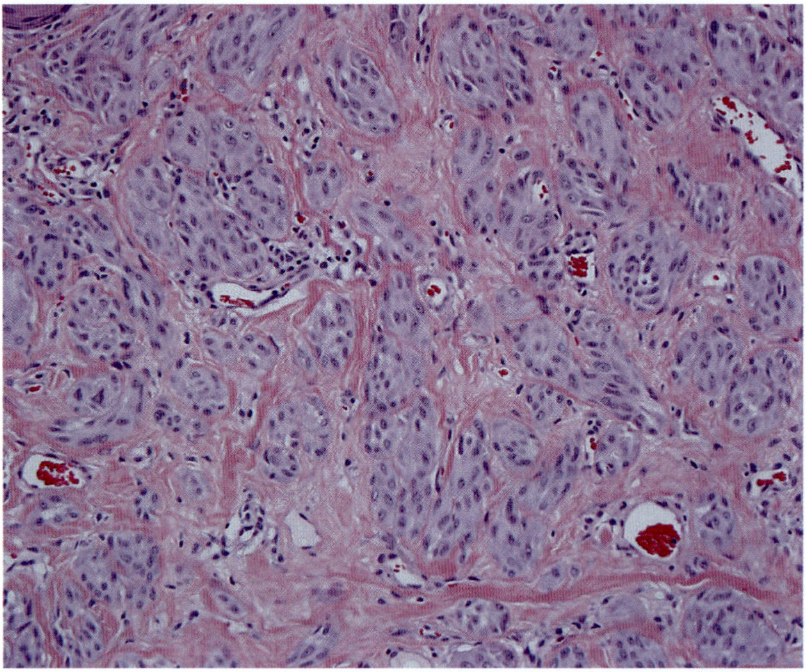

B

FIGURE 2.45 While the lesion is deep with an effacing growth pattern superficially **(A)**, there is evidence of maturation as defined by a reduction in cell size as the lesional base is approached **(B)**. While such findings may be a reasurring sign that the tumor is not melanoma, no criterion other than cytology is diagnostic. For example, maturation can be seen in nevoid melanoma but cytologically the cells exhibit fully evolved criteria of malignancy.

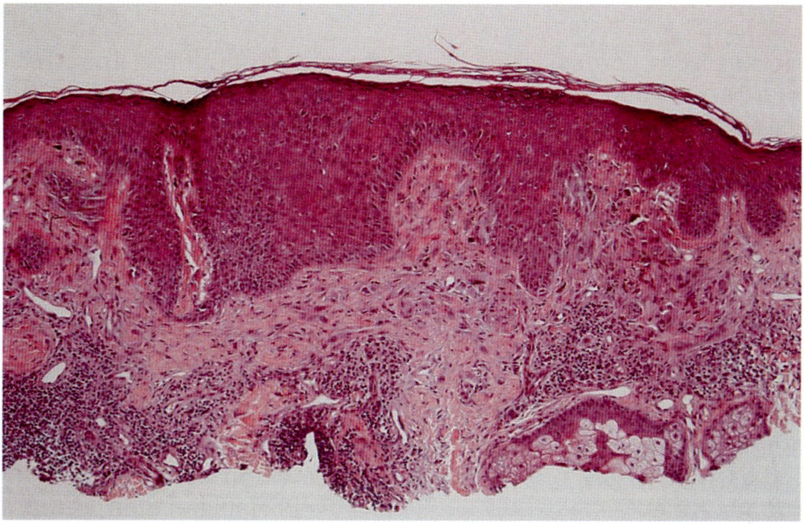

FIGURE 2.46 In the classic atypical Spitz tumor, the dominant cell population is a monoctypic appearing epithelioid cell and/or spindled cell typical of the conventional Spitz nevus. One exception is the superficial atypical Spitz tumor in which dysplastic features can be seen.

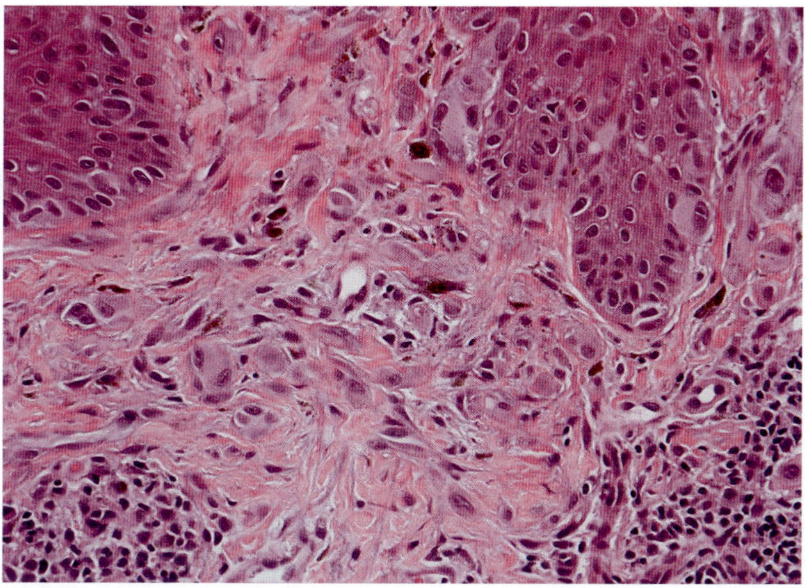

FIGURE 2.47 In the classic atypical Spitz tumor, the dominant cell population is a monoctypic appearing epithelioid cell and/or spindled cell typical of the conventional Spitz nevus. One exception is the superficial atypical Spitz tumor in which dysplastic features can be seen.

Differential Diagnosis

Distinction from vertical growth phase melanoma hinges upon recognition of a background population of epithelioid and spindled cells typical of the classic Spitz nevus. Effacement of dermal architecture and the malignant cytology seen with vertical growth phase melanoma is absent, as is an overlying melanoma in situ. The distinction of the atypical Spitz tumor from a minimal-deviation melanoma of Spitzian type is based on the melanoma having larger deforming nodules with minimal intervening stroma between individual tumor cells and greater numbers of mitoses including atypical forms.

Management

We advise a re-excision of atypical Spitz tumors to obtain a 1-cm margin. If a tumor is over 1 mm in depth, a sentinel lymph node biopsy is typically advised as well. These recommendations are empirically based. Gamblin et al.[118] identified 14 patients with controversial pigmented lesions that primarily fell under the designation of the so-called atypical Spitz tumor; 10 underwent sentinel lymph node biopsy. The lesions were between 1.22 and 4 mm in thickness and 50% of these patients were less than 17 years of age. A third of patients had lymph node metastases. In a study by Murali et al.,[119] cases of problematic Spitzoid neoplasms demonstrating incomplete maturation, 2 or more dermal mitoses per square millimeter (13 patients, 62%), and deep-dermal mitoses (11 patients, 52%) underwent sentinel lymph node biopsy; 30% of patients had sentinel lymph node metastasis. There were significant differences between those cases associated with metastatic disease versus those without any such association, including tumor thickness (3.38 mm versus 2.04 mm), incomplete maturation (83% versus 40%), median dermal mitotic rate (3.5/mm versus 2/mm), deep-dermal mitoses (83% versus 47%), and expansile dermal nodules (50% versus 13%).

The question arises regarding the biological significance of the nodal deposits observed in the setting of the atypical Spitz tumor: should these cases be recategorized as metastatic melanoma or are these simply nodal deposits of a tumor that remains biologically indolent? Since there is established literature precedent describing benign nevus cells within the cortical and medullary lymph node parenchyma, one might surmise that the presence of deposits within the lymph node parenchyma is not the sine qua non of aggressive metastatic melanoma.[120,121] Prior studies describing intraparenchymal deposits of nevus relied on cytology and certain aspects of the phenotypic profile, including the failure of the cells to label with Ki-67 and HMB-45.[120,121] In those cases held to reflect benign nevus cell rests, there was no apparent cutaneous lesion from which the deposits arose. At present, it seems logical to recategorize them as metastatic melanoma in such cases if the cytology of the cells in the lymph node is malignant; if the intraparenchymal deposits resemble the original borderline tumor, the biological import of the deposits in terms of predicting additional lymph node disease and/or distant metastasis is unclear. However, we still recommend completion lymphadenectomy in those patients whose sentinel lymph node biopsies are positive.

COMBINED NEVUS

The term *combined nevus* is applied to lesions with mixed patterns of nevomelanocytic proliferation that combine, in variable proportions, type A, type B, and type C nevomelanocytes with cells identical to those of Spitz and/or blue nevi. The mean age is 30 years, with the face and back being the most common sites.[122] Lesions are gray, brown, or black papules that average 5 mm in diameter[122] brought to the clinician's attention by virtue of a pigmentary change, increase in size, and/or alteration in surface morphology.

Histology

The following are the prototypic nevus cell combinations (Fig. 2.48): (i) type A and type B nevus cells, singly or in nests either along the dermoepidermal junction, in both the epidermis and dermis, or solely in the dermis; (ii) pigmented spindled cells arranged in well-defined fascicles; (iii) pigmented, slender dendritic cells typical of a blue nevus; and

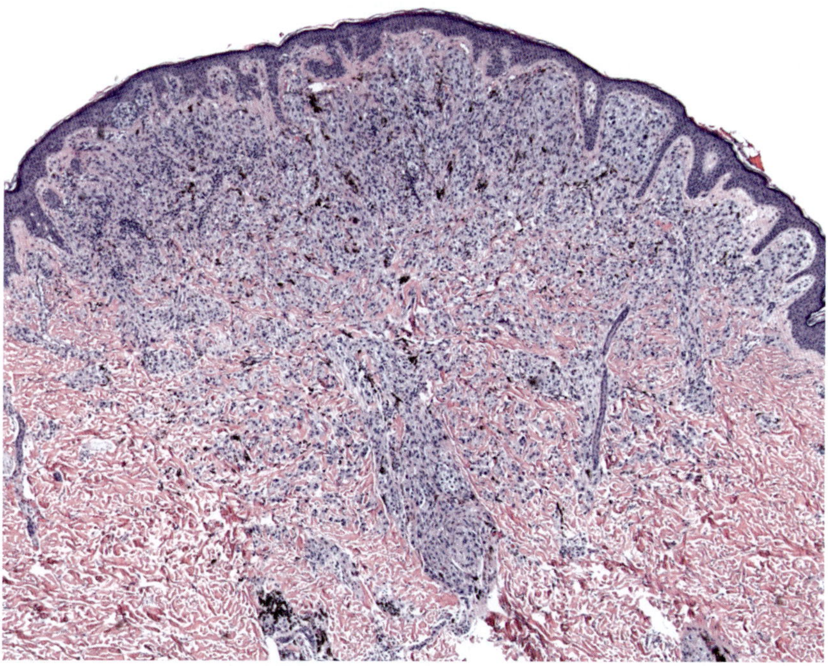

FIGURE 2.48 **Deep Penetrating Nevus.** There is an inverted wedge-shaped architecture with the critical cells extending along adnexal structures deep into the reticular dermis.

(iv) relatively amelanotic, plump, spindled cells arranged in fascicles characteristic of a Spitz nevus.[122] Eighty-five percent of such cases were found to be admixtures of ordinary nevus cells and either pigmented or nonpigmented spindle cells of Spitz nevus subtype. In our experience, the most common form comprises nests of type A nevomelanocytes admixed with dendritic melanocytes (Figs. 2.47 and 2.48). Up to 15% of the lesions are said to have concomitant features of dysplasia,[122] but in our view, this is an exceptional finding. Melanoma in situ has been described in a combined nevi.[123]

DEEP-PENETRATING NEVUS AND THE BORDER LINE TUMOR ARISING IN THE DEEP PENETRATING NEVUS

The deep-penetrating nevus is a lesion that occurs in the second to fourth decades of life on the proximal aspect of the upper or lower extremities, face, or trunk[124,125] as a variably colored, dome-shaped papule less than 1 cm and rarely more than 6 mm in diameter.[124,125] Clinicians often raise consideration of a blue nevus or a cellular blue nevus and sometimes of melanoma, but in the original series, no lesion recurred or metastasized.[124] Many such lesions have admixed dendritic cells and should be considered a form of combined nevus in our view.

Since the original description of that entity, there have been cases in which metastatic behavior has been described and has been recategorized as melanoma despite a morphologic resemblance to the deep-penetrating nevus. We have encountered atypical melanocytic proliferations occurring in the deep-penetrating nevus, which we consider to be a borderline or prognostically indeterminate melanocytic tumor. In our experience, these lesions have a significant incidence of intraparenchymal lymph node disease. One of our cases demonstrated progression to a deep-seated plexiform melanoma with widespread metastatic disease. The literature does not emphasize the biologically indeterminate character of some examples of deep-penetrating nevi. Conversely, there are reports describing patients with an initial diagnosis of deep-penetrating nevus whereby a subsequent lymph node biopsy performed due to adenopathy revealed metastatic melanoma.[126] It is possible that such cases are similar to those that we have encountered.

Histopathology

A wedge-shaped symmetrical lesion has a dominant composition of closely apposed, vertically oriented fascicles that assume an orderly pattern of infiltration within the dermis, closely following neurovascular bundles and the adventitia of the hair follicles and eccrine coil (Fig. 2.48). There is a minor interstitial component of pigmented cells that extend along reticular dermal collagen and elastic fibers, sometimes into the subcutis.[125] Fascicles tend to be confluent in the upper dermis and dissipate in size toward the base as an inverted triangle. The cells and fascicles may appear elongated or round, depending on whether they are examined en face or in cross-section. Pushing, nodular borders at the tumor base would be deemed an atypical feature, especially when such foci exceed the size of any superficially disposed nest. Junctional nests may be present. Cooper[125] recognized that in two thirds of deep-penetrating nevi, an ordinary nevus coexisted. Patterned periretal fibroplasia and perifascicular desmoplasia are unusual in the deep-penetrating nevus. The fascicles comprise spindle-shaped cells with variable melanization ranging from clear to heavily pigmented cytoplasms. Peripherally disposed melanophages delimit adjacent fascicles. The spindle cells show nuclear size and shape variability. There is a random disposition of pleomorphic hyperchromatic cells that are designated as tumor giant cells and may be uni- or multinucleated with dark, amorphous nucleoplasms and nuclear pseudoinclusions due to cytoplasmic invaginations. Prominent nucleoli may be observed. Mitoses, typical in morphology, are seen in some 10% of lesions, but are rare, and no more than one or two are seen in any given section. Their presence within the deeper aspects of the lesion should warrant concern. A mild lymphocytic infiltrate may be present.[124,125] The HMB-45 expression is usually extensively positive, a pattern useful to rule out a desmoplastic melanoma or atypical Spitzoid neoplasm. The atypical Spitzoid neoplasms can demonstrate some staining but never of the intensity seen with the deep-penetrating nevus. In our recent study, six patients had a background lesion exhibiting all of the typical features of a deep-penetrating nevus with supervening cellular proliferative areas, sometimes parallel to the long axis of the epidermis or as an expansile nodular growth pattern in the zones of vertically oriented melanocytic proliferation. Such foci had enhanced cytologic atypia with cellular enlargement and increased mitotic activity including marginal mitoses. Unlike the other subcategories of the borderline tumor, the abnormal proliferative foci could be superficially confined albeit still located in the reticular dermis, while the deeper aspect of the neoplasm could be within the spectrum of residual deep-penetrating nevus. Five of six patients demonstrated positive sentinel lymph nodes. In one of the cases, the lesion recurred 1.5 years after excision as a deeply invasive melanoma, ultimately with liver, lung, bone, and brain metastases, despite radiation and chemotherapy (Figs. 2.49 and 2.50).

Another patient had positive nonsentinel lymph node deposits; all save the aforementioned are alive and well without any clinical evidence of recurrent disease.

Management

We recommend a complete simple excision as we have seen cases in which the incisional biopsy was interpreted as a deep-penetrating nevus, and yet, at re-excision, the lesion proved to be a neurotropic melanoma. As the deep-penetrating nevus is a recently described entity,[124] long-term follow-up is still not available for patients in whom this diagnosis has been made. Time will establish whether the lesion has the potential for aggressive biological behavior.

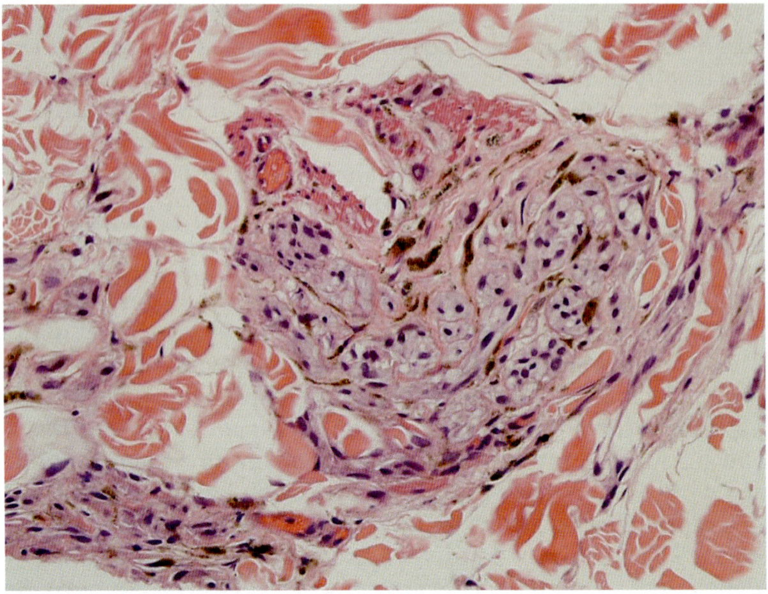

A

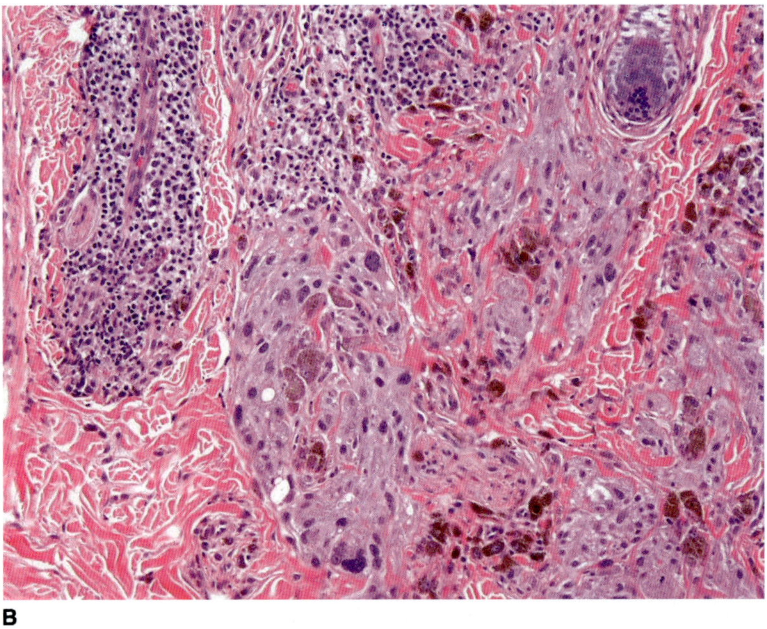

B

FIGURE 2.49 **Deep Penetrating Nevus: Cytology.** The fascicles show a characteristic adventitial dermal disposition. **A,B:** In the classic deep penetrating nevus, an element of pleomorphism is usually discernible with one of the most characteristic patterns being that of scattered, large atypical cells with prominent intranuclear inclusions and hyperchromasia.

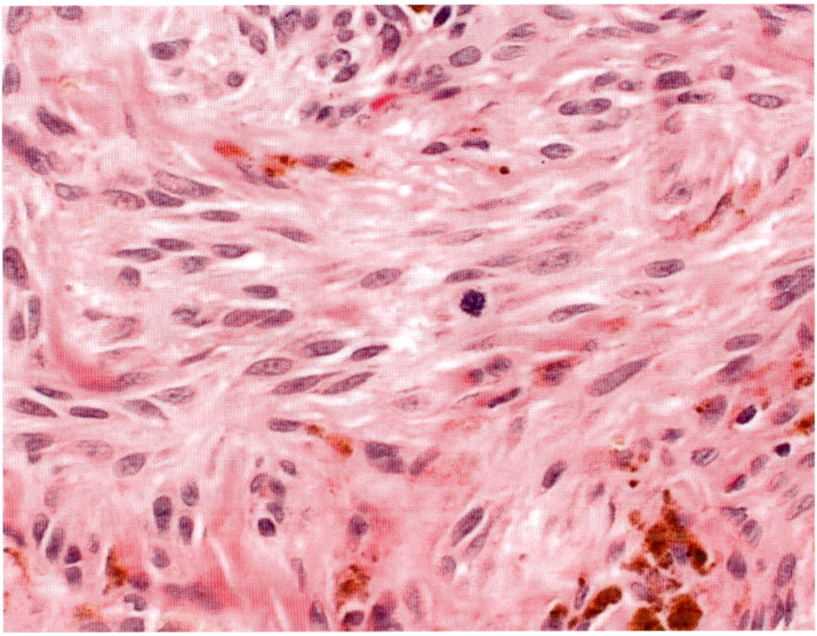

FIGURE 2.50 One must be cognizant of the borderline tumor, which may arise in the deep-penetrating nevus.The hallmarks are exemplified by this case and include zones of cellular effacing infiltratrion with enhanced atypia. Scattered mitoses can be seen.

PLEXIFORM SPINDLE CELL NEVUS

The plexiform spindle cell nevus shares with the deep-penetrating nevus,[127] and some feel that these diagnoses are interchangeable. There are in fact two variants of deep-penetrating nevus, one with an epithelioid cytomorphology (inverted type A nevus) and the other with a spindle cell morphology (inverted spindle cell nevus). The latter, due to its spindle cell morphology, has been the source of confusion. In point of fact, the plexiform spindle cell nevus has clinical and histologic features that are distinctive; the plexiform spindle cell nevus tracks along the superficial neurovascular bundles to generate the clinical appearance of a plaque.

DYSPLASTIC NEVUS AND DE NOVO INTRAEPIDERMAL EPITHELIOID MELANOCYTIC DYSPLASIA

In 1978, Lynch et al.[128] coined the term *familial multiple atypical mole melanoma syndrome* to describe a syndrome of multiple atypical nevi, which appeared to place family members at increased risk for developing melanoma. Clark et al.[129] characterized the dysplastic nevus as a defining element of the "B–K mole syndrome," so named for the first letters of the surnames of the kindreds affected by familial melanoma. Patients with dysplastic nevi of the familial type present with multiple large, atypical moles distributed everywhere on the body surface, including the scalp, the doubly covered areas, namely, breasts of women and the bathing trunk area of men and women, and the lower legs. In contrast, benign acquired nevi usually spare the scalp, the doubly covered areas, and the legs.[130] Dysplastic nevi can be diagnosed clinically because the lesions are highly characteristic. Unlike common acquired nevi, they are larger than 6mm in diameter, being typically in the 8 to 10mm size range with irregular borders and a variegated pattern of pigmentation.[131] There is great heterogeneity among the lesions in a given patient, a hallmark of the dysplastic nevus syndrome. In contrast, the common acquired nevi are symmetrical with round, regular borders, uniform pigmentation, and a diameter less than 6mm. The consensus conference on early melanoma hosted in January 1992 by the National Institutes of Health recommended supplanting the term dysplastic nevus with the appellation "nevus with architectural disorder and cytologic atypia."[132,133] We prefer the term dysplastic nevus as it is the term with which clinicians are most familiar, as there are subgroups of congenital and acquired nevi (such as those in acral and genital sites) that manifest architectural disorder and cytologic atypia but are not dysplastic nevi and are not associated with melanoma, and because the alternate terminology does not allow for grading, which is integral to the assessment of any dysplastic nevus. In short, the terminology adds nothing but confusion and has largely been abandoned. The incidence of dysplastic nevi is likely in the 5% to 10% range in North America and Europe.[134] The concern raised by the dysplastic nevus relates to the risk of its transformation to melanoma to its being a marker for the development of melanoma at other sites. Specifically, melanoma patients with two or more dysplastic nevi may be considered at increased risk for a second primary melanoma.[135,136] Up to 92% of melanomas occurring in patients with dysplastic nevus syndrome had evidence of a dysplastic nevus as a precursor lesion.[135] One study analyzing newly diagnosed cutaneous malignant melanomas estimated that 7% of malignant melanomas arise in prior dysplastic nevi,[137] whereas another study identified dysplastic nevi as precursors of 18% of all nonfamilial melanomas[138]; most melanomas arising in dysplastic nevi are of superficial spreading type.

Patients with two or more dysplastic nevi are said to suffer from the dysplastic nevus syndrome. An alternative term that more closely parallels the original one is *the melanoma-associated atypical multiple mole phenotype*. Multiple dysplastic nevi may occur sporadically or in a familial complex with an autosomal dominant pattern of inheritance. The gene that most commonly encodes the dysplastic nevus syndrome phenotype is found on chromosome 9.[139] The molecular basis of melanomagenesis in this syndrome is beyond the scope of this chapter and the reader is referred elsewhere.[140] The relative risk of developing melanoma in patients with sporadic dysplastic nevus syndrome is said to be 70 times greater than a person without dysplastic nevi.[141] People with a single dysplastic nevus are not considered to have sporadic dysplastic nevus syndrome, as they are said by some authorities to not be at increased risk for developing malignant melanoma[142,143]; there are epidemiologic studies to the contrary. There can be no doubt that dysplastic nevi differ from banal nevi from all of clinical, histologic, biochemical, and molecular standpoints.

Histology

The histology of the dysplastic nevus is so reproducible that a diagnosis can usually be rendered on scanning magnification (Figs. 2.51–2.54). Interobserver variability generally lies in the area of grading of atypia. The latter should not be done at scanning magnification as it requires an accurate assessment of cytologic features. The diagnosis is based on the application of criteria that are divided into those that must be present, i.e., major criteria, and those additional criteria that are not present in every case, so-called minor criteria. These major and minor criteria are outlined below and have been addressed in great detail by several authors over the years.[143–150]

Major Criteria for Diagnosis of a Dysplastic Nevus

There is an asymmetric basilar proliferation of nevomelanocytes along the dermoepidermal junction extending laterally beyond the confines of a pre-existing dermal component, if and when present, usually by three

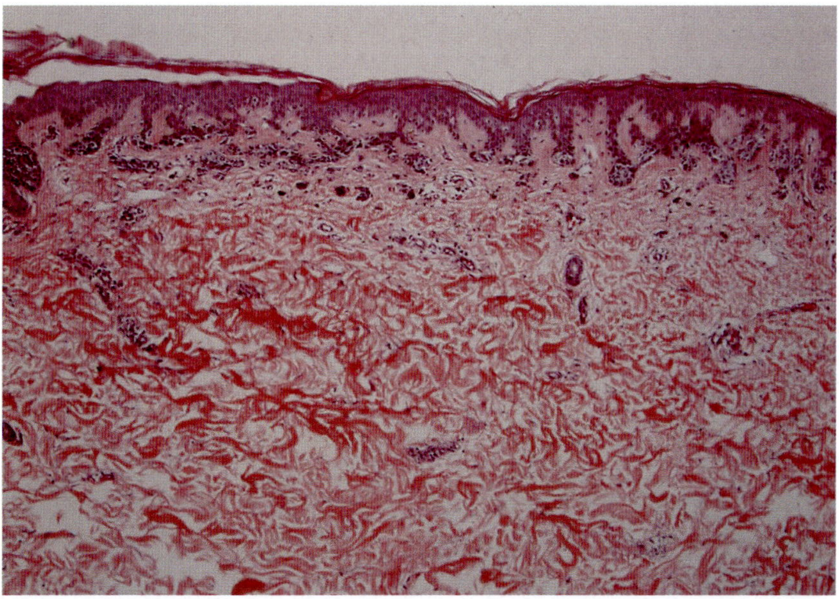

FIGURE 2.51 **Dysplastic Nevus.** There is an asymmetric basilar proliferation of nevomelanocytes along the dermoepidermal junction extending laterally beyond the confines of a pre-existing dermal component, if and when present, usually by three rete ridges or more.

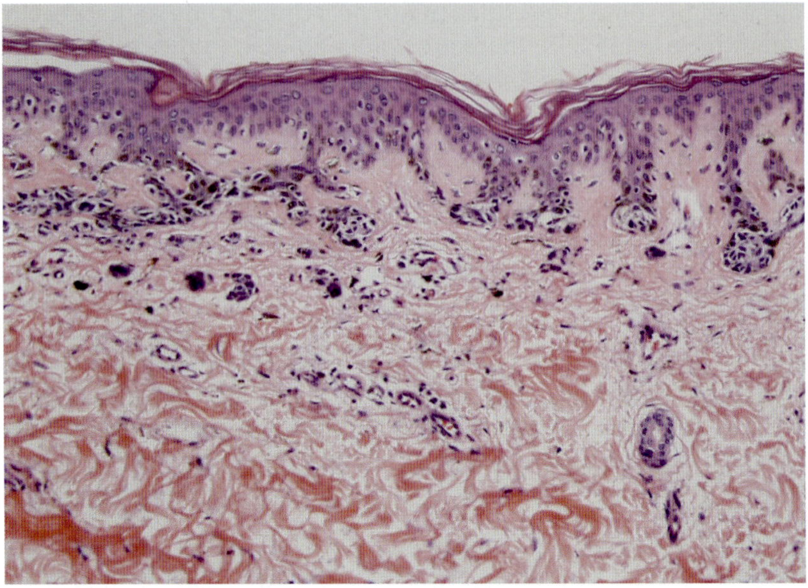

FIGURE 2.52 **Dysplastic Nevus.** There is an asymmetric basilar proliferation of nevomelanocytes along the dermoepidermal junction extending laterally beyond the confines of a pre-existing dermal component, if and when present, usually by three rete ridges or more.

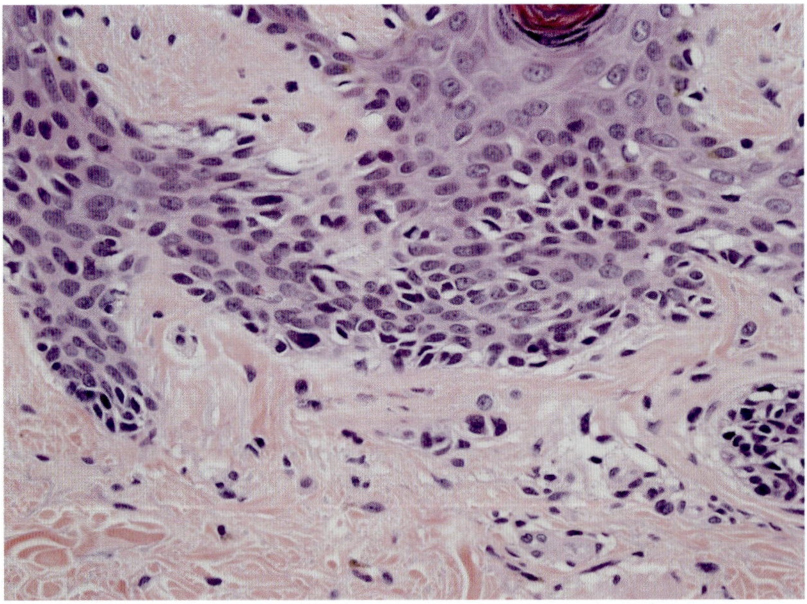

FIGURE 2.53 **Dysplastic Nevus.** There is an asymmetric basilar proliferation of nevomelanocytes along the dermoepidermal junction extending laterally beyond the confines of a pre-existing dermal component, if and when present, usually by three rete ridges or more.

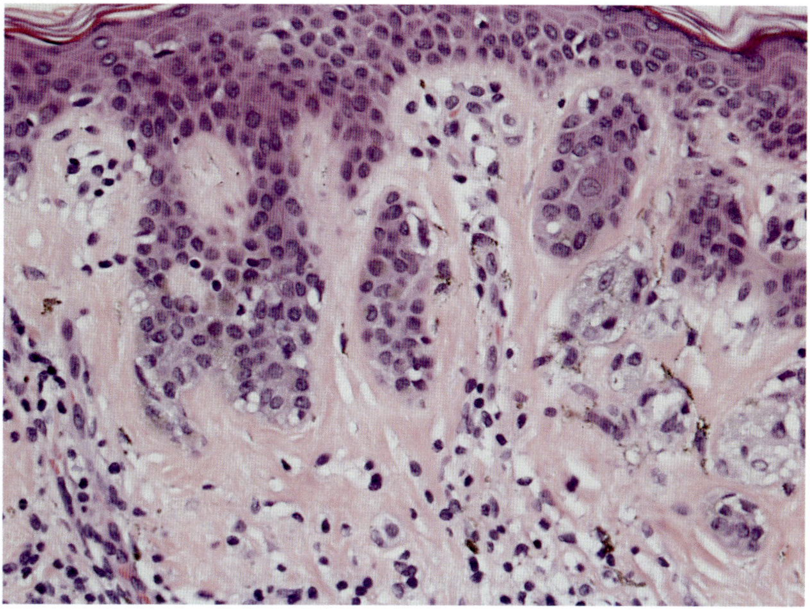

FIGURE 2.54 **Dysplastic Nevus.** There is an asymmetric basilar proliferation of nevomelanocytes along the dermoepidermal junction extending laterally beyond the confines of a pre-existing dermal component, if and when present, usually by three rete ridges or more.

rete ridges or more (Figs. 2.51 and 2.52). Cells have a characteristic cytomorphology and manifest a specific intraepidermal growth pattern. Two cytomorphologic subtypes are recognized, each corresponding to a specific pattern of intraepidermal growth:

1. Lentiginous melanocytic dysplasia: Randomly disposed single cells are located along and between the elongated rete and form nests of varying sizes. These cells show variability in nuclear size and appear hyperchromatic, imparting an "ink spot" quality to the nucleus. Nuclei are either similar in size to the adjacent keratinocytes or conspicuously enlarged. Nuclear contours are angulated. Cytoplasm borders may be spiculated (Figs. 2.53 and 2.55).
2. Epithelioid cell melanocytic dysplasia: Epithelioid melanocytes are disposed in variably sized junctional nests as well as in a single-cell array along the dermoepidermal junction of an often normal or hyperplastic epidermis. The cells have round to oval nuclei with open, delicate chromatin and rounded cytoplasmic contours. Cytoplasmic melanization is variable, with cytoplasms ranging from amelanotic to those that manifest coarse, irregular pigment granules. The cells are recognized as being dysplastic by virtue of cell-to-cell variability, conspicuous nucleolation, thick nuclear membranes, and nuclear diameters greater than those of adjacent keratinocytes (Figs. 2.54 and 2.56).

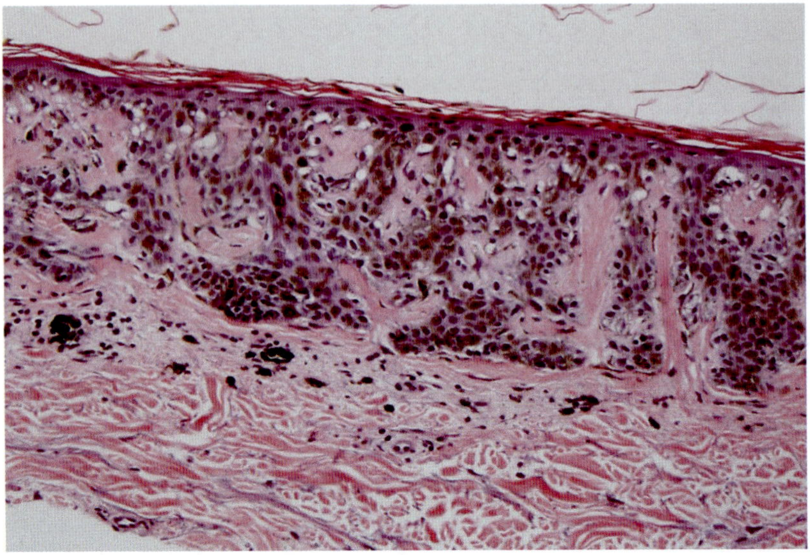

FIGURE 2.55 **Lentiginous Melanocytic Dysplasia.** Randomly disposed single cells are located along and between elongated rete and form nests of varying sizes. These cells show variability in nuclear size and appear hyperchromatic, imparting an "ink spot" quality to the nucleus. Nuclei are either similar in size to adjacent keratinocytes or sometimes enlarged. Nuclear contours are angulated. Cytoplasm borders may be spiculated.

Minor Criteria

1. Papillary dermal collagen shows two distinctive patterns: concentric eosinophilic fibrosis in which a dense zone of acellular, brightly eosinophilic collagen envelops rete ridges, and/or lamellar fibroplasia in which layers of collagen are interspersed with spindle-shaped cells of presumptive neural crest origin functioning as facultative fibroblasts laying down parallel arrays of collagen beneath hyperplastic retia (Figs. 2.55 and 2.56).
2. Lymphocytic infiltrates in the papillary dermis, being of maximal intensity beneath areas in which melanocytes show cytologic atypia.
3. Prominent vessels that may be newly formed or preexisting vessels that show endothelial cell activation and hyperplasia.
4. Fusion of retia by confluent growth between adjacent melanocytic nests (Fig. 2.57).

A diagnosis of dysplastic nevus is made when both the major and at least two minor criteria are met.

Grading Atypia

Many pathologists do not assign grades of atypia to dysplastic nevi, recognizing correctly that there is pronounced subjectivity associated with assigning a grade. Studies have shown, however, that criteria can be

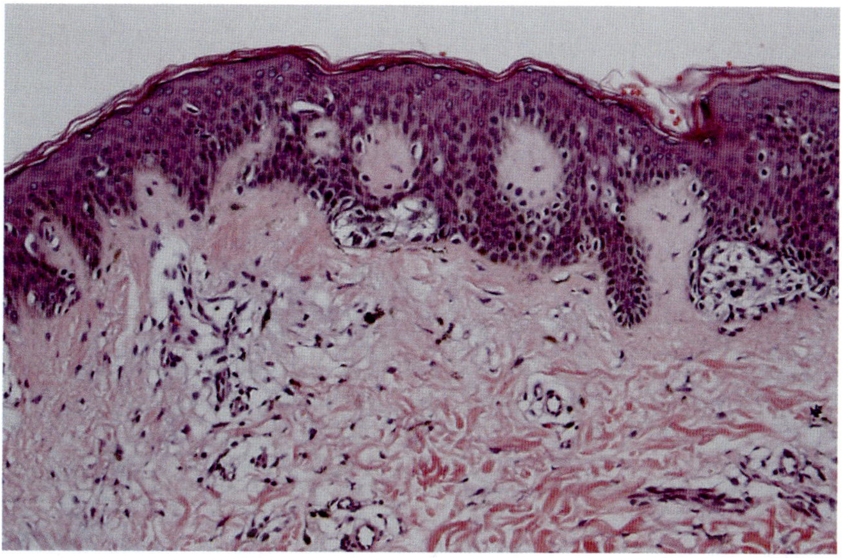

FIGURE 2.56 **Epithelioid Cell Melanocytic Dysplasia.** The cells are usually discernible in areas of junctional nested activity. The cells have and manifest round to oval nuclei with open, delicate chromatin and rounded cytoplasmic contours. Cytoplasmic melanization is variable, with cytoplasms ranging from amelanotic to those that manifest coarse, irregular pigment granules. The cells are recognized as being dysplastic by virtue of cell-to-cell variability, conspicuous nucleolation, thick nuclear membranes, and nuclear diameters greater than those of adjacent keratinocytes.

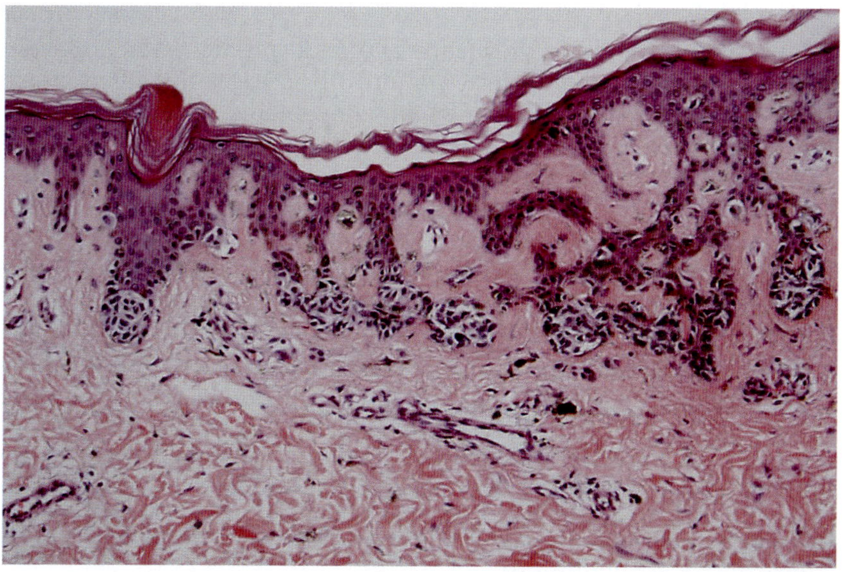

FIGURE 2.57 Papillary dermal collagen shows one and/or two distinctive patterns: Concentric eosinophilic fibrosis in which a dense zone of acellular brightly eosinophilic collagen envelops rete ridges and lamellar fibroplasia in which delicate layers of collagen are interspersed with spindle-shaped cells of presumptive neural crest origin, which function as facultative fibroblasts laying down collagen beneath the tips of hyperplastic retia in parallel arrays.

learned, applied, and reproduced by histopathologists for a variety of disease systems and a degree of consistency in grading atypia of dysplastic nevi can be achieved if a set of criteria is adhered to in the diagnostic assessment of the lesion. This consistency is maintained in both the three tier grading system which we employ, namely, mild, moderate, and severe, and the two tier system, namely, low- and high-grade dysplasia.[151–154] Some observers have found reasonable concordance in grading of architectural features, but not cytologic features, implying that the interpretation of cytology is more challenging.[155] We grade atypia on the basis of architecture and cytology; architectural and cytologic grades of atypia tend to show correlation.[154]

It is our belief that dysplastic nevi with mild degrees of atypia do not warrant a re-excision unless there is residual lesion apparent clinically. In contrast, a moderately or severely dysplastic nevus should likely be re-excised if it has not been completely excised regardless of whether a residual lesion is clinically apparent. It has been our experience that on a re-excision of incompletely excised severely atypical dysplastic nevi, foci of malignant melanoma can be found in the re-excision specimen. Most dermatologists and surgeons will re-excise moderately atypical nevi, which have been incompletely excised, even if there are no lesions left clinically. We are aware of at least two cases in which moderate atypia was present in the margins of the biopsy and melanoma subsequently developed at the biopsy site.

What is mild architectural atypia?

1. Fully evolved architectural features of a dysplastic nevus are present. Specifically, a highly orderly pattern of periretal fibrosis is present. The rete ridges are well formed and elongated.
2. Many of the junctional thèques are small and at the tips of the rete. A few of the thèques are aberrantly disposed. The nests are cohesive. The lateral borders of the intraepidermal component typically terminate in a nested array.
3. The overall density of the lentiginous component is mild, whereby the nested component is dominant over the lentiginous component.
4. If there is a dermal component, it comprises either single cells or small nests separated by paucicellular stroma.
5. Inflammation is slight.

What is mild cytologic atypia?

1. Either an epithelioid or a lentiginous pattern of dysplasia is present (see above for definition).
2. The cells have round or oval nuclear outlines if representing epithelioid dysplasia and hyperchromatic nuclei with polygonal or triangular outlines if representing lentiginous dysplasia.

3. The nucleus is the same size, smaller, or slightly larger than the adjacent keratinocyte nuclei depending, in part, on the type of dysplasia (lentiginous or epithelioid).
4. There is some minor variation in cell size and shape that is best appreciated by comparing cells within a specific nest; however, most of the cells within a nest appear similar in morphology compared to their adjacent neighbors.
5. Nucleoli may be discernible, manifesting as dotlike, usually solitary structures that are lightly eosinophilic, especially in the epithelioid form. Only a minority of cells show prominent nucleoli; if numerous cells show large nucleoli, it is likely that a higher grade of dysplasia is present.
6. In epithelioid cell dysplasia, the nuclear chromatinic rim is relatively inconspicuous and the chromatin is finely dispersed within the cell. The occasional large chromatin aggregate may be seen, as may the occasional cell with marked nuclear hyperchromasia; nonetheless the cell size is still small.
7. Spindled cells with oval nuclei containing linear grooves as seen with severe dysplasia are not observed or, if present, are few in number.
8. The cells usually have a small rim of eosinophilic cytoplasm. Because melanin synthesis is often not abundant, the cytoplasm may seem inconspicuous. If there is pigment deposition, the pigment granules are fine and evenly dispersed within the majority of the cells. Some cells with irregular and coarse pigment deposition are observed but are few in number. Giant melanin granules over 1 μm in diameter may be identified.

What is moderate architectural atypia?

1. Rete elongation is still present, and an organized pattern of periretal stroma fibroplasia is identified, although such changes may not be as conspicuous as those seen in the mildly dysplastic nevus.
2. The majority of nests are aberrantly disposed, with only a few nests appearing at the tips of retia. They manifest considerable variation is size, with some obscuring the normal epidermal contours. Nuclear overlap is conspicuous. There may be focal dyshesion of melanocytes within the nests.
3. The lentiginous component is of moderate density. In moderate density growths on nonsun-exposed skin, two to three keratinocytes should be interposed between each melanocyte. In sun-exposed skin of the face, in contrast, the normal density of melanocytes is one per three to four keratinocytes. In any event, areas of confluent growth are not seen in sun-protected or sun-exposed skin.
4. The dermal component may include a few large nests, although these do not exceed the size of those nests within the epidermis. The nests may show variation in size.
5. There is moderate inflammation.

What is moderate cytologic atypia?

1. The cells may show either an epithelioid or lentiginous pattern of dysplasia.
2. The epithelioid cells are larger than the adjacent keratinocytes, typically having nuclei 1.5 to 2 times the diameter of the adjacent keratinocyte nucleus. A moderate amount of cytoplasm is usually identified; the nuclear to cytoplasmic ratios are in the range of 1:1 to 1:2.
3. Chromatin is still relatively evenly dispersed. Nuclear chromatinic rims may be prominent. Nucleoli, while conspicuous, do not exceed one-third of the nuclear diameter.
4. Many of the cells are melanized, especially in the epithelioid form; the melanin granules vary in size and shape and some appear quite large. Giant melanin granules greater than 1 μm in diameter may be identified.
5. Many of the cells within a given nest show significant variability of size and shape when adjacent cells are compared.
6. In lentiginous melanocytic dysplasia, the cells are usually 1 to 1.5 times the size of adjacent keratinocytes and have jet black angulated nuclei.

What is severe architectural atypia?

1. There may be focal areas of rete elongation with condensed organized periretal stromal fibrosis; however, such areas may be obscured by the degree of melanocytic growth and/or inflammation.
2. Most of the nests assume an aberrant disposition within the epidermis. Variability of nest size and configuration may be striking. There may be a confluence of nests resulting in focal effacement of the epidermal architecture, although for the most part, the epidermal architecture is preserved. Such nests, rather than having an oval or rounded contour, may be oblong and assume a parallel arrangement to the epidermis. There is marked nest dyshesion.
3. Areas of marked single-cell lentiginous growth may be observed, resulting in broad zones of fused retia mainly comprising melanocytes; scattered residual keratinocytes may populate these fused retia but are few in number. Foci of confluent lentiginous growth may replace the lower layers of the epidermis; the melanocytes in these zones have less fully evolved atypia than does malignant melanoma in situ. Mitoses within the junctional nests may be observed but are few in number.
4. The striking intraepidermal melanocytic activity remains a junctional phenomenon, with only minimal upward migration of melanocytes. Areas of dominant upward migration by melanocytes showing severe cytologic atypia indicate differentiation toward melanoma in situ.

5. Large coalescing dermal thèques are present and may even exceed the size of those thèques within the epidermis. However, these nodules are devoid of mitotic activity and necrosis.
6. Inflammation may be prominent and can assume a lichenoid pattern.

What is severe cytologic atypia?

1. Cells with both an epithelioid and lentiginous pattern of dysplasia are present.
2. The epithelioid cell nucleus is conspicuously enlarged relative to the keratinocyte nucleus and is usually greater than twice its size.
3. The chromatin is irregularly disposed within the cells and appears as conspicuous aggregates of variable size. Chromatinic rims are thickened, often in an irregular fashion.
4. Distinctive nuclear grooves imparting a coffee bean-shaped appearance to the nucleus are present. Such grooves likely represent excessive nuclear infoldings and are manifested by cells within the nested component.
5. Nucleoli are prominent and may exceed one third of the nuclear diameter. Most of the cells have discernible nucleoli that may be multiple.
6. Cytoplasms may be abundant, typically with wispy borders enveloping oval nuclei, which impart a spindled morphology to the cell.
7. The cells show variable melanization. In those cells that are pigmented, there is marked heterogeneity of melanin pigment deposition; the melanin granules are coarse and show considerable variability in size; giant melanin granules over 1 μm in diameter may be identified.
8. The cells manifesting a lentiginous pattern of dysplasia by definition do not have a readily discernible chromatin pattern. Rather, the nuclei appear jet black with angulated contours. The nucleus occupies most of the cell; cytoplasm is scanty. Nucleoli may be seen but are rarely discernable. The nevomelanocytes manifest spiculated cytoplasmic borders and are often twice the size of the adjacent keratinocytes. Although the cytomorphology may not appear too dissimilar to those lentiginous dysplastic cells observed in the moderately atypical dysplastic nevus, they are more numerous and may be the dominant population of the lentiginous component.

DE NOVO INTRAEPIDERMAL EPITHELIOID MELANOCYTIC DYSPLASIA

De novo intraepidermal epithelioid melanocytic dysplasia is a name that we proposed for a distinct form of intraepidermal melanocytic dysplasia comprising an intraepidermal proliferation of atypical melanocytes distributed mainly in a single-cell array with foci of pagetoid growth pattern.[156] Regarding the distinction from the dysplastic nevus, de novo intraepidermal epithelioid melanocytic dysplasia cannot be so classified due to the dominant single-cell pattern of growth over a junctional nested one, the abundant pagetoid spread, the lack of epidermal hyperplasia, and the absence of stromal alterations of a dysplastic nevus, namely, concentric eosinophilic fibrosis or lamellar fibroplasia with attendant inflammation. Virtually all de novo intraepidermal epithelioid melanocytic dysplasia lesions represent high-grade intraepidermal melanocytic dysplasias, being moderately or severely atypical. In contrast, there is a greater range of architectural and cytologic atypia in the dysplastic nevus. A positive correlation arose between the lesion of de novo intraepidermal epithelioid melanocytic dysplasia and the presence of dysplastic nevus with higher grades of atypia. More challenging is the distinction from melanoma in situ, in which the higher density pagetoid dispersal of melanocytes comprises cells with fully transformed cytologic features of malignancy, and epidermal thinning and/or retiform effacement is common. While de novo intraepidermal epithelioid melanocytic dysplasia is usually unaccompanied by a stromal and/or inflammatory host response, in melanoma in situ, variable lymphocytic and plasmacellular infiltration with or without fibroplasia is seen.

We thus recommend complete lesional excision with a 5 mm margin of normal skin on all edges in those lesions of de-novo intraepidermal melanocytic dysplasia with severe atypia whereby the possibility of transition into early melanoma in situ cannot be excluded.

In our study, a significant percentage of patients had two or more biopsy proven dysplastic nevi and melanomas. If one accepts the older definition of the atypical mole phenotype, which is the presence of two or more variably pigmented moles in excess of 5 mm, then half of our patients would be defined as having an atypical mole phenotype. In our hands, patients had higher grades of dysplastic nevi indicating that not only did de novo epithelioid melanocytic dysplasia define part of the atypical mole phenotype but also it correlated with dysplastic nevi manifesting higher degrees of atypia; 20 of our 75 patients (26.6%) had a diagnosis of malignant melanoma in the time period of our study. One can reasonably infer that the diagnosis of de novo epithelioid melanocytic dysplasia is indicative of a patient who has a higher propensity to develop melanoma and therefore should be fully evaluated clinically and closely followed.

REFERENCES

1. Rhodes AR, Albert LS, Barnhill RL, Weinstock MA. Sun-induced freckles in children and young adults. A correlation of clinical and histopathologic features. *Cancer* 1991;67:1990–2001.
2. Barnhill, RL. *Pathology of Melanocytic Nevi and Malignant Melanoma*. Boston, MA: Butterworth-Heinemann, 1995.
3. Itin PH, Lautenschlager S, Meyer R, et al. Natural history of the Naegeli–Franceschetti–Jadassohn syndrome and further delineation of its clinical manifestations. *J Am Acad Dermatol* 1993;28:942–950.
4. Oriba HA, Lo JS, Dijkstra JWE, Bergfeld WF. Reticulate nonmelanocytic hyperpigmentation anomaly. A probable variant of Dowling Degos disease. *Int J Dermatol* 1991; 30:39–42.

5. Erel A, Guter MA, Edali N. Reticulate acropigmentation of Kitamura: Two case reports. *Int J Dermatol* 1993;32:726–727.
6. Bar Rahman S, Bhawan J. Lentigo. *Int J Dermatol* 1996;35:229–239.
7. Crowson AN, Magro CM, Mihm MC Jr. The freckles and lentigines. In: Crowson AN, Magro CM, Mihm MC Jr, eds. *The Melanocytic Proliferations: A Comprehensive Textbook of Pigmented Lesions*. New York, NY: John Wiley and Sons, 2001:49–72.
8. Stratakis CA. Genetics of Carney complex and related familial lentiginoses, and other multiple tumor syndromes. *Front Biosci* 2000;5:353–366.
9. Shapiro L, Zegarelli DJ. The solitary labial lentigo. A clinicopathologic study of twenty cases. *Oral Surg Oral Med Oral Pathol* 1971;31:87–92.
10. Gupta G, Williams RE, Mackie RM. The labial melanotic macule: A review of 79 cases. *Br J Dermatol* 1997;136:72–775.
11. Rudolph RI. Vulvar melanosis. *J Am Acad Dermatol* 1990;23(5 Pt 2):982–984.
12. Kanj LF, Rubeiz NG, Mroueh AM, Kibbi AG. Vulvar melanosis and lentiginosis: A case report. *J Am Acad Dermatol* 1992;27(5 Pt 1):777–778.
13. Estrada R, Kaufman R. Benign vulvar melanosis. *J Reprod Med* 1993;38:5–8.
14. Maize JC. Mucosal melanosis. *Dermatol Clin* 1988;6:283–293.
15. Roewert HJ, Ackerman AB. Large-cell acanthoma is a solar lentigo. *Am J Dermatopathol* 1992;14:122–132.
16. Rabinowitz AD, Inghirami G. Large-cell acanthoma. A distinctive keratosis. *Am J Dermatopathol* 1992;14:136–138.
17. Bolognia JL. Reticulated black solar lentigo ('ink spot' lentigo). *Arch Dermatol* 1992;128:934–940.
18. Robinson WA, Lemon M, Elefanty A, et al. Human acquired naevi are clonal. *Melanoma Res* 1998;8:499–503.
19. Maize JC, Foster G. Age-related changes in melanocytic naevi. *Clin Exp Dermatol* 1979;4:49–58.
20. Gallagher RP, McLean DI, Yang CP, et al. Anatomic distribution of acquired melanocytic nevi in white children. A comparison with melanoma: The Vancouver mole study. *Arch Dermatol* 1990;126:466–471.
21. Eady RA, Gilkes JJ, Jones EW. Eruptive naevi: Report of two cases, with enzyme histochemical, light and electron microscopical findings. *Br J Dermatol* 1977;97:267–278.
22. Mihm MC Jr, Crowson AN, Magro CM. The nondysplastic acquired nevi: Common acquired nevus and other benign acquired nevi. In: Crowson AN, Magro CM, Mihm MC Jr, eds. *The Melanocytic Proliferations: A Comprehensive Textbook of Pigmented Lesions*. New York, NY: John Wiley and Sons, 2001:73–96.
23. Kopf AW, Andrade R. A histologic study of the dermoepidermal junction in clinically "intraepidermal" nevi, employing serial sections: I. Junctional theques. *Ann NY Acad Sci* 1963;100:200–222.
24. Schrader WA, Helwig EB. Balloon cell nevi. *Cancer* 1967;20:1502–1514.
25. Goette DK, Doty RD. Balloon cell nevus. Summary of the clinical and histologic characteristics. *Arch Dermatol* 1978;114:109–111.
26. Akasaka T, Imamura Y, Kon S. Multiple agminated juvenile melanoma arising on a hyperpigmented macule. *J Dermatol* 1993;20:638–642.
27. Hofmann-Wellenhof R, Soyer HP, Smolle J, Kerl H. Spitz's nevus arising on a nevus spilus. *Dermatology* 1994;189:265–268.
28. Weinberg JM, Schutzer PJ, Harris RM, et al. Melanoma arising in nevus spilus. *Cutis* 1998;61:287–289.

29. Grinspan D, Casala A, Abulafia J, et al. Melanoma on dysplastic nevus spilus. *Int J Dermatol* 1997;36:499–502.
30. Takahasi M. Studies on cafe au lait spots in neurofibromatosis and pigmented macules of nevus spilus. *Tohoku J Exp Med* 1976;118:255–273.
31. Kiene P, Brodersen JP, Folster-Holst R. "Blue" variant of naevus spilus. *Hautarzt* 1995;46:349–351.
32. Betti R, Inselvini E, Palvarini M, Crosti C. Agminated intradermal Spitz nevi arising on an unusual speckled lentiginous nevus with localized lentiginosis: A continuum? *Am J Dermatopathol* 1997;19:524–527.
33. Bittencourt FV, Marghoob AA, Kopf AW, et al. Large congenital melanocytic nevi and the risk for development of malignant melanoma and neurocutaneous melanocytosis. *Pediatrics* 2000;106:736–741.
34. Swerdlow AJ, English JS, Qiao Z. The risk of melanoma in patients with congenital nevi: A cohort study. *J Am Acad Dermatol* 1995;32:595–599.
35. Lowes MA, Norris D, Whiteld M. Benign melanocytic proliferative nodule within a congenital naevus. *Australas J Dermatol* 2000;41:109–111.
36. Crowson AN, Magro CM, Mihm MC Jr. *The Nevomelanocytic Proliferations: A Comprehensive Textbook of Pigmented Lesions*. New York, NY: Wiley-Liss, 2001:550.
37. Sexton M, Sexton CW. Recurrent pigmented melanocytic nevus. A benign lesion, not to be mistaken for malignant melanoma. *Arch Pathol Lab Med* 1971;115:122–126.
38. Crowson AN, Magro CM, Mihm MC Jr. Recurrent melanocytic nevus. In: Crowson AN, Magro CM, Mihm MC Jr, eds. *The Melanocytic Proliferations: A Comprehensive Textbook of Pigmented Lesions*. New York, NY: John Wiley and Sons, 2001:195–207.
39. Blessing K. Benign atypical naevi: Diagnostic difficulties and continued controversy. *Histopathology* 1999;34:189–198.
40. Stern JB. Recurrent Spitz's nevi. A clinicopathologic investigation. *Am J Dermatopathol* 1985;7(Suppl.):49–50.
41. Kaye VN, Dehner LP. Spindle and epithelioid cell nevus (Spitz nevus). Natural history following biopsy. *Arch Dermatol* 1990;126:1581–1583.
42. Montgomery H. The blue nevus (Jaddasohn-Tieche): Its distinction from ordinary moles and malignant melanoma. *Am J Cancer* 1939;36:527–539.
43. Vidal S, Sanz A, Hernandez B, et al. Subungual blue naevus. *Br J Dermatol* 1997; 137:1023–1025.
44. Lovas GL, Wysocki GP, Daley TD. The oral blue nevus: Histogenetic implications of its ultrastructural features. *Oral Surg Oral Med Oral Pathol* 1983;55:145–150.
45. Heim K, Hopfl R, Muller-Holzner E, et al. Multiple blue nevi of the vagina. A case report. *J Reprod Med* 2000;45:42–44.
46. Lamovec J. Blue nevus of the lymph node capsule. Report of a new case with review of the literature. *Am J Clin Pathol* 1984;81(3):367–372.
47. Ro JY, Grignon DJ, Ayala AG, et al. Blue nevus and melanosis of the prostate. Electron-microscopic and immunohistochemical studies. *Am J Clin Pathol* 1988;90:530–535.
48. Casadei GP, Grigolato P, Cabibbo E. Blue nevus of the endocervix. A study of five cases. *Tumori* 1987;73:75–79.
49. Knoell KA, Nelson KC, Patterson JW. Familial multiple blue nevi. *J Am Acad Dermatol* 1998;39:322–325.
50. Pittman JL, Fisher BK. Plaque-type blue nevus. *Dermatology* 1976;112:1127–1128.
51. Busam KJ, Woodruff JM, Erlandson RA, Brady MS. Large plaque-type blue nevus with subcutaneous cellular nodules. *Am J Surg Pathol* 2000;24:920–929.
52. Del Rio E, Vasquez Viega HA, Suarez Penaranda JM. Blue nevus with satellitosis mimicking malignant melanoma. *Cutis* 2000;301–302.

53. Kamino H, Tam ST. Compound blue nevus: A variant of blue nevus with an additional junctional dendritic component. A clinical, histopathologic, and immunohistochemical study of six cases. *Arch Dermatol* 1990;126:1330–1333.

54. Carr S, See J, Wilkinson B, Kossard S. Hypopigmented common blue nevus. *J Cutan Pathol* 1997;24:494–498.

55. Harvell JD, White WL. Persistent and recurrent blue nevi. *Am J Dermatopathol* 1999;21:506–517.

56. Skelton HG III, Smith KJ, Barrett TL, et al. HMB-45 staining in benign and malignant melanocytic lesions. A reflection of cellular activation. *Am J Dermatopathol* 1991; 13:543–550.

57. Moreno C, Requena L, Kutzner H, et al. Epithelioid blue nevus: A rare variant blue nevus not always associated with the Carney complex. *J Cutan Pathol* 2000;27:218.

58. Carney JA, Ferreiro JA. The epithelioid blue nevus. A multicentric familial tumor with important associations, including cardiac myxoma and psammomatous melanotic schwannoma. *Am J Surg Pathol* 1996;20:259–272.

59. Temple-Camp CR, Saxe N, King H. Benign and malignant cellular blue nevus. A clinicopathological study of 30 cases. *Am J Dermatopathol* 1988;10:289–296.

60. Lach B, Russell N, Benoit B, Atack D. Cellular blue nevus (melanocytoma) of the spinal meninges: Electron microscopic and immunohistochemical features. *Neurosurgery* 1988;22:773–780.

61. Nakano S, Kinoshita K, Morita Y, et al. Cellular blue nevus of the scalp associated with intracranial involvement. *Surg Neurol* 1987;27:553–557.

62. Micali G, Innocenzi D, Nasca MR. Cellular blue nevus of the scalp infiltrating the underlying bone: Case report and review. *Pediatr Dermatol* 1997;14:199–203.

63. Michal M, Kerekes Z, Kinkor Z, et al. Desmoplastic cellular blue nevi. *Am J Dermatopathol* 1995;17:230–235.

64. Perez MT, Suster S. Balloon cell change in cellular blue nevus. *Am J Dermatopathol* 1999;21:181–184.

65. Tran TA, Carlson JA, Basaca PC, Mihm MC. Cellular blue nevus with atypia (atypical cellular blue nevus): A clinicopathologic study of nine cases. *J Cutan Pathol* 1998;25:252–258.

66. Mehregan DA, Gibson LE, Mehregan AH. Malignant blue nevus: A report of eight cases. *J Dermatol Sci* 1992;4:185–192.

67. Spatz A, Zimmermann U, Bachollet B, et al. Malignant blue nevus of the vulva with late ovarian metastasis. *Am J Dermatopathol* 1998;20:408–412.

68. Connelly J, Smith JL Jr. Malignant blue nevus. *Cancer* 1991;67:2653–2657.

69. Crowson AN, Magro CM, Mihm MC Jr. Malignant melanoma with prominent pigment synthesis: Animal type melanoma. *Hum Pathol* 1999;30:543–550.

70. Ota M, Tanino H. Nevus fusco-caeruleus opthalmomaxillaris and melanosis bulbi. *Tokyo Iji Shinshi* 1939;63:1243–1245.

71. Bisceglia M, Carosi I, Fania M, et al. Nevus of Ota. Presentation of a case associated with a cellular blue nevus with suspected malignant degeneration and review of the literature. *Pathologica* 1997;89:168–174.

72. Hidano A, Kajima H, Ikeda S, et al. Natural history of nevus of Ota. *Arch Dermatol* 1967; 95:187–195.

73. Hori Y, Kawashima M, Oohara K, Kukita A. Acquired, bilateral nevus of Ota-like macules. *J Am Acad Dermatol* 1984;10:961–964.

74. Nodl F, Kruger R. Malignant blue nevus in Ota's nevus. *Hautarzt* 1984;35:421–424.

75. Ito M. Nevus fusco-caeruleus acromio-deltoideus. *Tohoku Exp Med* 1954;60:10.

76. Sun CC, Lu YC, Lee EF, Nakagawa H. Naevus fusco-caeruleus zygomaticus. *Br J Dermatol* 1987;117:545–553.

77. Burkhart CG, Gohara A. Dermal melanocyte hamartoma. A distinctive new form of dermal melanocytosis. *Arch Dermatol* 1981;117:102–104.

78. Crowson AN, Magro CM, Mihm MC Jr. Dysplastic nevi, de novo intraepidermal epithelioid and lentiginous melanocytic dysplasias, and nevi at specific anatomic sites. In: Crowson AN, Magro CM, Mihm MC Jr, eds. *The Melanocytic Proliferations: A Comprehensive Textbook of Pigmented Lesions*. New York, NY: John Wiley and Sons, 2001:225–280.

79. Carlson JA, Mu XC, Slominski A, et al. Melanocytic proliferations associated with lichen sclerosus. *Arch Dermatol* 2002;138:77–87.

80. Blickstein I, Feldberg E, Dgani R, et al. Dysplastic vulvar nevi. *Obstet Gynecol* 1991;78(5 Pt 2):968–970.

81. Harris MN, Hurwitz RM, Buckel LJ, Gray HR. Congenital Spitz nevus. *Dermatol Surg* 2000;26:931–935.

82. Weedon D, Little JH. Spindle and epithelioid cell nevi in children and adults. A review of 211 cases of the Spitz nevus. *Cancer* 1977;40(1):217–225.

83. Akyurek M, Kayikcioglu A, Ozkan O, et al. Multiple agminated Spitz nevi of the scalp. *Ann Plast Surg* 199;43:459- 460.

84. Bullen R, Snow SN, Larson PO, et al. Multiple agminated Spitz nevi: Report of two cases and review of the literature. *Pediatr Dermatol* 1995;12:156–158.

85. Krakowski A, Tur E, Brenner S. Multiple agminated juvenile melanoma: A case with a sunburn history, and a review. *Dermatologica* 1981;163:270–275.

86. Onsun N, Saracoglu S, Demirkesen C, et al. Eruptive widespread Spitz nevi: Can pregnancy be a stimulating factor? *J Am Acad Dermatol* 1990;40(5 Pt 2):866–867.

87. Weimar VM, Zuehlke RL. Multiple agminate spindle and epithelioid cell nevi in an adult. *Arch Dermatol* 1978;114:1383–1384.

88. Binder SW, Asnong C, Paul E, Cochran AJ. The histology and differential diagnosis of Spitz nevus. *Semin Diagn Pathol* 1993;10:36–46.

89. Havenith MG, van Zandvoort EH, Cleutjens JP, et al. Basement membrane deposition in benign and malignant naevomelanocytic lesions: An immunohistochemical study with antibodies to type IV collagen and laminin. *Histopathology* 1989;15(2):137–146.

90. Kamino H, Jagirdar J. Fibronectin in eosinophilic globules in the Spitz nevus. *Am J Dermatopathol* 1984;6(Suppl. 1):313–316.

91. Howat AJ, Variend S. Lymphatic invasion in Spitz nevi. *Am J Surg Pathol* 1985; 9:125–128.

92. Crotty KA, McCarthy SW, Palmer AA, et al. Malignant melanoma in childhood: A clinicopathologic study of 13 cases and comparison with Spitz nevi. *World J Surg* 1992; 16:179–185.

93. Crotty KA. Spitz nevus: Histological features and distinction from malignant melanoma. *Australas J Dermatol* 1997;38(Suppl. 1):S49–S53.

94. Toussaint S, Kamino H. Dysplastic changes in different types of melanocytic nevi. A unifying concept. *J Cutan Pathol* 1999;26(2):84–90.

95. Harvell JD, Meehan SA, LeBoit PE. Spitz's nevi with halo reaction: A histopathologic study of 17 cases. *J Cutan Pathol* 1997;24:611–619.

96. Lee MW, Choi JH, Sung KJ, et al. Hyalinizing Spitz nevus. *J Dermatol* 2000;27:273.

97. Magro CM, Crowson AN, Mihm MC Jr. Spitz nevus. In: Crowson AN, Magro CM, Mihm MC Jr, eds. *The Melanocytic Proliferations: A Comprehensive Textbook of Pigmented Lesions*. New York, NY: John Wiley and Sons, 2001:121–181.

98. Diaz-Cascajo C, Borghi S, Weyers W. Angiomatoid Spitz nevus: A distinctive variant of desmoplastic Spitz nevus with prominent vasculature. *Am J Dermatopathol* 2000; 22:135–139.

99. Busam KJ, Barnhill RL. Pagetoid spitz nevus. Intraepidermal Spitz tumor with prominent pagetoid spread. *Am J Surg Pathol* 1995;19:1061–1067.

100. Han MH, Koh KJ, Choi JH, et al. Pagetoid Spitz nevus: A variant of Spitz nevus. *Int J Dermatol* 2000;39:555–557.
101. Reed RJ, Ichinose H, Clark WH Jr, Mihm MC Jr. Common and uncommon melanocytic nevi and borderline melanomas. *Semin Oncol* 1975;2:119–147.
102. Sau P, Graham JH, Helwig EB. Pigmented spindle cell nevus: A clinicopathologic analysis of ninety-five cases. *J Am Acad Dermatol* 1993;28:565–571.
103. Sagebiel RW, Chinn EK, Egbert BM. Pigmented spindle cell nevus. Clinical and histologic review of 90 cases. *Am J Surg Pathol* 1984;8:645–653.
104. Requena L, Sanchez Yus E. Pigmented spindle cell naevus. *Br J Dermatol* 1990; 123:757–763.
105. Wistuba I, Gonzalez S. Eosinophilic globules in pigmented spindle cell nevus. *Am J Dermatopathol* 1990;12:268–271.
106. Choi JH, Sung KJ, Koh JK. Pigmented epithelioid cell nevus: A variant of Spitz nevus? *J Am Acad Dermatol* 1993;28:497–498.
107. Murata H, Ashida A, Takata M, et al. Establishment of a novel melanoma cell line SMYM-PRGP showing cytogenetic and biological characteristics of the radial growth phase of acral melanomas. *Cancer Sci* 2007;98:958–963.
108. Carvalho L, Lipay M, Belfort F, et al. Telomerase activity in prognostic histopathologic features of melanoma. *J Plast Reconstr Aesthet Surg* 2006;59:961–968.
109. Bagheri S, Nostrati M, Li S, et al. Genes and pathways downstream of telomerase in melanoma metastasis. *Proc Natl Acad Sci USA* 2006;103:11306–11311.
110. Fulllen DR, Poynter JN, Lowe L, et al. BRAF and NRAS mutations in spitzoid melanocytic lesions. *Mod Pathol* 2006;19:1324–1332.
111. Barnhill RL, Argenyi ZB, From L, et al. Atypical Spitz nevi/tumors: Lack of consensus for diagnosis, discrimination from melanoma, and prediction of outcome. *Hum Pathol* 1999; 30:513–520.
112. Smith KJ, Barrett TL, Skelton HG III, et al. Spindle cell and epithelioid cell nevi with atypia and metastasis (malignant Spitz nevus). *Am J Surg Pathol* 1989;13(11):931–939.
113. Barnhill RL, Flotte TJ, Fleischli M, Perez-Atayde A. Cutaneous melanoma and atypical Spitz tumors in childhood. Cancer 1995;76:1833–1845.
114. Magro CM, Yaniv B, Mihm MC. The superficial atypical Spitz tumor and malignant melanoma of superficial spreading type arising in association with the superficial atypical Spitz tumor. A distinct form of dysplastic Spitzoid nevomelanocytic proliferation. *J Am Acad Dermatol* 2009;60:814–825.
115. Spatz A, Calonje E, Handfield-Jones S, Barnhill RL. Spitz tumors in children: A grading system for risk stratification. *Arch Dermatol* 1999;135:282–285.
116. Crotty KA, McCarthy SW, Palmer AA, et al. Malignant melanoma in childhood: A clinicopathologic study of 13 cases and comparison with Spitz nevi. *World J Surg* 1992;16:179–185.
117. McCarthy SW, Crotty KA, Palmer AA, et al. Cutaneous malignant melanoma in teenagers. *Histopathology* 1994;24:453–461.
118. Gamblin TC, Edington H, Kirkwood JM, Rao UN. Sentinel lymph node biopsy for atypical melanocytic lesions with spitzoid features. *Ann Surg Oncol* 2006 Dec;13(12):1664–1670.
119. Murali R, Sharma RN, Thompson JF, et al. Sentinel lymph node biopsy in histologically ambiguous melanocytic tumors with spitzoid features (so-called atypical spitzoid tumors). *Ann Surg Oncol* 2008 Jan;15(1):302–309.
120. Biddle DA, Evans HL, Kemp BL, et al. Intraparenchymal nevus cell aggregates in lymph nodes: A possible diagnostic pitfall with malignant melanoma and carcinoma. *Am J Surg Pathol* 2003 May;27(5):673–681.
121. Lohmann CM, Iversen K, Jungbluth AA, et al. Expression of melanocyte differentiation antigens and Ki-67 in nodal nevi and comparison of Ki-67 expression with metastatic melanoma. *Am J Surg Pathol* 2002;26:1351–1357.

122. Pulitzer DR, Martin PC, Cohen AP, Reed RJ. Histologic classification of the combined nevus. Analysis of the variable expression of melanocytic nevi. *Am J Surg Pathol* 1991;15:1111–1122.

123. Requena L, Barat A, Hasson A, et al. Malignant combined nevus. *Am J Dermatopathol* 1991; 13:169–173.

124. Seab JA Jr, Graham JH, Helwig EB. Deep penetrating nevus. *Am J Surg Pathol* 1989; 13:39–44.

125. Cooper PH. Deep penetrating (plexiform spindle cell) nevus. A frequent participant in combined nevus. *J Cutan Pathol* 1992;19:172–180.

126. Margo CM, Crowson AN, Mihm MC, et al. The dermal borderline melanocytic tumor. A categorical approach. *J Am Acad Dermatol* 2009 (in press).

127. Barnhill RL, Mihm MC Jr, Magro CM. Plexiform spindle cell naevus: A distinctive variant of plexiform melanocytic naevus. *Histopathology* 1991;18:243–247.

128. Lynch HT, Frichot B, Lynch JF. Familial atypical multi-mole melanoma syndrome. *J Med Genet* 1978 Oct;15(5):352–356.

129. Clark WH, Reimer RR, Greene M, et al. Origin of familial malignant melanomas from heritable melanocytic lesions. "The B-K mole syndrome." *Arch Dermatol* 1978 May;114(5):732–738.

130. Elder DE. Dysplastic nevi. Their significance and management. *Dermatol Clin* 1988; 6(2):257–269.

131. Knoell KA, Hendrix JD, Patterson JW, et al. Nonpigmented dysplastic melanocytic nevi. *Arch Dermatol* 1997;133(8):992–994.

132. National Institutes of Health Consensus Development Conference Statement on Diagnosis and Treatment of Early Melanoma, January 27–29, 1992. *Am J Dermatopathol* 1993;15(1):34–43.

133. Shea CR, Prieto VG. Recent developments in the pathology of melanocytic neoplasia. *Dermatol Clin* 1999;17(3):615–630.

134. Nordlund JJ, Kirkwood J, Forget BM, et al. Demographic study of clinically atypical (dysplastic) nevi in patients with melanoma and comparison subjects. *Cancer Res* 1985;45(4):1855–1861.

135. Clark WH Jr, Elder DE, Guerry D IV, et al. A study of tumor progression: The precursor lesions of superficial spreading and nodular melanoma. *Hum Pathol* 1984; 15(12):1147–1165.

136. Titus-Ernstoff. LT, Duray PH, Ernstoff MS, et al. Dysplastic nevi in association with multiple primary melanoma. *Cancer Res* 1988;48(4):1016–1018.

137. Hastrup N, Osterlind A, Drzewiecki KT, Hou-Jensen K. The presence of dysplastic nevus remnants in malignant melanoma. *Am J Dermatopathol* 1991;13(4):378–385.

138. Grob JJ, Andrac L, Romano MH, et al. Dysplastic naevus in non-familial melanoma. A clinicopathological study of 101 cases. *Br J Dermatol* 1988;18(6):745–752.

139. Cannon-Albright LA, Meyer LJ, Lewis CM, et al. Penetrance and expressivity of the chromosome 9p melanoma susceptibility locus (MLM). *Cancer Res* 1994;54(23):6041–6044.

140. Crowson AN, Magro C, Miller A, et al. The molecular basis of melanomagenesis and the metastatic phenotype. *Semin Oncol* 2007;34:476–490.

141. Rhodes AR, Harrist TJ, Day CL, et al. Dysplastic melanocytic nevi in histologic association with 234 primary cutaneous melanomas. *J Am Acad Dermatol* 1983;9(4):563–574.

142. Elder DE, Goldman LI, Goldman SC, et al. Dysplastic nevus syndrome: A phenotypic association of sporadic cutaneous melanoma. *Cancer* 1980;46(8):1787–1794.

143. Ahmed I, Piepkorn MW, Rabkin MS, et al. Histopathologic characteristics of dysplastic nevi. *J Am Acad Dermatol* 1990;22(5pt1):727–733.

144. Steijlen PM, Bergman W, Herman J, et al. The efficacy of histopathological criteria required for diagnosing dysplastic naevi. *Histopathology* 1988;12:289–300.

145. Rhodes AR, Mihm MC, Weinstock MA. Dysplastic melanocytic nevi: A reproducible histologic definition emphasizing cellular morphology. *Mod Pathol* 1989;2(4):306–319.

146. Barnhill RL, Roush GC, Duray PH. Correlation of histologic architectural and cytoplasmic features with nuclear atypia in atypical (dysplastic) nevomelanocytic nevi. *Hum Pathol* 1990;21(1):51–58.

147. Rivers JK, Cockerall CJ, McBride A, Kopf AW. Quantification of histologic features of dysplastic nevi. *Am J Dermatopathol* 1990;12(1):42–50.

148. Black WC, Hunt WC. Histologic correlations with the clinical diagnosis of dysplastic nevus. *Am J Surg Pathol* 1990;14(1):44–52.

149. Roth ME, Grant-Kels JM, Ackerman AB, et al. The histopathology of dysplastic nevi. *Am J Dermatopathol* 1991;13(1):38–51.

150. Clemente C, Cochran AJ, Elder DE, et al. Histopathologic diagnosis of dysplastic nevi: Concordance among pathologists convened by the World Health Organization Melanoma Programme. *Hum Pathol* 1991;22:313–319.

151. Roush GC, Barnhill RL, Duray PH, et al. Diagnosis of dysplastic nevus in different populations. *J Am Acad Dermatol* 1986;14(3):419–425.

152. Duncan LM, Berwick M, Bruijn JA, et al. Histopathologic recognition and grading of dysplastic melanocytic nevi: An interobserver agreement study. *J Invest Dermatol* 1993;100(3):318S–321S.

153. Piepkorn M, Barnhill RL, Cannon-Albright LA, et al. A multiobserver, population-based analysis of histologic dysplasia in melanocytic nevi. *J Am Acad Dermatol* 1994;30(5 Pt 1):707–714.

154. Shea CR, Vollmer RT, Prieto VG. Correlating architectural disorder and cytologic atypia in Clark (dysplastic)melanocytic nevi. *Hum Pathol* 1999;30(5):500–505.

155. Hastrup N, Clemmenson OJ, Spaun E, Sondergaard K. Dysplastic naevus: Histopathologic criteria and their inter-observer reproducibility. *Histopathology* 1994;24(6): 503–509.

156. Sachdeva M, Frambach GE, Crowson AN, et al. De novo intraepidermal epithelioid melanocytic dysplasia as a marker of the atypical mole phenotype–a clinical and pathological study of 75 patients. *J Cutan Pathol* 2005;32(9):622–628.

3

MELANOMA: CLASSIC SUBTYPES

The incidence of melanoma has been rapidly increasing over the last 30 years, especially among Caucasians. This chapter presents a concise summary of the basic criteria that are critical to the histological diagnosis of melanoma. Melanomas in humans were divided by Clark et al.[1,2] into several subtypes including superficial spreading melanoma, lentigo maligna melanoma, and nodular melanoma. Acral lentiginous melanoma was an additional subtype subsequently characterized by Reed.[3] Other less common forms of melanoma have since been described. Melanoma equally affects men and women, and is uncommon in children of either sex. The average age at diagnosis is in the fourth decade of life. In one typical study, the most common location was the trunk (43.5%), followed by extremities (33.9%), head and neck (10.7%), and acral locations (11.9%).[4]

Melanoma has clinically and histologically distinctive steps in tumor progression.[5] These include (i) melanoma confined above the epidermal basement membrane, termed *radial growth phase-confined melanoma in situ* (e-figs. 3.1–3.3); (ii) melanoma which penetrates the delimiting basement membrane to enter the superficial papillary dermis, a phase termed *radial growth phase-confined microinvasive melanoma* (e-figs. 3.4 and 3.5); and (iii) melanoma which invades the dermis as a tumorigenic nodule that has acquired the capacity for metastatic growth, which is termed *vertical growth phase melanoma* (e-figs. 3.6–3.10).

The identification of its presence in any given lesion is essential for accurate subclassification and also for a critical analysis of its potential to cause harm to the patient. Melanoma often begins as an intraepidermal proliferation of neoplastic melanocytes that, sometimes for decades, remains confined to the epidermis or superficial dermis. In this stage of development, known as the radial or horizontal growth phase, the melanoma is virtually always completely curable by surgical excision. For example, all of 161 patients whose pure, radial growth phase-confined melanoma showed no histological evidence of regression in the primary excision specimen and were followed for a median of 13.7 years had a metastasis-free survival.[5] Tumors may develop expansile nodules, or significantly invade the reticular dermis or subcutaneous fat. At this time, the lesion has acquired the capacity to metastasize and is said to be in vertical growth phase wherein its prognosis is directly related to the measured depth of invasion[6] along with other histological parameters.[2,7–15] One type of melanoma, termed "nodular melanoma," has no pre-existing radial or horizontal growth phase and is presumptively in vertical growth phase from its inception (e-figs. 3.11 and 3.12). The five basic subtypes of melanoma are superficial spreading melanoma, nodular melanoma, lentigo maligna melanoma, acral lentiginous melanoma,[16] and mucosal lentiginous melanoma. Other types of melanoma include minimal deviation melanoma,[17,18] malignant cellular blue nevus,[19] desmoplastic melanoma,[20] nevoid melanoma,[21] and a form of malignant melanoma with prominent pigment syntheses termed "animal type melanoma" by some observers.[22]

From the standpoint of the pathobiology of these cancers, substantial advances have been made in our understanding of the molecular basis of melanomagenesis.[23,24] Although beyond the scope of a textbook on skin biopsy morphology such as this one, the aforementioned molecular advances underscore the idea that melanoma is not a single integrated disease, but heterogeneous groups of lesions that arise from complex molecular changes. In part, these molecular alterations may be site dependent; differences in the expression of *BRAF* and *NRAS* genes have been shown in melanomas arising in sun-exposed versus sun-protected sites, with intermittently exposed skin bearing the highest mutation rates in these two genes.[25,26] These advances offer the promise of novel therapeutic strategies targeted at the specific molecular profile of a given tumor in an individual patient. For example, tumors that bear *KIT* mutations, which are apparently more frequent in mucosal than in acral melanomas, are more likely to respond to imatinib.[27] The expression of MAPK pathway anomalies such as *NRAS* and *BRAF* mutations can be impacted by sorafenib, a protein kinase inhibitor, and in concert with other chemotherapeutic drugs, this agent may inhibit melanoma growth.[26] It seems that epigenetic factors may impact gene expression in melanoma. For example, the expression of a stem cell protein termed Nodal is limited to vertical growth phase and metastatic melanoma; inhibition of Nodal signaling causes reversion to a nonmetastasizing phenotype.[28] Presumably, epigenetic events in the microenvironment also impact the expression of cortactin and other surface proteins involved in the assembly and regulation of the actin cytoskeleton and the production of invadopodia, the cell pseudopodia critical to motility in melanoma and in basal cell carcinoma[29] and also to the vascular ingress and egress of melanoma.[30] Emerging strategies for gene transfer are aimed at repairing the cell signaling pathways perturbed by specific mutations.[31] In short, novel advances confirm that melanoma has a molecular heterogeneity that mirrors its morphologic heterogeneity and correlates with its biological characteristics.

SPECIFIC SUBTYPES OF MALIGNANT MELANOMA

Superficial Spreading Melanoma

CLINICAL FEATURES. Superficial spreading melanoma constitutes approximately 70% to 75% of all melanomas, and, though mainly found on the trunk and the sun-exposed areas of the upper arms and the lower legs, it may occur anywhere on the body surface.[32,33] Therapeutic ultraviolet (UV) irradiation and use of tanning bed may play an etiological role.[34] A Norwegian melanoma project carried out between 1989 and 1993 revealed that persons with red hair and skin type I/II were at increased risk of developing melanoma.[35,36] Intermittent intense exposure to UV irradiation as in the context of beach vacation in adolescence, prior sun burns, or exposure to sunbeds and sunlamps is associated with increased risk, while chronic sun exposure may be protective (Table 3.1).[37]

Clinically, the incipient lesion is a dark-brown macule, a few millimeters in size, that gradually enlarges to reach an average size of 2.5 cm. However, marked variation in size may be noted with some lesions being as small as 4 mm and others as large as 8 to 10 cm. When fully evolved, the lesion has variegated color and irregular borders. The onset of the vertical growth phase is associated with the presence of a distinctive nodule. Superficial spreading melanoma arises de novo in approximately 75% of the cases and, in the remainder, it is associated with a pre-existing nevus, including those of congenital and dysplastic nevus subtypes. Melanoma arising in a pre-existing dysplastic nevus is usually of superficial spreading type.[38]

HISTOPATHOLOGY. By definition, a superficial spreading melanoma must have a radial growth phase.[5] At its inception, this radial growth phase is confined to the epidermal compartment (i.e., "in situ" melanoma of superficial spreading type; Fig. 3.1), manifesting an epithelioid cytomorphology and a pagetoid (i.e., single cell or "buckshot") architecture.

Epithelioid melanoma cells have round-to-oval nuclei with thick nuclear chromatinic rims, macronucleoli, and abundant quantities of eosinophilic cytoplasm within which variably sized and variably shaped melanin granules are identified (e-figs. 3.13 and 3.14). The epidermis is frequently hyperplastic. The second intraepidermal growth pattern is one of contiguous proliferation of singly disposed cells along the dermoepidermal junction with retiform effacement. These atypical cells have angulated, hyperchromatic nuclei that often lack internal nuclear detail and exceed the size of adjacent keratinocyte nuclei (e-fig. 3.15). The third pattern is one of confluent oblong nests composed of hyperchromatic spindle-shaped cells with distinct nuclear grooves, prominent nuclear chromatinic rims, eosinophilic nucleoli, and variable melanization (e-fig. 3.16). In most cases, a hybrid pattern of intraepidermal growth is observed with a combination of these three patterns. Dermal lymphocytic inflammation may be observed and may herald the onset of incipient microinvasive melanoma.

TABLE 3.1 Histological Precis of Five Major Subtypes of Melanoma

	SSM	NM	LMM	ALM	MLM
Pattern of radial growth phase (RGP)	Diffuse pagetoid	Absent	Lentiginous	Lentiginous	Lentiginous
Epidermis of RGP	Normal or hyperplastic		Atrophic	Often hyperplastic	Often hyperplastic
Usual cell type of RGP	Epithelioid		Spindle, epithelioid, sometimes dendritic	Spindle, epithelioid, often dendritic	Epithelioid; often dendritic
Papillary dermis of RGP	Variable inflammation, thickening, and fibrosis		Usually inflamed	Almost always inflamed, with papillary dermal fibrosis	Variable inflammation and fibrosis
Frequency of regression	Frequent partial	Uncommon	Common	Variable	Common
Solar elastosis of dermis	Often absent	Often absent	Characteristic feature	Absent	Absent
Usual cell type of vertical growth phase	Epithelioid	Epithelioid	Spindled and epithelioid	Spindled and epithelioid, often highly pleomorphic	Epithelioid or spindled
Desmoplasia	Rare	Uncommon	Common	Common	Common
Neurotropism	Rare	Uncommon	Common	Common	Variable
Precursor nevus or melanosis	Common (nevus) (25%–40%)	Uncommon	Uncommon	Uncommon	Common (melanosis)

SSM, superficial spreading malignant melanoma; NM, nodular malignant melanoma; LMM, lentigo maligna melanoma; ALM, acral lentiginous malignant melanoma; MLM, mucosal lentiginous melanoma.

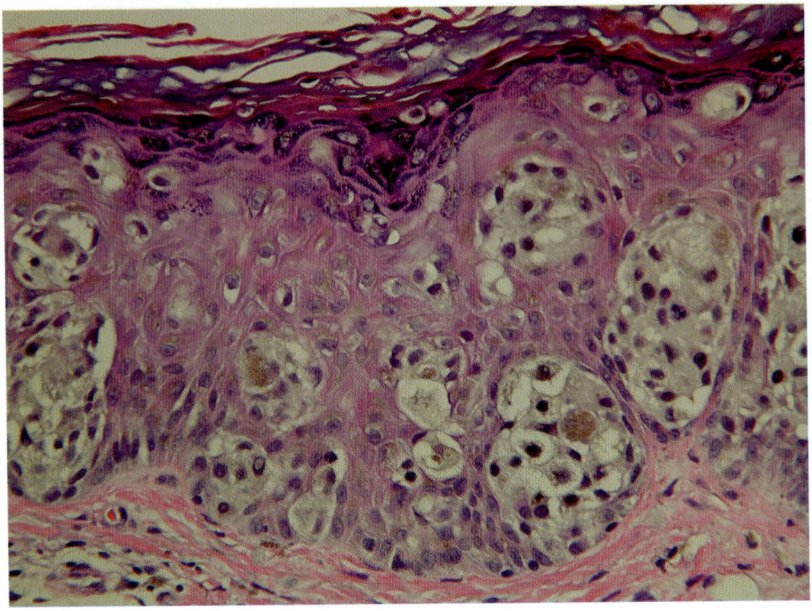

FIGURE 3.1 **Superficial Spreading Melanoma In Situ: Epithelioid Pattern of Melanocytic Dysplasia.** Cells with an epithelioid cytomorphology grow in a haphazard, pagetoid fashion with single-cell dispersal through the epidermis to the cornified layer. The cells exhibit prominent nucleolation and high nuclear to cytoplasmic ratios. There is significant variability with respect to nuclear size and shape.

An organized periretal stromal response is only seen if areas of residual dysplastic nevus are present. If a vertical growth phase is seen, the radial growth phase can be identified as an asymmetric growth above and lateral to the nodule(s) of vertical growth phase tumor in the epidermis or in the papillary dermis (Fig. 3.2).

The next phase in the progression of radial growth phase melanoma is the development of a microinvasive component (Fig. 3.3) confined to the papillary dermis with nested and dispersed single-cell growth in the upper dermis that has a similar cytomorphology to the intraepidermal component.

The nests, by definition, do not exceed the size of any nest along the dermoepidermal junction. By historical convention, extension of the intraepidermal component for more than three rete ridges past the confines of the dermal component has been used to define the subtype of melanoma designated as superficial spreading melanoma,[2] but, in our view, any discernible lateral invasion within the epidermis beyond the confines of the dermal component defines superficial spreading melanoma. Regression or a vertical growth phase component (Figs. 3.4–3.6) implies a risk of metastasis even in radial growth phase-confined

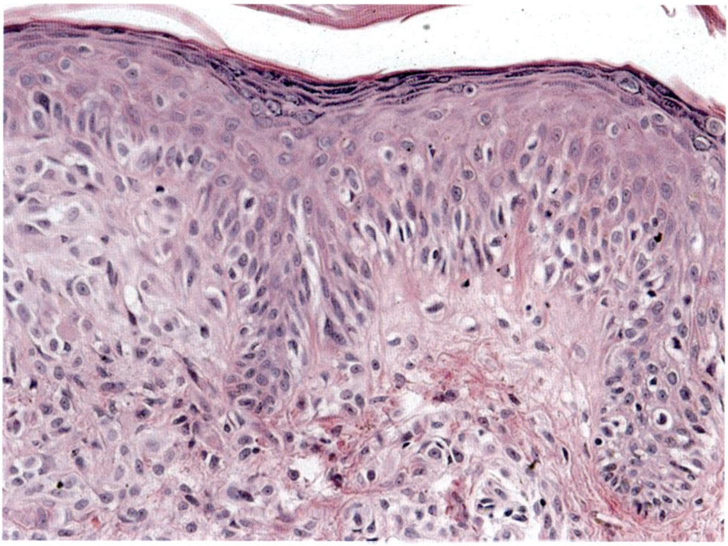

FIGURE 3.2 **Superficial Spreading Melanoma: Radial Growth Phase.** Integral to the definition of superficial spreading malignant melanoma is the identification of a radial growth phase component which extends laterally, as demonstrated in the right hand of the panel, beyond the invasive component noted in the left hand of the figure. These changes are best appreciated, as this figure illustrates, at scanning (i.e., 4× objective) magnification.

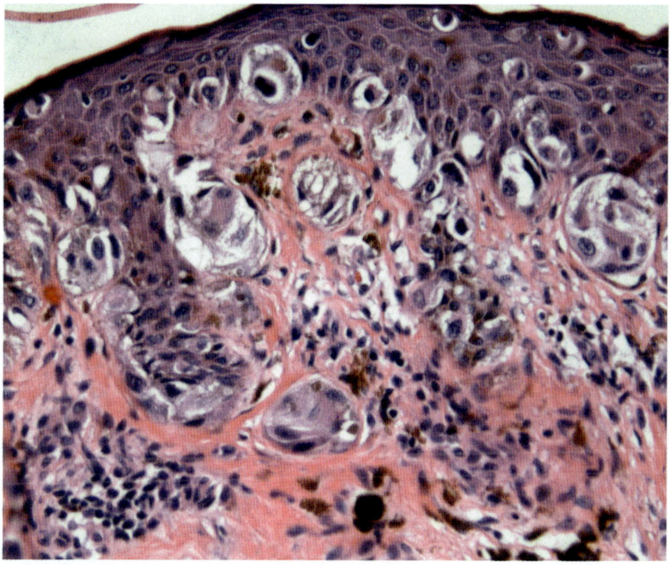

FIGURE 3.3 **Superficial Spreading Melanoma: Microinvasive Melanoma.** The progression of radial growth phase malignant melanoma encompasses the development of a component of microinvasive melanoma confined to the papillary dermis. This will comprise both nested and dispersed single cells with a cytomorphology similar to the intraepidermal component. Dominant nests which exceed the size of junctional nests are not observed; if present, they are a clue to vertical growth phase melanoma.

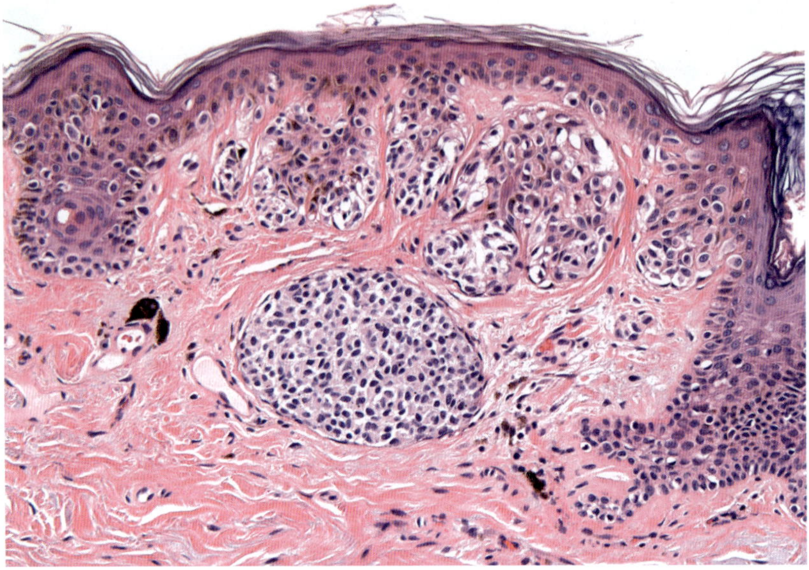

FIGURE 3.4 **Superficial Spreading Melanoma—Early Vertical Growth Phase.** One of the characteristic hallmarks of early vertical growth phase melanoma is the presence of a dominant nest within the papillary dermis which exceeds the size of any junctional thèque.

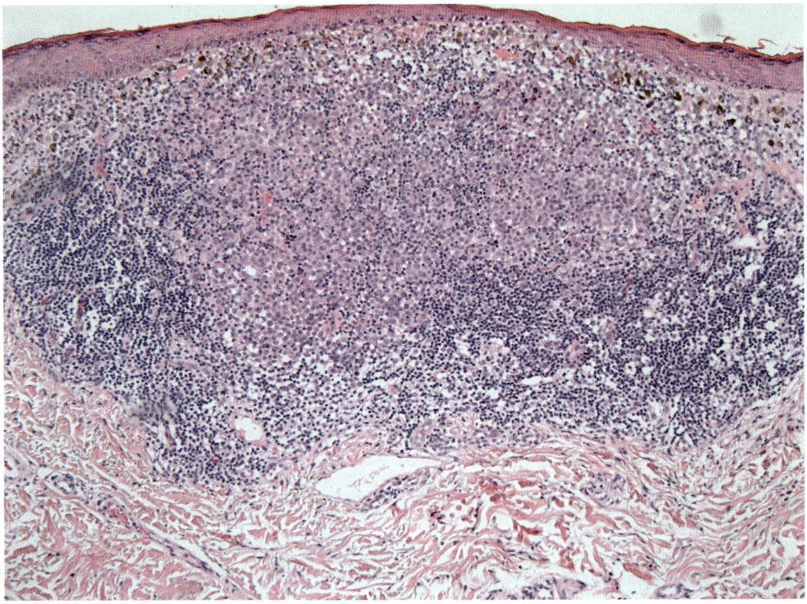

FIGURE 3.5 **Superficial Spreading Melanoma: Fully Evolved Vertical Growth Phase, Level III.** Filling the papillary dermis are fully transformed malignant epithelioid melanocytes, forming a confluent mass. The overlying retiform pattern is bowed and effaced by the dermal tumor nodule.

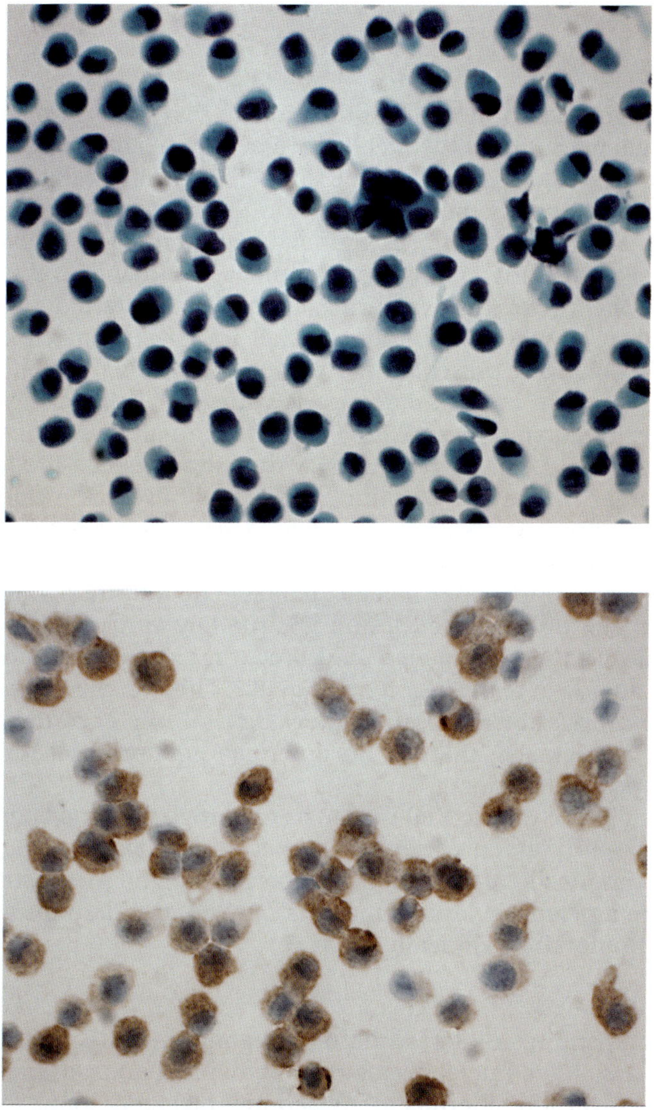

FIGURE 3.6 **Metastatic Melanoma to Supraclavicular Lymph Node from Case in Figure 3.5. A:** The fine needle aspiration biopsy shows noncohesive malignant cells. An immunostain with antibody to Melan-A **(B)** confirms a melanocyte histogenesis of the metastatic tumor deposit.

melanoma; hallmarks of regression include delicate fibroplasia, vertically oriented telangiectatic vessels within the fibrous zone, accumulation of melanophages, absence of neoplastic melanocytes in the dermis and in the overlying epidermis, and infiltrate of lymphocytes and plasma cells (e-figs. 3.17–3.25).

LENTIGO MALIGNA

Clinical Features

Lentigo maligna is a form of melanoma in situ that occurs on sun-exposed skin and thus predominantly affects the face, the head and neck, and, less often, other sun-exposed areas of the body.[39,40] Lentigo maligna melanoma of the head and neck is most common on the face in women and on the scalp, neck, and ears in men.[41] Extrafacial lentigo maligna melanoma constitutes 18% of all lentigo maligna melanomas, occurring on the forelegs of women and the forelegs and forearms of men.[41,42] The term lentigo maligna melanoma is used when the tumor assumes invasive properties.

Lentigo maligna presents as a pigmented macule that initially may measure 0.5 to 1 cm in size; the color is variegated tan to brown and the borders are irregular (e-figs. 3.26–3.28). The initial presentation may be in the fourth decade of life or earlier, with a slight female preponderance. From its initial size at presentation, it gradually evolves, sometimes to a size of 15 to 20 cm, covering large areas. During the entire course of its intraepidermal phase, which can last from 10 to 50 years, confinement of the lesion is as a nonpalpable macule; palpable nodularity signifies invasion most often. The fully evolved lesion is strikingly variegated in color and may extend into the conjunctiva, oral mucosa, or external auditory canal, depending upon where the lesion originated.[40] The average size of the lesion at the time of invasion is approximately 6 cm. If one controls for level of invasion and thickness, there is no difference in survival with respect to other subtypes of melanoma.[43]

Clinically, the differential diagnosis of lentigo maligna encompasses a dysplastic nevus, pigmented seborrheic keratosis, solar lentigo, pigmented superficial basal cell carcinoma, and superficial pigmented actinic keratosis. The rare amelanotic lentigo maligna may be mistaken for a squamous epithelial proliferation clinically.[44]

Histology of Radial Growth Phase Lentigo Maligna Melanoma

The characteristic histology is one of polygonal melanocytes with hyperchromatic, angulated nuclei dispersed as individual units, initially confined to the basal layer of epidermis in a discontiguous lentiginous fashion with extension down the basal layer of adnexae (e-figs. 3.29–3.33). Another characteristic feature is the multinucleated giant melanocyte containing more than 30 nuclei (Figs. 3.7–3.9; e-figs. 3.34 and 3.35).[45,46] Termed a "starburst giant cell," this is disposed along the basal layer of the epidermis[47] in up to 85% of cases. The epidermis is characteristically atrophic, manifesting thinning and loss of the retiform pattern overlying elastotic dermal collagen (e-fig. 3.36). As the lesion progresses, continuity of single-cell basilar melanocytic proliferation is observed, followed by a nested pattern of junctional activity; such nests assume a parallel disposition to the long axis of the epidermis in what is referred to as "the swallow nest sign" (e-fig. 3.37). Pagetoid infiltration and nesting are the harbingers of the next phase of lesional evolution, namely, dermal invasion. When pagetoid spread occurs, the cytomorphology is characteristically that of an epithelioid cell type similar to that observed in a superficial spreading melanoma (e-fig. 3.38). The presence of a lichenoid infiltrate with admixed melanophages in a papillary dermis which exhibits laminated sclerosis warrants careful scrutiny of the inflamed papillary dermis for singly disposed neoplastic melanocytes that signify microinvasion. Regressive stromal changes, neovascularization, and an inflammatory host response may be a clue to an antecedent microinvasive component.[48] Distinction of microinvasive melanoma from activated melanophages may be difficult, requiring the use of HMB-45, Melan-A, and/or CD68 preparations. An S100 preparation is generally of little use as many antigen-presenting dendritic cells stain positively in the dermis.

Unfortunately, not all cases of lentigo maligna have this prototypic morphology. In particular, in some cases the epidermis appears hyperplastic, with rete elongation and some degree of fibrotic condensation around rete ridges, mimicking a dysplastic nevus (e-figs. 3.39 and 3.40). The distinction is made by identifying concomitant interposed foci that are more typical of lentigo maligna. The patterned, festooned fibrosis seen in dysplastic nevi is not present. A dermal component that comprises benign nevus cells would not be present unless there was a concomitant dermal nevus. The atypia is worse in lentigo maligna by virtue of striking pleomorphism, wide

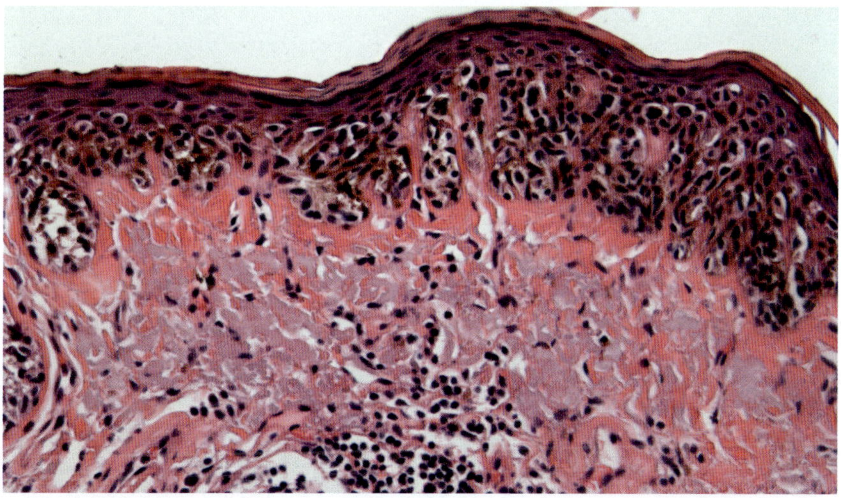

FIGURE 3.7 **Lentigo Maligna.** The characteristic histomorphological appearance of lentigo maligna (i.e., precursor to invasive lentigo maligna melanoma) comprises polygonal-shaped melanocytes with enlarged hyperchromatic, angulated nuclei dispersed primarily as individual units initially along the basal layer in a discontiguous lentiginous fashion; the epidermis is attenuated. The nuclei are larger than adjacent keratinocyte nuclei. While the dominant pattern is single cells, focally nests comprising 5 to 10 hyperchromatic "lentiginous dysplastic" cells may be observed.

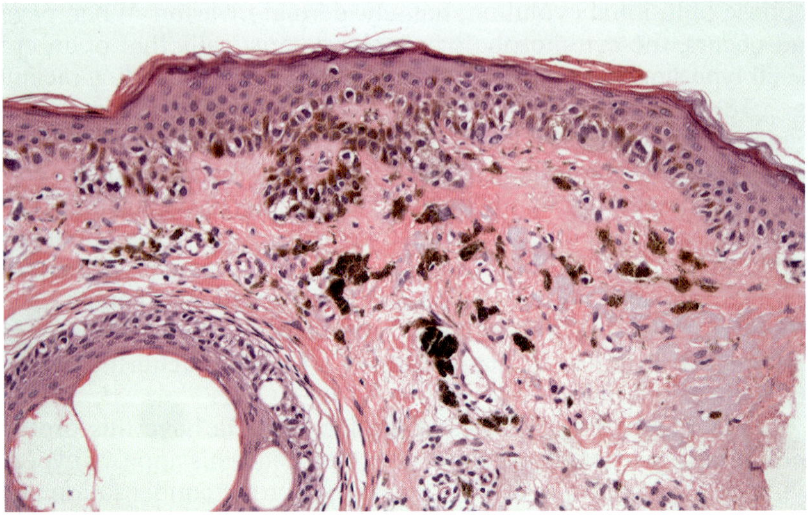

FIGURE 3.8 **Lentigo Maligna: Abnormal Melanization as a Clue to the Diagnosis.** The pattern of melanization in the epidermis is abnormal; specifically there is irregular deposition of melanin pigment within individual melanocytes as well as adjacent keratinocytes. Prominent dendritic processes extending into the mid and upper layers of the stratum malpighii may be observed and are, in our view, a feature of phototransformation and thus a clue to UV light exposure.

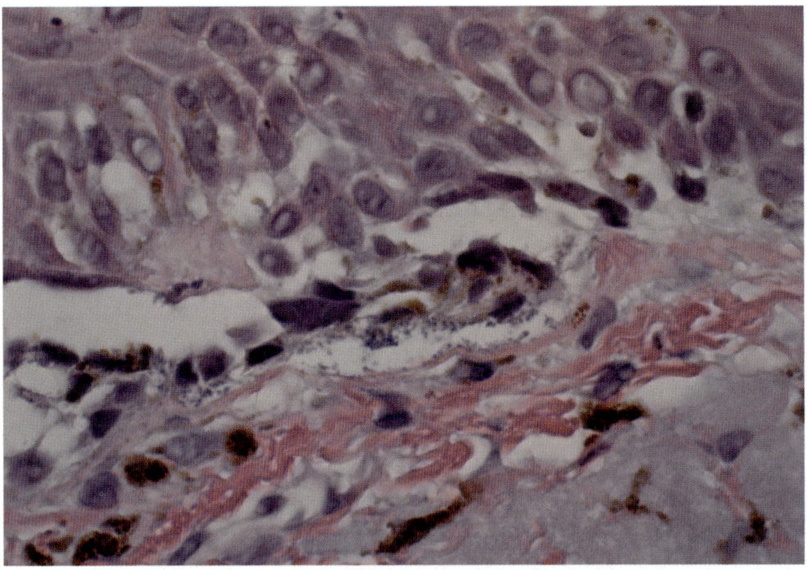

FIGURE 3.9 **Lentigo Maligna: The "Star Burst" Giant Cell.** Multiple neoplastic multinucleated giant cells are seen along the dermoepidermal junction; these have fallen under the designation of "star burst" giant cell and are held to be characteristic of lentigo maligna. Note that the multinucleated giant cells characteristically show fully transformed malignant cells in the nuclei which constitute the giant cell: they are hyperchromatic, contain spiculated chromatin, and are overlaid one upon another.

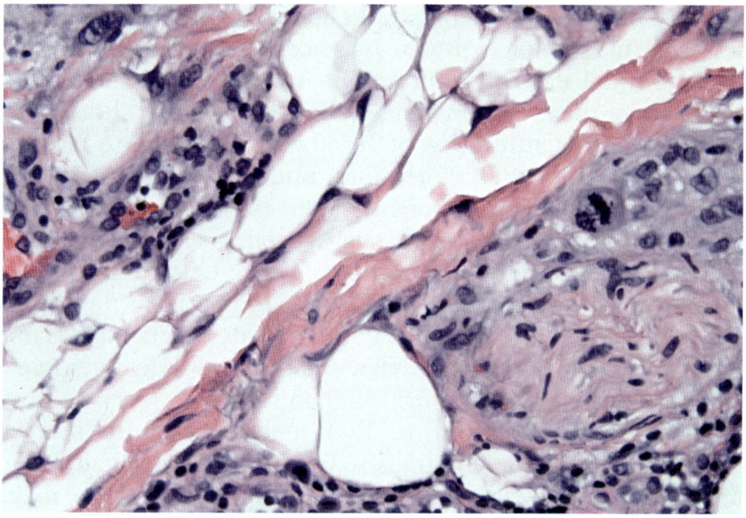

FIGURE 3.10 **Lentigo Maligna Melanoma—Neurotropism** Endoneurial and perineural invasion is more frequent in melanomas with a spindle cell or a desmoplastic vertical growth phase in any site and can extend deeply with permeation of the subcutaneous fat as in this case. Neurotropism can be marked by nothing more than subtle endoneurial hypercellularity or, as in this case, overtly malignant cells encasing the nerve. As with adventitial dermal invasion, a separate measurement for the depth and level of the neurotropic component should be given. Neurotropism is mediated by expression of p75 neurotrophin receptor in the melanoma cells and portends stubborn local recurrence.

variations in size and shape, and marked nuclear hyperchromasia; unlike the random atypia of a dysplastic nevus, virtually all cells disposed along the basal layer in lesions of lentigo maligna appear atypical. Bizarre, multinucleated giant cells are not part of the cytology of the dysplastic nevus.

The hallmark of vertical growth phase lentigo maligna melanoma is the formation of a nodule or fascicle within the dermis that exceeds the size of any thèque within the dermis (e-figs. 3.41 and 3.42). The cells in vertical growth phase melanoma often assume a spindled morphology and may be similar to the spindled cells which comprise the nested intraepidermal component. There is a variable stromal response. At times, prominent desmoplasia may be observed, warranting a designation of desmoplastic melanoma. Neurotropism frequently accompanies tumors that evoke prominent desmoplasia (Fig. 3.10).

Assessment of Depth and Level of Invasion in Lentigo Maligna

The assessment of level and depth of invasion in lentigo maligna melanoma can be difficult for a few reasons. Due to abundant elastotic material, demarcation between papillary and reticular dermis is often ill defined, making the designation of a precise Clark level difficult. Invasion of the adventitial dermis of a follicle situated in the reticular dermis may be misinterpreted as level IV melanoma if the follicular epithelium is not apparent in the sections examined. The maximum depth of invasion should not be based on the depth of adventitial dermal involvement unless that is the only invasion discernible. Under these circumstances, the measurement should be the distance from the point of infiltration of the adventitial dermis to the inner most layer of the outer root sheath epithelium. Endoneurial invasion can extend deeply, with permeation of the subcutaneous fat (e-figs. 3.43 and 3.44). As with adventitial dermal invasion, we suggest giving a separate measurement for the depth and level of the neurotropic component; the Breslow depth is still determined by the depth of invasive melanoma from the granular cell layer of the interfollicular epidermis. Photoactivated melanocytes mimic the cells of lentigo maligna but often have enlarged, spherical cytoplasm with low nucleocytoplasmic ratios (e-figs. 3.45 and 3.46).

Quantitative studies confirm that melanocytes are increased up to twofold in facial solar lentigines.[49] We frequently utilize Melan-A or HMB-45 preparations with a red chromogen to quantitate melanocyte density to enable the distinction of an actinic lentigo from lentigo maligna (e-fig. 3.47); melanocyte nesting is not seen in actinic lentigo or pigmented actinic keratosis, and typically, the lesional diameters are smaller than those of lentigo maligna. Additional biopsies or complete removal of the lesion for full pathologic assessment may be indicated.

The foregoing begs the question: "When should one interpret a margin as positive for subtle lentigo maligna as opposed to representing non-neoplastic photoactivated melanocytes at a margin?" It is our recommendation to focus on areas of the slide that represent unequivocal lentigo maligna. If the cytomorphology and density of proliferation are maintained or if an atypical nested melanocytic proliferation extends to the margin, then that margin is interpreted as being positive for malignancy. If the cytomorphology is maintained but the density is reduced to a moderately dense single-cell proliferation, defined as there being at least one abnormal melanocyte for every three to five keratinocytes, then the margin is reported as being probably positive (or suspicious for) malignancy. Clinical follow-up is recommended if a re-excision would prove too disfiguring, as is often the case in a large facial lesion of lentigo maligna. If the atypical cytomorphology is maintained but the density of proliferation is low, defined as less than one abnormal melanocyte for every five or more keratinocytes, the margin is interpreted as not being diagnostic of lentigo maligna. It is indicated in the note that the significance of the finding is unclear but does warrant clinical follow-up with rebiopsy in the event of repigmentation at the surgical site.

In fibrous papules, an exuberant hyperplasia of melanocytes can be observed along the basal layer of the epidermis.[50,51] The cells are primarily in a single-cell array but can aggregate to form occasional nests. The atypical cytomorphology is one which characterizes photoactivation overlying a dermal-based lesion, namely, plump oval, nuclei with smooth contours and small, rounded nucleoli accompanied by expanded variably melanized cytoplasm. The dermis is characteristic of a fibrous papule, manifesting organized dermal fibroplasia with accentuation around the adventitial dermis and vessels within which stellate fibroblasts are identified. These lesions are almost invariably recognized as fibrous papules clinically.

Management of Lentigo Maligna and Lentigo Maligna Melanoma

Treatment includes conventional surgery, Mohs micrographic surgery,[47] cryotherapy,[52] radiation therapy, and application of topical imiquimod.[53] In one study, a 91% cure rate was obtained with conventional surgery, with a recurrence rate of 9%.[54] By contrast, recurrence rates of 20% to 25% are reported following treatment by electrodessication and curettage, 38% for X-radiation, 50% for cryotherapy, and 100% for 5-fluorouracil.[52,55] Recurrences tend to develop within 14 months.[45] In 1992, the National Institutes of Health Consensus Development Conference advised 0.5 cm margins for melanoma in situ and 1 cm margins for melanomas less than 1 mm in thickness.[56,57] Lentigo maligna routinely extends beyond the clinically evident margin, and hence the recurrence rate is higher than that for other forms of melanoma[58]; application of imiquimod roughly 1 cm past the clinically evident margin has been advocated as a therapeutic option.

ACRAL LENTIGINOUS MELANOMA

Clinical and Histological Features

Acral lentiginous melanoma occurs predominantly on the palms, soles, subungual regions, and digits (Figs. 3.11 and 3.12).[59–61] This lesion, constituting less than 5% of malignant melanomas, presents characteristically on the palms and soles as a rapidly spreading, darkly pigmented patch with an irregular border[59]; rare examples are amelanotic.[62] Though uncommon in Caucasians, it is the most common subtype of cutaneous melanoma in Asians.[61,63] Areas of invasive melanoma may be associated with papules and hyperkeratotic plaques, nodules, and in late lesions, ulceration.

Foci of regression manifest as areas of gray-white discoloration and invasion is marked by the onset of a raised area. If melanoma invades the perieccrine adventitial dermis, the clinical lesion may remain flat despite the presence of tumor in the subcutaneous fat. Not all melanomas in acral sites are acral lentiginous melanomas; of 62 cases of plantar melanoma in one series from Japan, 14.5% were classified as nodular melanoma, and 3.2% as superficial spreading melanoma histologically.[64] Subungual melanoma presents in Caucasians as irregular streaks of pigmentation in the nail plate, sometimes with extension of pigmentation around the cuticle (*Hutchinson sign*).[60] In one study, 68% of subungual melanomas occurred on the fingers while 32% occurred on the toes; the great toe and the thumb were the most common sites.[65] The tumor usually arises from the proximal nail fold, which is the site from where the biopsy must be procured; biopsy

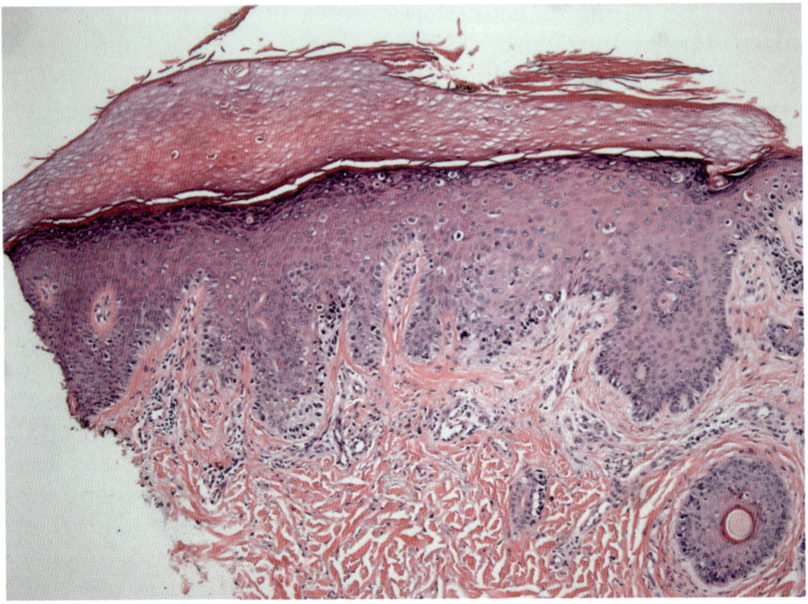

FIGURE 3.11 **Acral Lentiginous Melanoma In Situ.** The early phase of acral lentiginous melanoma may be one of atypical melanocytes dispersed singly in a lentiginous array with foci of confluent basilar growth. Note the stromal lymphocytic response, which is almost an invariable accompaniment of acral nevomelanocytic dysplasia. With further progression of the radial growth phase, nested pagetoid infiltration of the epidermis may comprise the dominant pattern of intraepidermal growth. This lesion shows pagetoid upward spread, an immediate precursor to dermal invasion in this setting.

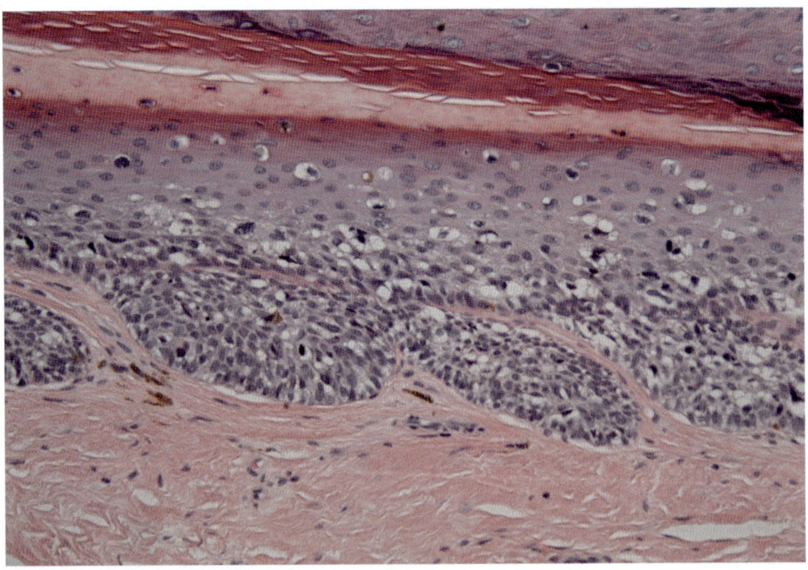

FIGURE 3.12 **Acral Lentiginous Melanoma of Subunguum.** There is a lentiginous (single-cell) array of neoplastic melanocytes in the basal layer of the epidermis, accompanied by nesting and pagetoid spread.

methods include an incisional biopsy, cutting the nail plate and proximal nail fold, or a punch biopsy of the proximal nail fold. Invasion is associated with thickening of the cuticular area and eventual deformity of the nails. Acral lentiginous melanoma has a propensity to metastasize to the central nervous system, liver, lungs, bone, and lymph nodes.[59] This subtype of melanoma has proven to be an independent negative prognostic factor,[66] though there are conflicting data.[67,68] In one study, the median survival was 32 months, with a 26% 5-year survival rate. Delayed diagnosis and advanced disease at presentation may contribute to the poor prognosis in nail bed melanoma (Fig. 3.12).[65,69] A review of 84,836 cases of melanoma in the National Cancer Data Base (1985–1994), the largest study of which we are aware, showed nodular melanoma and acral lentiginous melanoma to be associated with decreased survival as independent prognostic variables.[70]

The clinical differential diagnosis of radial growth phase acral lentiginous melanoma is a flat congenital nevus of the foot, which may have irregular borders but usually is uniform in coloration (Fig. 3.13).

Tinea nigra, a form of superficial dermatophytosis, is commonly mistaken for acral lentiginous melanoma as it manifests as a darkly pigmented macule with irregular borders. Other diagnostic considerations

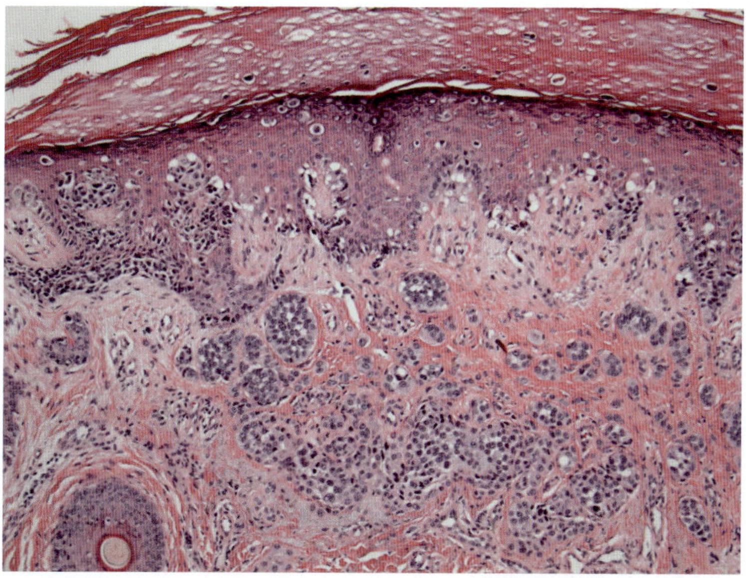

FIGURE 3.13 **Acral Lentiginous Melanoma.** When in a pagetoid array, the neoplastic melanocytes typically have an epithelioid morphology. They extend randomly into the epidermis independent of the nested junctional component. The presence of a lentiginous pattern of dysplasia, in terms of both its architectural and its cytological features, defines this lesion as an acral lentiginous malignant melanoma. A single-cell pattern typically predominates over a nested pattern, whereas the converse is true in benign nevi. There is a vertical growth phase of epithelioid cell type in this lesion.

include a traumatically induced subungual hematoma, the *talon noir*. This discoloration, which is usually purple and subungually includes a zone of hemorrhage that will move with the growth of the nail plate, has no associated cuticular spread of pigmentation as in Hutchinson sign. The term talon noir can also be applied to other acral hemorrhages mimicking melanocytic proliferations. A subungual common acquired nevus often presents as a pigmented longitudinal dark-brown or black nail plate streak termed *melanonychia stria*, as is seen in subungual melanoma as well. Other presentations of subungual melanoma include pain, bleeding, or shedding of the nail.[71]

The incipient lesion of acral lentiginous melanoma manifests as atypical melanocytes dispersed singly in a lentiginous array with foci of confluent basilar growth in an epidermis that shows hyperplasia alternating with zones of epidermal effacement and an overlying dense orthohyperkeratotic scale as typifies acral skin (e-figs. 3.48–3.50). Transepithelial pigment elimination is a characteristic and assumes a haphazard pattern, unlike the organized vertical pigment columns that overlie the junctional nests of acral nevi (e-figs. 3.51 and 3.52). A mononuclear cell inflammatory response is present in the superficial dermis, a finding which is uniformly lacking in banal acral nevi. With further progression of the radial growth phase, pagetoid infiltration of the epidermis may constitute the dominant pattern of intraepidermal growth (e-fig. 3.53). The cytology of the lentiginous component is one of large cells with hyperchromatic angulated large nuclei and scant cytoplasm. Prominent dendritic processes from lentiginously disposed neoplastic melanocytes may extend into the upper layers of the stratum spinosum. When in a pagetoid array, the neoplastic melanocytes typically have an epithelioid morphology, and so mimic superficial spreading melanoma, extending randomly into the epidermis independent of the nested junctional component. Tropism to adnexal structures may be prominent. A single-cell pattern predominates over a nested pattern, while the converse is true in banal nevi. The nests are variable in size and shape, manifest dyshesion, and are composed of cells with either an epithelioid or spindled morphology. While large and variably sized and variably disposed nests may be seen in the prototypic benign acral nevus, the cells of acral melanoma show severe nuclear atypia. The invasive component of the radial growth phase comprises cells in a single-cell or nested disposition with a cytomorphology similar to those cells within the epidermis. The invasive single cells usually exhibit more abundant cytoplasm, often with fine pigmentation. Mitoses are common in the intraepidermal component. Dominant thèques with dermal mitoses signify progression to vertical growth phase melanoma.

MUCOSAL MELANOMA

The mucosal melanomas encompass those of the mouth, esophagus, anal canal, penis, nasal mucosa, and vulva.[72,73] In one study, the most common mucosal sites in decreasing order of frequency were vulva/vagina, oral cavity, anus/rectum, nasal cavity, and penis.[73] The National Cancer Data Base of the American Cancer Society indicates that mucosal melanomas occur in the head and neck area, female genital tract, anal/rectal region, and urinary tract in 55%, 18%, 24%, and 3%, respectively.[70]

Melanoma of the Vulva

CLINICAL FEATURES. Melanoma is the second most common form of vulvar cancer representing 3% to 8% of all primary vulvar malignancies.[74] Vulvar melanomas are most commonly located on the labia minora, and account for 3% to 7% of all melanomas in women.[75] Roughly 35% of women present with a polypoid mass lesion, while in one quarter of patients, the tumor is amelanotic.[76] Ragnarsson-Olding et al.[77] found the mucosal lentiginous type to be the most common form of vulvar melanoma (e-figs. 3.54–3.56). The morphology is analogous to acral lentiginous melanoma and, like the latter, is less dependent on UV-induced mutagenesis than are other forms of melanoma.[75] Although the mean age of patients with vulvar melanoma is 61.4 years (range 43 to 82 years),[78] the disease has been reported in childhood,[79] including in the setting of lichen sclerosus.[80] The atypical melanocytic proliferation occurring in the setting of lichen sclerosus closely mimics melanoma (e-figs. 3.57 and 3.58)[81]; we believe that many of the lesions formerly reported as vulvar melanoma in childhood may have represented atypical melanocytic proliferations in the setting of lichen sclerosus. Only long-term follow-up and close scrutiny of previously reported patients will resolve this question.

The great majority of vulvar melanomas have a radial growth phase; only 10% of vulvar melanomas present as nodular melanoma. The Swedish workers quoted above found that 22% of tumors in their series were of nodular subtype.[76] The radial growth phase of vulvar melanoma clinically presents as a flat, irregularly colored lesion with borders that are highly irregular in contour. Most occur in the labia minora (80%) and a few in the labia majora (13%); only rarely is the clitoris involved (7%).[82] Metastatic disease to lymph nodes is present in some 30% of patients at presentation.[83] With respect to the latter, the high-risk melanomas are those which are greater than 3 mm in thickness with or without ulceration. The low-risk vulvar melanoma patient has a nonulcerated tumor less than 3 mm in thickness without clinical evidence of inguinal lymph node metastasis.[84] Pre-existing nevi are associated in the vulva with superficial spreading melanoma, but not with the other histological types.[76] Mucosal lentiginous melanoma can arise in a precursor lesion, namely vulvar melanosis, when a high density lentiginous proliferation with cytologic atypia is present. When fully evolved, vulvar malignant melanoma may extend across the clitoris from one labia to the other; vaginal involvement is common in advanced lesions. Vulvar skin lacks a clear distinction between the papillary and reticular dermis.

DIFFERENTIAL DIAGNOSIS OF VULVAR MELANOMA. The differential diagnosis clinically includes vulvar melanosis (e-fig. 3.59), which can be clinically alarming, manifesting as an area of irregular pigmentation with skip areas, at times several centimetres in size; borders are well-defined and pigmentation is uniform. Pigmented Bowen's disease (e-figs. 3.60 and 3.61) is associated with hyperkeratosis while extramammary Paget's disease presents with discomfort, including itching and burning. However, these symptoms are not useful discriminators of vulvar melanoma as pruritus occurs in 27% of patients with vulvar melanoma; other common clinical manifestations of melanoma include ulceration and bleeding.[72]

Melanoma of the Penis

Melanoma of the penis may occur around the glans as an irregularly discolored macule with irregular borders, or may take origin around the urethra where it manifests as pigmentary discoloration of the urethral meatus. One symptom of urethral melanoma is melanuria. The neoplasms are rare, and thus, prognostication is difficult; high vascularity, multiple lymphatic drainage sites, and late diagnosis all contribute to poor survival.[73]

Melanoma of the Oral Mucosa

CLINICAL FEATURES. Melanoma of oral mucosa presents as an irregularly colored brown patch that commonly extends into the gingival margins. Areas of gray-white color reflect regression, while induration may indicate invasion. It may be completely amelanotic. Two thirds of patients with oral mucosal melanoma are men whose common presentation is a mass lesion.[85] The differential diagnosis of in situ disease includes the lower labial macule (e-figs. 3.62 and 3.63), which is a discrete, midline to off-midline, dark, round discoloration of the lower lip that is usually stationary; it is 1 to 1.5 cm in size. The amalgam tattoo can enter into the differential diagnosis, if extensive, because of its bluish-gray discoloration. Its proximity to areas of dental repair is helpful. Melanomas of the esophagus and nasal mucosa are usually occult and are found because of symptoms of obstruction or nasal bleeding.[86]

Histology of Radial Growth Phase-confined Mucosal Melanoma

In 50% of cases, radial growth phase vulvar melanoma may assume a pattern similar to superficial spreading melanoma or nodular melanoma,[80] while in most of the remainder a lentiginous pattern is observed (Fig. 3.14); a mixed pattern is also described.

When the intraepidermal component is predominantly in a pagetoid array, there is often coexisting papillary dermal invasion characterized by single-cell permeation of the dermis. When a lentiginous pattern of radial growth phase dominates, prominent atypical dendritic melanocytes are observed, which are heavily laden with melanin pigment. There is transepidermal elimination of melanin pigment, which typically manifests as irregular pigment columns within the stratum corneum. Radial growth phase-confined

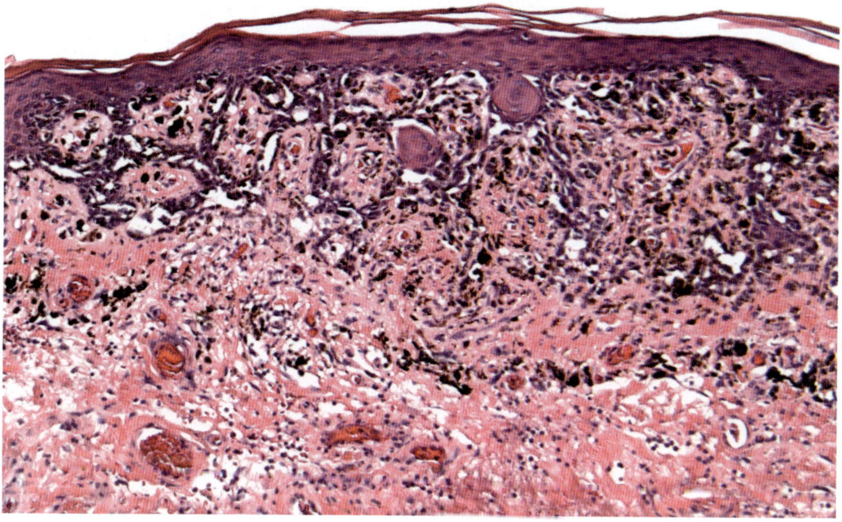

FIGURE 3.14 **Mucosal Melanoma: Vulvar Melanoma of Mucosal Lentiginous Type.** In 50% of cases, the radial growth phase of vulvar malignant melanoma may assume a pattern similar to that of either superficial spreading melanoma while in most of the remainder the pattern mimics acral lentiginous melanoma; these figures vary in different populations. In this photomicrograph, the presence of a high-density, lentiginous array indicates the lentiginous pattern.

melanoma of the esophageal, urethral, oral, and nasal mucosae usually demonstrates a lentiginous pattern and cytology. A conspicuous dendritic cell component may be observed. The invasive component usually assumes a spindled morphology and may be associated with a desmoplastic stromal response. Osteoid formation is characteristic of nasal melanomas.[87,88]

VERTICAL GROWTH PHASE OF MELANOMA

Introduction and Clinical Features

The vertical growth phase, regardless of the subtype of melanoma from which it takes origin, signifies the acquisition by the neoplasm of the capability to metastasize. The vertical growth phase appears typically as a pigmented nodule supervening on a pre-existing macule or plaque, the one exception being nodular melanoma which exhibits the rapid appearance of a nodule in clinically normal skin. In nodular melanoma, there is, by definition, no radial growth phase component.[89] The histological description which follows for vertical growth phase melanoma arising in a radial growth phase lesion of lentigo maligna melanoma, mucosa lentiginous melanoma, acral lentiginous melanoma, or superficial spreading melanoma could equally be applied to nodular melanoma (Figs. 3.15 and 3.16). It is critical for therapy and prognostication to accurately identify by light

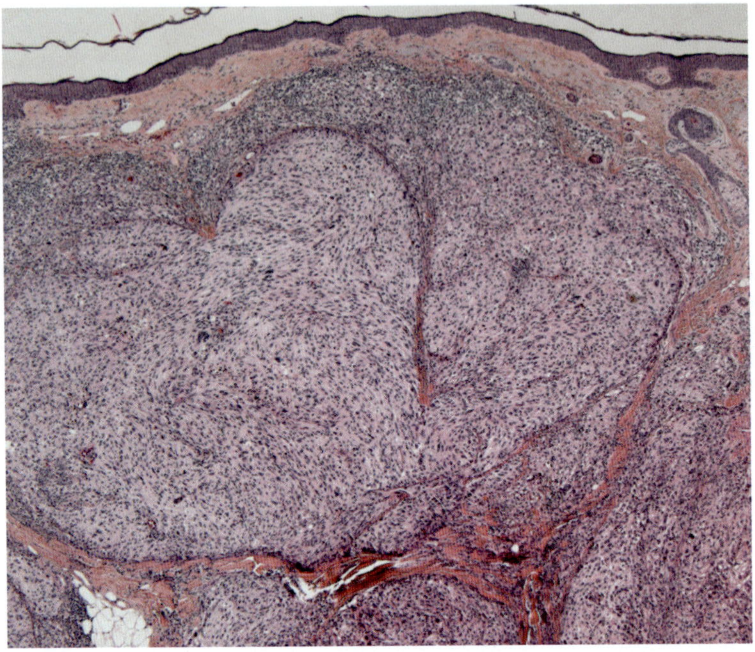

FIGURE 3.15 **Nodular Melanoma.** An expansile nodular growth is present within the dermis. There is no radial growth phase component. A vertical growth phase in the absence of a discernible radial growth phase component is the defining feature of nodular melanoma. Any radial growth phase component would obligate reclassification of the lesion. A brisk lymphocytic host response is present along the base of the tumor (i.e., along >90% of the tumor circumference).

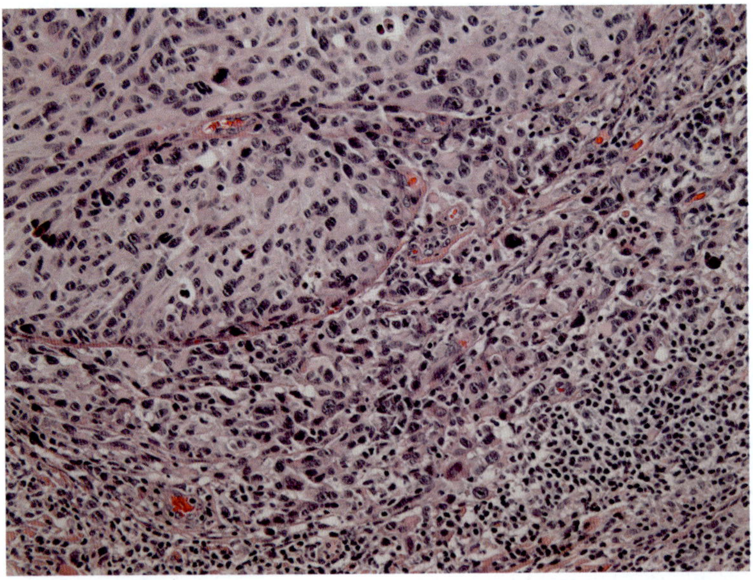

FIGURE 3.16 **Nodular Melanoma.** The lymphocytic host response is a useful discriminating feature that helps separate nodular melanoma from metastatic malignant melanoma.

microscopy the vertical growth phase, as its presence indicates a melanoma that has acquired the ability to metastasize and kill the patient.

Histology

Clark et al.[90] defined the early vertical growth phase, distinguished from the radial growth phase by the presence of a dominant nest within the papillary dermis that is conspicuously larger than any nest within the epidermis or surrounding dermis and forms an expansile nodule. The cells forming this nodule are cytologically different from those of the intraepidermal component, showing conspicuous nucleolation, coarse heterochromatin, and prominent, irregularly thickened, notched nuclear chromatinic rims. Tumor cell necrosis and mitoses may be observed. This distinctiveness represents a form of clonal selection. When associated with extensive regression (i.e., >75% of the lesion), this early phase of vertical growth phase melanoma may be associated with metastatic behavior. Coalescence of several such nodules indicates progression to fully evolved vertical growth phase melanoma. Incipient vertical growth phase melanoma typically does not fill the papillary dermis and correlates with level II or level III invasion. It has been shown that the presence of the early vertical growth phase infers a risk for metastasis of roughly 10% at 8 years' follow-up, in contrast to the radial growth phase in which the patients are cured by surgery, provided regression is not identified in the primary tumor.[5,91]

Epithelioid Vertical Growth Phase

The prototype of the vertical growth phase of melanoma comprises an expansile nodule of epithelioid melanocytes: loosely cohesive round-to-cuboidal cells with round or oval nuclei containing coarse, spiculated chromatin, prominent and often spiculated nucleoli, and chromatinic rims which are irregularly thickened and irregularly contoured (e-figs. 3.64 and 3.65). Modest cytoplasms have an eosinophilic or amphophilic granular staining quality with variable melanization and rounded or polygonal cytoplasmic contours that are often distinct. Unlike squamous cell carcinoma or eccrine porocarcinoma, no intercellular bridges are identified. These balls or nodules of cells distort the architecture of the papillary dermis with or without extension into the reticular dermis. Mitotic figures are usually seen; their morphology includes both typical and atypical division figures, the latter defined by tri-, tetra-, or penta-polar mitoses, signifying an aneuploid DNA content with a high DNA index, or chromosomal lags, which may signify the presence of double minutes, near-diploid aneuploidy, or aberrancy of the centromere/spindle apparatus. Multinucleated tumor giant cells may be observed. An inflammatory response is variable.

Spindle Cell Vertical Growth Phase

The spindle cell vertical growth phase is usually observed in lentigo maligna melanoma, mucosal melanoma, or acral lentiginous melanoma. Fascicles of markedly hyperchromatic fusiform cells extend at various angles from the epidermis into the dermis (e-figs. 3.66 and 3.67).

Differential Diagnosis

The differential diagnosis of spindle cell vertical growth phase melanoma, particularly in sun-damaged skin of the elderly, includes the atypical fibroxanthoma (e-figs. 3.68–3.75). The atypical fibroxanthoma, whose histology is described elsewhere, does not decorate with antibodies to cytokeratins, S100 protein or HMB-45, but does show strong expression of vimentin, as does melanoma.[92] The use of procollagen-1 to identify atypical fibroxanthoma is in our view problematic, as desmoplastic melanoma will also express this marker. Cytokeratin expression in a spindle cell malignancy of the skin correlates strongly with spindle cell squamous cell carcinoma. Leiomyosarcoma also enters into the differential diagnosis of spindle cell melanoma and often shows diffuse weak expression of S100 protein; however, leiomyosarcoma is HMB-45 negative and the individual cells contain abundant particulate cytoplasmic glycogen, demonstrable with a PAS preparation. It is prudent to establish the histogenesis of any spindle cell malignancy. The profile which we typically utilize for this purpose employs immunohistochemical studies for expression of S100 protein, gp100 (HMB-45) and/or A103 (Melan A), cytokeratins (typically an antibody to pankeratins such as DAKO AE1/3), and vimentin, with a histochemical study for glycogen. Antibodies to desmin and smooth muscle-specific actin can be added if suspicion of a leiomoysarcoma is high. Usually, the whorled, storiform pattern of dermatofibrosarcoma protuberans, in concert with its inverted mushroom-cap-shaped architecture extending as a horizontal shelf along the dermal–subcutaneous junction, permits easy distinction from desmoplastic melanoma. When in doubt, the expression by dermatofibrosarcoma protuberans of CD34 and the absence of S100 protein expression permit easy distinction.[93] Other benign fibrous histiocytomas manifest secondary elements such as foamy histiocytes which are absent in desmoplastic melanoma.

METASTATIC MELANOMA

Clinical and Histological Features

Metastatic melanoma prototypically presents as a nodule within the dermis and/or subcutaneous fat[94] which may or may not be contiguous with the epidermis; the majority of metastatic melanomas are not epidermotropic (Fig. 3.17, e-figs. 3.76 and 3.77).

The most common cell type is epithelioid. When metastatic melanoma manifests tropism to the epidermis, the distinction from a secondary primary melanoma or multiple primary melanomas, the latter accounting for 3.9% of all cases of melanoma,[95] becomes very difficult.[96] Some cases of epidermotropic metastatic melanoma may have no dermal component and thus may mimic melanoma in situ.[97] Some authors feel that histological criteria are not, by themselves, adequate for the distinction, and that a clinical history is needed.[98] In contradistinction to superficial spreading melanoma, the dermal component of a metastatic deposit typically extends laterally beyond the confines of the epidermal component.[99] The cytology

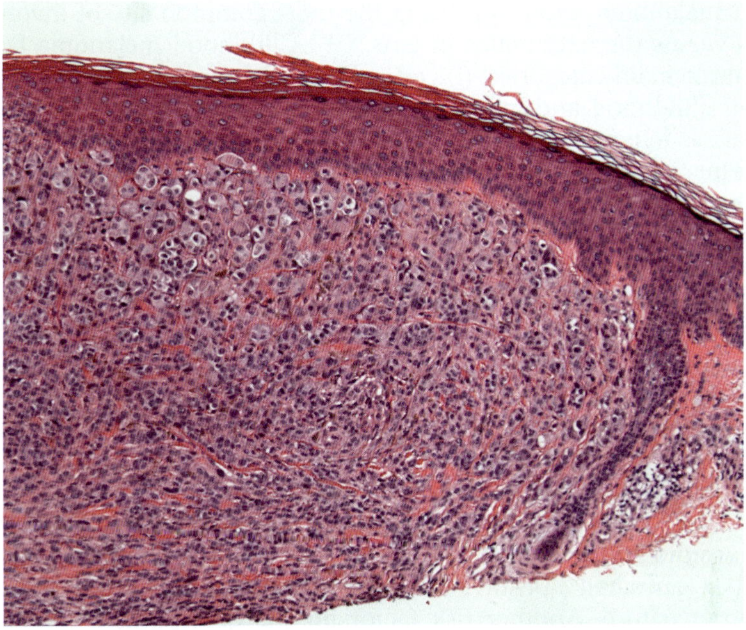

FIGURE 3.17 **Metastatic Melanoma.** The absence of a lymphocytic host response is a useful discriminating feature that helps separate this metastatic tumor deposit from a primary nodular melanoma; note also that the retiform pattern is bowed around the deposit.

of metastatic melanoma cells in the epidermal and dermal compartments is similar, whereas in primary melanoma, the vertical growth phase component typically has a disparate morphology to the intraepidermal component. In metastatic melanoma, the presence of an inflammatory host response is uncommon,[100] though it may be seen, as may regressive stromal changes and tumoral melanosis. In epidermotropic metastatic melanoma the epidermis is classically attenuated while the dermal papillae are widened by an intradermal metastatic deposit whose lateral extent is demarcated by a clawlike deformity of the epidermis. Aggregates of tumor cells within vascular channels are characteristic of metastatic melanoma (e-figs. 3.78–3.80).[100]

MELANOMA IN CHILDHOOD

Introduction and Clinical Features

Melanoma in childhood is uncommon, accounting for 1% to 3% of all pediatric malignancies; most occur between the ages of 12 and 15 years, with melanoma in children less than 10 years of age being rare.[101] Less than 5% of all melanomas occur in patients who are less than 20 years of age. The highest incidence is in Australia. In individuals younger than 20 years, there is no sex predilection and the body distribution is no different from that observed in adult melanoma, the trunk being the most common site of involvement in boys versus the extremities in girls.[102,103] Childhood melanoma falls into one of three main categories: (i) congenital melanoma; (ii) melanoma developing in childhood and infancy which arise de novo; and (iii) melanoma which arises in a pre-existing lesion such as a congenital nevus or dysplastic nevus. The cases of congenital melanoma which either represent transplacental metastatic disease or arise from a giant nevus are invariably fatal. In one study of 22 cases of childhood melanoma, 2 children died of disease at 1 and 7 years following diagnosis and 6 additional patients developed metastatic disease but are still alive. Five lesions were classified as superficial spreading type and one was a nodular melanoma, while the other two melanomas were unclassifiable. When thickness and level were known, tumors were either of Clark level III or level IV and the average thickness was 1.15 mm. Based on this study, prognosis is less closely associated with tumor thickness, as relatively thin melanomas can be associated with aggressive behavior.[101] In another series, 15% of patients died as a result of their disease, with a median survival of 3 years. Many of the patients in this large epidemiologic study died at around 20 years of age.[103] One third of childhood melanoma patients in another series had a positive family history of melanoma[104]; 21 cases were sporadic in nature. Another risk factor for the development of childhood melanoma is treatment of another childhood cancer wherein genetics, chemotherapy, and radiation therapy may all play a role.[105] Congenital melanoma may represent transplacental transmission of metastatic melanoma of maternal derivation; rare cases of spontaneous regression have been reported. Congenital melanoma may arise de novo with no evidence of melanoma in the mother. It appears as a black nodule ranging in size from 1 to 3 cm with a tendency to ulcerate and bleed and have an unpredictable course. Congenital melanoma may develop in a pre-existing giant nevus and is then associated with a very poor prognosis; in children less than 12 years of age, the history is one of a rapid increase in lesional size, bleeding or color change in a nodular lesion, pruritus, and lymph node enlargement. The clinical appearance of melanoma in an adolescent is no different from that in an adult.

In the study by Scalzo et al.,[101] the majority of childhood melanomas (14 out of 22 cases) arose in pre-existing lesions, with the other 8 cases apparently arising de novo. The precursor lesion falls into one of five categories: (i) giant congenital nevus (>20 cm in diameter); (ii) small congenital nevus (<2 cm in diameter); (iii) intermediate-sized congenital nevus (2 to 20 cm in diameter); (iv) dysplastic nevus; and (v) other types of nevus such as nevus spilus.

Histology

In the study by Scalzo et al.,[101] of 22 primary cutaneous melanomas, lesions were classified as superficial spreading melanoma in 10, borderline or minimal deviation melanoma in 3, nodular melanoma in 2, and melanoma in situ in 1, the remainder being unclassifiable.[101] Of these tumors, 47% of the melanomas were level IV. In one study of childhood melanoma, 60%

were of level IV or level V, while 80% of the children had lesions, which were greater than 1.5 mm in thickness.[106] Another group found 45% of childhood melanomas to be greater than 1.5 mm in thickness.[107] It would appear that melanoma in children and adolescents tends to be diagnosed at a more advanced stage than in adults.

Although the histological features are often similar to those encountered in adults, at times, lesions of melanoma in children are composed of spindle and epithelioid cells and present difficult problems in diagnosis, the obvious differential diagnosis being that of Spitz's nevus. The mean thickness of Spitz's nevi is in the range of 0.7 to 1.2 mm. Lesions that measure several millimeters in depth are therefore suspicious for melanoma. In childhood melanoma, the variation in the size of the nests at any given level in the tumor is usually great. Furthermore, there is striking side-by-side nuclear pleomorphism at any level. Deep-seated marginal mitoses, that is, mitotic activity identified in the periphery or deep margins, may be indicative of metastatic potential. There is no evidence of maturation in the vast majority of melanomas and, in fact, cells in the deeper portion of the tumor are often more cytologically atypical than those located more superficially. Furthermore, in melanomas of the teenage years, the presence of melanin pigmentation in the deeper atypical cells is a worrisome sign. The presence of angioinvasion is not indicative of malignancy, as intravascular nevus cells aggregates were identified in 14.3% of all Spitz's nevi procured from children in one series.[108] The most striking differences between melanomas and Spitz's nevi in one series were a higher degree of pagetoid spread, cellular pleomorphism, nuclear hyperchromasia, and mitotic activity in the melanomas.[109] When one applies a rigorous statistical approach to the retrospective analysis of metastasizing lesions with a Spitzlike histomorphology, only diagnosis at age greater than 10 years, lesional surface diameter over 10 mm, ulceration, involvement of the subcutaneous fat, and mitotic activity of at least 6/mm^2 emerge as significant variables predictive of aggressive behavior.[110] In an Australian series with large patient numbers, the presence of the so-called marginal mitotic activity, defined as mitoses within 0.25 mm of the lesional edge, was associated with statistically higher risk of metastatic events.[111] We thus examine the peripheral margin of all putative Spitz's nevi with a high dry (40×) objective in order to assess this criterion. In addition to marginal and/or atypical mitoses, the presence of fine dusty cytoplasmic melanization, atypical epithelioid intraepidermal melanocytes beneath mounds of parakeratin, a high mitotic rate in the papillary dermis, and dermal nests larger than overlying junctional nests are features favoring melanoma over Spitz's nevus in epithelioid cell melanocytic proliferations in adolescence.[112] A diagnosis of Spitz nevus is favored over melanoma in the presence of Kamino bodies, especially if numerous or clustered, diffuse maturation, spindle cells, and spindled nuclei.[112] Although patient age, sharp demarcation, symmetry, melanocytic maturation, and epithelial hyperplasia are all helpful predictors of benign behavior, 6% to 8% of cases defy confident classification as Spitz's nevi versus malignant melanoma.[113] All Spitz's nevi, irrespective of histology or patient age, require complete lesional excision in our view.

In melanomas arising in congenital nevi, a poorly differentiated small cell melanoma has been described whereby monotonous sheets of small, round undifferentiated cells with nuclear moulding arise in the dermal component of an otherwise typical congenital nevus. Extensive myxoid areas can be seen and malignant heterologous elements have been described in such lesions, including the presence of lipoblasts and rhabdomyoblasts.[114] Nodules of melanoma in congenital nevi have several distinctive characteristics. Each nodule tends to comprise a monotonous population of atypical cells sharply demarcated from the surrounding nevus cell component and showing no evidence of maturation. Mitoses are frequent and often atypical, while single-cell or zonal necrosis is usually present. There is often a lymphocytic infiltrate.

Differential Diagnosis

Certain histological features considered valuable in establishing a diagnosis of melanoma in adults are not applicable to lesions of children. Specifically, various benign pigmented lesions in children manifest pagetoid infiltration of the epidermis by melanocytes in a fashion, which, unlike malignant melanoma, are confined to the central portion of the lesion. When such a distinction concerning the epidermal component is problematic, examination of the lateral borders of the lesion is helpful, as the benign nevus cell proliferations manifest sharp lateral circumscription. Mitotic figures in congenital nevi are a frequent finding, being identified in 60% of large congenital nevi or of congenital nevi of any size in newborns. The mitoses are usually confined to the superficial dermis or to proliferation nodules and do not have an atypical morphology and do not efface architecture as does vertical growth phase melanoma.[115] Unlike fully evolved cytologic criteria for malignancy, the cells of these proliferative nodules in children is one of a reactive/proliferative type with nuclei that are round to oval with regular contours–there is only slight variability of size and shape–nucleoli that are round and lack spiculated contours, and chromatin that is evenly distributed (e-figs. 3.81 and 3.82).

SUMMARY

A diagnosis of melanoma in childhood cannot be based on any one single criterion but is rather based on a multifactorial assessment of varied cytologic and architectural features in concert with the clinical setting.[116–122] The occasion will arise when it is impossible to predict the biological behavior of a given neoplasm on histomorphological grounds alone. When this occurs, the pathologist must refrain from stating a diagnosis unequivocally, expressing his degree of uncertainty and liberally obtaining additional expert opinions.

REFERENCES

1. Clark WH Jr. A classification of malignant melanoma in man correlated with histogenesis and biological behaviour. In: Montagna W, Hu F, eds. *Advances in the Biology of the Skin*. Vol. VIII. New York: Pergamon Press; 1967:621–647.
2. Clark WH Jr, From L, Bernardino EA, Mihm MC. Histogenesis and biologic behavior of primary human malignant melanomas of the skin. *Cancer Res* Mar 1969;29(3):705–726.
3. Reed RJ. Acral lentiginous melanoma. In: Reed RJ, ed. *New Concepts in Surgical Pathology of the Skin*. New York: John Wiley and Sons; 1976:89–90.
4. Radovic-Kovacevic V, Pekmezovic T, Adanja B, et al. Survival analysis in patients with cutaneous malignant melanoma. *Srp Arh Celok Lek* May–June 1997;125(5–6):132–137.
5. Guerry D IV, Synnestvedt M, Elder DE, Schultz D. Lessons from tumor progression: The invasive radial growth phase of melanoma is common, incapable of metastasis, and indolent. *J Invest Dermatol* Mar 1993;100(3):342S–345S.
6. Breslow A. Thickness, cross-sectional areas and depth of invasion in the prognosis of cutaneous melanoma. *Ann Surg* Nov 1970;172(5):902–908.
7. Day CL, Harrist TJ, Gorstein F, et al. Malignant melanoma. Prognostic significance of "microscopic satellites" in the reticular dermis and subcutaneous fat. *Ann Surg* Jul 1981;194(1):108–112.
8. Day CL, Mihm MC Jr, Sober AJ, et al. Prognostic factors for melanoma patients with lesions 0.76–1.69 mm in thickness. An appraisal of "thin" level IV lesions. *Ann Surg* Jan 1982;195(1):30–34.
9. Day CL, Mihm MC Jr, Lew RA, et al. Prognostic factors for clinical stage I melanoma of intermediate thickness (1.51–3.39 mm). A conceptual model for tumor growth and metastasis. *Ann Surg* Jan 1982;195(1):35–43.
10. Day CL, Lew RA, Mihm MC Jr, et al. A multivariate analysis of prognostic factors for melanoma patients with lesions greater than or equal to 3.65 mm in thickness. The importance of revealing alternate Cox models. *Ann Surg* Jan 1982;195(1):44–49.
11. Day CL, Harrist TJ, Lew RA, Mihm MC Jr. Classification of malignant melanomas according to the histologic morphology of melanoma nodules. *J Dermatol Surg Oncol* Oct 1982; 8(10):874–875.
12. Balch CM, Wilkerson JA, Murad TM, et al. The prognostic significance of ulceration of cutaneous melanoma. *Cancer* Jun 1980;45(12):3012–3017.
13. Harrist TJ, Rigel DS, Day CL Jr, et al. "Microscopic satellites" are more highly associated with regional lymph nodes metastases than is primary melanoma thickness. *Cancer* May 1984;53(10):2183–2187.
14. Balch CM, Milton GW, eds. Cutaneous melanoma: Clinical management and treatment results worldwide. Philadelphia, PA: JB Lippincott Co., 1985:329.
15. Leon P, Daly JM, Synnestvedt M, et al. The prognostic implications of microscopic satellites in patients with clinical stage I melanoma. *Arch Surg* Dec 1991; 126(12):1461–1468.
16. Jelfs PL, Giles G, Shugg D, et al. Cutaneous malignant melanoma in Australia, 1989. *Med J Aust* Aug 1994;161(3):182–187.
17. Reed R, Ichinose H, Clark WC, Mihm M. Common and uncommon melanocytic nevi and borderline melanomas. *Semin Oncol* June 1975;2(2):119–147.
18. Reed RJ. Minimal deviation melanoma. *Hum Pathol* Dec 1990;21(12):1206–1211.
19. Merkow LP, Burt RC, Hayeslip DW, et al. A cellular and malignant blue nevus: A light and electron microscopic study. *Cancer* Nov 1969;24(5):888–896.
20. Conley J, Lattes R, Orr W. Desmoplastic malignant melanoma (a rare variant of spindle cell melanoma). *Cancer* Oct 1971;28(4):914–936.

21. Schmoeckel C, Castro CE, Braun-Falco O. Nevoid malignant melanoma. *Arch Derm Res* Sep 1985;277(5):362–369.
22. Crowson AN, Magro CM, Mihm MC Jr. Malignant melanoma with prominent pigment synthesis: "Animal type" melanoma. *Hum Pathol* May 1999;30(5):543–550.
23. Crowson AN, Magro C, Miller A, et al. The molecular basis of melanomagenesis and the metastatic phenotype. *Semin Oncol* Dec 2007;34:476–490.
24. Sekulic A, Haluska P Jr, Miller AJ, et al. Malignant melanoma in the 21st century: The emerging molecular landscape. *Mayo Clin Proc* Jul 2008;83:825–846.
25. Curtin JA, Fridlyand J, Kagashita T, et al. Distinct sets of genetic alterations in melanoma. *New Engl J Med* Nov 2005;353:2104–2107.
26. Fecher LA, Amaravidi RK, Flaherty KT. The MAPK pathway in melanoma. *Curr Opin Oncol* Mar 2008;20:183–189.
27. Curtin JA, Busam K, Pinkel D, et al. Somatic activation of KIT in distinctive subtypes of melanoma. *J Clin Oncol* Sep 2006;24:4340–4346.
28. Postovit LM, Margararyan NV, Seftor EA, Hendrix MJ. Role of nodal signaling and the microenvironment underlying melanoma plasticity. *Pigment Cell Melanoma Res* June 2008;21:348–357.
29. Crowson AN. The future of dermatopathology. *Mod Pathol* Jan 2006;19:S155–S163.
30. Ayala I, Baldassarre M, Giacchetti G, et al. Multiple regulatory inputs converge on cortactin to control invadopodia biogenesis and extracellular matrix degradation. *J Cell Sci* Jan 2008;121:369–378.
31. Han SY, Gai W, Yancovitz M, et al. Nucleofection is a highly effective gene transfer technique or human melanoma cell lines. *Exp Dermatol* Feb 2008;17:405–411.
32. Holman CD, Armstrong BK, Heenan PJ. A theory of the etiology and pathogenesis of human cutaneous malignant melanoma. *J Natl Cancer Inst* Oct 1983;71(4):651–656.
33. Holman CD, Armstrong BK. Cutaneous malignant melanoma and indicators of total accumulated exposure to the sun: An analysis separating histogenetic types. *J Natl Cancer Inst* Jul 1984;73(1):75–82.
34. Bergner T, Przybilla B. Malignant melanoma in association with phototherapy. *Dermatology* 1992;184(1):59–61.
35. Selvaag E, Loeb M, Larsen TE, Thune P. Prevention and early diagnosis of malignant melanoma. *Tidsskr Nor Laegeforen* June 1998;118(15):2316–2318.
36. Selvaag E, Loeb M, Larsen TE, et al. Cutaneous malignant melanoma in Norway: Experiences from the Norwegian Melanoma Project. *Melanoma Res* Feb 1999;9(1): 92–95.
37. Walter SD, King WD, Marrett LD. Association of cutaneous malignant melanoma with intermittent exposure to ultraviolet radiation: Results of a case–control study in Ontario, Canada. *Int J Epidemiol* June 1999;28(3):418–427.
38. Clark WH, Reimer RR, Greene M, Mihm MC. Origin of familial malignant melanomas from heritable melanocytic lesions. 'The B-K mole syndrome'. *Arch Dermatol* May 1978; 114(5):732–738.
39. Dubreuilh MW. Lentigo malin des vieillards. *Ann Dermatol Syphil* (*Paris*) 1894; 5:1092–1099.
40. Clark WH, Mihm MC. Lentigo maligna and lentigo maligna melanoma. *Am J Pathol* Apr 1969;55(1):39–54.
41. Cox NH, Aitchison TC, MacKie RM. Extrafacial lentigo maligna melanoma: Analysis of 71 cases and comparison with lentigo maligna melanoma of the head and neck. *Br J Dermatol* Sep 1998;139(3):439–443.
42. Cox NH, Aitchison TC, Sirel JM, et al. Comparison between lentigo maligna melanoma and other histogenetic types of malignant melanoma of the head and neck. Scottish Meanoma Group. *Br J Cancer* Apr 1996;73(7):940–944.

43. Koh HK, Michalik E, Sober AJ, MacKie RM. Lentigo maligna melanoma has no better prognosis than other types of melanoma. *J Clin Oncol* Sep 1984;2(9):994–1001.
44. Allan SJ, Dicker AJ, Tidman MJ, et al. Amelanotic lentigo maligna and amelanotic lentigo maligna melanoma: A report of three cases mimicking intraepidermal squamous carcinoma. *J Eur Acad Dermatol Venereol* July 1998;11(1):78–81.
45. Cohen LM. Lentigo maligna and lentigo maligna melanoma. *J Am Acad Dermatol* Dec 1995;33(6):923–936.
46. Cohen LM. The starburst giant cell is useful for distinguishing lentigo maligna from photodamaged skin. *J Am Acad Dermatol* Dec 1996;35(6):962–968.
47. Cohen LM, McCall MW, Hodge SJ, et al. Successful treatment of lentigo maligna and lentigo maligna melanoma with Mohs micrographic surgery by rush permanent sections. *Cancer* June 1994;73(12):2964–2970.
48. Trotter MJ, Tron VA. Dermal vascularity in lentigo maligna. *J Pathol* Aug 1994;173(4): 341–345.
49. Andersen WK, Labadie RR, Bahwan J. Histopathology of solar lentigines of the face: A quantitative study. *J Am Acad Dermatol* Mar 1997;36(3 Pt 1):444–447.
50. Rosen LB, Suster S. Fibrous papules: A light microscopic and immunohistochemical study. *Am J Dermatopathol* Apr 1988;10(6):109–115.
51. Zimarowski MJ, Harrist TJ, Crowson AN, et al. Atypical melanocytic hyperplasia in fibrous papules mimicking lentigo maligna [abstract]. *Lab Invest* Jan 1994;70:51A.
52. Kuflik EG, Gage AA. Cryosurgery for lentigo maligna. *J Am Acad Dermatol* July 1994;31(1):75–78.
53. Naylor M, Crowson N, Kuwahara R, et al. Treatment of lentigo maligna with topical imiquimod. *Br J Dermatol* Nov 2003;149(Suppl. 66):66–70.
54. Pitman GH, Kopf AW, Bart RS, et al. Treatment of lentigo maligna and lentigo maligna melanoma. *J Dermatol Surg Oncol* Sep 1979;5(9):727–737.
55. Petratos MA, Kopf AW, Bart RS, Casson PR. Treatment of melanotic freckle with x-rays. *Arch Dermatol* Aug 1972;106(2):189–194.
56. National Institutes of Health Consensus Development Conference Statement on Diagnosis and Treatment of Early Melanoma, January 27–29, 1992. *Am J Dermatopathol* Feb 1993;15(1):34–43; discussion 46–51.
57. Day CL Jr, Mihm MC Jr, Sober AJ, et al. Narrower margins for clinical stage I malignant melanoma. *N Engl J Med* Feb 1982;306(8):478–482.
58. Urist MM, Black CM, Soong S, et al. The influence of surgical margins and prognostic factors predicting the risk of local recurrence in 3445 patients with primary cutaneous melanoma. *Cancer* Mar 1985;55:1398–1402.
59. Harmelin ES, Holcombe RN, Goggin JP, et al. Acral lentiginous melanoma. *J Foot Ankle Surg* Nov–Dec 1998;37(6):540–545.
60. Kato T, Suetake T, Sugiyama Y, et al. Epidemiology and prognosis of subungual melanoma in 34 Japanese patients. *Br J Dermatol* Mar 1996;134(3):383–387.
61. Kato T, Kumasaka N, Suetake T, et al. Clinicopathological study of acral melanoma in situ in 44 Japanese patients. *Dermatology* 1996;193(3):192–197.
62. Yusuoka N, Ueda M, Ohgami Y, et al. Amelanotic acral lentiginous malignant melanoma. *Br J Dermatol* Aug 1999;141(2):370–372.
63. Cho KH, Han KH, Minn KW. Superficial spreading melanoma arising in a longstanding melanocytic nevus on the sole. *J Dermatol* May 1998;25:337–340.
64. Kato T, Suetake T, Tabata N, et al. Epidemiology and prognosis of plantar melanoma in 62 Japanese patients over a 28-year period. *Int J Dermatol* July 1999;38(7): 515–519.
65. Kridge JE, Hudson DA, Johnson CA, et al. Subungual melanoma. *S Afr J Surg* Mar 1995;33(1):10–14.

66. Massi D, Franchi A, Borgognoni L, et al. Thin cutaneous malignant melanomas (< or = 1.5 mm): Identification of risk factors indicative of progression. *Cancer* Mar 1999;85(5):1067–1076.
67. Ridgeway CA, Hieken TJ, Roonan SG, et al. Acral lentiginous melanoma. *Arch Surg* Jan 1995;130(1):88–92.
68. Cascinelli N, Zurrida S, Galimberti V, et al. Acral lentiginous melanoma. A histological type without prognostic significance. *J Dermatol Surg Oncol* Dec 1994;20(12):817–822.
69. Jimbow K, Takahashi H, Miura S, et al. Biological behaviour and natural course of acral malignant melanoma. *Am J Dermatopathol* Summer 1984;6(Suppl. 1):43–53.
70. Chang AE, Karnell LH, Menck HR. The National Cancer Data Base report on cutaneous and noncutaneous melanoma: A summary of 84,836 cases from the past decade. The American College of Surgeons Commission on Cancer and the American Cancer Society. *Cancer* Oct 1998;83(8):1664–1678.
71. Barnhill RL. *Pathology of Melanocytic Nevi and Malignant Melanoma.* Boston, MA: Butterworth-Heinemann; 1995:214–217.
72. Pandey M, Mathew A, Abraham EK, et al. Primary malignant melanoma of the mucous membranes. *Eur J Surg Oncol* Aug 1998;24(4):303–307.
73. Larrson KB, Shaw HM, Thompson JF, et al. Primary mucosal and glans penis melanomas: The Sydney Melanoma Unit experience. *Aust N Z J Surg* Feb 1999; 69(2):121–126.
74. Gonzalez-Bosquet J, Garcia Jimenez A, Moreno G, et al. Malignant vulvo-vaginal melanoma: A report of 7 cases. *Eur J Gynaecol Oncol* 1997;18(1):63–67.
75. Dunton CJ, Berd D. Vulvar melanoma, biologically different from other cutaneous melanomas. *Lancet* Dec 1999;354(9195):2013–2014.
76. Ragnarsson-Olding BK, Kanter-Lewensohn LR, Lagerlof B, et al. Malignant melanoma of the vulva in a nationwide, 25-year study of 219 Swedish females: Clinical observations and pathological features. *Cancer* Oct 1999;86(7):1273–1284.
77. Ragnarsson-Olding BK, Nilsson BR, Kanter-Lewensohn LR, et al. Malignant melanoma of the vulva in a nationwide, 25-year study of 219 Swedish females: Predictors of survival. *Cancer* Oct 1999;86(7):1285–1293.
78. DeMatos P, Tyler D, Seigler HF. Mucosal melanoma of the female genitalia: A clinicopathologic study of forty-three cases at Duke University Medical Center. *Surgery* July 1998;124(1):38–48.
79. Raber G, Mempel V, Jackish C, et al. Malignant melanoma of the vulva. Report of 89 patients. *Cancer* Dec 1996;78(11):2353–2358.
80. Egan CA, Bradley RR, Logsdon VK, et al. Vulvar melanoma in childhood. *Arch Dermatol* Mar 1997;133(3):345–348.
81. Carlson JA, Mihm MC. Vulvar nevi, lichen sclerosis et sclerosis, and vitiligo [letter]. *Arch Dermatol* Oct 1997;133(10):1314–1316.
82. Piura B, Rabinovich A, Dgani R. Malignant melanoma of the vulva: Report of six cases and review of the literature. *Eur J Gynaecol Oncol* 1999;20(3):182–186.
83. Ragnarsson-Olding B, Johansson H, Rutqvist LE, et al. Malignant melanoma of the vulva and vagina. Trends in incidence, age distribution, and long-term survival among 245 consecutive cases in Sweden 1960–1984. *Cancer* Mar 1993;171(5):1893–1897.
84. Tasseron EW, van der Esch EP, Hart AA, et al. A clinicopathological study of 30 melanomas of the vulva. *Gynecol Oncol* Aug 1992;46(2):170–175.
85. Gorsky M, Epsein JB. Melanomas arising from the mucosal surfaces of the head and neck. *Oral Surg Med Oral Pathol Oral Radiol Endod* Dec 1998;86(6):715–719.
86. Regauer S, Anderhuber W, Richtig E, et al. Primary mucosal melanomas of the nasal cavity and paranasal sinuses. A clinicopathological analysis of 14 cases. *APMIS* Mar 1998;106:403–410.

87. Hoorweg JJ, Loftus BM, Hilgers FJ. Osteoid and bone formation in a nasal mucosal melanoma and its metastasis. *Histopathology* Nov 1987;31(5):465–468.

88. Friedman I. Osteoid and bone formation in a nasal mucosal melanoma and its metastasis [letter]. *Histopathology* July 1988;33(1):88.

89. Kato T, Suetake T, Kumasaka N, et al. Nodular melanoma in 62 Japanese patients: Influence of initial surgical treatment of local recurrence and prognosis. *J Dermatol* Oct 1995;22(10):723–728.

90. Clark WH Jr, Elder DE, Guerry D IV, et al. A study of tumor progression: The precursor lesions of superficial spreading and nodular malignant melanoma. *Hum Pathol* Dec 1984;15(12):1147–1165.

91. Elder DE, Guerry D IV, Epstein MN, et al. Invasive melanomas lacking competence for metastasis. *Am J Dermatopathol Summer* 1984;6(Suppl. 1):55–61.

92. Silvis NG, Swanson PE, Manivel JC, et al. Spindle-cell and pleomorphic neoplasms of the skin. A clinicopathologic and immunohistochemical study of 30 cases, with emphasis on "atypical fibroxanthomas". *Am J Dermatopathol* Feb 1988;10(1):9–19.

93. Haycock CL, Odland PB, Olbricht SM, Piepkorn MP. Immunohistochemical characterization of dermatofibrosarcoma protuberans with practical applications for diagnosis and treatment. *J Am Acad Dermatol* Sep 1997;37(2 Pt 1):438–444.

94. Elder DE. Metastatic melanoma. In: Elder DE, ed. *Pathobiology of Malignant Melanoma*. Basel: Karger, 1987:182–204.

95. Beardmore GL, Davis NC. Multiple primary cutaneous melanomas. *Arch Dermatol* May 1975;111(5):603–609.

96. White WL, Hitchcock MG. Dying dogma: The pathological diagnosis of epidermotropic metastatic malignant melanoma. *Semin Diagn Pathol* Aug 1998;15(3):176–188.

97. Abernathy JL, Soyer HP, Kerl H, et al. Epidermotropic metastatic malignant melanoma simulating melanoma in situ. A report of 10 examples from two patients. *Am J Surg Pathol* Nov 1994;18(11):1140–1149.

98. Bengoechea-Beeby MP, Velasco-Oses A, Mourino Fernandez F, et al. Epidermotropic metastatic melanoma. Are the current criteria adequate to differentiate primary from metastatic melanoma? *Cancer* Sep 1993;72(6):1909–1913.

99. Kornberg R, Harris M, Ackerman AB. Epidermotropically metastatic malignant melanoma. Differentiating malignant melanoma metastatic to the epidermis from malignant melanoma primary in the epidermis. *Arch Dermatol* Jan 1978;114(1):67–69.

100. Heenan PJ, Clay CD. Epidermotropic metastatic melanoma simulating multiple primary melanomas. *Am J Dermatopathol* Aug 1991;13(4):396–402.

101. Scalzo DA, Hida CA, Toth G, et al. Childhood melanoma: A clinicopathological study of 22 cases. *Melanoma Res* Feb 1997;7(1):63–68.

102. Temple WJ, Mulloy RH, Alexander F, et al. Childhood melanoma. *J Pediatr Surg* Feb 1991;26(2):135–137.

103. Berg P, Lindelof B. Differences in malignant melanoma between children and adolescents. *Arch Dermatol* Mar 1997;133(3):295–297.

104. Whiteman D, Milligan A, Welch J, et al. Germline CDKN2A mutations in childhood melanoma. *J Natl Cancer Inst* Oct 1997;89:1460.

105. Corpron C, Black T, Ross M, et al. Melanoma as a second malignant neoplasm after childhood cancer. *Am J Surg* Nov 1996;172(5):459–462.

106. Rao BN, Hayes FA, Pratt CB, et al. Malignant melanoma in children: Its management and prognosis. *J Pediatr Surg* Feb 1990;25(2):198–203.

107. Melnik MK, Urdaneta LF, Al-Jurf AS, et al. Malignant melanoma in childhood and adolescence. *Am Surg* Mar 1986;52(3):142–147.

108. Howat AJ, Variend S. Lymphatic invasion in Spitz nevi. *Am J Surg Pathol* Feb 1985;9(2):125–128.

109. Peters MS, Goellner JR. Spitz naevi and malignant melanomas of childhood and adolescence. *Histopathology* Dec 1986;10(12):1289–1302.
110. Spatz A, Calonje E, Handfield-Jones S, et al. Spitz tumors in children: A grading system for risk stratification. *Arch Dermatol* Mar 1999;135(3):282–285.
111. Crotty KA, McCarthy SW, Palmer AA, et al. Malignant melanoma in childhood: A clinicopathologic study of 13 cases and comparison with Spitz nevi. *World J Surg* Mar–Apr 1992;16(2):179–185.
112. McCarthy SW, Crotty KA, Palmer AA, et al. Cutaneous malignant melanoma in teenagers. *Histopathology* May 1994;24(5):453–461.
113. Rapini RP. Spitz nevus or melanoma? *Semin Cutan Med Surg* Mar 1999;18(1):56–63.
114. Hendrickson MR, Ross JC. Neoplasms arising in congenital giant nevi: Morphological study of seven cases and a review of the literature. *Am J Surg Pathol* Mar 1981;5(2):109–135.
115. Ceballos PI, Ruiz-Maldonado R, Mihm MC. Melanoma in children. *N Engl J Med* Mar 1995;332(10):656–662.
116. Spitz S. Melanomas in childhood. *Am J Pathol* 1948;24:591–609.
117. Skov-Jensen T, Hastrup J, Lambrethsen F. Malignant melanoma in prepubertal children. *Cancer* May 1966;19(5):620–626.
118. Weedon D, Little JB. Spindle and epithelioid cell naevi in children and adults. *Cancer* Jul 1977;40(1)217–225.
119. Reintgen DS, Vollmer R, Seigler HF. Juvenile malignant melanoma. *Surg Gynecol Obstet* Mar 1989;168(3):249–253.
120. Tate PS, Ronan SG, Feucht KA, et al. Melanoma in childhood and adolescence: Clinical and pathological features of 48 cases. *J Pediatr Surg* Feb 1993;28:217–222.
121. Chun K, Vazquez M, Sanchez JL. Malignant melanoma in children. *Int J Dermatol* Jan 1993;32(1):41–43.
122. Sander B, Karlsson P, Rosdahl I, et al. Cutaneous malignant melanoma in Swedish children and teenagers 1973–1992: A clinico-pathological study of 130 cases. *Int J Cancer* Mar 1997;80(5):646–651.

4

HISTOLOGICAL AND PHENOTYPIC VARIANTS OF MELANOMA AND OF THE BORDERLINE MELANOCYTIC TUMOR

A potential diagnostic pitfall in the histologic assessment of melanoma is the inability to recognize unusual melanoma variants. Of these, the more treacherous examples include the desmoplastic melanoma, the nevoid melanoma, the so-called minimal-deviation melanoma, melanoma with prominent pigment synthesis or animal type melanoma, and the malignant blue nevus. Also problematic are the unusual phenotypic profiles seen in vertical growth phase melanomas; these include those tumors whose morphological peculiarities mimic cancers of nonmelanocytic lineage and those melanomas that express aberrant antigenic profiles not commonly associated with a melanocytic histogenesis. Metaplastic change in melanoma, balloon cell melanoma, signet ring cell melanoma, myxoid melanoma, small cell melanoma, and rhabdoid melanoma all have the potential to mimic metastatic and primary neoplasms of different lineage derivations. Abnormal immunohistochemical expression of CD34, cytokeratins (CKs), epithelial membrane antigen, and smooth muscle markers as well as the deficient expression of S100 protein and melanocyte lineage-specific markers such as gp100 protein (i.e., HMB-45 antibody) and A103 (i.e., Melan-A antibody) also present confusing diagnostic challenges.

In this chapter, we will discuss in some detail certain of these novel clinicopathologic types of melanoma, as the abnormal phenotypic expressions of the vertical growth phase, and expand upon the concept of the borderline melanocytic tumor.

DESMOPLASTIC MELANOMA

Introduction and Clinical Features

Demoplastic melanoma is a rare variant of malignant melanoma first recognized in 1971.[1] Desmoplastic and neurotropic melanoma may be mistaken clinically for a scar, a fibroma, a basal cell carcinoma, or a fibromatosis.

Sometimes there is pronounced mucin deposition that imparts a boggy quality to the lesion.[2,3] The clinical clue to the diagnosis, when present, is cutaneous or mucosal pigmentation overlying a palpable dermal or submucosal nodule. That said, only half of desmoplastic melanomas are clinically pigmented.[3] Desmoplastic melanomas tend to occur in the head and neck area and the upper back,[4–7] but are also seen in mucosal sites such as the vulva or gingiva[8] and in acral locations. Typically, they occur in older patients, with mean ages in the larger series falling into the sixth to eighth decades of life.[4,6,9–15] Larger series show a male preponderance of 1.75 to 1.[15] Although any given desmoplastic melanoma can be deeply invasive, when matched for a given depth of invasion, they are associated with a lesser risk of metastatic disease than conventional melanomas of similar depth. The classical clinical finding is that of a pale or fleshy firm nodule reminiscent of a scar, which tends to delay clinical diagnosis and biopsy. Carlson et al.[6] who reported an equal distribution in men and women, found most tumors to be located in the head and neck area (75%) and to be nonpigmented (57%); they concluded that most desmoplastic melanomas took origin in neoplasms that were of lentigo maligna subtype. The lesions show a high recurrence rate, with recurrent tumors typically being amelanotic and presenting as an area of scarring or induration with palpable, ill-defined margins. In patients with multiple recurrences, invasion of adjacent structures such as salivary gland, periosteum, glenoid fossa, and cranial cavity can be seen.[9] Local recurrences were seen in 29% of patients in one series of 58 desmoplastic and/or neurotropic melanomas, with a malignant cranial neuropathy occurring in four patients and death from metastatic disease in 19% of cases.[16] Neurotropism strongly enhances the statistical likelihood of local recurrence.[15] The probability of a 5-year survival for tumors greater than 4 mm in thickness is higher than that for other types of melanomas that are of similar thickness,[6,17] as alluded to above.

Histology

Desmoplastic melanoma is a form of vertical growth phase melanoma in which the invasive tumor cells have a spindled morphology and are associated with a striking desmoplastic stromal response (Figs. 4.1–4.6, e-figs. 4.1–4.6). There appears to be a morphologic continuum between desmoplastic melanoma and vertical growth phase spindle cell melanoma, the latter being the most frequent type of invasive melanoma seen in lentigo maligna melanoma. In desmoplastic melanoma, the neoplasm tends to extend deeply into the reticular dermis. The average depth of invasion at the time of first excision is 4.1 mm.[6] Desmoplastic melanoma is poorly circumscribed, with the deep and lateral margins of the tumor being ill defined (Fig. 4.1).[3] Reactive fibroblasts, the presumptive source of matrix production, are intimately admixed with the tumor cells, although there is some controversy about the source of stromal collagenization in these neoplasms. The neoplastic melanocytic component may either assume a single-cell dispersal pattern within the sclerotic dermis or be disposed in long fascicles in a fashion reminiscent of a fibrosarcoma, sometimes assuming a whorled or storiform pattern. The fascicles may be ensheathed by a mucinous matrix (e-figs. 4.7 and 4.8), imparting an appearance resembling a peripheral nerve sheath tumor such as a neuroma, schwannoma, or neurofibroma[2] and prompting misdiagnosis as a form of peripheral nerve sheath tumor[18] (Fig. 4.3). The spindle cell and collagenous process may lie in intimate apposition to the epidermis, which usually appears attenuated, or there may be a grenz zone (e-fig. 4.9).[6] When the tumor is contiguous with the epidermis, a significantly thinner depth of invasion is the rule. Within the epidermis in up to 80% of lesions in some series, but in only half of cases in our hands, there is a proliferation of atypical melanocytes (Figs. 4.2 and 4.4). Most often, this atypical proliferation is present in a lentiginous array; the density and degree of cytologic atypia is consonant with lentigo maligna in 25% to 50% of cases.[6] Rarely, a pagetoid pattern of epithelioid melanocytes consistent with superficial spreading malignant melanoma is seen. Because an intraepidermal component tends not to be identifiable in deeper lesions,[6] it may be that migration from an intraepidermal to an intradermal location occurs during the evolution of desmoplastic melanoma. Not infrequently, the most superficial aspect of the invasive component may show a nested

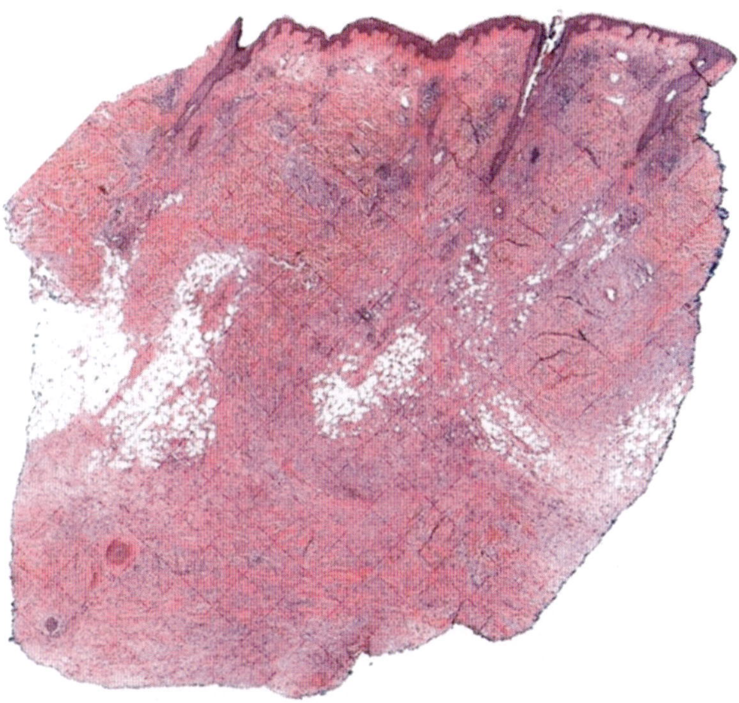

FIGURE 4.1 **Desmoplastic Melanoma.** The biopsy has a square contour due to the presence of abundant stromal collagen deposition. It also appears vaguely hypercellular at scanning magnification with extension of a process in and around the subcutaneous fat lobules accompanied by fatty atrophy and extension into the subcutaneous fascia.

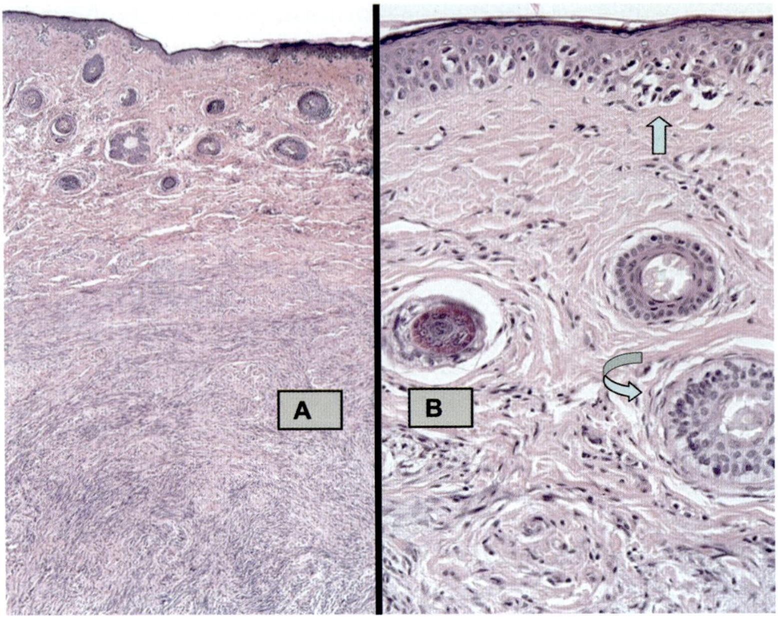

FIGURE 4.2 **Desmoplastic Melanoma.** The dermis appears hypercellular in a diffuse, ill-defined fashion **(A)**. There is lentiginous melanocytic hyperplasia and atypia **(B)** (*straight arrow*), an important criterion for desmoplastic melanomas arising in the setting of lentigo maligna, mucosal lentiginous, or acral lentiginous melanoma. This finding is, unfortunately, seen in only roughly half of cases. There is an invasion by atypical spindle cells into the adventitia of adnexal structures (*curved arrow*), another important criterion for this diagnosis which distinguishes desmoplastic melanoma from blue nevi and other melanocytoses that spare the adventitia.

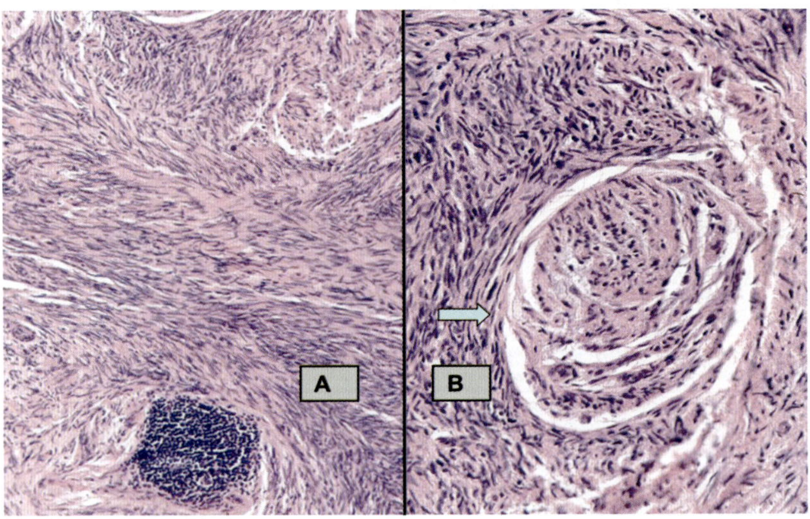

FIGURE 4.3 **Desmoplastic Melanoma.** Nidi of chronic inflammation **(A)** in any hypercellular, collagenized spindle cell lesion should merit extra scrutiny for other features of desmoplastic melanoma. These would include neurotropism **(B)** (*arrow*).

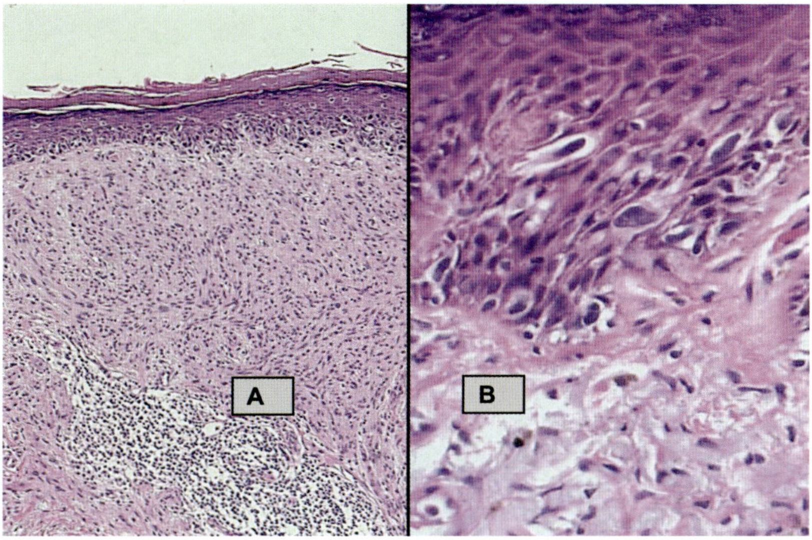

FIGURE 4.4 **Desmoplastic Melanoma.** In addition to lentiginous melanoma in situ (**A** and **B**) this diffusely cellular dermis is heavily infiltrated by small lymphoid forms (**A**). Note the dermal solar elastosis in this lesion which has arisen in the setting of lentigo maligna (**B**).

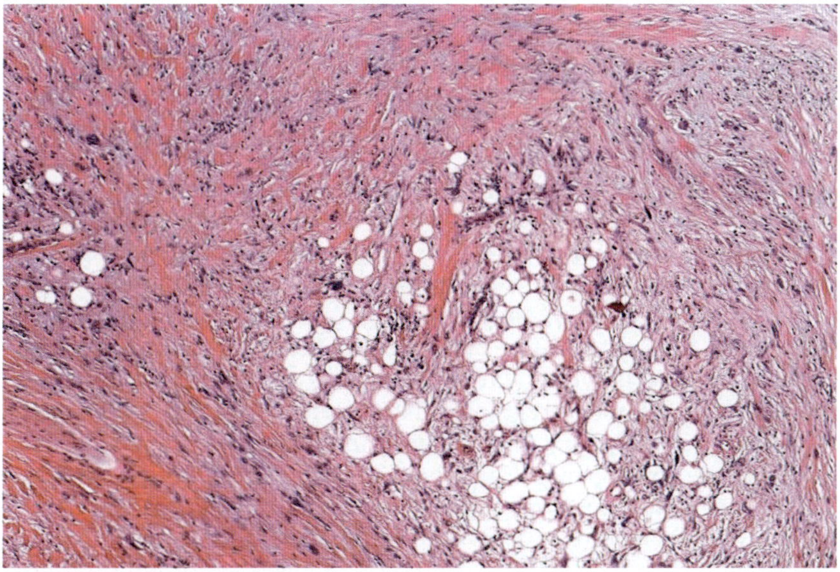

FIGURE 4.5 **Desmoplastic Melanoma.** Hyperchromatic spindle cell forms extend between and around the fat lobules that are associated with fatty atrophy in this tumor which extends into the subcutaneous fascia.

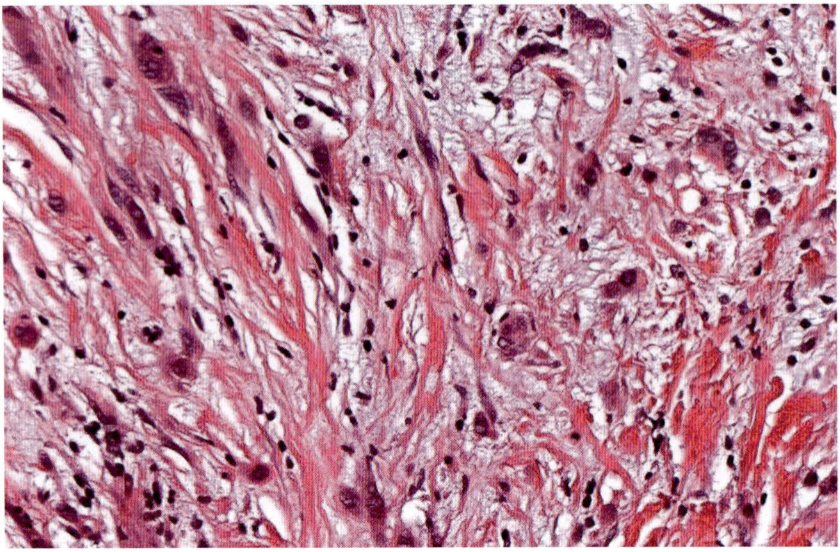

FIGURE 4.6 **Desmoplastic Melanoma.** Note the hyperchromatic fusiform neoplastic cells, the abundant quantity of mature eosinophilic collagen fiber deposition and stromal mucinosis which is pronounced in this example. Lymphocytes diffusely percolate the dermis.

pattern of dermal infiltration in which the superficial nests are at varying angles to the long axis of the epidermis (e-figs. 4.10–4.12). In addition, an occasional nest may be seen amidst the dominant spindled sclerotic component. There is usually infiltration of nerves by tumor, which tends to surround and permeate cutaneous nerve trunks, resulting in an endoneurium that appears hypercellular. These infiltrated nerves may be found at significant distances from the main tumor mass including within the subcutaneous fat.[19] It is prudent to study the nerve trunks in any invasive melanoma, but particularly in those neoplasms of lentigo maligna melanoma or acral lentiginous melanoma subtypes. Desmoplastic melanomas may also manifest considerable pagetoid infiltration of the straight eccrine ducts and glands. The cytomorphology of the spindled populace is one of large cells with oval to elongated nuclei that appear hyperchromatic with coarse, irregularly distributed chromatin and conspicuous nucleoli (e-figs. 4.13–4.15). The attenuated cytoplasmic processes merge with the background stroma (Fig. 4.5). There may be individual cell necrosis. Mitoses are identified throughout the tumor, although the mitotic index is usually low, averaging approximately two mitoses per 10 high-power fields. In one series, 10 of 28 cases exhibited no mitoses[6]; this has been our experience as well. The tumor cells are usually devoid of pigment, although there are often occasional melanophages scattered through the stroma. There are rare reports, however, of heavily melanized neurotropic melanomas in which perineural collections of pigment-containing cells were seen. The presence of nodular chronic inflammatory cell infiltrates along with mucinotic zones[2] (see Figs. 4.3 and 4.6, e-figs. 4.16 and 4.17), the latter in rare cases so extensive as to lead to a misdiagnosis of focal cutaneous mucinosis, completes the picture. The presence of a lymphocytic infiltrate in a sclerosing nevomelanocytic proliferation ought to prompt careful consideration of desmoplastic melanoma, in our view. Osteoid and bone formation may be seen, particularly in subungual desmoplastic melanomas.[20]

A recent study of 131 desmoplastic melanomas showed a pure desmoplastic morphology in 93 cases versus a mixed pattern in 39 cases, where the second component was nondesmoplastic and often epithelioid in character.[21]

Differential Diagnosis

Misdiagnosis at initial biopsy is common in our experience and that of others and may be the basis for inadequate initial local therapy that underlies the high rates of local recurrence of this neoplasm.[4,22] Early lesions of desmoplastic melanoma may be difficult to distinguish from sclerosing nevi of spindle and/or epithelioid cell (i.e., Spitz) type (e-figs. 4.18 and 4.19), sclerosing type A nevi, and sclerosing blue nevi. The latter lesions show a central zone of fibrosis with a well-circumscribed perimeter comprising typical blue nevus cells and macrophages that tend to spare the adventitial dermis of the hair follicle. The desmoplastic Spitz nevus has an inverted wedge-shaped pattern, manifesting an admixture of spindle cells with delicate elongate nuclei and bizarre ganglion-like cells, the dual population of cell components that also typifies the nonsclerotic Spitz nevus variant. The critical cell of the sclerosing type A nevus has a characteristic banal elongate or cigar-shaped nuclear morphology with rounded or blunt nuclear contours and modest quantities of clear or lightly melanized cytoplasm. By contrast, early desmoplastic melanoma shows a haphazard, highly infiltrative pattern of growth in which large atypical hyperchromatic spindle cells deform the dermal architecture and invade the adventitial dermis of hair follicles. Neurotropism and foci of chronic inflammation typify desmoplastic melanoma,[2] but are usually absent in Spitz nevi. The nucleocytoplasmic ratios of desmoplastic melanoma are higher than the cells of the Spitz nevus, the cytoplasms are more sparse, and usually, but not always, melanin pigment is absent in the cytosol of the melanocytes in desmoplastic melanoma. None of the aforementioned benign nevi manifest zones of mucinotic stromal change, as are often present in the desmoplastic melanoma.[2] Furthermore, most inverted type A nevi and most blue nevi lack a lentiginous junctional component, and although over one half of Spitz nevi do have an intraepidermal melanocytic proliferation, this is more often nested than lentiginous in character and has a distinctive cytomorphology.

Metastatic melanoma may provoke a desmoplastic stromal response to generate a morphology that resembles the pattern of classical desmoplastic primary melanoma; neurotropism is said not to be seen in metastatic desmoplastic melanoma, however.[9]

Nonmelanocytic neoplasms that enter the differential diagnosis include leiomyosarcoma, neurothekeoma and its cellular variant spindle cell squamous cell carcinoma, and, of course, scars and dermatofibromata.[22–24] Neurotropism may be seen in a number of benign and malignant neoplasms; as congenital and Spitz nevi may show this feature, it is certainly not pathognomonic of the malignant melanocytic phenotype.[25] Neurotropism is also a feature of squamous cell carcinoma, basal cell carcinoma, keratoacanthoma, and adenoid cystic carcinoma, but these lesions should not pose a diagnostic dilemma when the appropriate immunohistochemical workup has been performed.

Histogenesis

The source of the collagen matrix in the desmoplastic melanoma is a subject of considerable controversy. According to one hypothesis, that the tumor cells evoke a host response characterized by a proliferation of fibroblasts, the collagen production is of fibroblastic origin. The alternative hypothesis is that the tumor cells are dedifferentiated neoplastic melanocytes that function as facultative fibroblasts.[26] Supportive of the latter hypothesis are ultrastructural studies showing fibroblastic qualities in the neoplastic cells[11] and macular desmosomes between adjoining neoplastic cells, held to be evidence that the tumor populace constitutes a modified or dedifferentiated melanocyte with fibroblastic attributes.[27,28] Macular desmosomes are a characteristic feature of melanoma and likely account for the tendency for nesting of dermal melanocytes seen in a minority of desmoplastic melanomas. The concomitant fibroblastlike features identified in the tumor cells include the presence of dilated rough endoplasmic reticulum.[27,28] The tumor cells of desmoplastic melanoma decorate with antibodies to S100 protein in an almost ubiquitous fashion (e-figs. 4.20 and 4.21),[6] with antibodies to neuron-specific enolase in 40% to 96% of cases,[6,17] and with HMB-45 in roughly 20% of cases[6] (Fig. 4.7). Typically, lesions either give negative results[29] or show differential staining patterns in which tumor cells are weakly positive, superficially with negative results in the deep portions of the tumor.[30] As previously mentioned, this staining pattern is different from that observed in the blue nevus with atypia seen in elderly patients. Similarly, sclerosing Spitz nevi tend to show high HMB-45 expression superficially, which tapers off to negativity in the lesional base; the finding of an HMB-45-negative sclerosing nevomelanocytic proliferation ought to prompt careful scrutiny for criteria of desmoplastic melanoma. Longacre et al.[31] established that lesional melanocytes decorated with S100 protein in 94% of 32 studied cases of desmoplastic and spindle cell melanoma, of which two S100-positive cases showed decoration in fewer than 5% of the critical cells. Using a two-color system, they demonstrated that 32% of cases contained a significant number of smooth muscle actin-positive cells, interpreted by them as representing myofibroblasts, admixed with the neoplastic spindled melanocytes and

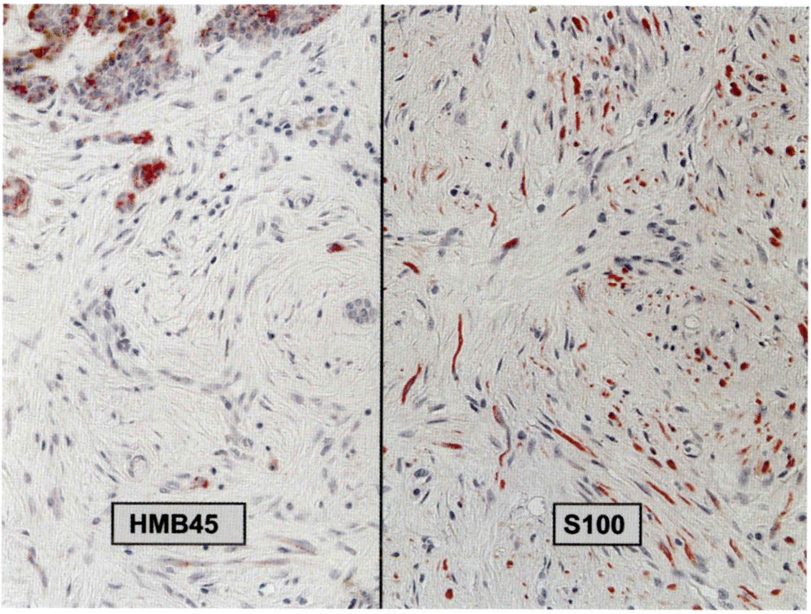

FIGURE 4.7 **Desmoplastic Melanoma: Immunohistochemical Profile.** HMB-45 and other markers of melanocyte lineage-specific differentiation, are either negative in desmoplastic melanoma or focally positive and then only in the more superficial aspects of the neoplasm **(left panel)**. Immunohistochemical studies for S100 protein, by contrast, diffusely decorate the neoplasm in the great majority of cases **(right panel)**. These stains were kindly provided by Dr HR Wightman of Grace General Hospital in Winnipeg, Canada.

representing the putative source of the desmoplasia in these neoplasms.[31] This study would support the first construction concerning the histogenesis of desmoplastic melanoma, that is, that a biphasic populace is present and that the melanocytes and the collagen-producing myofibroblastic cells are two distinct and phenotypically separable populations.

The tendency for desmoplastic melanoma to manifest neurotropism and stromal collagenization can be explained at the molecular level by gene expression profiling that shows activation of genes encoding for neurotrophic factors and for extracellular matrix elaboration,[32] expressed at the protein level in fixed tissues by immunohistochemical assay for p75 nerve growth factor receptor,[33] basic fibroblast growth factor (b-FGF),[34] and the fibroblastic markers CD90 and CD13.[35] The expression of genes for melanocytic differentiation was reduced in desmoplastic melanoma as compared to conventional melanoma; the reduced melanocyte differentiation gene expression has its counterpart at the tissue level by virtue of absent expression of melanocyte lineage-specific markers such as HMB-45 and Melan-A,[6] tyrosinase and D5, an antibody to microphthalmia transcription factor (Mit-f).[36,37] More recently, a similar lack of immunoreactivity has been described with the novel monoclonal antibody PNL2.[38]

Therapy

Because the lesions are often amelanotic, and so mimic scars and basal cell and squamous cell carcinomas clinically, initial biopsy may be delayed,[39] compounding the problem of histologic misdiagnosis mentioned above and so delaying proper surgical therapy.[4,22] Deep excision to encompass fascia, where possible, is often advised owing to the deeply invasive nature of the neurotropic component.[39] Great care must be taken to ensure that there is no evidence of perineural infiltration in the margins, the commonest cause of recurrence. Survivorship at 5 years approaches 75% and in thin lesions less than 2 mm in thickness, 90%.[39] It has been suggested that those desmoplastic melanomas having foci of conventional vertical growth phase melanoma manifest a significantly worse prognosis, with regional lymph node metastases in 10% of cases as opposed to only 1% of patients with pure desmoplastic melanoma.[21] Disease-specific 5-year mortality in one study was 11% for pure desmoplastic vertical growth phase tumors versus 31% for those neoplasms having the aforementioned hybrid morphology.[21] There is little doubt that desmoplastic melanoma manifests up to a threefold greater thickness at presentation, but nonetheless has better survivorship than conventional melanomas of similar thickness.[21]

NEVOID MELANOMA

Introduction and Clinical Features

The term nevoid melanoma was first proposed by Schmoeckel et al.[40] to describe a heterogeneous group of lesions showing histologic features closely recapitulating a benign nevus including a symmetrical, dome-shaped or verrucous and papillomatous silhouette and a cell populace manifesting apparent maturation of cells with descent in the dermis.[40–45] The clinical setting in our experience is that of a tan nodule typically greater than 1 cm in size on the trunk or proximal limbs of a young adult. Our experience is thus similar to that of Blessing et al.,[43] but is at variance with that of Kossard and Wilkinson.[46] This is, fortunately for pathologists, a rare form of malignant melanoma comprising less than 1% of all lesions seen in consultation. The lesions behave like invasive melanoma including in the context of local recurrence and metastatic disease.[40,45] However, in our opinion, many of the cases so designated were, in fact, small epithelioid melanomas in which the pleomorphic confluent growth and high mitotic rate distinguished the lesions from nevoid melanoma. Previous reports describing a similar entity under a different nomenclature antedated the report of Schmoekel et al.[41,42]; Levene described such deceptively bland appearing lesions as "verrucous pseudonevoid melanoma," and, indeed, the lesions clinically resemble benign nevi. In a series of 33 cases, 15 patients developed metastatic disease and eight died of disseminated melanoma.[40] In the series of 15 patients reported by McNutt et al.,[47] recurrent disease was observed in three patients; local nodal metastases developed in three patients, cutaneous metastatic disease in three patients, and disseminated disease in one patient, a 32-year-old man who succumbed to his cancer. There was a 2:1 male predominance and the average age was 43 years. In the series by Wong et al.,[45] regional metastases developed in one patient and local recurrence in three, and three were reported to be alive and well with no evidence of disease after excision. The average age at presentation in the latter series was 40 years; there was a similar slight male predominance. In a series of 20 patients with nevoid melanoma, the mortality and metastasis rate at 3 years was 37.5%.[48] These lesions are not to be confused with minimal-deviation melanoma, which is considered a borderline tumor whose biological behavior is difficult to predict on the basis of the histology of the primary lesion.

Histology

Low-power architectural examination reveals either a verrucoid (Figs. 4.8–4.10) or a dome-shaped pattern (Fig. 4.11, e-figs. 4.22–4.25). In a series of 20 patients with nevoid melanoma, 13 had dome-shaped surface contours while seven were verrucous in character.[48] There is a circumscribed subjacent proliferation of mitotically active melanocytes (see Fig. 4.10) that extends to lie in direct apposition to either a smooth, papillomatous or verrucous epidermis. The lesions manifest sharp lateral circumscription (e-figs. 4.26 and 4.27).[45,47] With respect to the intraepidermal component, prominent pagetoid infiltration is notably absent. Junctional activity is uncommon but can be observed in some cases of verrucoid forms of nevoid melanoma. The superficial dermal component is composed of nests of epithelioid-appearing melanocytes (Fig. 4.12); a discernible spindle-cell component is not identified. In the verrucous variant, the superficial nests can be quite large with confluence. There may be a gradual diminution in cell size toward the base.[44,47] In addition, the cells are arranged in smaller units including short cords, small nests,[44] and a single-cell dispersion[47] (Fig. 4.13, e-figs. 4.28 and 4.29). The base is not well demarcated. The dermal component typically extends into the superficial reticular dermis for a depth of anywhere from 0.67 to 1.2 mm from the epidermal surface.[44] Although the cells at the base are smaller, they show atypical features including conspicuous nucleolation, nuclear membrane irregularity, hyperchromasia, increased nuclear-to-cytoplasmic ratios, and mitotic activity, all of which are unusual in the banal common acquired nevus (Figs. 4.14 and 4.15, e-figs. 4.30 and 4.31). Features that allow easy recognition of the process as malignant melanoma, such as a pushing border, high mitotic activity, and striking pleomorphism, are usually absent, which compounds the risk of misdiagnosis of such lesions as benign dermal nevi. Foci consistent with a residual dermal nevus are not usually present. Lymphatic invasion can be observed and may be a sign of more aggressive behavior.[44]

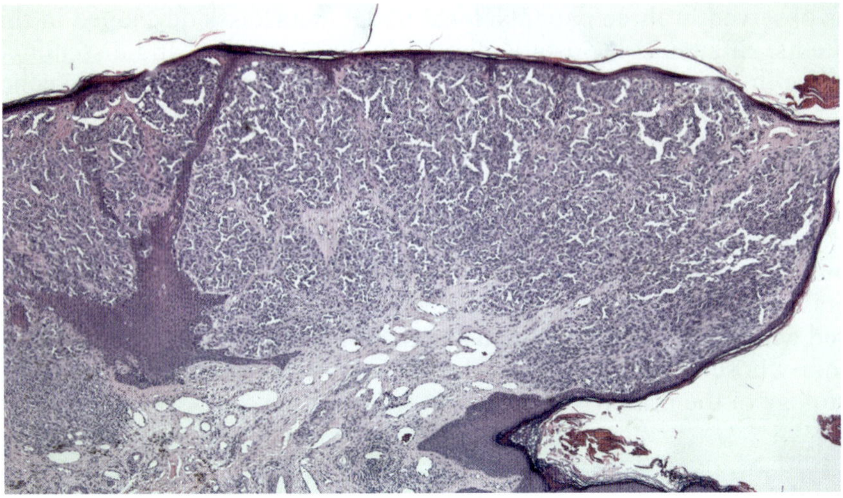

FIGURE 4.8 **Nevoid Melanoma: Verrucous Variant.** This verrucous nevoid melanoma shows a polypoid surface contour with a confluent and nodular growth of neoplastic melanocytes causing an asymmetric expansile dermal population.

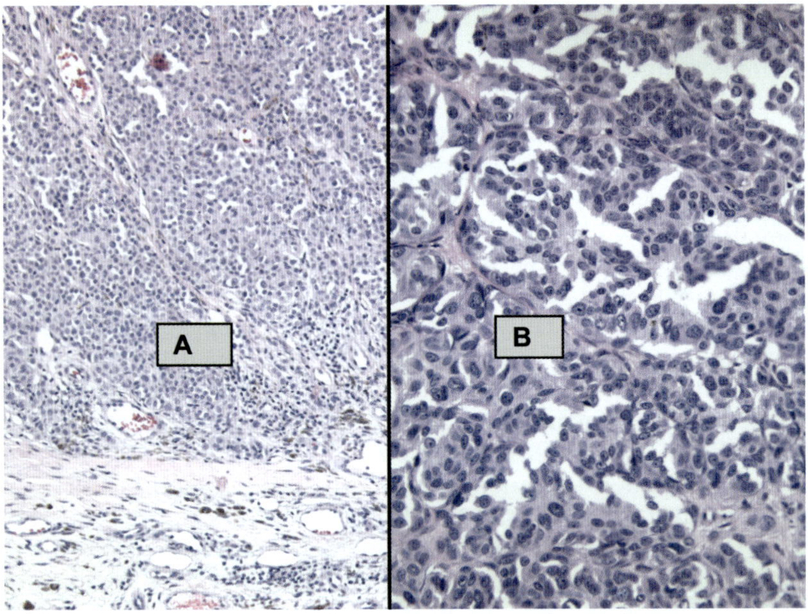

FIGURE 4.9 **Nevoid Melanoma.** The tumor cells form confluent expansile nodules and sheets **(A)** of monotonous melanocytes **(B)**.

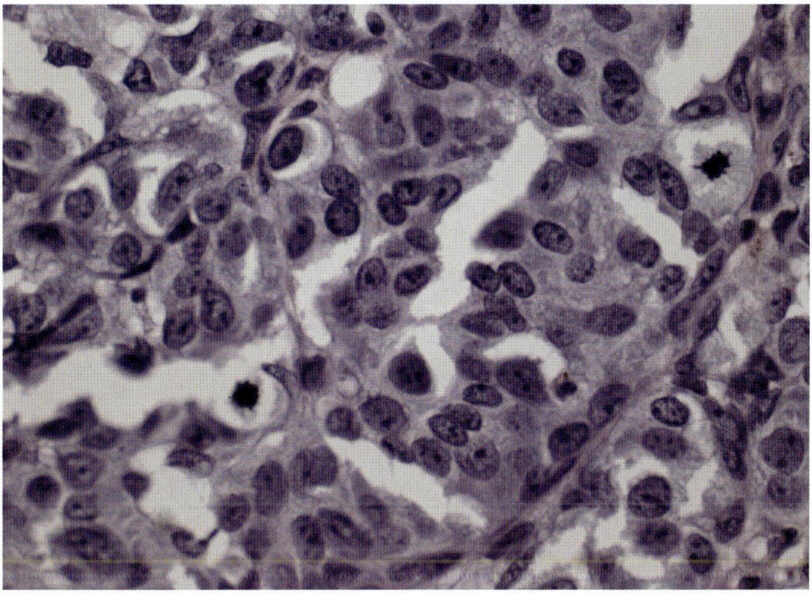

FIGURE 4.10 **Nevoid Melanoma.** Two mitotic figures are demonstrated in this single 60× high dry objective magnification image. Note that the neoplastic cells are monotonous, manifesting prominent nucleoli and occasional bean-shaped grooved nuclei.

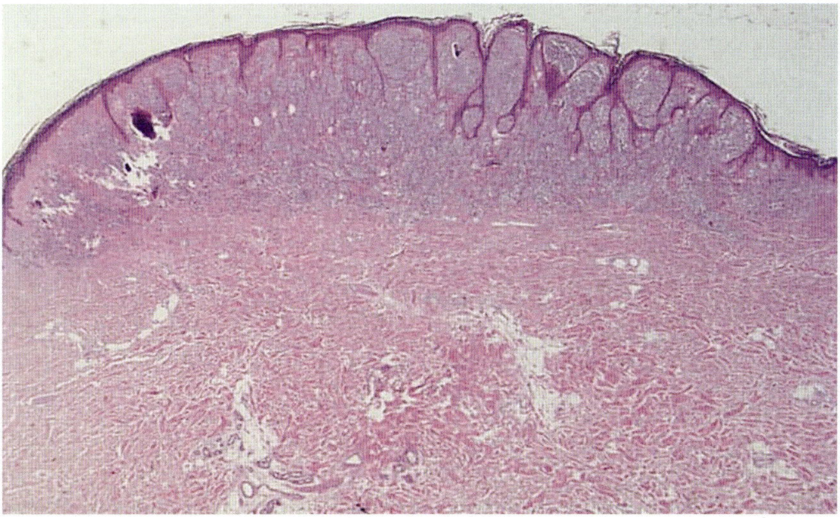

FIGURE 4.11 **Nevoid Melanoma: Smooth Contoured Variant.** The upper dermis is diffusely replaced by neoplastic melanocytes in this example of a nevoid melanoma which has generated a smooth surface contour.

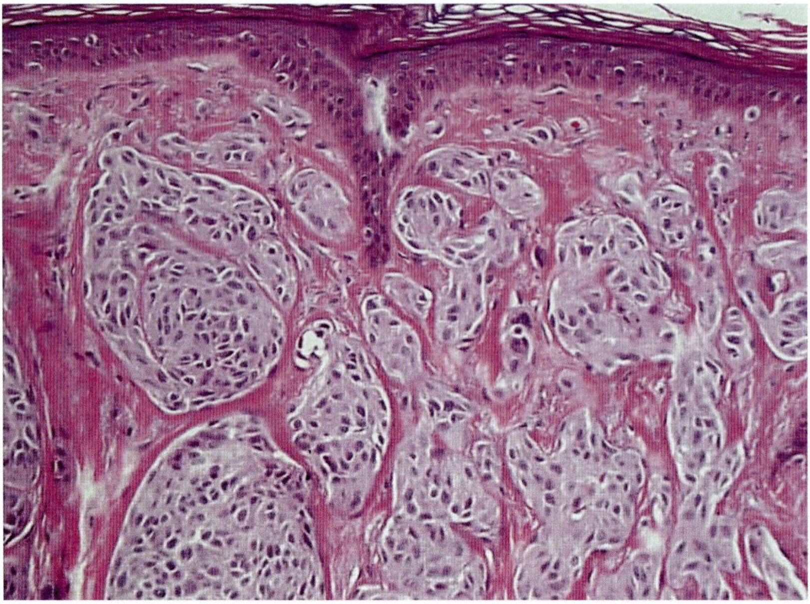

FIGURE 4.12 **Nevoid Melanoma.** There are expansile nodules deforming the papillary dermis.

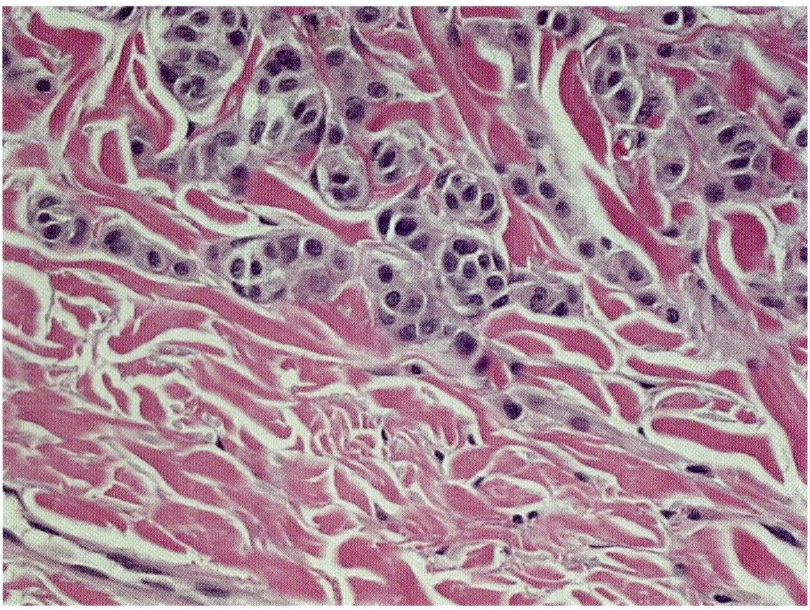

FIGURE 4.13 **Nevoid Melanoma.** At the base, the neoplastic cells manifest little or no maturation in this example; rather, the tumor cells show prominent nucleoli and large nuclei. Pseudomaturation may be seen due to presumptive compression of neoplastic cells by the collagen table, a deceptive finding in nevoid melanoma that mimics closely a benign melanocytic nevus.

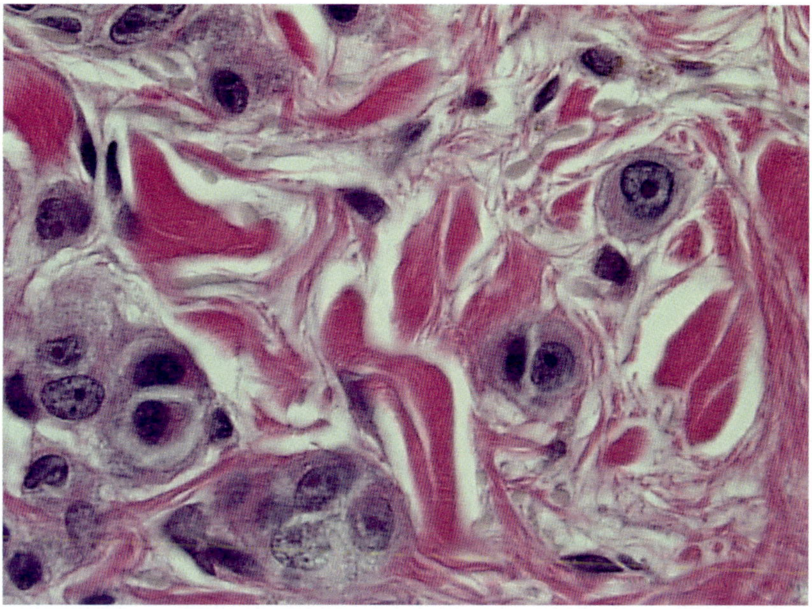

FIGURE 4.14 This oil immersion (1000× magnification) image shows the fully transformed malignant cytomorphology of nevoid melanoma. In particular, the chromatinic rims of the neoplastic melanocytes are irregularly thickened, the nucleoli are prominent, and the chromatin is spiculated.

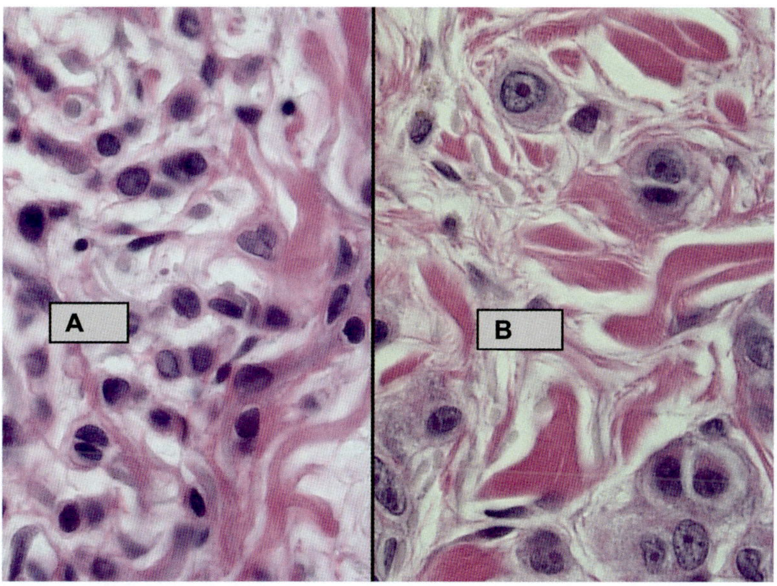

FIGURE 4.15 **Nevoid Melanoma: High Power Morphology.** The contrast between banal nevomelanocytes at the base of a benign intradermal nevus **(A)** with the neoplastic, fully transformed melanocytes of nevoid melanoma **(B)** is evident when seen at identical high power magnification.

Differential Diagnosis

The differential diagnosis of such lesions includes nevoid borderline tumors, nodular melanoma, and melanoma arising in a dermal nevus.[49,50] With respect to the first two considerations, the pattern of growth is not nevoid but rather is an expansile nodule distorting and effacing the dermal architecture. Other features such as high-grade nuclear atypia and intra-epidermal melanocytic atypia consistent with melanoma in situ are further differentiating points of nodular melanoma from nevoid melanoma. In minimal-deviation melanoma, the disposition of the cells within the dermis should allow distinction.[49,50] The expansile growth pattern displaces surrounding structures, and there are frequently remnants of the pre-existing benign nevus, be it a Spitz nevus, a congenital nevus, a common acquired nevus, or a pigmented spindle cell nevus. The minimal-deviation melanoma is equivalent to at least a level III melanoma with respect to the extent of dermal invasion.[51] The cells are relatively monotypic, manifesting mild to moderate atypia in contrast to the more fully evolved atypia seen in nevoid melanoma. The latter manifests more hyperchromatic nuclei and higher nuclear-to-cytoplasmic ratios. Mitoses are typically more scarce in minimal-deviation melanoma than in nevoid melanoma.[49–52] In melanomas arising in dermal nevi, by definition, there is a residual nevus, a feature not typical of nevoid melanoma. In addition, there is extension into the deep

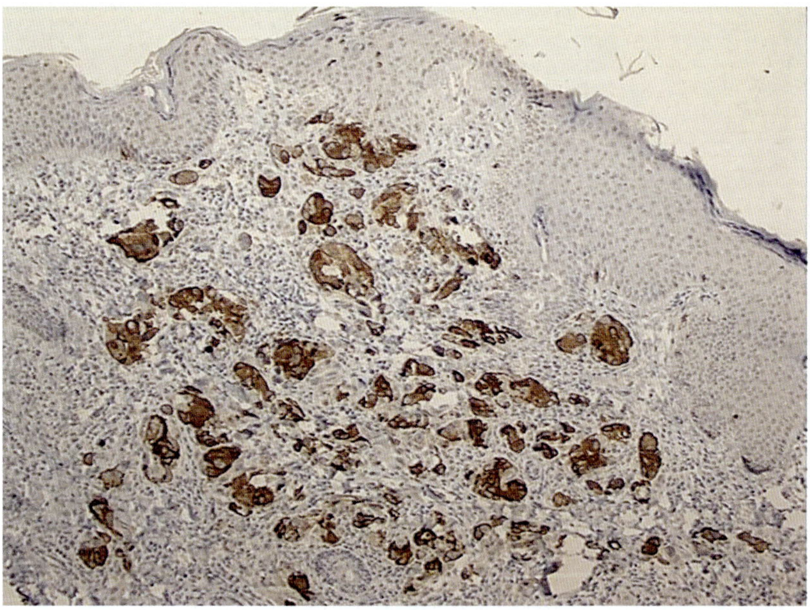

FIGURE 4.16 **Nevoid Melanoma: Loss of Differential HMB-45 Expression.** Most nevi show progressive diminution of HMB-45 and Melan-A expression in the deeper dermis. Note that this nevoid melanoma shows diffuse expression of HMB-45 in the neoplastic population.

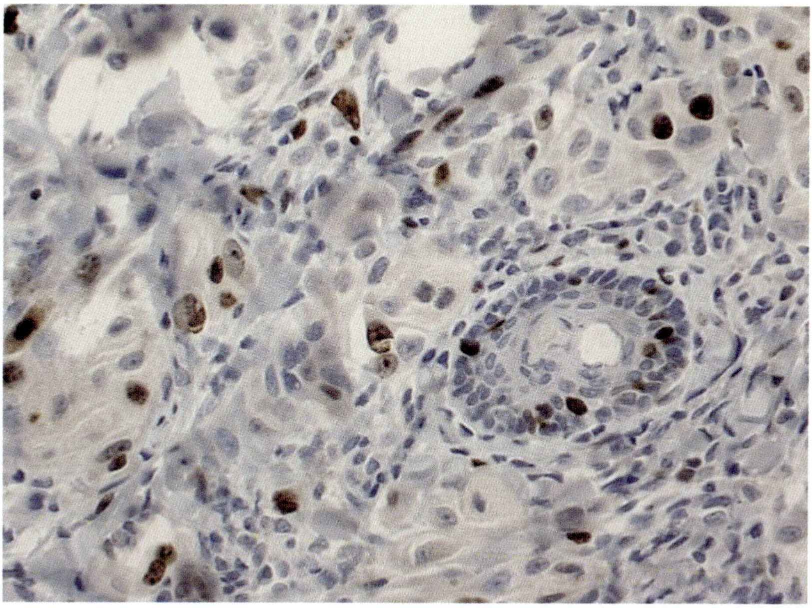

FIGURE 4.17 **Nevoid Melanoma: Ki-67 Decoration.** In nevoid melanoma, the Ki-67 expression level is higher than that seen in benign, common acquired, and Spitz nevi, where less than 10% and often less than 5% of the critical cells decorate with this nuclear marker of proliferation. In nevoid melanoma, greater than 10% and often greater than 20% of neoplastic cells decorate. Furthermore, there is no differential decoration pattern. That is, the neoplastic melanocytes diffusely express Ki-67 in a patternless fashion.

reticular dermis and fat accounting for depths greater than those reported in nevoid melanoma.[53]

There are ancillary studies that can be used to further differentiate nevoid melanoma from either dermal nevi or more common forms of melanoma. The average number of nucleolar organizing regions (AgNORs) and their nuclear area and perimeter are significantly smaller for nevoid melanoma compared to those of superficial spreading melanoma and significantly greater than those of banal dermal nevi. Digital image analysis has shown that the nuclear area in nevoid melanoma is similar to that of benign nevi; however, it is significantly less than that of conventional melanoma.[54] The differential superficial expression of HMB-45 and Ki-67 which characterizes benign nevomelanocytic proliferations is characteristically lost in nevoid melanoma (Figs. 4.16 and 4.17, e-figs. 4.32–4.35).

MINIMAL-DEVIATION MELANOMA/NEVOID BORDERLINE MELANOCYTIC TUMOR

Introduction and Clinical Features

The concept of minimal-deviation melanoma as introduced by Richard Reed is not one that is universally accepted. We feel that what Dr Reed described does, indeed, represent a distinct clinicopathologic entity. All such tumors shared an architectural growth pattern that simulates vertical growth phase melanoma, but lacked the cytologic features diagnostic of malignant transformation.[19,52] The prognosis of "minimal-deviation melanoma" is uncertain, but it has been imputed in limited series to be better when compared with other melanomas at a similar depth and level of invasion.[55] The prefered term today is *nevoid borderline melanocytic tumor*.

The nevoid borderline melanocytic tumor presents either as a nodule or a plaque that varies from flesh-colored to dark brown or blue-black, most often ranging in size from 0.5 to 1.0 cm, and is characteristically located on the trunk. Young adults in the third and fourth decades of life are most frequently affected. Often demonstrated histologically is a preexisting acquired nevus or a congenital nevus. When present in a congenital nevus, the minimal-deviation melanoma may manifest as a subcutaneous nodule; such a nodule is commonly misdiagnosed as an epidermal cyst. The histopathology of the prototypic nevoid borderline melanocytic tumor is discussed below, followed by a consideration of the entity formely known as minimal-deviation melanoma of Spitzian type. The mean age was 27 years in a recent study from Irvine, California.[56] The behavior of such lesions is unpredictable. Although in most cases the behavior appears indolent,[56] nonetheless aggressive behavior as defined by metastatic disease has been reported[57] and we have encountered it. Reed himself has suggested that minimal-deivation melanoma of less than 1.5 mm in thickness might better be classified as a "melanocytic neoplasm of indeterminate malignant potential."[58] Our prefered diagnosis, *nevoid borderline melanocytic tumor*, has thus supplanted the term *minimal deviation melanoma* in our practices.[59]

Histology

Nevoid borderline melanocytic tumor is characterized by an expansile nodule either confined to the papillary dermis (for which the

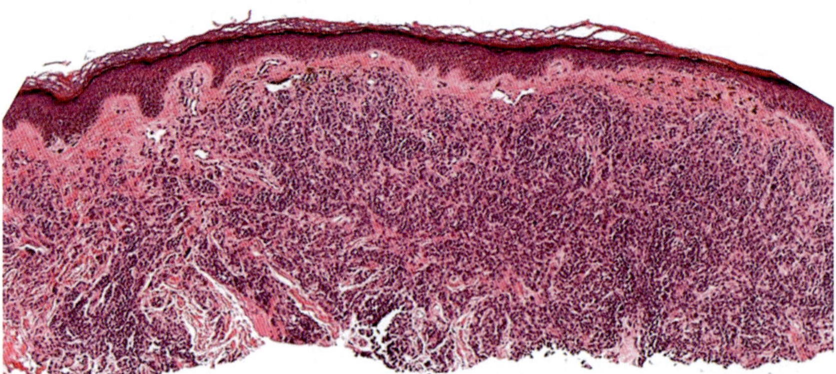

FIGURE 4.18 **Nevoid Borderline Melanocytic Tumor: Low Power Architecture.** The minimal-deviation melanoma manifests either a diffuse replacement of papillary and reticular dermal collagen or an asymmetric, expansile nodule of rather monotonous cells.

appellation "borderline melanoma" was applied by Reed) or permeative of the reticular dermis, hence resembling at scanning magnification fully evolved level III or IV vertical growth phase melanoma (Fig. 4.18). What Reed termed minimal-deviation melanoma averaged 3.4 mm in thickness, whereas what he termed "borderline melanomas" averaged 1.24 mm in thickness. There is usually no infiltration of the subcutaneous fat except in those lesions that arose in congenital nevi or in the Spitzian variants. Perineural invasion can be observed. Although the prototypic low-power architecture is one of an expansile nodule, one report describes a spindle cell form of minimal-deviation melanoma that assumed a diffusely infiltrative pattern within the dermis.[58] Mitoses are infrequently observed, and necrosis is absent. Inflammation with desmoplasia may be noted but is usually absent.[49,51,60]

These neoplastic melanocytic proliferations are composed of a relatively uniform population of moderately atypical-appearing nevuslike cells; such cells may resemble type A, B, or C nevomelanocytes or have a predominantly spindle cell morphology resembling a pigmented spindle cell nevus.[23,55,58,61] Within a given lesion, there is monotypism of cell type (Fig. 4.19). The usual prognostic variables that apply to invasive melanoma are not assigned to such a lesion, as its biological behavior cannot be predicted in the same fashion as the more aggressive conventional melanoma. The cells of nevoid borderline tumor resemble nevus cells but exhibit moderately enlarged nuclei, irregular chromatin distribution, and

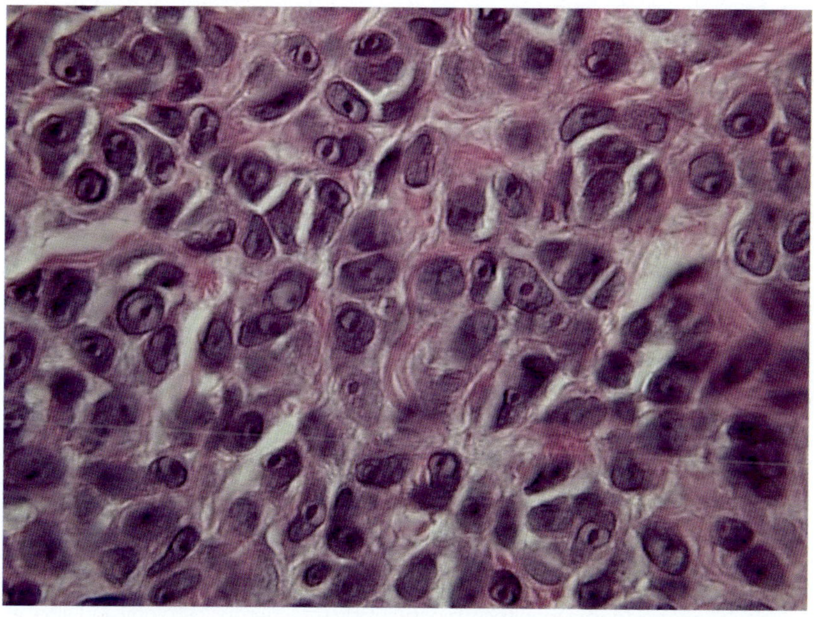

FIGURE 4.19 **Nevoid Borderline Melanocytic Tumor: High Power Microscopy.** In this oil immersion (1000× objective magnification) micrograph, the cells are monotonous, show prominent nucleoli and, frequently, irregular nuclear contours.

increased nuclear-to-cytoplasmic ratios relative to benign nevus cells (Fig. 4.20). Conspicuous nucleoli are identified. There is no apparent maturation either with respect to diminution in cell or nest size. The cells comprising the nodules are arranged in uniform, rounded nests of epithelioid pigmented cells, closely aggregated cohesive nests of small cells, or as fascicles of pigmented spindle cells resembling the patterns of type A and B nevomelanocytes and pigmented spindle cell nevi, respectively. However, the nests and/or fascicles are closely apposed with narrow bands of intervening collagenous matrix, and are irregular in size, outline, and aggregation. Mitotic activity is usually quite low; up to 6 mitoses per 100 high-power fields are observed. Corresponding studies of Ki-67 labelling show a proliferation index greater than that of Spitz or common compound nevi, but less than that of superficial spreading melanoma.[62]

The distinction of a nevoid borderline tumor arising in a congenital nevus from the proliferation nodule of the congenital nevus may be difficult. There is little difference architecturally, as both manifest a nodular pattern of growth that results in distortion of the dermal silhouette. However, in the proliferation nodule the cells are cytologically bland with inconspicuous nucleoli and merge with the background nevus cell population.

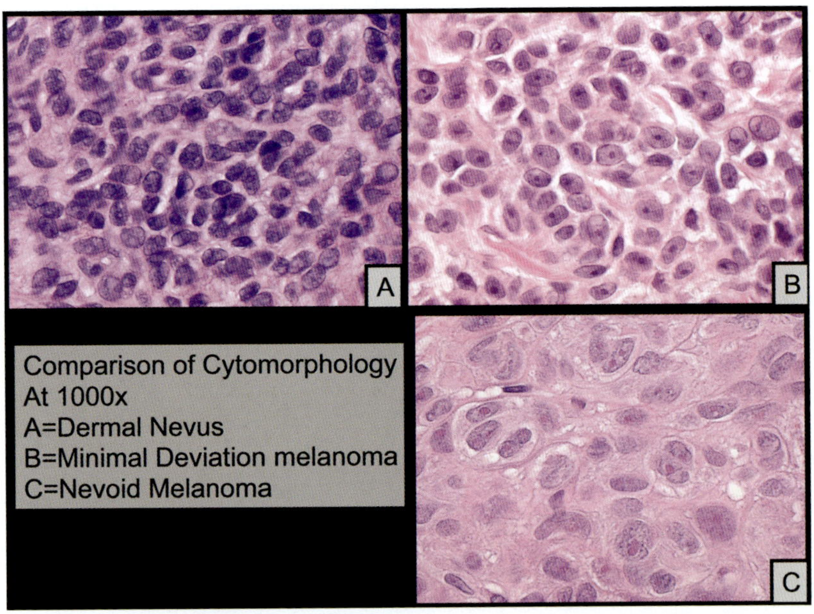

FIGURE 4.20 This illustration demonstrates the comparative morphology of the melanocytes at 1000× objective magnification in a banal intradermal nevus **(A)**, a nevoid borderline tumor **(B)**, and a nevoid melanoma **(C)**. As can be easily appreciated, the minimal-deviation melanoma manifests a particularly treacherous cytology and also, at least in the hands of some observers, has a lower risk of metastasis than nevoid and other more conventional vertical growth phase melanomas of epithelioid type.

Collagen surrounds the individual nevomelanocytes within proliferation nodules, whereas tumor cells in melanomas are not surrounded by collagen or basement membrane material. This likely relates to certain biological properties of vertical growth phase melanoma, specifically, the expression of transmembrane metalloproteinases which digest basement membrane material and facilitate the growth and spread of tumor. In nevoid borderline tumor, cellular atypia and rare mitoses are seen. The cells have a cytomorphology disparate from the remainder of the lesion. Mitoses are uncommon in both the proliferation nodule and the minimal-deviation melanoma, but, because mitoses can be seen in either, their presence is not a distinguishing criterion.

ANIMAL-TYPE MELANOMA IN HUMANS (MELANOMA WITH PROMINENT PIGMENT SYNTHESIS) AND THE PIGMENTED EPITHELIOID MELANOCYTOMA

Introduction

The existence in horses of skin neoplasms comprising nodules of heavily melanized cells has been recognized for centuries and is termed equine melanotic disease.[63–65] These common neoplasms classically develop in old gray horses and are also described in nonequine animal models such as those induced via cutaneous application of topical carcinogens.[66–69] The similarities between these lesions and a similar process in humans were first recognized by Darier in 1925.[70] As only a few human cases are described, the biological behavior of these heavily pigmented "animal-type" melanomas is unclear.[71] In one series, patients seemed to manifest a long indolent phase,[72] although in our hands two of six patients developed metastases and one died of disease.[71] There is one case report where metastasis to a regional lymph node occurred without widespread dissemination, another case report describing a local cutaneous metastasis 1 year after excision,[65] and a third case report of a patient who developed widespread metastatic disease.[73]

Animal-type melanoma manifests a common theme, namely, a tumorous proliferation of melanocytes with striking pigment synthesis. The differential diagnosis encompasses benign cellular pigment-synthesizing melanocytic tumors, but there is sufficient distinctiveness to the histomorphology and to the biological behavior to preclude other diagnoses such as cellular blue nevus or deep-penetrating nevus. Pigmented epithelioid melanocytoma is a more recent term applied to these borderline melanocytic tumors.

Clinical Features

The lesions present as blue-black plaques or nodules averaging 1 cm in diameter (e-fig. 4.36), but with some lesions measuring several centimeters, without a predilection for site or sex. In our own series, four of the patients were in the first or second decades of life, suggesting an incidence skewed to a younger population. There was no association with familial dysplastic nevus syndrome, sun exposure, or family history of malignant melanoma disease.[71] Tuthill et al. reported an 18-year-old woman with a 10-year history of a shoulder plaque that reached a size of 10 cm before excision; the lesion was of variegated shades of brown, blue, and black comprising beaded rows of papules and macules. One year after the initial excision, a cutaneous metastasis developed at the graft site. Levene described a progressive punctate dermal melanocytosis that started in childhood and terminated in the fifth decade as disseminated melanoma.[72] Pathy et al. described a 65-year-old man who developed numerous nodules in the periphery of a giant blue nevus of the scalp that had been present since childhood. His subsequent course was one of local satellite metastases and of subsequent spread to cervical lymph nodes and parotid gland.[73]

Histology

These tumors are heavily pigmented neoplasms that extend to the dermal subcutaneous interface and often lack a grenz zone of papillary dermal sparing (Figs. 4.21 and 4.22, e-figs. 4.37–4.39). Pagetoid infiltration of a hyperplastic epidermis may be seen (e-fig. 4.40). Tumor cell cytoplasms manifest pigment deposition that ranges from fine granular deposits of light brown melanin to dark brown coarse deposits that obscure nuclear detail (e-figs. 4.40 and 4.41). The latter, when manifesting polygonal or rounded cytoplasmic contours, are difficult to distinguish from the melanophages present in variable numbers in all cases. The tumor cells have either a spindled morphology or a polygonal morphology, the spindled cells frequently being disposed in fascicles. The population with a rounded or polygonal contour often assumes a nodular disposition within the dermis. Areas of confluent melanocytic growth are invariably present and typically dissipate in cellularity at the periphery of the lesion where the cells manifest a dendritic appearance that may be mistaken for a blue nevus. Mitotic activity is usually very low, a host response is negligible, ulceration is never seen, and intravascular invasion is not identified. The dominant cytomorphology in most cases is that of cells that show some nuclear atypia, namely, regular oval to round nuclear shapes, with moderate anisonucleosis, small nucleoli, and delicate, evenly distributed chromatin; characteristically, these do not fulfill the cytologic criteria of malignancy (Figs. 4.23–4.25, e-figs. 4.42–4.45). In our series, roughly half of cases had a cytomorphology was recognizably malignant. The tumors with overt cytologic anaplasia have in the past been termed "animal type melanoma" or "melanoma with prominent pigment synthesis," terms which some authors continue to apply today. An important clue to the diagnosis is effacement of dermal architecture by areas of confluent melanocytic growth. There is a propensity for tumor cells to infiltrate the adventitial dermis of follicular and adnexal structures. The close association of the tumor cells to the follicular sheaths has prompted an alternative appellation for this neoplasm, namely, pilar neurocristic hamartoma.[65,71,73,74] The latter is apparently a hamartomatous lesion in which melanoma with

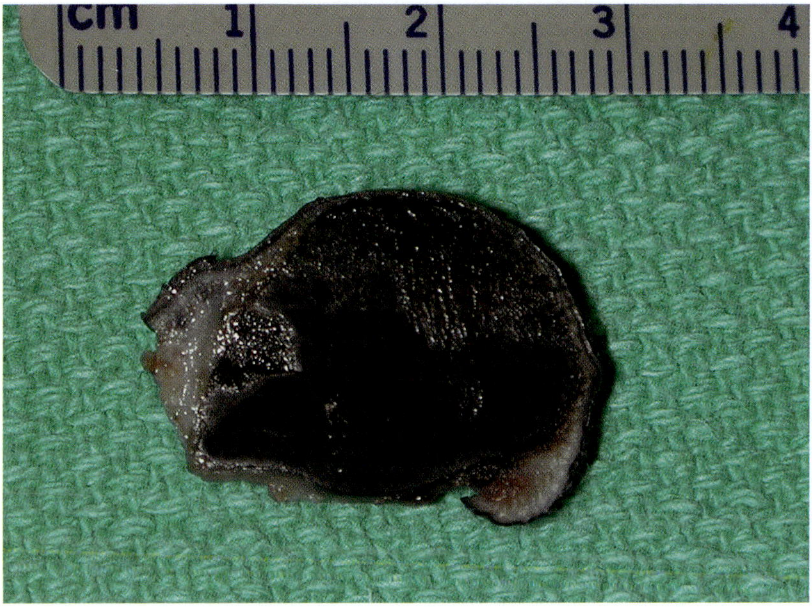

FIGURE 4.21 **Pigmented Epithelioid Melanocytoma ("Animal Type Melanoma").** This particular tumor shows a 2.5 cm diameter black nodule extensively replacing the dermis and upper subcutis.

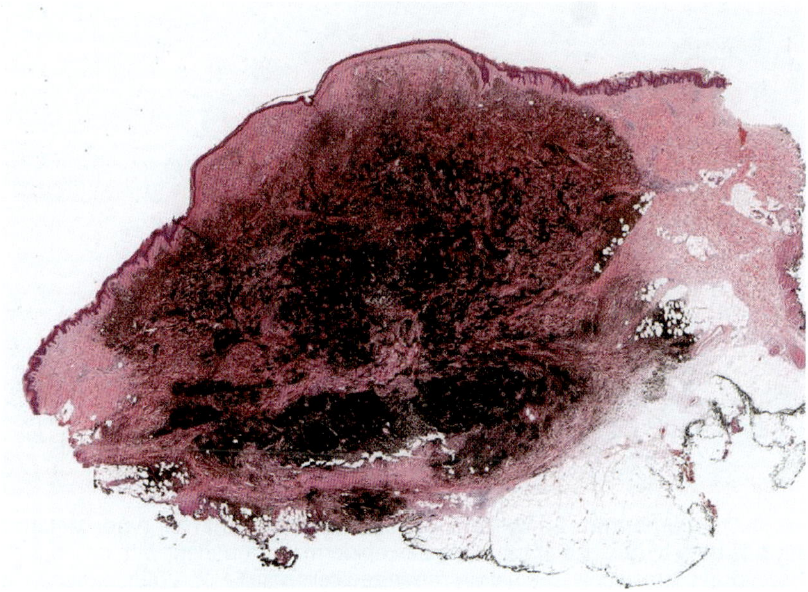

FIGURE 4.22 **Pigmented Epithelioid Melanocytoma ("Animal Type Melanoma").** The tumor diffusely replaces the dermis and the upper subcutis and manifests prominent pigment deposition which obscures nuclear detail.

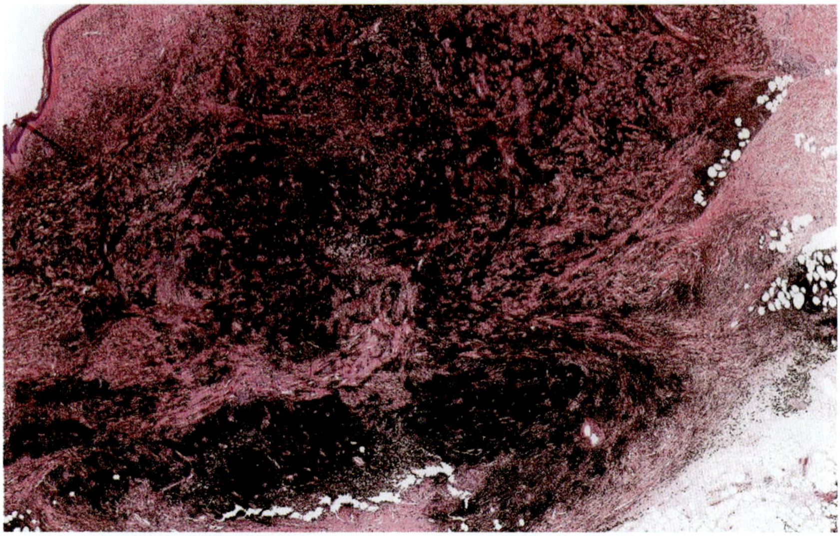

FIGURE 4.23 **Pigmented Epithelioid Melanocytoma ("Animal Type Melanoma").** Heavy melanin pigment obscures nuclear detail.

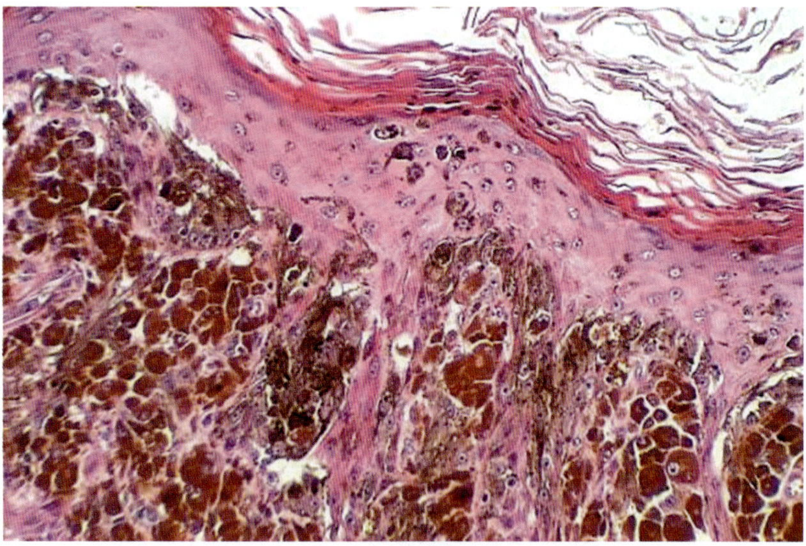

FIGURE 4.24 **Pigmented Epithelioid Melanocytoma ("Animal Type Melanoma").** Roughly one third to one half of cases have an epidermal component with prominent pagetoid spread. In this example, the heavily melanized cells manifest prominent dendritic processes within the epidermis.

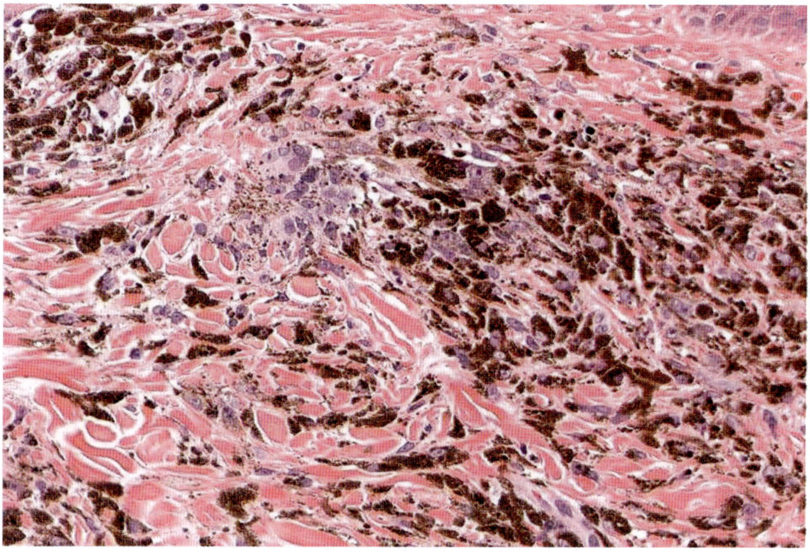

FIGURE 4.25 **Pigmented Epithelioid Melanocytoma ("Animal Type Melanoma").** Where nuclear details can be discerned, the nuclei are clearly atypical and large with high nucleocytoplasmic ratios and prominent nucleoli. Melanin bleach preparations can be employed to remove the pigment, and thus to identify mitotic activity.

prominent melanin synthesis may arise; some cases of animal-type melanoma develop in the setting of a hybrid pattern of blue nevus with a background perifollicular and perieccrine population of well-differentiated pigment-laden cells which seem to give rise to the foci of melanoma. Metastases have a variable morphology in this scenario, whereby some deposits resemble pilar neurocristic hamartoma and others are typical of melanoma. Malignancy developing in other prominent pigment-synthesizing tumors is described for cellular blue nevi,[75,76] extrasacral mongolian spots, and the nevi of Ota and Ito.[77] Precursor dysplastic, common acquired, or congenital nevi have not been identified. The typical case lacks melanoma in situ; rather, like nodular melanoma, there may be pagetoid spread centrally overlying massive dermal involvement. One case in our series had a precursor lesion suggestive of a cellular blue nevus, whereas three other cases had areas recapitulating the morphology of a common blue nevus.[71] Other authors have reported an apparent relationship with blue nevi, suggesting a common histogenetic precursor, namely, the dermal dendritic melanocyte. Perhaps these tumors should be considered a form of aggressive dermal melanocytosis with a potential to metastasize.[78] In our experience, those cases with bland cytomorphology did not manifest aggressive behavior, whereas, of those cases with overtly anaplastic nuclei, one showed intracutaneous metastatic disease and one led to death from metastasis. The term "pigmented epithelioid melanoma" without qualification is used only for those cases that have banal cytology or show low-grade nuclear atypia. They have a propensity for sentinal lymph node metastasis but only rarely extend into non-sentinal lymph nodes in the drainage basin. These appear to represent the great majority of the heavily pigmented lesions.

Differential Diagnosis

The differential diagnosis of such lesions includes cellular blue nevus, blue nevus with hypercellularity, the heavily pigmented epithelioid cell nevus, and regressed melanoma with prominent melanophage accumulation.[79–82] Cellular blue nevus manifests nests of cells with monotonous round to oval nuclei, bland, evenly dispersed chromatin, and abundant quantities of clear cytoplasm with well-defined cell margins arranged in discrete nodules. There is an interposition by components typical of a common blue nevus and nests of melanophages in the stroma between tumor nodules. The cellular blue nevus typically assumes a "dumbbell"-shaped configuration that is vertically oriented. The cellular foci may be relatively devoid of pigment synthesis, the foci of prominent pigment synthesis being identified in the more hypocellular blue nevuslike areas. The blue nevus with hypercellularity resembles a common blue nevus, but also contains cellular fascicles of relatively amelanotic spindled cells. The blue nevus with hypercellularity is not as large as a cellular blue nevus and fails to demonstrate the dumbbell-shaped configuration that is typical of the cellular blue nevus. The heavily pigmented epithelioid cell nevus is usually well circumscribed, with either a rounded or wedge-shaped lower border, and the cells, where visible, have a bland cytomorphology. Although we have encountered a case of animal-type melanoma with a whorled, or storiform, low-power architecture, we do not consider the Bednar tumor (pigmented dermatofibrosarcoma protuberans) to be a realistic differential diagnostic consideration. The reason for this is that the dendritic pigmented cells scattered throughout the Bednar tumor are incapable of producing a sufficient quantity of melanin to obscure nuclear features. If in doubt, the critical cells in the Bednar tumor mark, as expected, with antibody to CD34.[83]

Features of regressed vertical growth phase melanoma include a distinctive pattern of delicate fibrosis comprising fine collagen fibers amidst an edematous matrix that contains scattered mononuclear cells. Prominent elongated venules are present, often with a perpendicular arrangement to the epidermis. Amidst these stromal alterations are accumulations of pigment-laden macrophages that can assume a globular architecture similar to animal-type melanoma, but lack nuclear atypia. The nuclei of the critical cells of animal-type melanoma are variable in size and shape but never include those with the reniform contour of a histiocyte. In regressed melanoma, the melanin pigment is coarse and irregularly distributed within the cytoplasms of melanophages, which contrasts with the fine granular pattern of deposition seen in the neoplastic melanocytes in animal-type melanoma. Immunohistochemical stains would be confirmatory of the dominant histiocytic composition of the infiltrate in regressed melanoma; the dominant cell type in lesions of equine melanoma is a spindled melanocyte. We recommend the use of an alternate chromagen to diaminobenzidene (DAB), because the brown reaction product of this chromagen may be difficult to visualize in the melanized tumor. One alternative choice for a chromagen is aminoethylcarbazole (AEC), which decorates the reaction product with a distinct reddish-brown color. Another would be a streptavi din-alkaline-phosphatase system followed by new fuschin chromagen (Bio Genex Laboratories, San Ramon, California), which imparts a distinctive purplish hue to the reaction product. A third alternative that we employ is the alkaline phosphatase system using Fast Red chromagen (Ventana Medical Systems, Inc, Tucson, Arizona). We do not recommend the use of permanganate–oxalate bleach methods to remove the melanin pigment, as their use causes loss of decoration with antibodies Melan-A and HMB-45. Although S100 protein antigenicity is maintained in permanganate–oxalate bleach methods, the specificity of S100 expression as an indicator of melanocytic differentiation is, of course, less.

Management and Prognosis

The biological behavior of animal-type melanoma is hard to predict, given the small series in the literature. There is some evidence that tumors with banal cytologic characteristics behave in a more indolent fashion. Although the tumor can be lethal, given the depth and level of reported lesions and the lack of a host response, it would seem that in most instances the course is less aggressive than that of nodular or superficial spreading vertical growth phase melanomas with similar histologic parameters. Lesions of animal-type melanoma manifest a low mitotic index and lack regression, vascular invasion, or ulceration. As there is a potential for aggressive behavior that cannot be reliably predicted on the basis of histologic criteria, we advise re-excision of all animal-type melanomas with 1 to 2 cm margins. Sentinel lymph node biopsies are also probably of value and should be performed in cases where this procedure is available. A recent study of heavily pigmented epithelioid melanocytic neoplasms, lumped together under the common term "pigemented epithelioid melanocytoma," showed regional lymph node metastases in 46% of cases in which lymph node biopsies were performed. Only 24 of 40 patients in that series underwent lymph node biopsies, however, suggesting that this grouping of lesions included those known or thought most likely to have no metastatic potential.[84] In an earlier study, seven of 10 patients with pigment synthesizing tumors who underwent sentinel lymph node biopsies were found to have metastatic tumor deposits.[85] Follow-up, as in any case of invasive malignant melanoma, should be conducted. Our recent study showed a low incidence of regional lymph node metastasis, and no reported deaths attributable to diseases.[59]

MALIGNANT BLUE NEVUS

Introduction and Clinical Features

The malignant blue nevus is a rare lesion first described by Allen and Spitz,[86] that usually arises in a background of cellular blue nevus.[87–97] These lesions are most common on the scalp, although they have been reported at other sites such as the arm (Figs. 4.26 and 4.27).[98] In only rare cases will a malignant blue nevus arise de novo with no apparent benign precursor, and in

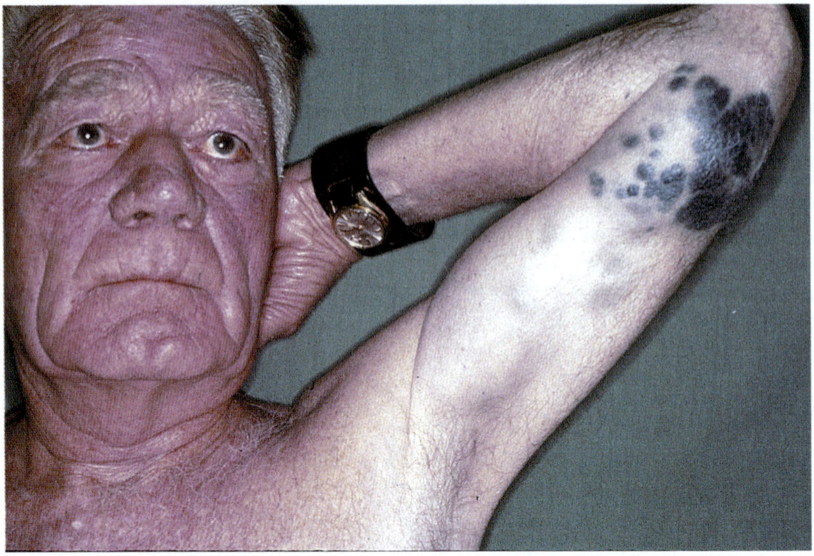

FIGURE 4.26 **Malignant Blue Nevus.** This elderly man's longstanding blue nevus underwent progressive expansion to a size of over 12 cm and developed multiple blue-black satellite nodules within it. (Case courtesy of Dr Mirek Stranc, Winnipeg, Manitoba.)

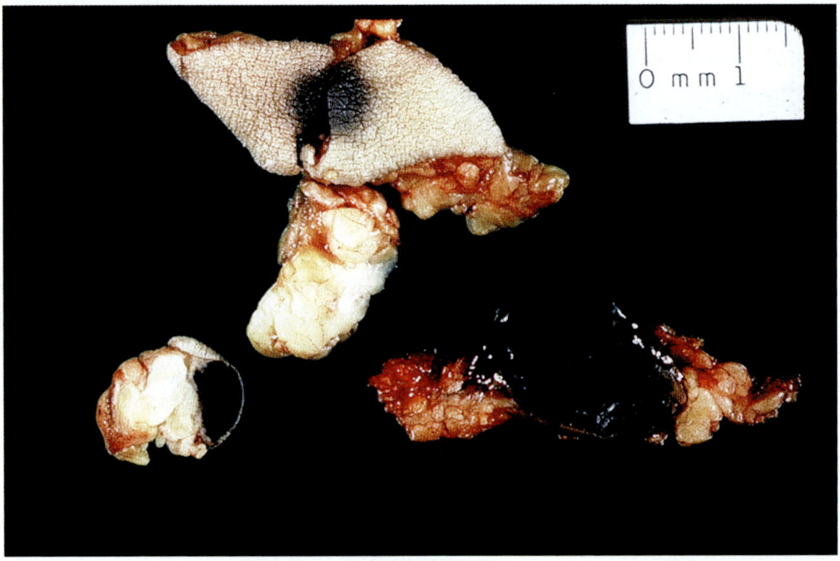

FIGURE 4.27 **Malignant Blue Nevus.** Note the blue-black nodule with a surface diameter in excess of 1 cm and a superoinferior dimension of 1.5 cm, as the tumor infiltrates the subcutaneous tissue. (Case courtesy of Dr Mirek Stranc, Winnipeg, Manitoba.)

such circumstances, an alternate label or diagnosis should be considered. Although the precursor lesion has invariably been present since birth or early childhood, malignant transformation occurs in an age group typically greater than 45 years,[94] with a male preponderance. The clinical hallmarks of malignant cellular blue nevus include rapid enlargement, ulceration, and change in color. The lesions may attain a large size (3 to 13 cm). The tumor is thought to have an aggressive behavior and metastasizes in the majority of patients.[98-100] Molecular analysis following microdissection has failed to show loss of heterozygosity for a number of genes operative in melanomagenesis, such as MTS1, MX11, CMM1, p53, NF1, L-myc, hOCG1, and MCC.[97]

Histology

There is typically a background lesion consistent with a cellular blue nevus (Fig. 4.28),[90,95,96,97] usually situated laterally to the malignant component. Occasional examples have been seen superimposed upon pre-existing nevi of Ito or Ota.[77,101] An exceptional case may arise in the background of a dermal melanocytosis in other settings, such as in a nevus spilus.[102] In most cases, a moderately dense inflammatory cell infiltrate is present at the base. The histologic features of the benign component, be it a blue or cellular blue nevus, are prototypic for the respective entity. Amidst this precursor lesion are fascicles and nodules of markedly pleomorphic spindle and epithelioid

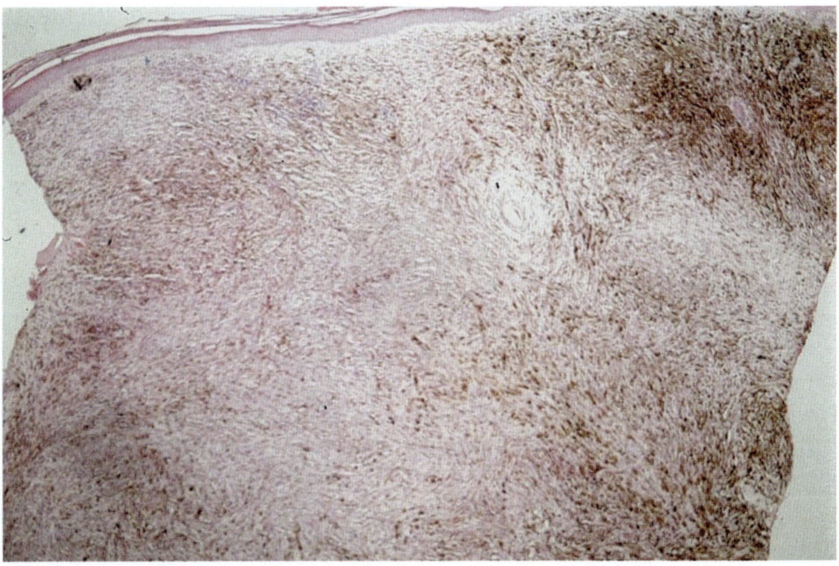

FIGURE 4.28 **Malignant Blue Nevus.** In this example, there is heavy pigment synthesis within the dermis. The central area of depigmentation represents a zone of confluent necrosis which is characteristic of malignant blue nevus; the peripheral aspects show more typical blue nevus and/or cellular blue nevus.

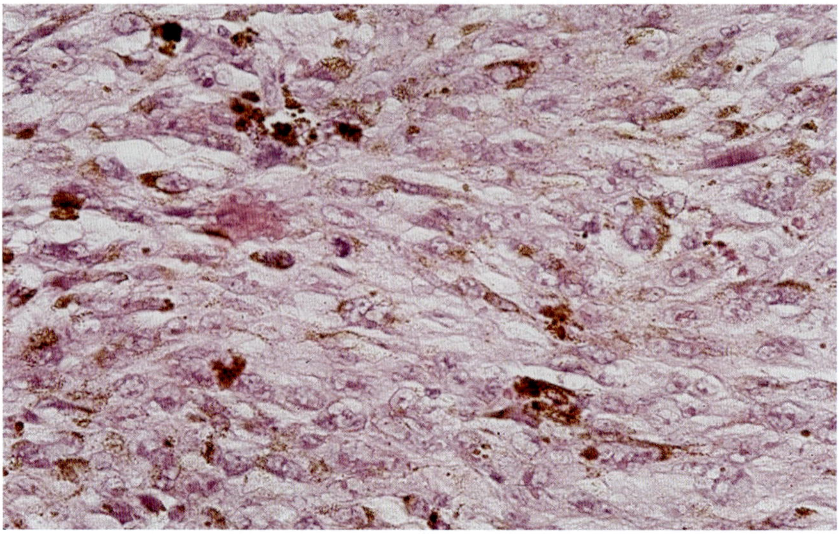

FIGURE 4.29 **Malignant Blue Nevus.** Where nuclear preservation is optimal, mitotic figures can be seen and the fully transformed malignant cytology of this lesion can be appreciated.

cells, the former cell type dominating in the fascicular component and the latter being primarily found within the nodular areas. The fascicles and nodules coalesce, resulting in effacement of the dermal architecture (e-figs. 4.46–4.52). This form of malignant melanoma frequently exhibits extension into the subcutis. There are interspersed bizarre tumor giant cells. Numerous abnormal mitotic figures are observed, averaging 8 to 9 per mm^2 (Fig. 4.29).[92] Zones of tumor cell necrosis are observed. There may be blood vessel invasion. A junctional component is typically absent.[94]

Differential Diagnosis

The differential diagnosis is primarily with a cellular blue nevus with atypia[92,103,104] versus the pigmented epithelioid melanocytoma.[71] In the atypical cellular blue nevus there is a minor component that appears very similar to a malignant cellular blue nevus as manifested by marked pleomorphism, the presence of bizarre giant cells, and atypical mitoses. Such atypical cells are the dominant component in malignant cellular blue nevus, but by contrast comprise only a small component of the cellular blue nevus with atypia. Possibly, the latter represents a cellular blue nevus in transition to a malignant cellular blue nevus. The main differentiating points, in addition to the extent of the cytologic atypism in the lesion, are large areas of necrosis, a high mitotic rate, blood vessel invasion, and cytologic atypia with nucleolar prominence. The animal-type melanoma typically has less atypical cytology and a lower mitotic rate, and it does not manifest confluent necrosis as does the malignant blue nevus.[19,71] The diagnosis of malignant blue nevus should be considered when a lesion that has arisen in a pre-existing blue or cellular blue nevus exhibits highly atypical epithelioid melanocyte with bizarre tumor giant cells and numerous abnormal mitotic figures averaging 8 to 9 per mm^2.

It should be remembered that cellular blue nevi can be associated with rests within lymph nodes,[81] mimicking metastatic disease.

UNUSUAL CYTMORPHOLOGIC AND PHENOTYPIC VARIANTS OF MELANOMA (METAPLASATIC, BALLOON, SIGNET RING, MYXOID, SMALL CELL, AND RHABDOID MELANOMA)

The spectrum of abnormal phenotypes which can be encountered in melanoma includes the expression of morphologies and antigens more commonly encountered in the lesions of epithelial, fibrohistiocytic, rhabdoid, smooth muscle, and osteocartilagenous derivation. Conversely, some melanomas do not express markers commonly associated with melanocytic phenotypes (i.e., S100 protein or HMB-45) and thus prove to be particularly treacherous diagnostic pitfalls.

METAPLASTIC CHANGE IN MALIGNANT MELANOMA

Metaplastic foci mimicking osteogenic sarcoma have been described in the lesions of malignant melanoma. Some of these cases were associated with external iatrogenic procedures, suggesting the role of trauma as an inducing factor (Fig. 4.30).[105–111]

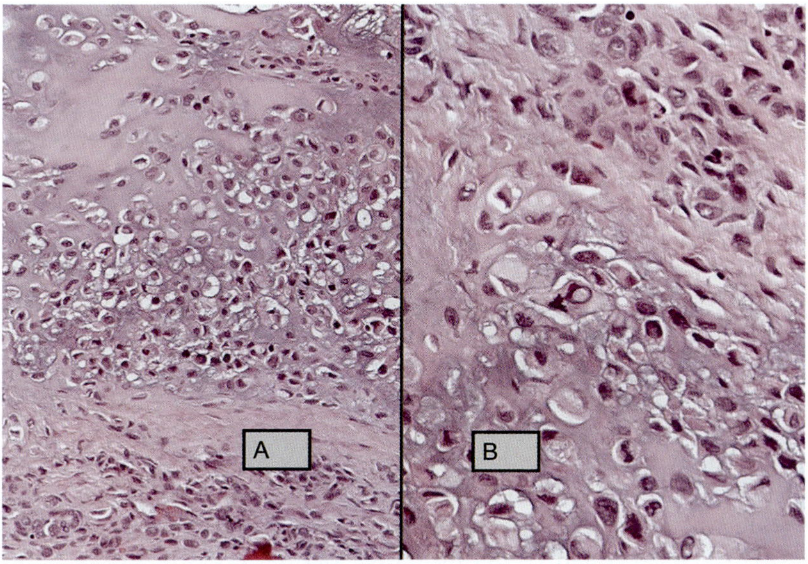

FIGURE 4.30 **Metaplastic Melanoma.** In this subungual melanoma, extensive cartilaginous matrix is produced by the neoplastic melanocytes **(A)**. Malignant cytologic features are visible at intermediate and high power microscopy **(B)**.

Osteosarcomatous metaplasia in a malignant melanoma may be the sequela of an alteration in benign stromal fibroblasts as a host response to the tumor, or it could represent a divergent differentiation pattern, whereby melanoma cells acquire the machinery necessary for the production of malignant osteoid. Cartilaginous metaplasia has also been described,[106,110,112] often combined with bone formation to yield a form of osteocartilaginous metaplasia, such as that reported in one case of a nasal mucosal primary and its metastasis[110] and in cases of subungual melanoma.[111,112] Mesenchymal elements with rhabdomyoblastic, lipoblastic, and neurogenous features have been described in those malignant melanomas that arise in giant congenital nevus.[113]

BALLOON CELL MELANOMA

Clinical Features

Balloon cell melanoma is a rare form of vertical growth phase malignant melanoma characterized by a nodular proliferation of neoplastic balloon cells; the background lesion is typically one of a superficial spreading melanoma.[114] Clinically, lesions appear as soft, rubbery, or firm nodules with a polypoid or papillomatous contour whose cut surfaces are grayish white or brown.[115] The prognosis is similar to that of other types of malignant melanoma matched for depth of invasion, with tumor thickness being of greatest importance and the poor patient-survival statistics usually reflecting the deep extent of the tumor at the time of presentation. In the largest series on record, 57.5% of patients died with metastatic disease 2 months to 12 years after initial surgery.[115] Primary balloon cell melanoma in brain arising from melanoblastic meningeal (or diffuse meningeal) nevus has been described.[116] Amelanotic balloon cell melanoma represents a common histologic variant in the spectrum of feline malignant melanoma[117] and has also been described in humans.[118] This unusual neoplasm has been reported in the choroids.[119,120]

Histology

The tumor is characterized by nests and sheets of large cells that exhibit an abundant quantity of clear or finely vacuolated cytoplasm (Fig. 4.31). The lesion resembles a balloon cell nevus, although there are important distinguishing features. In particular, there is effacement of dermal architecture by sheets of neoplastic cells with no intervening stroma. Cytologic atypia and mitotic activity are present, and necrosis, when visible, is a helpful sign. The nuclei are large and exhibit prominent nucleoli and highly irregular chromatin patterns. The clearness of cytoplasms in some cases appears to be due to the intracellular accumulation of glycogen as characterized by strong diastase-sensitive periodic acid-Schiff (PAS) positivity.[121] In the majority of ultrastructural studies, however, the vacuoles either appear empty or are held to represent degenerating melanosomes in a fashion

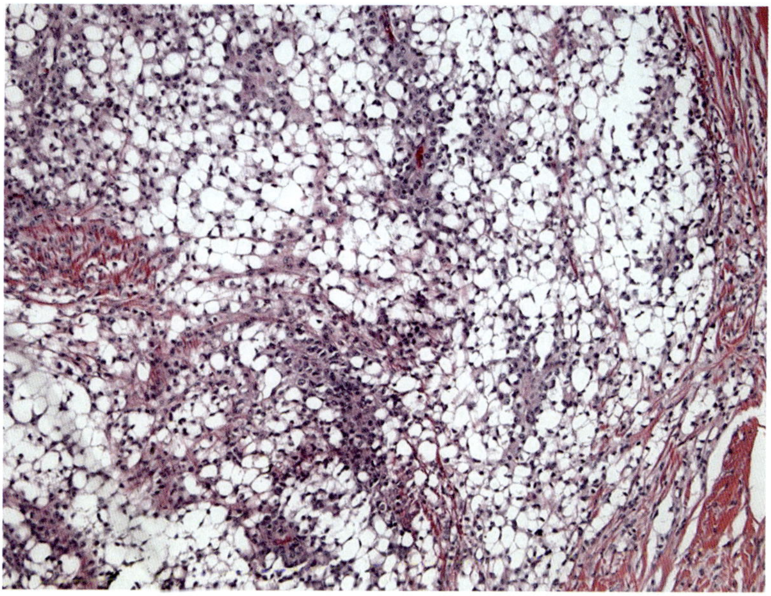

FIGURE 4.31 **Balloon Cell Melanoma.** The vertical growth phase of balloon cell melanoma is characterized by clear or empty cytoplasmic spaces, which indent and displace the nucleus to the peripheral margin of the cell. In some areas, conventional epithelioid vertical growth phase melanoma can be identified.

analogous to the balloon cell change of benign nevi.[115,120,122] This is also likely true of most metastases from balloon cell melanomas, which in one report, did not contain glycogen, fat, or melanin.[118] In another case of metastatic balloon cell melanoma, however, the tumor cells were shown by electron microscopy to contain lipid.[123] Immunohistochemical studies with antibodies to S100 protein, Melan-A, and HMB-45 are positive in balloon cell melanoma and its metastases (Fig. 4.32),[115,118,124,125] whereas neuron-specific enolase preparations tend to decorate the cells weakly.[115]

Differential Diagnosis

The differential diagnosis encompasses balloon cell change in benign nevi including blue nevi[122] and common acquired nevi, with which balloon cell melanoma may coexist,[125] as well as other malignant clear cell neoplasms. The latter include clear cell sarcoma of soft parts, atypical fibroxanthoma and granular cell carcinoma with clear cell change, metastatic renal cell carcinoma, clear cell basal cell carcinoma, and malignant clear cell acrospiroma[115] as well as sebaceous carcinoma and clear cell squamous cell carcinoma. Benign nonmelanocytic lesions that merit consideration include lepromatous leprosy, xanthomata and hibernomas,[115] and clear cell dermatofibroma.[126] Regarding the latter, overlying epidermal hyperplasia and a storiform arrangement of spindle cells amidst sclerotic stroma typical of a benign fibrohistiocytic neoplasm are characteristic. The critical cells in

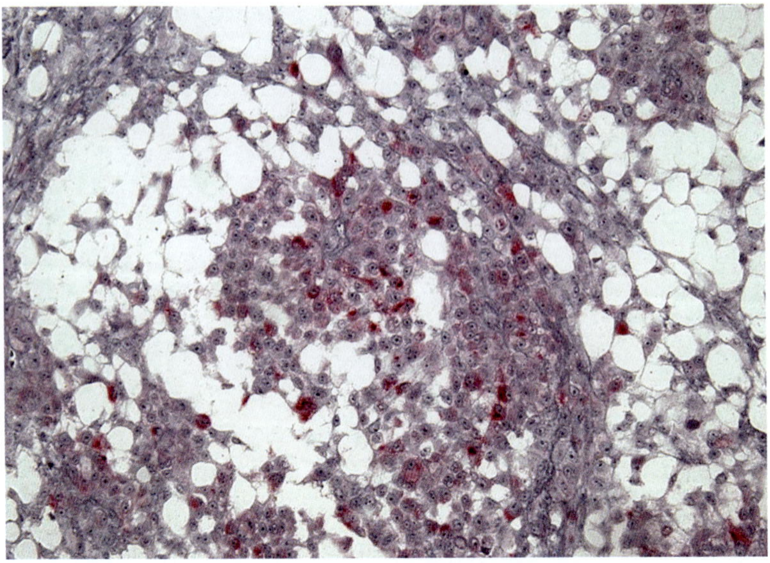

FIGURE 4.32 **Balloon Cell Melanoma: Melan-A Immunohistochemical Preparation.** Although the balloon cell areas typically are Melan-A and HMB-45 negative, the more conventional epithelioid vertical growth phase zones show cytopasmic expression of Melan-A in this figure, attesting to their melanocytic derivation. The balloon cell change is largely attributed to degeneration of melanosomes and their phagocytosis within lysosomal structures, thus perhaps explaining the relative lack of expression of Melan-A and HMB-45.

clear cell dermatofibroma are factor XIII positive.[126] Balloon cell melanoma cells can mimic foamy histiocytes at fine needle aspiration biopsy.[127]

SIGNET RING CELL MELANOMA

A signet ring morphology may be observed in lesions of melanoma and most commonly reflects metastatic or recurrent lesions (Fig. 4.33).[128,129] The finding of signet ring differentiation in malignant melanoma is an unusual event, being seen in some 0.5% of melanomas.[128] Such findings raise diagnostic consideration of metastatic adenocarcinoma, particularly in metastatic sites[129,130] and in pleural or peritoneal effusion cytology.[131] The signet ring cells may have a small cell, large cell, or giant cell morphology. Ultrastructural examination reveals that the vacuolated appearance is most often imparted by the intracytoplasmic accumulation of intermediate filaments, specifically, vimentin.[132,133] The cells characteristically decorate with antibodies to S100 protein and are HMB-45 positive; however, exceptions to this profile exist. For example, cases of S100-positive, HMB-45-negative signet ring melanoma are described[134,135] as are cases of HMB-45-positive, S100-negative signet ring melanoma.[136] In rare examples, intracytoplasmic neutral mucin may be observed. The differential diagnosis of signet ring melanoma includes neoplasms with prominent cytoplasmic vacuolation;

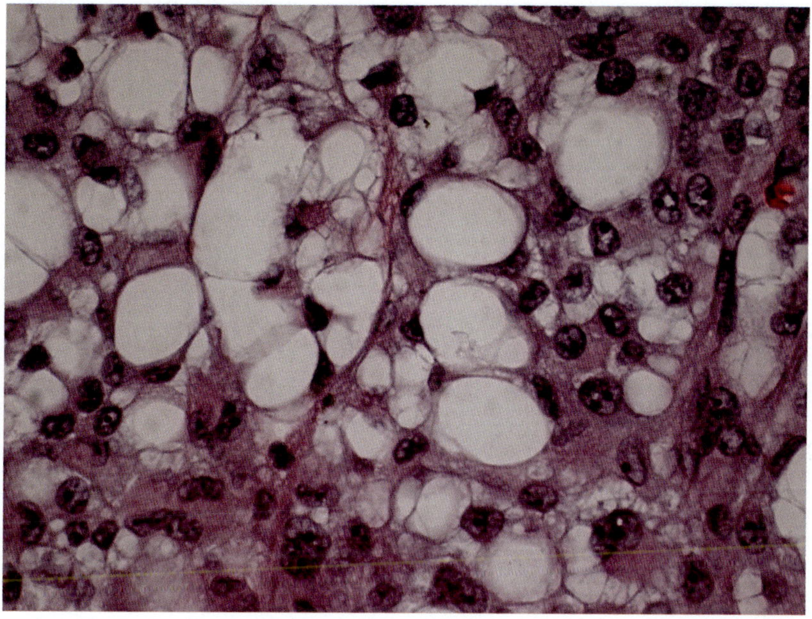

FIGURE 4.33 **Signet Ring Melanoma.** In signet ring melanoma, as in balloon cell melanoma, a large vacuole displaces the nucleus to the periphery of the cell; however, the tumor cells may also have a bubbly or physaliferous morphology. In this case, the bubbly morphology and the cytoplasmic vacuolization are attributable to the accumulation of aggregates of vimentin filaments, as proven at the ultrastructural level.

tumors of vascular endothelium or adipose tissue, signet ring lymphoma,[137] and epithelioid smooth muscle lesions as well as the obvious signet ring adenocarcinoma are thus considered.[138] This is a common histologic variant in malignant melanoma in animal models.[117]

MYXOID MELANOMA

Introduction and Clinical Features

Most often, the myxoid melanoma presents as a metastatic tumor deposit that is associated with a primary neoplasm that does not manifest a myxoid morphology.[139] However, primary myxoid melanoma has also been described in the skin[128,140–147] and in extracutaneous sites including the sinonasal passages.[148]

Histology

The rare myxoid melanoma manifests large malignant cells amidst a basophilic mucinous matrix. In all cases, the myxoid stroma comprises mesenchymal acidic mucopolysaccharides, as opposed to neutral epithelial mucins (Fig. 4.34). Thus, epithelial mucin preparations such as mucicarmine and PAS-diastase are negative, whereas stains for acidic

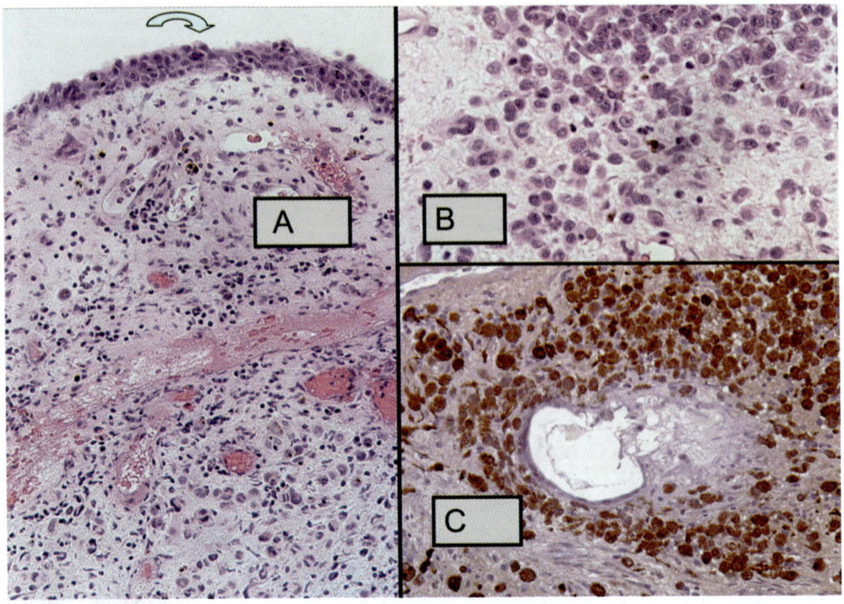

FIGURE 4.34 **Myxoid Melanoma.** In this mucosal melanoma from the nasopharynx, there is lentiginous melanocytic hyperplasia with fully transformed malignant cells within the epithelial compartment **(A)** (*curved arrow*). The myxoid change is seen in the epithelioid vertical growth phase areas where an abundant quantity of acid mucosubstances is deposited in the subepithelial stroma **(B)**. The tumor cells show strong decoration with antibody to S100 protein **(C)**.

mucosubstances (i.e., Alcian blue at low pH) are positive. The tumors are essentially amelanotic, although by Fontana Masson preparations some manifest evidence of melaninogenesis. Melanosomes, including aberrant variants, are demonstrable by electron microscopy.[139,146] As there is no cytoplasmic localization of the mucinous material within the tumor cells, it is likely that the myxoid matrix is produced as a response of the stromal cells to the tumor rather than being a product of the tumor cells per se. Such lesions should prompt evaluation for a primary malignant melanoma because they most often represent metastatic tumor deposits.[128,139,149–154] Recently, a myxoid variant of clear cell sarcoma, the soft tissue counterpart of cutaneous melanoma, has been described.[155]

Distinction of primary from secondary myxoid melanoma rests on the demonstration in the primary lesions of an atypical intraepidermal melanocytic proliferation.[141] The pattern of intraepidermal melanocyte proliferation can be subtle, with irregular nesting that is only focal.[146] The lesions are usually sparsely melanized or amelanotic; some show neurotropism.[146] Typically, ubiquitous S100 decoration can be demonstrated. Decoration with HMB-45 is less uniform, however, with both positive[139] and negative[146] results reported. In our hands, S100 protein was ubiquitously expressed in myxoid melanomas, while only two third expressed lineage-specific markers Melan-A or HMB-45.[156] One group found that labeling of primary myxoid melanomas with E9, an antimetallothionein marker, was predictive of rapid progression.[146]

Differential Diagnosis

The differential diagnosis of myxoid melanoma is broad, encompassing as it does other benign and malignant myxoid neoplasms. With respect to the latter, the spectrum includes soft tissue malignancies as well as epithelial cancers. The soft tissue malignancies include myxoid liposarcoma,[157] myxoid malignant fibrous histiocytoma[158] and its allied lesions, low-grade fibromyxoid sarcoma[159,160] and low-grade myofibroblastic sarcoma,[161] myxoid chondrosarcoma,[158,162] myxoid peripheral nerve sheath tumors,[139] myxoid rhabdomyosarcoma,[163] malignant myoepithelioma,[164] myxoid synovial sarcoma,[165] myxoid follicular dendritic cell sarcoma,[166] myxoid dermatofibrosarcoma protuberans,[167] metastatic chordoma and its benign mimic parachordoma.[168–170] The epithelial cancers that may mimic myxoid melanoma include metastatic adenocarcinomas, discussed under the differential diagnosis of signet-ring melanoma, and malignant sweat duct tumors including malignant mixed tumor. The very rare sarcomatoid variant of anaplastic large cell Ki-1 lymphoma[171] can also produce areas strikingly similar to myxoid melanoma at the light microscopic level.

Myxoid melanoma lacks the arborizing, delicate vasculature of the myxoid liposarcoma and, although the latter may rarely present as a primary skin neoplasm,[172] it usually has a manifestly different clinical presentation that should enable easy distinction. In any event, liposarcomas manifest weak cytoplasmic membrane rim staining with S100 protein quite unlike that seen in a melanocytic neoplasm. The myxoid malignant fibrous histiocytoma and other soft tissue cancers of myofibroblastic derivation are generally S100 negative and, like the liposarcoma, have a different pattern of clinical presentation in most cases. The atypical fibroxanthoma, a superficial cutaneous variant of malignant fibrous histiocytoma arising in the sun-damaged skin of the elderly, can also have a myxoid morphology. The low-grade fibromyxoid sarcoma might be confused with myxoid melanomas having a high content of spindled cells and manifests strong vimentin immunoreactivity[159,160]; however, all other melanocyte-related immunohistochemical markers, including S100 protein, are not expressed.[160] Similarly, S100 protein is not expressed in low-grade myofibroblastic sarcoma,[161] which may be closely allied to the fibromyxoid sarcoma in any event.

Extraskeletal myxoid chondrosarcoma has long been considered a distinctive form of low-grade sarcoma occurring in the deeper soft tissues of proximal extremities, limb girdle, and trunk. Larger series show the estimated 10-year survivorship to be only 70%.[162] Neoplasms tend to be weakly positive for antibodies to S100 protein in only a minority of cases (38%), and CK preparations are negative.[162] Myxoid malignant nerve sheath tumors may arise de novo or in the setting of neurofibromatosis.[173,174]

Rhabdomyosarcomas characteristically are glycogen rich and manifest an immunohistochemical profile (desmin +ve/S100 –ve) unlikely to be confused with melanoma. Malignant myoepithelioma manifests myxoid, spindled, epithelioid, and plasmacytoid zones in a solid or partly cystic lesion; cells tend to have an epithelioid/rhabdoid cytomorphology and to decorate with antibodies to S100 protein, smooth muscle actin, and CK.[164] Myxoid synovial sarcoma tends to manifest as lacy cords of monophasic spindled cells embedded in a myxoid stroma.[165] Some examples manifest a biphasic morphology. Synovial sarcoma, arising as it does in an undifferentiated mesenchymal precursor, can rarely present as a primary skin neoplasm.[175] Roughly half of such lesions express S100 protein, whereas most also express CK and/or epithelial membrane antigen.[165] A myxoid variant of the follicular dendritic cell sarcoma exists; these are malignant tumors of the follicular dendritic cell apparatus that may occur in extranodal sites.[166] The tumor cells, dispersed as cords of slightly atypical spindled cells, manifest immunoreactivity for S100 protein and epithelial membrane antigen, as well as CD21 and CD35, respectively, as the Epstein Barr virus receptor on B lymphocytes and a monocyte marker.[166] Myxoid dermatofibrosarcoma protuberans is a challenging diagnosis as the lesion is CD34 negative, unlike its conventional counterpart.[167] However, antibody to S100 protein does not decorate this lesion, which should make distinction from myxoid melanoma simple. Chordoma metastatic to the skin, classically from a primary tumor of sacrum or clivus, can produce an appearance quite like myxoid melanoma. Chains of cells are enmeshed in a myxoid stroma; the cells manifest physalliferous (i.e., spongelike or bubbly) cytoplasmic vacuolation. Coexpression of S100 protein and CK enables distinction from myxoid melanoma.[176–181] Histologically identical to chordoma at the light microscopic level is the parachordoma, a benign cutaneous neoplasm that most often is seen in the extremities adjacent to synovia, tendons, or osseous structures.[169] The immunohistochemical profile may be similar to chordoma, which more frequently manifests expression of CK (98% vs. 66%) and epithelial membrane antigen (90% vs. 20%).[169] This distinction is an important one, however, as the diagnosis of chordoma implies a metastatic malignant neoplasm. Correlation with clinical history and imaging studies is thus of paramount importance.

The malignant neoplasms of the sweat gland and duct manifest keratin positivity in most cases, as do malignant mixed tumors and metastatic carcinomas such as those of breast and lung. Furthermore, epithelial mucins are the rule in these scenarios. One can discern the very rare sarcomatoid variant of anaplastic large cell lymphoma from malignant melanoma based on S100 negativity as well as its expression of CD30 and, focally, of epithelial membrane antigen.[171]

Benign lesions that merit consideration in the differential diagnosis of myxoid melanoma include soft tissue myxoma,[182] myxoid common acquired nevi,[183] myxoid cellular blue nevi,[184] myxoid neurothekeoma,[185] and hyaline-cell rich chondroid syringoma.[186] The soft tissue myxoma manifests bland stellate or spindled cells lacking cytologic criteria for malignancy and can so be distinguished from myxoid malignant melanoma.[182] Similarly, the myxoid cellular blue nevus lacks cytologic features of malignancy. With regard to the myxoid neurothekeoma, this lesion tends to decorate with antibody to S100 protein,[185] as does the hyaline cell-rich chondroid syringoma[186]; the latter will also show keratin decoration in the modified myoepithelia that make up the cell populace, thus enabling distinction when the appropriate immunohistochemical cocktail is applied.

SMALL CELL MELANOMA

Undifferentiated small cell melanomas are most frequently encountered in the setting of a malignant melanoma that has arisen in a giant congenital nevus (Fig. 4.35), the characteristic clinical herald of which is the development of a protuberant and/or ulcerating nodule.[19] The small cell foci may show nuclear molding reminiscent of small cell carcinoma or exhibit a strikingly dyshesive growth pattern resembling the morphology of a lymphoblastic lymphoma. Melanomas manifesting this morphology are invariably in vertical growth phase and have an aggressive course.

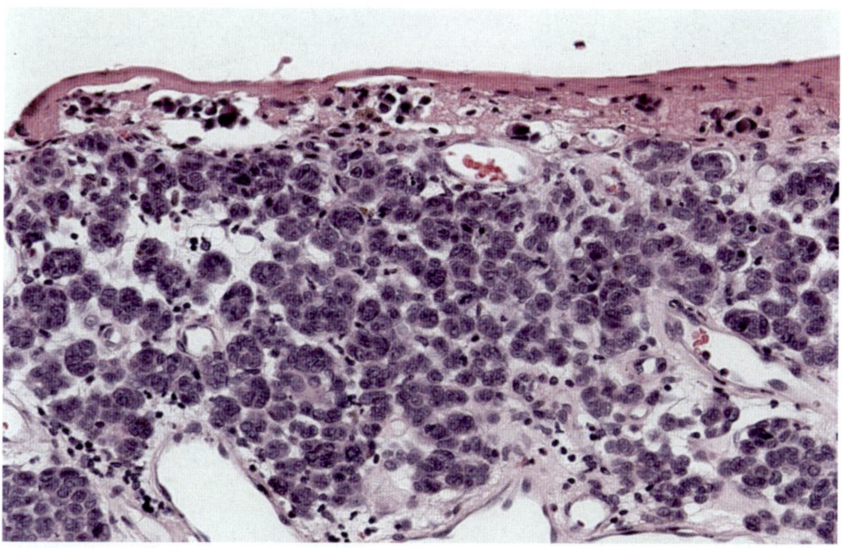

FIGURE 4.35 **Small Cell Melanoma.** In this small cell melanoma, which has arisen in the setting of a giant congenital nevus in an infant, the neoplastic melanocytes have nuclei only two to three times the diameter of red blood cells (i.e., roughly 20μ in size). They show nuclear contact molding and coarse heterochromatin cognate to a neuroendocrine cell carcinoma.

In addition to being a cytomorphologic mimic of lymphoblastic lymphoma, other small round cell tumors of childhood, including Ewing's sarcoma, peripheral neuroectodermal tumors, and Merkel cell carcinoma enter the differential diagnosis of small cell malignant melanoma.

RHABDOID MELANOMA

The presence of rhabdoid features in melanoma has been described and is not uncommon in metastatic melanoma; however, it is quite rare in primary lesions with only a few cases reported. Rhabdoid tumors are characterized by large sheets of polygonal cells with abundant cytoplasm containing eosinophilic inclusions and a peripherally displaced vesicular nucleus (Fig. 4.36). Ultrastructural anaylsis of one case showed cytoplasmic whorls of intermediate filaments with entrapped rough endoplasmic reticulum, mitochondiria, and lipid.[187] They have diverse patterns of immunoreactivity, reacting with antibodies to S100 and vimentin as well as, in some cases, keratins and desmin, and have been reported to frequently lose HMB-45 expression.[188]

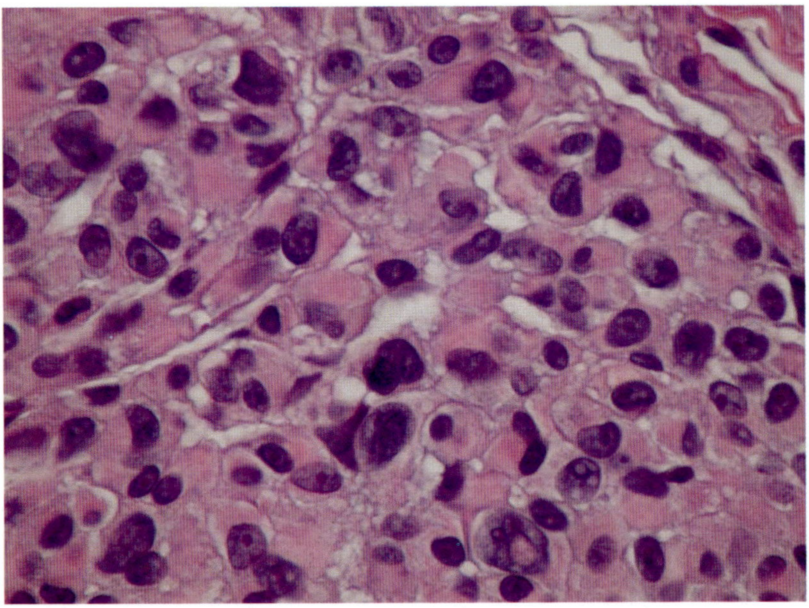

FIGURE 4.36 **Rhabdoid Melanoma.** In this example of rhabdoid vertical growth phase melanoma, there are large eosinophilic inclusions in the cytoplasm in a fashion that mimics rhabdomyoblasts of rhabdomyosarcoma. At the ultrastructural level, these filaments are aggregates of vimentin; on occasion, muscle-type intermediate filaments may also be seen.

CD34 EXPRESSION IN MALIGNANT MELANOMA

The CD34 antigen is a 110kDa protein encoded by a gene located on chromosome 1q and expressed on the surface of hemopoietic stem cells in bone marrow.[189] It was first used as a means to isolate stem cells for transplantation and to identify subgroups of acute leukemia. It is also found in vascular and spindle cell tumors as well as tumors of neural and myofibroblastic derivation including dermatofibrosarcoma protuberans, solitary fibrous tumors, and pleomorphic fibromas.

Melanocytic neoplasms have long been held to be CD34 negative, but there is a limited literature precedent regarding CD34 expression in lesions of melanoma (Fig. 4.37). Hoang et al. described a case of a desmoplastic malignant melanoma, resembling dermatofibrosarcoma protuberans (DFSP) histologically, which expressed CD34 strongly in the tumor spindle cells.[190] This further complicates an already difficult challenge of distinguishing a DFSP from desmoplastic melanoma, as CD34 is often used as a marker of DFSP.[191] Chen et al. described CD34 expression in uveal melanoma cells.[192] The authors speculate that CD34 expression may be a marker of aggressive behavior. CD34 expression has also been described in a cellular blue nevus.[193] CD34 is often used to calculate microvascular density in uveal tumors, one indicator of prognosis,[194] owing to its expression in endothelia.[195]

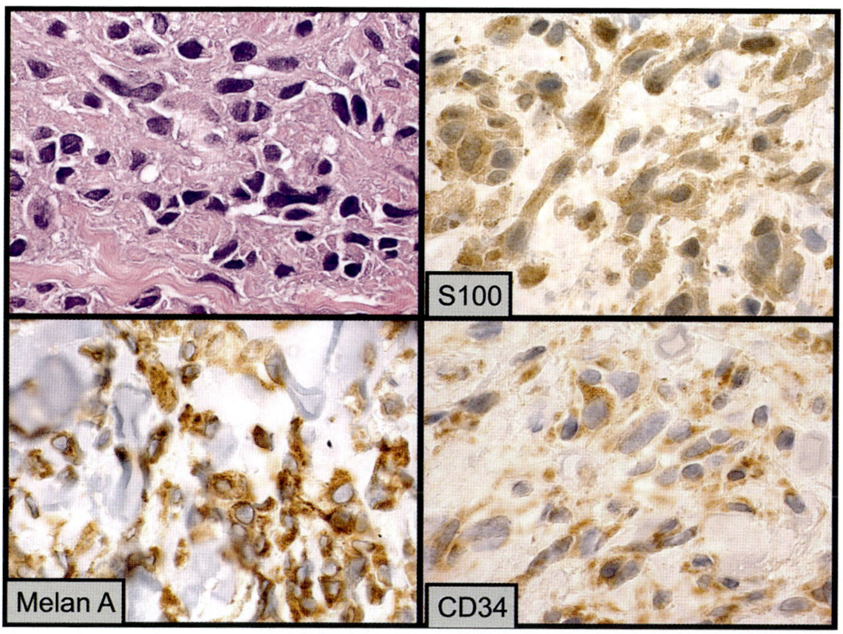

FIGURE 4.37 **Aberrant CD34 Expression in Melanoma.** This melanoma expresses S100 protein and Melan-A immunohistochemically, but also shows florid expression of CD34.

The expression of CD34 in melanoma may be explained by genetic dysregulation. It has been shown that aggressive melanoma cells express inappropriate markers that would not be expected of normal melanocytes.[196] Specifically, Hendrix et al. showed expression of vascular endothelial (VE)-cadherin in aggressive melanoma cells which correlated with their ability to form vascular channels.[196] The authors speculate that the expression of VE-cadherin may represent a reversion to a more primitive, embryonal phenotype. The expression of CD34 in melanoma may also be indicative of a similar state of dedifferentiation, as other cells of neural crest origin such as peripheral nerve cells and Schwann cells have been shown to express CD34.[197]

The Bednar tumor has also been shown to express a mixed immunophenotype (CD34-positive or Mart-1-positive) in dispersed dermal spindle cells within a DFSP-like lesion suggesting a common cell of origin, namely, a putative neuromesenchymal cell, the potential cell of origin of all neural crest-derived dermal tumors including DFSP.[198] This overlap of histologic and immunohistochemical phenotypes may indicate the existence of a spectrum of neuromesenchymal conditions that range from purely melanocytic lesions (dermal melanocytosis and blue nevi), to varied proportions of melanocytic and neuromesenchymal elements (cellular blue nevi, desmoplastic melanomas, and Bednar tumors), to purely mesenchymal lesions (DFSP).

EPITHELIAL MARKER EXPRESSION

Some melanomas have been observed to express CK which had been considered a specific marker for epithelial differentiation. One restrospective study described expression of CK in five of 19 melanomas analyzed.[199] Other studies have shown similar results, including in the context of the demonstration of proteins by Western blot analysis that migrated to positions correlating with CK.[200] This suggests that such melanomas are actually expressing CKs rather than some other explanation for spurious expression, such as impure polyclonal antibodies or cross-reactivity attributed to specific monoclonal antibodies.[200] This epithelial differentiation may be important, as keratins coexpressed with vimentin have been correlated to invasive and metastatic potential.[201] Epithelial membrane antigen is expressed in some 2% to 10% of melanomas studied (Fig. 4.38).

FIBROHISTIOCYTIC DIFFERENTIATION

Fibrohistiocytic differentiation is demonstrated in desmoplastic melanoma. This variant of melanoma shows features in common with the DFSP as discussed earlier, being composed of elongated spindle-shaped cells resembling fibroblasts, and surrounded by mature collagen bundles. Desmoplastic melanomas have been reported to be misdiagnosed as other soft tissue tumors such as malignant fibrous histiocytoma, atypical fibroxanthoma, and myxofibrosarcoma. They can be differentiated from these soft tissue tumors by the presence of S100. A rare example of melanocytic tumors such as the Spitz nevus expresses CD68 (Fig. 4.39).

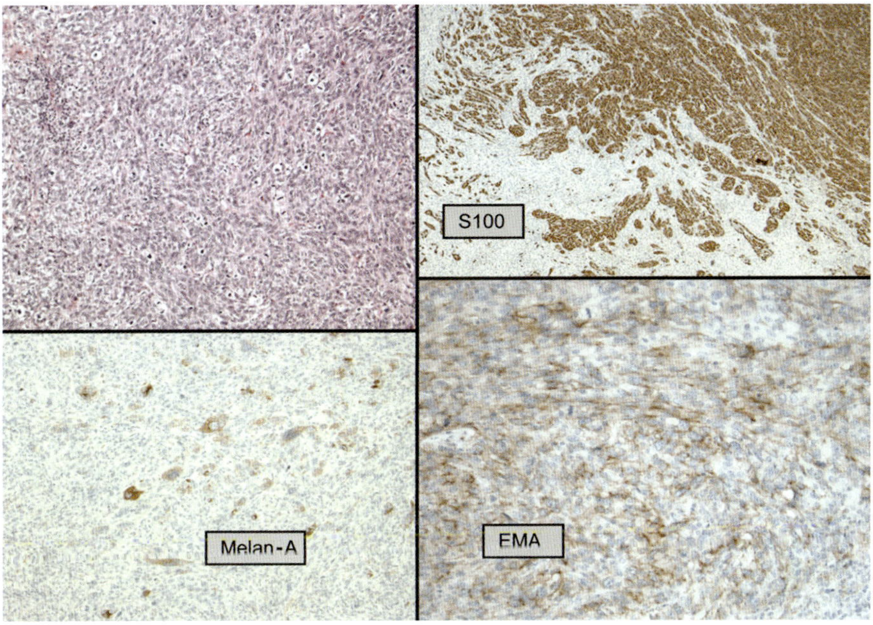

FIGURE 4.38 **Aberrant Expression of Epithelial Membrane Antigen (EMA) in Melanoma.** This melanoma shows florid S100 protein expression; only some 1% to 5% of cells express Melan-A. A larger number of cells express epithelial membrane antigen.

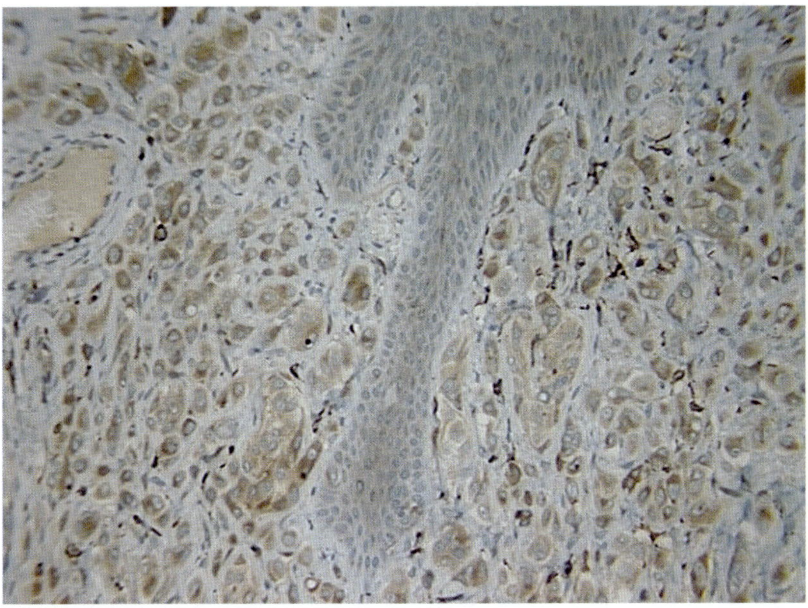

FIGURE 4.39 **CD68 Expression in a Spitz Nevus.** There is diffuse expression of the histiocyte marker CD68 in this example of a Spitz nevus. The tumor also expressed Melan-A and S100 protein, however, and had a more or less classical histomorphology, enabling diagnosis.

SMOOTH MUSCLE DIFFERENTIATION

Smooth muscle and osteocartilagenous differentiation are exceedingly rare phenotypes exhibited by melanoma.[112,202] There have been several studies showing expression of muscle actin proteins in melanoma with up to 52% of desmoplastic melanomas being positive. However, there has been only one study showing ultrastructural smooth muscle differentiation with fine filaments and focal densities. These cells, interestingly, lost reactivity to HMB-45 and S100.[202] Osteocartilagenous differentiation usually occurs in acral, particularly subungual, lesions. They typically show osteoid matrix and occasionally chrondroblastic differentiation. They are S100 and HMB-45 positive.

ABSENCE OF MELANOCYTE DIFFERENTIATION MARKERS

Occasionally, melanomas may not express certain of the melanocyte lineage-specific markers. For example, S100 protein is widely misconstrued to be ubiquitously expressed by melanomas. However, in one study, 17 cases of melanoma that previously tested negative for S100 protein expression were re-evaluated by light microscopy, a broad panel of immunohistochemical reagents including monoclonal and polyclonal antibodies to S100 protein, and electron microscopy.[203] On re-examination, 4 of the 17 cases repeatedly tested negative for S100 protein despite various antigen enhancement methods, but they were positive for HMB-45 antigen and contained premelanosomes or melanosomelike structures by electron microscopy. Two of these repeatedly S100 negative melanomas were acrally located; although the numbers are small, a possible relationship to a specific anatomic location was suggested. These findings suggested that in a small subset of melanomas S100 protein is either not fully expressed or is expressed at a level below that which can be detected by routine immunohistochemistry. In our hands, we have seen several cases of lentigo maligna in which the neoplastic melanocytes expressed Melan-A but not S100 protein. HMB-45 and Melan-A detect, respectively, the tyrosinosome matrix-related protein gp100 and the tyrosinase pathway antigen A103.[19] Both markers, like microphthalmia transcription factor (mit-f), are much less sensitive than S100 protein expression and are often negative in melanoma. Orchard suggests that 25% of conventional melanomas are negative for HMB-45 so are as many as 50% of metastatic melanomas.[204] Desmoplastic melanomas are often negative for HMB-45 unless a junctional component is present. In regard to tyrosinase and Melan-A, both have been reported to lose expression progressively in melanoma from clinical stages I to IV.

REFERENCES

1. Conley J, Lattes R, Orr W. Desmoplastic malignant melanoma (a rare variant of spindle cell melanoma). *Cancer* 1971;28:914–936.
2. Bruijn JA, Mihm MC Jr, Barnhill RL. Desmoplastic melanoma. *Histopathology* 1992;20:197–205.

3. Wharton JM, Carlson JA, Mihm MC Jr. Desmoplastic malignant melanoma: Diagnosis of early clinical lesions. *Hum Pathol* 1999;30:537–542.
4. Egbert B, Kempson R, Sagebiel. Desmoplastic malignant melanoma. A clinicopathologic study of 25 cases. *Cancer* 1988;62:2033–2041.
5. Skelton HG, Smith KJ, Laskin WB, et al. Desmoplastic malignant melanoma. *J Am Acad Dermatol* 1995;32:717–725.
6. Carlson JA, Dickersin GR, Sober AJ, Barnhill RL. Desmoplastic neurotropic melanoma. A clinicopathologic analysis of 28 cases. *Cancer* 1995;75:478–494.
7. Mulvany NJ, Sykes P. Desmoplastic melanoma of the vulva. *Pathology* 1997;29: 241–345.
8. Kurihara K, Sanada E, Yasuda S, Yamasaki H. Desmoplastic melanoma of the gingiva. *Oral Surg Med Oral Pathol* 1992;74:201–205.
9. Reed R, Leonard D. Neurotropic melanoma. A variant of desmoplastic melanoma. *Am J Surg Pathol* 1979;3:301–311.
10. Reiman HM, Goellner JR, Woods JE, Mixter RC. Desmoplastic melanoma of the head and neck. *Cancer* 1987;60:2269–2274.
11. Walsh NM, Roberts JT, Orr W, Simon GT. Desmoplastic malignant melanoma. A clinicopathological study of 14 cases. *Arch Pathol Lab Med* 1988;112:922–927.
12. Jain S, Allen PW. Desmoplastic malignant melanoma and its variants. *Am J Surg Pathol* 1989;13:358–373.
13. Beenken S, Byers R, Smith JL, et al. Desmoplastic melanoma. Histological correlation with behaviour and treatment. *Arch Otolaryngol Head Neck Surg* 1989;115:374–379.
14. Smithers BM, McLeod GR, Little JH. Desmoplastic, neural transforming and neurotropic melanoma: A review of 45 cases. *Aust NZ J Surg* 1990;60:967–972.
15. Quinn MJ, Crotty KA, Thompson JF, et al. Desmoplastic and desmoplastic neurotropic melanoma: Experience with 280 patients. *Cancer* 1998;83:1128–1135.
16. Smithers BM, McLeod GR, Little JH. Desmoplastic melanoma: Patterns of recurrence. *World J Surg* 1992;16:186–190.
17. Tsao H, Sober AJ, Barnhill RL. Desmoplastic neurotropic melanoma. *Semin Cutan Med Surg* 1997;16:131–136.
18. Sangueza OP, Requena L. Neoplasms with neural differentiation: A review. *Am J Dermatopathol* 1998;20:89–102.
19. Crowson AN, Magro CM, Mihm MC Jr. *The Melanocytic Proliferations: A Comprehensive Textbook of Pigmented Lesions.* New York: John Wiley and Sons, 2001:281–397.
20. Moreno A, Lamarca J, Martinez R, Guix M. Osteoid and bone formation in desmoplastic malignant melanoma. *J Cutan Pathol* 1986;13:128–134.
21. Hawkins WG, Busam KJ, Ben-Porat L, et al. Desmoplastic melanoma: A pathologically and clinically distinct form of cutaneous melanoma. *Ann Surg Oncol* 2005; 12:197–199.
22. Barnhill RL. *Pathology of Melanocytic Nevi and Malignant Melanoma.* Boston, MA: Butterworth-Heinemann, 1995:216–224.
23. Mihm MC Jr, Googe PB. *Problematic Pigmented Lesions. A Case Method Approach.* Philadelphia, PA: Lea & Febiger, 1990:279–370.
24. Barnhill RL, Mihm MC. Cellular neurothekeoma: A distinctive variant of neurothekeoma mimicking nevomelanocytic tumors. *Am J Surg Pathol* 1990;14:113–120.
25. Ackerman AB, Godomski J. Neurotropic malignant melanoma and other neurotropic neoplasms in the skin. *Am J Dermatopathol* 1984;6(Suppl. 1):63–80.
26. From L, Hanna W, Kahn HJ, et al. Origin of the desmoplasia in desmoplastic malignant melanoma. *Hum Pathol* 1983;14:1072–1080.
27. Valensi QJ. Desmoplastic malignant melanoma. A light and electron microscopic study of two cases. *Cancer* 1979;43:1148–1155.

28. Valensi QJ. Desmoplastic malignant melanoma. Study of a case by light and electronmicroscopy. *J Dermatol Surg Oncol* 1979;5:31–35.

29. Wick MR, Swanson PE, Rocamora A. Recognition of malignant melanoma by monoclonal antibody HMB-45: An immunohistochemical study of 200 paraffin-embedded cutaneous tumors. *J Cutan Pathol* 1988;15:201–207.

30. Anstey A, Cerio R, Ramnarain N, et al. Desmoplastic malignant melanoma. *Am J Dermatopathol* 1994;16:14–22.

31. Longacre TA, Egbert BM, Rouse RV. Desmoplastic and spindle cell melanoma. An immunohistochemical study. *Am J Surg Pathol* 1996;20:1489–1500.

32. Busam KJ, Zhao H, Coit DG, et al. Distinction of desmoplastic melanoma from non-desmoplastic melanoma by gene expression profiling. *J Invest Dermatol* 2005; 124:412–833.

33. Iwamoto S, Odland PB, Piepkorn M, Bothwell M. Evidence that the p75 neurotrophin receptor mediates perineural spread of desmoplastic melanoma. *J Am Acad Dermatol* 1996; 35(5 Pt 1):725–731.

34. Al-Alousi S, Carlson JA, Blessing K, et al. Expression of basic fibroblast growth factor in desmoplastic melanoma. *J Cutan Pathol* 1996;23:118–125.

35. Winnepenninckx V, De Vos R, Stas M, van den Ooord JJ. New phenotypic and ultrastructural findings in spindle cell (desmoplastic/neurotropic) melanoma. *Appl Immunohistochem Mol Morphol* 2003;11:319–325.

36. King R, Googe PB, Weilbaecher KN, et al. Microphthalmia transcription factor expression in cutaneous benign, malignant melanocytic, and non-melanocytic tumors. *Am J Surg Pathol* 2001;25:512–557.

37. Busam KJ, Iversen K, Coplan KC, Jungbluth AA. Analysis of microphthalmia transcription factor expression in normal tissues and tumors, and comparison of its expression with S100 protein, gp100, and tyrosinase in desmoplastic melanoma. *Am J Surg Pathol* 2001;25:197–204.

38. Busam KJ, Kucukgol D, Sato E, et al. Immunohistochemical analysis of novel monoclonal antibody PNL2 and comparison with other melanocyte differentiation markers. *Am J Surg Pathol* 2005;29:400–406.

39. Sagebiel RW. Unusual variants of melanoma: Fact or fiction? *Semin Oncol* 1996; 23:703–708.

40. Schmoeckel C, Castro CE, Braun-Falco O. Nevoid malignant melanoma. *Arch Derm Res* 1985;277:362–369.

41. Levene A. On the histological diagnosis and prognosis of malignant melanoma. *J Clin Pathol* 1980;33:101–124.

42. Suster S, Ronnen M, Bubis JJ. Verrucous pseudonevoid melanoma. *J Surg Oncol* 1987;36:134–137.

43. Blessing K, Grant JJ, Sanders DS, et al. Small cell malignant melanoma: A variant of naevoid melanoma. Clinicopathological features and histological differential diagnosis. *J Clin Pathol* 2000;53:591–595.

44. Wong TY, Duncan LM, Mihm MC Jr. Melanoma mimicking dermal and Spitz's nevus ("nevoid melanoma"). *Semin Surg Oncol* 1993;9:188–193.

45. Wong TY, Suster S, Duncan LM, Mihm MC Jr. Nevoid melanoma: A clinicopathological study of seven cases of malignant melanoma mimicking spindle and epithelioid cell nevus and verrucous dermal nevus. *Hum Pathol* 1995;26:171–179.

46. Kossard S, Wilkinson B. Small cell (naevoid) melanoma: A clinicopathologic study of 131 cases. *Australas J Dermatol* 1997;38(Suppl. 1): S54–S58.

47. McNutt NS, Urmacher C, Hakimian J, et al. Nevoid malignant melanoma: Morphologic patterns an immunohistochemical reactivity. *J Cutan Pathol* 1995;22:502–517.

48. Zembowicz A, McCusker M, Chiarelli C, Reed R. Morphological analysis of nevoid melanoma: A study of 20 cases with a review of the literature. *Am J Dermatopathol* 2001;23:167–175.

49. Muhlbauer J, Margolis R, Mihm MC, et al. Minimal deviation melanoma: A histologic variant of cutaneous malignant melanoma in vertical growth phase. *J Invest Dermatol* 1983;80:63s–65s.

50. Philips ME, Margolis RJ, Merot Y, et al. Common and uncommon melanocytic nevi and borderline melanomas. *Semin Oncol* 1975;2:119–147.

51. Reed RJ. Minimal deviation melanoma. *Hum Pathol* 1990;21:1206–1211.

52. Reed RJ, Martin P. Variants of melanoma. *Semin Cutan Med Surg* 1997;16:137–158.

53. Okun MR, DiMattia A, Thompson J, Pearson SH. Malignant melanoma developing from intradermal nevi. A clinicopathologic entity. *Arch Dermatol* 1974;110:559–601.

54. Kossard S, Wilkinson B. Nucleolar organizer regions and image analysis nuclear morphometry of small cell (nevoid) melanoma. *J Cutan Pathol* 1995;22:132–136.

55. Philips ME, Margolis RJ, Merot Y, et al. The spectrum of minimal deviation melanoma: A clinicopathologic study of 21 cases. *Hum Pathol* 1986;17:796–806.

56. Podnos YD, Jimenez JC, Zainabadi K, et al. Minimal deviation melanoma. *Cancer Treat Rep* 2002;28:219–221.

57. Becker DW Jr, Miller CJ, Keller HB. Metastatic minimal-deviation melanoma. *Ann Plast Surg* 1980;4:230–237.

58. Reed RJ. Minimal deviation melanoma. Borderline and intermediate melancoytic neoplasia. *Clin Lab Med* 2000;20:745–758.

59. Magro CM, Crowson AN, Gupta K, et al. The dermal borderline melanocytic tumor. A categorial approach. *J Am Acad Dermatol* (in press).

60. Reed R, Ichinose H, Clark WC, Mihm M. Common and uncommon melanocytic nevi and borderline melanomas. *Semin Oncol* 1975;2:119–147.

61. Merot Y, Mihm MC. Unusual and unknown aspect of cutaneous malignant melanoma: Minimal deviation malignant melanoma. Retrospective study of 45 cases. *Ann Dermatol Venereol* 1985;112:325–336.

62. Chorny JA, Barr RJ, Kyshtoobayeva A, et al. Ki-67 and p53 expression in minimal deviation lesions as compared with other nevomelanocytic lesions. *Mod Pathol* 2003;16:525–529.

63. Levene A. Equine melanotic disease. *Tumori* 1971;57:133–168.

64. Lerner AB, Cage GW. Melanomas in horses. *Yale J Biol Med* 1973;46:646–649.

65. Tuthill RJ, Clark WH, Levene A. Pilar neurocristic hamartoma. Its relationship to blue nevus and equine melanotic disease. *Arch Dermatol* 1982;118:592–596.

66. Rappaport H, Pietra G, Shubick P. The induction of melanotic tumors resembling cellular blue nevi in the Syrian hamster by cutaneous application of 7,12-dimethylbenz-(a)-anthracene. *Cancer Res* 1961;21:661–666.

67. Walters MA, Roe FJC, Levene A. The induction of tumors and other lesions in hamsters by a single subcutaneous injection of 9,10-dimethyl-1,2-benzanthracene or urethane on the first day of life. *Br J Cancer* 1967;21:184–189.

68. Nakai T, Rappaport H. A study of the histogenesis of experimental melanocytic tumors resembling cellular blue nevi: The evidence in support of their neurogenic origin. *Am J Pathol* 1963;43:175–199.

69. Epstein JH, Epstein WL, Nakai T. Production of melanomas from DMBA-induced "blue nevi" in hairless mice with ultraviolet light. *J Nat Cancer Inst* 1967;38:19–30.

70. Darier J. Le melanome malin mesenchymateaux ou melano-sarcome. *Bull Assoc Fr Cancer* 1925;14:221–249.

71. Crowson AN, Magro CM, Mihm MC Jr. Malignant melanoma with prominent pigment synthesis: "animal type" melanoma. *Hum Pathol* 1999;30:543–550.

72. Levene A. Disseminated dermal melanocytosis terminating in melanoma: A human condition resembling equine melanotic disease. *Br J Dermatol* 1979;101:197–205.

73. Pathy AL, Helm TN, Elston D, et al. Malignant melanoma arising in a blue nevus with features of pilar neurocristic hamartoma. *J Cutan Pathol* 1993;20:459–464.

74. Crowson AN, Magro CM, Clark WH. Pilar neurocristic hamartoma [letter]. *J Am Acad Dermatol* 1996;34:715.

75. Kopf AW, Bart RS. Malignant blue (Ota's?) nevus. *J Dermatol Surg Oncol* 1982; 8:442–445.

76. Mehregan DA, Gibson LE, Mehregan AH. Malignant blue nevus: A report of eight cases. *J Dermatol Sci* 1992;4:185–192.

77. Van Krieken JH, Boom BW, Scheffer E. Malignant transformation in a naevus of Ito: A case report. *Histopathology* 1988;12:100–102.

78. Levene A. On the natural history and comparative pathology of the blue naevus. *Ann R Coll Surg Engl* 1980;62:327–334.

79. Rodriguez HA, Ackerman LV. Cellular blue nevus: Clinicopathologic study of forty-five cases. *Cancer* 1968;21:393–405.

80. Silverberg GD, Kadin ME, Dorfman RF, et al. Invasion of the brain by a cellular blue nevus of the scalp. A case report with light and electron microscopic studies. *Cancer* 1971;27:349–355.

81. Sterchi JM, Muss HB, Weidner N. Cellular blue nevus simulating metastatic melanoma: Report of an unusually large lesion associated with nevus-cell aggregates in regional lymph nodes. *J Surg Oncol* 1987;36:71–75.

82. Lach B, Russell N, Benoit B, et al. Cellular blue nevus ("melanocytoma") of the spinal meninges: Electron microscopic and immunhistochemical features. *Neurosurgery* 1988;22:773–780.

83. Kaburagi Y, Hatta N, Kawara S, Takehara K. Pigmented dermatofibrosarcoma protuberans (Bednar tumor) occurring in a Japanese patient. *Dermatology* 1998;197:48–51.

84. Zembowicz A, Carney JA, Mihm MC. Pigmented epithelioid melanocytoma: A low grade melanocytic tumor with metastatic potential indistinguishable from animal-type melanoma and epithelioid blue nevus. *Am J Surg Pathol* 2004;28:31–40.

85. Zembowicz A, Mihm MC. Pigment synthesizing melanocytic tumor: A low grade melanocytic tumor with frequent lymph node metastases [Abst]. *Lab Invest* 2002;112A.

86. Allen AC, Spitz S. Malignant melanoma: A clinicopathologic analysis of the criteria for diagnosis and prognosis. *Cancer* 1953;6:1–45.

87. Merkow LP, Burt RC, Hayeslip DW, et al. A cellular and malignant blue nevus: A light and electron microscopic study. *Cancer* 1969;24:888–896.

88. Mishima Y. Cellular blue nevus: Melanogenic activity and malignant transformation. *Arch Dermatol* 1970;101:104–110.

89. Okun MR. Malignant blue nevus [letter]. *Arch Dermatol* 1973;108:726–727.

90. Hernandez FJ. Malignant blue nevus: A light and electron microscopic study. *Arch Dermatol* 1973;107:741–744.

91. Reiss RF, Gray GF Jr. Malignant blue nevus. Occurrence with aggressive behavior. *NY State J Med* 1975;75:1749–1751.

92. Temple-Camp CRE, Saxe N, King H. Benign and malignant cellular blue nevus: A clinicopathological study of 30 cases. *Am J Dermatopathol* 1988;10:289–296.

93. Goldenhersh MA, Savin RC, Barnhill RL, et al. Malignant blue nevus. Case report and literature review. *J Am Acad Dermatol* 1988;19:712–722.

94. Connelly J, Smith JL. Malignant blue nevus. *Cancer* 1991;67:2653–2657.

95. Aloi F, Pich A, Pippione M. Malignant cellular blue nevus: A clinicopathological study of 6 cases. *Dermatology* 1996;192:36–40.

96. Duteille F, Duport G, Larregue M, et al. Malignant blue nevus: Three new cases and a review of the literature. *Ann Plast Surg* 1998;41:674–678.
97. Ariyanayagam-Baksh SM, Baksh FK, Finkelstein SD, et al. Malignant blue nevus. A case report and molecular analysis. *Am J Dermatopathol* 2003;25:21–27.
98. Ozgur F, Akyurek M, Kayikcioglu A, et al. Metastatic malignant blue nevus: A case report. *Ann Plast Surg* 1997;39:411–415.
99. Biernat W, Kordek R, Arkuszewska C, et al. Malignant blue nevus with neurosarcoma-like lymph node metastases. *Pol J Pathol* 1995;46:51–54.
100. English JC III, McCollough ML, Grabski WJ. A pigmented scalp nodule: Malignant blue nevus. *Cutis* 1996;58:40–42.
101. Nödl F, Krüger R. Maligner blauer Navus bei Navus Ota. *Hautartz* 1984;35:421–424.
102. Yoneyama K, Kamada N, Mizoguchi M, et al. Malignant melanoma and acquired dermal melanocytosis on congenital nevus spilus. *J Dermatol* 2005;32:454–458.
103. Avidor I, Kessler E. "Atypical" blue nevus-a benign variant of cellular blue nevus. Presentation of three cases. *Dermatologica* 1977;154:39–44.
104. Tran TA, Carlson JA, Basaca PC, Mihm MC. Cellular blue nevus with atypia (atypical cellular blue nevus): A clinicopathologic study of nine cases. *J Cutan Pathol* 1998;25:252–258.
105. Urmacher C. Unusual stromal patterns in truly recurrent and satellite metastatic lesions of malignant melanoma. *Am J Dermatopathol* 1984,6(suppl):331–335.
106. Grunwald MH, Rothem A, Feuerman EJ. Metastatic malignant melanoma with cartilaginous metaplasia. *Dermatologica* 1985;170:249–252.
107. Weidner N, Flanders DJ, Jochimsen PR, Stamler FW. Neurosarcomatous malignant melanoma arising in a neuroid giant congenital melanocytic nevus. *Arch Dermatol* 1985;121:1302–1306.
108. Moreno A, Lomarca J, Martinez R, et al. Osteoid and bone formation in desmoplastic malignant melanoma. *J Cutan Pathol* 1986;13:128–134.
109. Nakagawa H, Imakado S, Nogita T, Ishibashi Y. Osteosarcomatous changes in malignant melanoma. *Am J Dermatopathol* 1990;12:162–168.
110. Hoorweg JJ, Loftus BM, Hilgers FJ. Osteoid and bone formation in a nasal mucosal melanoma and its metastasis. *Histopathology* 1987;31:465–468.
111. Toda S, Heasley DD, Mihm MC. Osteogenic melanoma: Stromal metaplasia in association with subungual melanoma. *Histopathology* 1997;31:293–295.
112. Cachia AR, Kedziora AM. Subungual melanoma with cartilaginous differentiation. *Am J Dermatopathol* 1999;21:165–169.
113. Hendrickson MR, Ross JC. Neoplasms arising in congenital giant nevi: Morphological study of seven cases and a review of the literature. *Am J Surg Pathol* 1981;5:109–135.
114. Perniciaro C. Dermatopathologic variants of malignant melanoma. *Mayo Clin Proc* 1997;72:273–279.
115. Kao GF, Helwig EB, Graham JH. Balloon cell malignant melanoma of the skin. A clinicopathologic study of 34 cases with histochemical, immunohistochemical, and ultrastructural observations. *Cancer* 1992;69:2942–2952.
116. Adamek D, Kaluza J, Stachura K. Primary balloon cell malignant melanoma of the right temporo-parietal region arising from meningeal nevus. *Clin Neuropathol* 1995;14:29–32.
117. Van der Linde-Sipman JS, de Wit MM, van Garderen E, et al. Cutaneous malignant melanomas in 57 cats: Identification of (amelanotic) signet-ring and balloon cell types and verification of their origin by immunohistochemistry, electron microscopy, and in situ hybridization. *Vet Pathol* 1997;34:31–38.
118. Mowat A, Reid R, Mackie R. Balloon cell metastatic melanoma: An important differential in the diagnosis of clear cell tumors. *Histopathology* 1994;24:469–472.

119. Riley FC. Balloon cell melanoma of the choroid. *Arch Ophthalmol* 1974;92:131–133.

120. Khalil MK. Balloon cell malignant melanoma of the choroid: Ultrastructural studies. *Br J Ophthalmol* 1983;67:579–584.

121. Nowak M, Fatteh S, Campbell T. Glycogen-rich malignant melanomas and glycogen-rich balloon cell malignant melanomas: Frequency and pattern of PAS positivity in primary and metastatic melanomas. *Arch Pathol Lab Med* 1998;122:353–360.

122. Perez MT, Suster S. Balloon cell change in cellular blue nevus. *Am J Dermatopathol* 1999;21:181–184.

123. Martinez F, Merenda G, Bedrossian CW. Lipid-rich metastatic balloon-cell melanoma: Diagnosis by a multimodal approach to aspiration biopsy cytology. *Diagn Cytopathol* 1990;6:427–433.

124. Aloi FG, Coverlizza S, Pippione M. Balloon cell melanoma: A report of two cases. *J Cutan Pathol* 1988;15:230–233.

125. Gregel C, Wolter M, Kaufmann R. Co-existence of balloon cell melanoma with balloon cells in a dermal nevus. *Pathologe* 1998;19:151–153.

126. Wambacher-Gaser B, Zelger B, Zelger BG, Steiner H. Clear cell dermatofibroma. *Histopathology* 1997;30:64–69.

127. Terayama K, Hirokawa M, Shimizu M, et al. Balloon melanoma cells mimicking foamy histiocytes. *Acta Cytol* 1999;43:325–326.

128. Nakleh RE, Wick MR, Rocamora A, et al. Morphological diversity in malignant melanomas. *Am J Clin Pathol* 1990;93:731–840.

129. Tsang WY, Chan JK, Chow LT. Signet-ring melanoma mimicking adenocarcinoma. A case report. *Acta Cytol* 1983;37:559–562.

130. Simmons TJ, Martin SE. Fine-needle aspiration biopsy of malignant melanoma: A cytologic and immunocytochemical analysis. *Diagn Cytopathol* 1991;7:380–386.

131. Neimann TH, Thomas PA. Melanoma with signet-ring cells in a peritoneal effusion. *Diagn Cytopathol* 1995;12:241–244.

132. Al-Talib, Theaker JM. Signet-ring melanoma: Light microscopic, immunohistochemical and ultrastructural features. *Histopathology* 1991;18:572–575.

133. Eckert F, Baricevic B, Landthaler M, Schmid U. Metastatic signet-ring melanoma in a patient with an unkown primary tumor. Histologic, immunohistochemical and ultrastructural findings. *J Am Acad Dermatol* 1992;26(5 Pt 2):870–875.

134. Sheibani K, Battifora H. Signet-ring cell melanoma. A rare morphologic variant of malignant melanoma. *Am J Surg Pathol* 1988;12:28–34.

135. Rutten A, Huschka U, Requena C, et al. Primary cutaneous signet-ring melanoma: A clinicopathologic and immunohistochemical study of two cases. *Am J Dermatopathol* 2003;25:418–422.

136. Bonetti F, Colombari R, Zamboni G, Chilosi M. Signet ring melanoma, S-100 negative. *Am J Surg Pathol* 1989;13:522–523.

137. Hanna W, Kahn HJ, From L. Signet ring lymphoma of the skin: Ultrastructural and immunohistochemical features. *J Am Acad Dermatol* 1986;14(2 Pt 2):344–350.

138. LiVolsi VA, Brooks JJ, Soslow R, et al. Signet ring melanocytic lesions. *Mod Pathol* 1992;5:515–520.

139. Collina G, Losi L, Taccagni GL, Maiorana A. Myxoid metastases of melanoma: Report of three cases and review of the literature. *Am J Dermatopathol* 1997;19:52–57.

140. Nottingham JF, Slater DN. Malignant melanoma: A new mimic of colloid adenocarcinoma. *Histopathology* 1988;13:576–578.

141. Urso C, Giannotti B, Bondi R. Myxoid melanoma of the skin. *Arch Pathol Lab Med* 1990;114:527–528.

142. Garcia-Caballero T, Fraga M, Antunez JR, et al. Myxoid metastatic melanoma. *Histopathology* 1991;18:371–373.

143. Sarode VR, Joshi K, Ravichandran P, et al. Myxoid variant of primary cutaneous malignant melanoma. *Histopathology* 1992;20:186–187.

144. Prieto VG, Kanik A, Salob S, McNutt NS. Primary cutaneous myxoid melanoma: Immunohistologic clues to a difficult diagnosis. *J Am Acad Dermatol* 1994;30(2 Pt 2):335–339.

145. McCluggage WG, Shah V, Toner PG. Primary cutaneous myxoid malignant melanoma. *Histopathology* 1996;28:179–182.

146. Zelger BG, Steiner H, Wambacher B, Zelger B. Malignant melanomas simulating various types of soft tissue tumors. *Dermatol Surg* 1997;23:1047–1054.

147. Hitchcock MG, McCalmont TH, White WL. Cutaneous melanoma with myxoid features. *Am J Surg Pathol* 1999;23:1506–1513.

148. Chetty R, Slavin JL, Pitson GA, Dowling JP. Melanoma botryoides: A distinctive myxoid pattern of sino-nasal melanoma. *Histopathology* 1994;24:377–379.

149. Rocamora A, Carrillo R, Vives R, Solera JC. Fine needle aspiration biopsy of myxoid metastasis of malignant melanonma. *Acta Cytol* 1988;32:94–100.

150. Lindholm K, de la Torre M. Fine needle aspiration cytology of myxoid metastatic melanoma. *Acta Cytol* 1988;32:719–721.

151. Olinici CD, Vasiu R. Myxoid malignant melanoma. Report of three cases and review of the literature. *Morphol Embryol (Bucur)* 1989;35:285–287.

152. Lodding P, Kindblom LG, Angervall L. Metastases of malignant melanoma simulating soft tissue sarcoma. A clinico-pathological, light- and electron microscopic and immunohistochemical study of 21 cases. Virchows *Arch A Pathol Anat Histopathol* 1990;417:377–388.

153. Auger M, Caraway NP, Wojcik EM, Ordonez NG. Fine needle aspiration biopsy of metastatic myxoid melanoma. *Cytopathology* 1994;5:118–122.

154. Hitchcock MG, White WL. Malicious masquerade: myxoid melanoma. *Semin Diagn Pathol* 1998;15:195–202.

155. Kim YC, Vandersteen DP, Juang HG. Myxoid clear cell sarcoma. *Am J Dermatopathol* 2005;27:51–55.

156. LaMar WL, Crowson AN. Malignant melanoma with prominent myxoid stroma ("myxoid melanoma"). *Melanoma Res* 2001;11(Suppl. 1):S58.

157. Patel SR, Burgess MA, Plager C, et al. Myxoid liposarcoma. Experience with chemotherapy. *Cancer* 1994;74:1265–1269.

158. Patel SR, Burgess MA, Papadopoulos NE, et al. Extraskeletal myxoid chondrosarcoma. Long-term experience with chemotherapy. *Am J Clin Oncol* 1995;18:161–163.

159. Shidham VB, Ayala GE, Lahaniatis JE, Garcia FU. Low grade fibromyxoid sarcoma: Clincopathologic case report with review of the literature. *Am J Clin Oncol* 1999;22: 150–155.

160. Lindberg GM, Maitra A, Gokaslan ST, et al. Low grade fibromyxoid sarcoma: Fine-needle aspiration cytology with histologic, cytogenetic, immunohistochemical and ultrastructural correlation. *Cancer* 1999;87:75–82.

161. Mentzel T, Dry S, Katenkamp D, Fletcher CDM. Low grade myofibroblastic sarcoma. Analysis of 18 cases in the spectrum of myofibroblastic tumors. *Am J Surg Pathol* 1998;22:1228–1238.

162. Meiss-Kindblom JM, Bergh P, Gunterberg B, et al. Extraskeletal myxoid chondrosarcoma: A reappraisal of its morphological spectrum and prognostic factors based upon 117 cases. *Am J Surg Pathol* 1999;23:636–650.

163. Bhuta S, Mirra J, Cochran A. Myxoid malignant melanoma. A previously undescribed histologic pattern noted in metastatic lesions and a report of four cases. *Am J Surg Pathol* 1986;10:203–211.

164. Hinze P, Feyler S, Berndt J, et al. Malignant myoepithelioma of the vulva resembling a rhabdoid tumour. *Histopathology* 1999;35:50–54.

165. Krane JF, Bertoni F, Fletcher CD. Myxoid synovial sarcoma: An underappreciated morphological subset. *Mod Pathol* 1999;12:456–462.

166. Fisher C, Magnusson B, Hardarson S, Smith ME. Myxoid variant of follicular dendritic cell sarcoma arising in the breast. *Ann Diagn Pathol* 1999;3:92–98.

167. Orlandi A, Bianchi L, Spagnoli LG. Myxoid dermatofibrosarcoma protuberans: Morphological, ultrastructural and immunohistochemical features. *J Cutan Pathol* 1998; 25:386–393.

168. Fisher C, Miettinen M. Parachordoma: A clinicopathological and immunohistochemical study of four cases of an unusual soft tissue neoplasm. *Ann Diagn Pathol* 1997;1:3–10.

169. Imlay SP, Argenyi ZB, Stone MS, et al. Cutaneous parachordoma. A light microscopic and immunohistochemical report of two cases and review of the literature. *J Cutan Pathol* 1998;25:279–284.

170. Folpe AL, Agoff SN, Willis J, Weiss SW. Parachordoma is immunohistochemically and cytogenetically distinct from axial chordoma and extraskeletal myxoid chondrosarcoma. *Am J Surg Pathol* 1999;23:1059–1067.

171. Chan JK, Buchanan R, Fletcher CD. Sarcomatoid variant of anaplastic large-cell Ki-1 lymphoma. *Am J Surg Pathol* 1990;14:983–988.

172. Dei Tos AP, Mentzel T, Fletcher CD. Primary liposarcoma of the skin: A rare neoplasm with unusual high grade features. *Am J Dermatopathol* 1998;20:332–338.

173. Sakaguchi N, Sano K, Ito M, et al. A case of von Recklinghausen's disease with bilateral pheochromocytoma-malignant peripheral nerve sheath tumors of the adrenal and gastrointestinal autonomic nerve tumors. *Am J Surg Pathol* 1996;20:889–897.

174. Rao UN, Surti U, Hoffner L, Yaw K. Cytogenetic and histologic correlation of peripheral nerve sheath tumors of soft tissue. *Cancer Genet Cytogenet* 1996;88:17–25.

175. Flieder DB, Moran CA. Primary cutaneous synovial sarcoma: A case report. *Am J Dermatopathol* 1998;20:509–512.

176. Gagne EJ, Su WP. Chordoma involving the skin: An immunohistochemical study of 11 cases. *J Cutan Pathol* 1992;19:469–475.

177. Su WP, Louback JB, Gagne EJ, Scheithauer BW. Chordoma cutis: A report of nineteen patients with cutaneous involvement of chordoma. *J Am Acad Dermatol* 1993;29:63–66.

178. Jones B, Ghosh BC, Skelton HG. Chordoma with cutaneous metastasis. *Cutis* 1994; 54:250–252.

179. Ogi H, Kiryu H, Yori Y, Fukui M. Cutaneous metastasis of CNS chordoma. *Am J Dermatopathol* 1995;17:599–602.

180. Cesinaro AM, Maiorana A, Annessi G, Collina G. Cutaneous metastasis of chordoma. *Am J Dermatopathol* 1995;17:603–605.

181. Miller SD, Vinson RP, McCullough ML, Keeling JH III. Multiple smooth skin nodules. Chordoma cutis. *Arch Dermatol* 1997;133:1579–1580, 1582–1583.

182. Nielsen GP, O'Connell JX, Rosenberg AE. Intramuscular myxoma. A clinicopathologic study of 51 cases with emphasis on hypercellular and hypervascular variants. *Am J Surg Pathol* 1998;22:1222–1227.

183. Michal M. Mucinous naevoacellular nevi. *Dermatopathology* 1994;188:232–235.

184. Michal M, Baumrunk L, Skalova A. Myxoid change within cellular blue nevi a diagnostic pitfall. *Histopathology* 1992;20:527–530.

185. Husain S, Silvers DN, Halperin AJ, Mc Nutt NS. Histologic spectrum of neurothekeoma and the value of immunoperoxidase staining for S-100 protein in distinguishing it from melanoma. *Am J Dermatopathol* 1994;16:496–503.

186. Ferreiro JA, Nascimento AG. Hyaline-cell rich chondroid syringioma. A tumor mimicking malignancy. *Am J Surg Pathol* 1995;19:912–917.
187. Abbott JJ, Amirkhan RH, Hong MP. Malignant melanoma with a rhabdoid phenotype: Histologic, immunohistochemical, and ultrastructural study of a case and review of the literature. *Arch Pathol Lab Med* 2004;128:686–688.
188. Borek B, McKee P, Freeman J, et al. Primary malignant melanoma with rhabdoid features: A histologic and immunocytochemical study of three cases. *Am J Dermatopathol* 1998;20:123–127.
189. Molgaard H, Spurr N, Greaves M. The hemopoietic stem cell antigen, CD34, is encoded by a gene located on chromosome 1. *Leukemia* 1989;3:773–776.
190. Hoang M, Selim M, Bentley R, et al. CD34 expression in desmoplastic melanoma. *J Cutan Pathol* 2001;28:508–512.
191. Aiba S, Tabata N, Ishii H, et al. Dermatofibrosarcoma protuberans is a unique fibrohistiocytic tumour expressing CD34. *Br J Dermatol* 1992;127:79–84.
192. Chen X, Maniotis A, Majumdar D. Uveal melanoma cell staining for CD34 and assessment of tumor vascularity. *Invest Ophthalmol Vis Sci* 2002;43:2533–2539.
193. Smith K, Germain M, Williams J, et al. CD34-positive cellular blue nevi. *J Cutan Pathol* 2001;28:145–150.
194. Maniotis A, Folberg R, Hess A, Skelton H. Vascular channel formation by human melanoma cells in vivo and in vitro: Vasculogenic mimicry. *Am J Pathol* 1999;155:739–752.
195. Nickoloff, B. The human progenitor cell antigen (CD34) is localized on endothelial cells, dermal dendritic cells, and perifollicular cells in formalin-fixed normal skin, and on proliferating endothelial cells and stromal spindle-shaped cells in Kaposi's sarcoma. *Arch Dermatol* 1991;127:523–529.
196. Hendrix M, Seftor E, Meltzer P, et al. Expression and functional significance of VE-cadherin in aggressive human melanoma cells: Role in vasculogenic mimicry. *Proc Natl Acad Sci USA* 2001;98:8018–8023.
197. Weiss S, Nickoloff B. CD-34 is expressed by a distinctive cell population in peripheral nerve, nerve sheath tumors, and related lesions. *Am J Surg Pathol* 1993;17:1039–1045.
198. Goncharuk V, Mulvany M, Carlson A. Bednar tumor associated with dermal melanocytosis: Melanocytic colonization or neuroectodermal multidirectional differentiation? *J Cutan Pathol* 2003;30:147–151.
199. Banks E, Jansen J, Oberle E, Davey D. Cytokeratin positivity in fine-needle aspirates of melanomas and sarcomas. *Diagn Cytopathol* 1995;12:230–233.
200. Zarbo RJ, Gown A, Nagle R, et al. Anomalous cytokeratin expression in malignant melanoma: One and two-dimensional western blot analysis and immunohistochemical survey of 100 melanomas. *Mod Pathol* 1990;3:494–501.
201. Hendrix M, Seftor E, Chu Y, et al. Coexpression of vimentin and keratins by human melanoma tumor cells: Correlation with invasive and metastatic potential. *J Natl Cancer Inst* 1992;84:165–174.
202. Banerjee S, Bishop P, Nicholson C, Eyden D. Malignant melanoma showing smooth muscle differentiation. *J Clin Pathol* 1996;49:950–951.
203. Argenyi Z, Cain C, Bromley C, et al. S-100 protein-negative malignant melanoma: Fact or fiction? A light-microscopic and immunohistochemical study. *A J Dermatopathol* 1994;16:233–240.
204. Orchard GE. Comparison of immunohistochemical labeling of melanocyte differentiation antibodies Melan-A, tyrosinase and HMB-45 with NKIC3 and S100 protein in the evaluation of benign naevi and malignant melanoma. *Histochem J* 2000;32:475–481.

5

PROGNOSTICATORS OF MELANOMA, THE MELANOMA REPORT, AND THE SENTINEL LYMPH NODE

Clark et al.[1,2] recognized the importance of anatomic compartment of invasion to the prognosis of melanoma. In 1970, Breslow[3] described the use of an ocular micrometer to specifically measure primary tumor thickness. These two parameters became the recognized prognostic variables available to histopathologists in predicting the biologic behavior of melanoma.[4] Throughout the 1980s, advances in comprehension of the biology and pathology of melanoma made it apparent that tumors undergo specific growth phases. In particular, neoplasms confined to a histologically defined radial growth phase were proven incapable of generating metastatic events unless regression was seen histologically at the primary site. Subsequent to this, further work done by the pigmented lesion clinics of Massachusetts General Hospital and the University of Pennsylvania established that the presence of microscopic satellites within tumors, the presence of brisk mitotic activity, the absence of an inflammatory infiltrate and in some circumstances, the presence of vascular invasion could modify the behavior of a neoplasm.

More recently, the American Joint Committee on Cancer (AJCC) Melanoma Committee, representing the expertise of major melanoma centers in the United States, Europe, and Australia and cancer co-operative groups in several countries, recommended a major revision of the TNM staging system following the analysis of prognostic and staging data of 17,654 prospectively enrolled melanoma patients.[5–7] In all, 13 cancer centers and co-operative groups registered data on 30,450 patients for whom full staging information was available for the aforementioned 17,654. Most had follow-up in excess of 10 years. Prognostic variables accounted for included tumor thickness, ulceration, level of invasion, anatomic site, satellites, in-transit metastases (defined clinically), gender, age, sentinel lymph node (SLN) status, elective lymph node status, therapeutic lymph node status, number of positive nodes, and sites of distant metastasis, correlated to dates of relapse and disease specific survival. The results of a complex multivariate statistical analysis showed through a Cox regression model that thickness was the most powerful predictor of biological behavior, followed by ulceration, age (over 60 years), anatomic site (trunk), Clark level, and gender. These factors all had p values ranging from 0.00001 to 0.001.[5–7]

PROGNOSTICATION INCLUDING MICROSTAGING OF MELANOMA

The prognosis of patients with invasive melanoma in vertical growth phase can be predicted by specific light microscopic parameters including the measured depth, mitotic count, host response, sex, anatomic site, and presence or absence of regression, angioinvasion, or ulceration. All of this information should appear in the pathology report.[8]

VERTICAL GROWTH PHASE MELANOMA

Introduction and Clinical Features

The presence of the vertical growth phase signifies the acquisition by a melanoma of the capacity for metastasis. The vertical growth phase usually manifests as a pigmented or amelanotic nodule supervening on a pre-existing macule or plaque, the sole exception being nodular melanoma that results from the rapid appearance of a malignant neoplasm in previously unremarkable skin. Nodular melanoma lacks a radial growth phase by definition.[2,8–11] The histologic descriptions that follow for vertical growth phase melanoma apply whether one is considering the acquisition of a vertical growth phase arising in a radial growth phase lesion of lentigo maligna melanoma, acral lentiginous melanoma, or superficial spreading melanoma, or to the de novo vertical growth phase of nodular melanoma. Therapy and prognostication depend on the pathologist's ability to accurately identify by light microscopy the vertical growth phase, as it defines the point in lesional evolution when a melanoma acquires the ability to metastasize and to kill the patient.[12–15]

Radial Versus Vertical Growth Phase

The radial growth phase comprises neoplastic melanocytes growing in a horizontal array as single cells and small nests predominantly in an intraepidermal location. The radial growth phase may also involve the papillary dermis (i.e., Clark level II) (Fig. 5.1).

The latter phenomenon describes a microinvasive melanoma and is similar to other concepts of early microinvasive cancer of diverse types. The work of Guerry et al.[16] in Philadelphia showed that radial growth phase neoplasms, in the absence of regression, were biology indolent and lacked a metastatic capacity. Others have emphasized the uniformly excellent

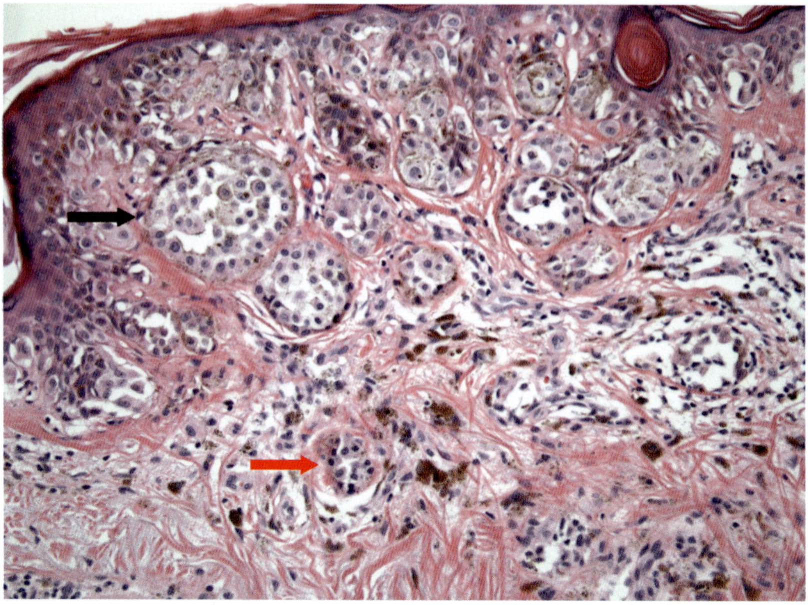

FIGURE 5.1 **Radial Growth Phase Melanoma.** The radial growth phase is biologically incapable of generating metastatic events, save for specific and uncommon circumstances. In this example, there is pagetoid spread of fully transformed malignant epithelioid melanocytes within the epidermis above the basement membrane zone (*black arrow*) in concert with a level 2 component in the papillary dermis. Note that the dermal component comprises small nests of neoplastic melanocytes (*red arrow*) with a similar cytology to those seen above the basement membrane zone which separates them from the overlying epidermal component (*black arrow*). The dermal nests of radial growth phase melanoma are smaller than those seen in the overlying epidermal component.

survivorship–approaching 100%–for patients with thin melanomas (≤1.0 mm in thickness) when confined to the radial growth phase.[9,10] An Australian study of 1,716 patients with radial growth phase melanoma showed metastases in only 67 (3.9%), all of whom had regression in their primary tumors.[17] Another series showed acquisition of early vertical growth phase to be associated with mortality in 12 patients with thin melanomas less than 0.76 mm at Clark level II.[18] In summation, the radial growth phase melanoma is virtually always curable by complete local excision with rare and specific exceptions. The radial growth phase is usually accompanied by a dermal lymphocytic inflammatory response that has no prognostic significance in this setting.

Early Vertical Growth Phase

Clark et al.[10] described the early vertical growth phase and distinguished it from the radial growth phase by criteria that included, most importantly, the presence of a dominant nest within the papillary dermis. This expansile nest is larger than any nest within the epidermis or the surrounding dermis (Fig. 5.2).

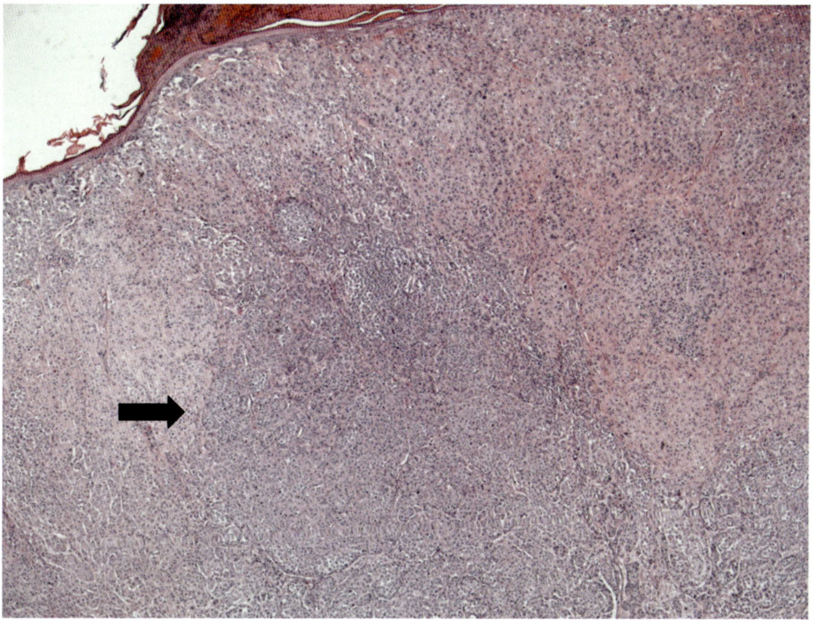

FIGURE 5.2 **Vertical Growth Phase Melanoma.** The vertical growth phase signifies the point at which the melanoma becomes biologically capable of producing metastatic events. Note that there is a dominant expansile dermal nest of neoplastic melanocytes (*arrow*) which is larger than any of the overlying thèques at the dermal–epidermal junction or within the epidermis. Furthermore, the cytology is typically distinctive in the dominant nest. Mitoses are often present. In the fully evolved vertical growth phase, these dominant nodules are noted at level III or level IV, while the incipient vertical growth phase tumor would be confined to the papillary dermis (i.e., Clark level II).

Clark suggested that the nodule should have 25 to 50 cells to aid in its identification, and that the cells comprising this nodule are cytologically distinct from those of the intraepidermal component by virtue of their different characteristics, be they of shape, size, nuclear or cytoplasmic features, or the presence or absence of pigment. The presence of regression, especially if extensive (i.e., >75% of tumor volume), may signal an enhanced capacity for metastatic behavior.[19,20] Incipient vertical growth phase melanoma typically does not fill the papillary dermis and manifests level II or incipient level III invasion. The presence of the early vertical growth phase imputes a risk for metastasis of roughly 10% at 8 years' follow-up.[21] A recent study showed that a mitotic rate of greater than zero or a thickness greater than 0.76 mm can be associated with positive SLNs in up to 12% of patients.[22] Patients with lesions of similar thickness which were not mitotically active had virtually no metastatic disease. In summation, patients with level II tumors less than 0.76 mm in thickness with an early vertical growth phase, ulceration of the primary tumor, extensive regression, or mitotic activity are at risk for metastatic disease.

FULLY EVOLVED VERTICAL GROWTH PHASE MELANOMA

Fully evolved vertical growth phase melanoma is defined by the following criteria: (i) the presence of a dominant nest within the dermis filling and widening the papillary dermis and extending to the papillary–reticular dermal interface or into the reticular dermis and/or subcutaneous fat (Clark levels IV and V) comprising (ii) cells with a distinct cytomorphology different from the intraepidermal radial growth phase component when present, often with (iii) mitoses. This defining expansile nest is larger than any nest within the epidermis or surrounding dermis and is classified by the cell type in order to avoid the potentially fatal error of overlooking a sometimes subtle phenomenon and also because certain of the subtypes have specific biological characteristics.[8] An inflammatory response is usually present and is of prognostic significance.

Cell Types of Vertical Growth Phase

EPITHELIOID VERTICAL GROWTH PHASE. Most often the vertical growth phase comprises epithelioid melanocytes with a round or cuboidal cytoplasmic

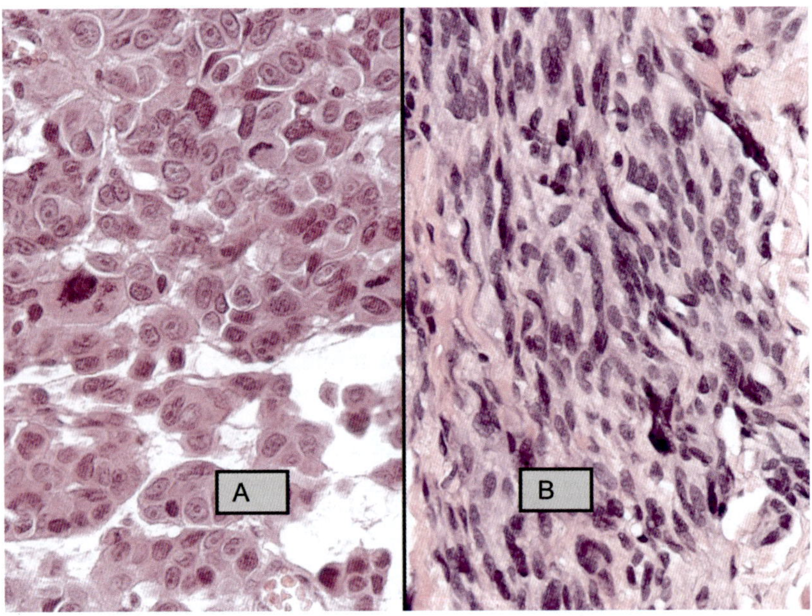

FIGURE 5.3 **Vertical Growth Phase Phenotypes, Classic. (A)** demonstrates classic epithelioid vertical growth phase melanoma. This is the form of vertical growth phase most commonly associated with widespread metastases. **(B)** shows a spindle cell vertical growth phase with wavy or fusiform, hyperchromatic nuclei, mimicking those of Schwann cell derivation. This form of vertical growth phase is prone to stubborn local recurrence and neurotropism, but less frequently causes widespread metastatic disease.

profile, round or oval nuclei with coarse, spiculated chromatin, prominent nucleoli, and chromatinic rims that are irregular in thickness and contour (Fig. 5.3).

Cytoplasms are often abundant with an eosinophilic staining quality and variable melanization. Cell cohesion is variable. Vertical growth phase nodules typically distort the architecture of the papillary or papillary and reticular dermis. Mitotic figures of both typical and atypical types are often apparent. The latter manifest as tri-, tetra- or pentapolar mitoses that reflect an aneuploid DNA content or chromosomal lags that signify the presence of double minutes (i.e., extra pieces of DNA that represent small chromosomelike structures from amplified proto-oncogenes), near-diploid aneuploidy, or aberrancy of the centromere/spindle apparatus. A variant of epithelioid vertical growth phase is the nevoid melanoma. Some studies have shown a significant tendency for the epithelioid vertical growth phase melanoma to manifest metastases preferentially over other vertical growth phase morphologies.[23]

SPINDLE CELL VERTICAL GROWTH PHASE. The spindle cell vertical growth phase is a form of vertical growth phase usually observed in lentigo maligna melanoma, acral lentiginous melanoma, or in other melanomas arising in acral or mucosal sites (i.e., mucosal lentiginous melanoma). Fascicles of hyperchromatic fusiform cells extend at various angles from the epidermis into the dermis (Fig. 5.3B). One observes no progressive diminution in cell size or in the overall size of the fascicles as one approaches the base of the lesion from above. There is evidence that the spindle cell vertical growth phase has a better prognosis than the epithelioid vertical growth phase.[14] A variant of spindle cell melanoma, the desmoplastic melanoma, tends to recur locally but uncommonly metastasizes.[24–30] It has been suggested that those desmoplastic melanomas having foci of conventional vertical growth phase melanoma manifest a significantly worse prognosis, with regional lymph node metastases in 10% of cases as opposed to only 1% of patients with pure desmoplastic melanoma.[31] Disease-specific 5-year mortality in one study was 11% for pure desmoplastic vertical growth phase tumors, versus 31% for those neoplasms having the aforementioned hybrid morphology.[31] The tendency for desmoplastic melanoma to manifest neurotropism and striking stromal collagenization can be explained at the molecular level by gene expression profiling that shows activation of genes encoding for neurotrophic factors and for extracellular matrix elaboration,[30] demonstrated at the protein level in fixed tissues by immunohistochemical assay for p75 nerve growth factor receptor[32] and basic fibroblast growth factor (b-FGF).[33] The expression of genes for melanocytic differentiation is reduced in desmoplastic melanoma as compared to conventional melanoma. This reduced expression of melanocyte differentiation genes has as its counterpart at the tissue level the absent expression of melanocyte lineage-specific markers such as HMB-45 and Melan-A.[28] There is little doubt that desmoplastic melanoma manifests up to a threefold greater thickness at presentation, but nonetheless has better survivorship than conventional melanomas of similar thickness.[31]

Histologic Type of Melanoma

Since the 1970s, melanomas have been histologically subclassified as belonging to four major groups: superficial spreading, lentigo maligna, acral lentiginous, and nodular melanoma.[2,34,35] The significance of these different melanoma subtypes remains a controversial subject. Some observers suggest that the relatively greater survivorship seen in lentigo maligna melanoma versus the other histologic subtypes is reflective of lesser thickness at the time of diagnosis.[10,36,37] It is apparent that the thickness of primary melanoma at the time of initial diagnosis shows progressive diminution in nodular versus superficial spreading versus lentigo maligna melanoma.[38] However, our contention is that this reflects reproducible differences in the biology of each process, thus, nodular melanoma, which manifests a vertical growth phase de novo would naturally be expected to have the greatest thickness and also to contain, by definition, a clone or clones of neoplastic cells capable of metastatic progression. By contrast, lentigo maligna melanoma, arising in a lentigo maligna manifesting as a persistent pigmented macule or plaque years prior to invasion,[39] would be obvious clinically and so potentially treatable at an early and curable stage. The lifetime risk for developing invasive disease in a lesion of lentigo maligna has been estimated to be only in the 5% range.[39] The worse prognosis of acral lentiginous melanoma[40] has been attributed not to its histomorphology, but to its location in acral glabrous skin.[41,42] The thinner dermis in acral sites lends itself to greater Clark levels of invasion despite lesser Breslow thickness, and so to access to larger-caliber blood vessels early in evolution. The early work of Fidler[43] suggests that those are the blood vessels capable of accommodating the large tumor bolus conducive to the establishment of the metastatic seed and so suggests that this is a critical factor in the lethality of any given acral melanoma. Although the significance of histologic type may be diminished in multivariate analysis,[44] it seems to us that common sense trumps statistics when assiduously applied.

LEVEL AND DEPTH OF INVASION. A critical factor is the extent of invasion into the dermis.[45] Tumor invasion may be qualitatively expressed according to the anatomic compartment of invasion (i.e., the papillary or reticular dermis or subcutis), which is referred to as the Clark level, or quantitatively assessed as the Breslow measurement, the thickness of the melanoma from the most superficial aspect of the granular cell layer to the deepest point of invasion into the dermis. Adventitial dermal invasion is not measured unless it is the only site of dermal invasion, and one then measures from the inner luminal surface of the eccrine gland or duct or the inner aspect of the outer root sheath epithelium of the hair follicle.[3]

Thickness (Breslow)

In the accumulated experience of numerous investigators over a long period of time, tumor thickness as measured by ocular micrometer has emerged as the most powerful predictor of outcome in primary cutaneous melanoma.[3,6,10,11,46–54] The Breslow measurement is taken from the epidermal surface or, in the event that the surface is ulcerated, from the base of the ulcer and is made with a calibrated ocular micrometer.[3] Long clinical follow-up indicates that melanoma thickness is a continuous variable associated with the dropout of survivors beyond 10 years. Thus, while formerly a tumor of 0.76 mm thickness was held to have a 99% survival rate at 5 years (and thus a virtual statistical certainty of "cure"), a large cohort of patients with tumors of that thickness, when followed out to 10 years, shows only a 90% to 92% survivorship. Patients with tumors 1 mm in thickness have a 20% likelihood of mortality at 10 years for reasons discussed earlier, while those with tumors over 4 mm in thickness have roughly a 50% mortality at 10 years. The Breslow measurement is the most important means of prognosticating mucosal melanomas that lack the anatomic compartmentalization seen in the skin.[20] In most prognostic studies, the measured depth emerges as the most powerful independent factor for prediction of lymph nodes metastasis and survival.[55]

Anatomic Compartment of Invasion ("Clark Level")

Clark levels are defined as follows[2]:

Level I: Malignant melanocytes are confined to the epidermis.
Level II: Partial infiltration of the papillary dermis by single cells or small nests of cells.
Level III: Tumor cells fill and expand the papillary dermis with extension of tumor to the papillary–reticular dermal interface, the latter identifiable through the routine use of a polarizer and compensator to take advantage of the birefringence patterns of the dermal collagen; the papillary dermal collagen fibers are oriented vertically whereas the reticular dermal collagen bundles have a more horizontal orientation. In level III invasion, a few cells may infiltrate the superficial reticular dermis, but the growth is not permeative. Level III penetration usually signifies vertical growth phase melanoma.[8,56]
Level IV: Melanoma cells infiltrate the reticular dermis in a significant fashion.
Level V: Melanoma cells infiltrate the subcutaneous fat.

Although the measured thickness emerges as a more powerful prognosticator than the anatomic compartment of invasion in most series, for thin melanomas ≤1.0 mm in depth, the Clark level remains a powerful independent prognostic variable, second only in importance to ulceration.[6] One German database showed that a Clark level III tumor had a 3.5 times greater risk of disease progression than did a level II tumor in melanomas ≤1.0 mm in thickness.[57]

MITOTIC RATE. Several large studies have emphasized the prognostic importance of the mitotic rate. The mitotic rate should be reported in any melanoma showing a vertical growth phase component, and is expressed as a mitotic index, namely, the number of mitoses in a square millimeter. About 3 to 10 high-power fields is equivalent to 1 mm^2, depending upon the nature of optical equipment used. There is a wide variance between different microscope makes and models, and we recommend calibration using a stage micrometer.[8,56] In Clark's original work on mitotic activity, 0 versus 1 to 6 versus greater than 6 mitoses/mm^2 were the breakpoints of analysis.[58] It is important to recognize that mitotic "hot spots" occur in tumors and that sampling can therefore be an issue. Clark advised studying sections for a few minutes to identify the areas of highest mitotic activity and beginning the formal count at that location. Mitotic rate links to tumor thickness in multivariate analysis,[37] but remains an independent variable in several studies.[10] Some authors have advocated the use of a "prognostic index" defined by a combination of mitotic rate and tumor thickness.[59,60]

In 3,661 patients from Australia, the mitotic rate was the most statistically powerful prognosticator of survival after thickness.[61] A mitotic rate of one or more per square millimeter was associated with a significant reduction in survivorship,[61] although in this data stepwise increases in mitotic activity did not show significant proportionate reduction in survival.[62] The Philadelphia group has shown a 10-year metastatic rate in men with vertical growth phase melanoma of 31% when a mitotic rate of greater than 0 was identified, versus a 4% mortality rate when the mitotic rate was 0.[63] Barnhill et al.[58] studied the impact of mitotic rate upon survival for 650 consecutive primary cutaneous melanoma patients in a logistic regression model. Using 0 versus 1 to 6 versus greater than 6 mitoses/mm^2 as their discriminative categories, they found that both moderate (1 to 6/mm^2) and high (>6/mm^2) mitotic activities were independent prognostic variables.[58] In particular, the highest mitotic index category was associated with an 11.6-fold increase in relative mortality at 5-year follow-up.[58]

A surrogate marker for mitotic activity can be found in those nuclear factors that serve as indicators of proliferative activity, several of which have been used in an attempt to distinguish benign from malignant melanocytic proliferations. MIB-1 is a monoclonal antibody that recognizes a Ki-67 epitope, but unlike Ki-67 antibody, which until recently required fresh or frozen tissue, MIB-1 antibody has been available for over a decade in formalin-fixed paraffin-embedded material. Ramsay et al.[64] found a significant reduction in cause-specific survival in thick, (>4.0 mm Breslow depth) stage I melanomas with high MIB-1 reactivity (defined as >20% of tumor cells decorating). A similar analysis in a small series of thin melanomas showed a statistically insignificant correlation with behavior, perhaps reflecting the small sample size.[65] The same observers did find a progressive increase in MIB-1 expression from benign nevi through primary melanomas to metastases, as well as a significant correlation with Clark level of invasion and Breslow depth.[65] Proliferating cell nuclear antigen (PCNA) is a polymerase accessory protein expressed during the cell cycle from G_1 to G_2, peaking at the G_1/S phase. A monoclonal antibody to PCNA that reacts in formalin-fixed paraffin-embedded tissue has been developed. The PCNA index, as defined by the number of positive staining cells per 1,000 tumor cells, is different in benign nevi versus melanoma; averaging 7.2 in nevi and 248.5 in melanoma.[66] In one study, the PCNA index proved more efficacious than the Breslow depth in predicting locoregional recurrences and metastases.[67] The predictive value of Ki-67 correlated more closely in one study of uveal melanoma with S phase, shorter survival, histological type, and tumor size than did PCNA expression.[68] Others found both Ki-67 and PCNA markers to correlate with survivorship in a study of 93 consecutive melanomas[69]; there was a correlation of metastatic behavior to PCNA expression in a study of 143 melanomas in which Ki-67 expression was not assessed.[70] One study of level III and IV melanomas found no correlation of survivorship with PCNA or Ki-67 expression; however, in that study, flow cytometric analysis showing an aneuploid DNA content was associated with a higher risk of metastatic progression.[71]

TUMOR INFILTRATING LYMPHOCYTES/INFLAMMATORY HOST RESPONSE. A lymphocytic response to the vertical growth phase component influences prognosis in some studies. The presence of tumor infiltrating lymphocytes (TILs) was shown to be a significant prognostic factor by Clemente et al.,[72] confirming Clark's observation from 1989 concerning the significance of TILs in melanoma prognosis.[8,10,56] A brisk infiltrate was defined as either a diffuse infiltrate of lymphocytes throughout the vertical growth phase or the presence of infiltrating lymphocytes along 90% of the circumference of the lesional base (Fig. 5.4). The nonbrisk infiltrate comprised only focal infiltration. An absent lymphoid infiltrate was one in which there were no lymphocytes admixed with melanoma cells, even if they were present in a perivascular array within the tumor or in a perivascular disposition beyond the tumor border but not abutting the tumor cells. Survival differences were highly significant, being 77% at 8 years for patients whose tumors showed brisk infiltration, 53% for those with nonbrisk infiltration, and 37% for those whose tumors were designated as having absent TILs.[72] Not surprisingly, the assessment of the intensity and distribution of the host lymphocytic infiltrate has a significant subjective component. This impacts the reproducibility of this criterion and lowers its predictive power in the hands of some authors.[73] Image analysis has been employed to reduce the impact of subjectivity and in one study was found to generate statistically significant prognostic data.[74] The presence of plasma cells[75] and macrophages[76] has been suggested to impact prognosis as well.

REGRESSION. Complete regression, characterized by an area of absent melanocytic growth in the epidermis and dermis, often bordered on one

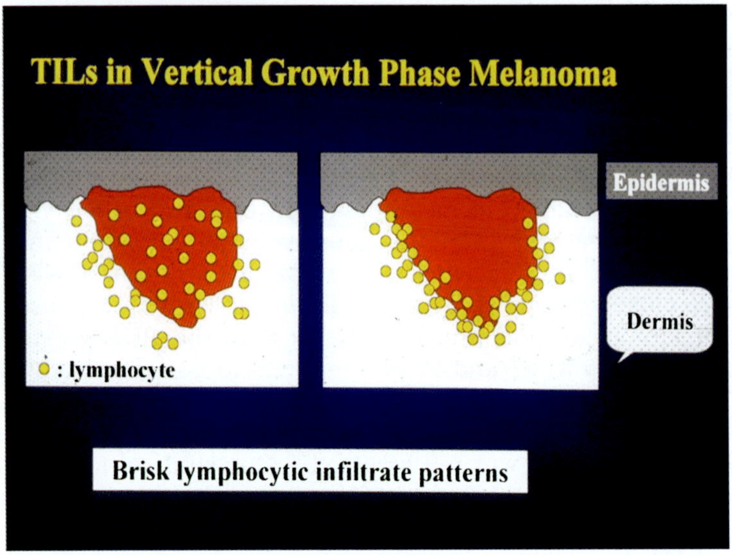

FIGURE 5.4 **Tumor Infiltrating Lymphocytes (TILs).** Depicted are the two patterns of TILs which would be designated as "brisk" and which would be a positive prognostic sign. In the left panel, lymphocytes diffusely infiltrate the melanoma mass and break up the neoplastic melanocytes into groups and single cells. In the right half of the panel, TILs surround 90% of the peripheral margin of the melanoma nodule. Either of these two patterns constitutes a "brisk" lymphocytic infiltrate.

or both sides by melanoma, may signify a worse prognosis.[19,41,77–80] The epidermis is often attenuated with loss of the retiform pattern. The subjacent dermis shows a nonlaminated fibroplasia containing a few inflammatory cells and melanophages with variable edema and telangiectasia, with the vessels typically assuming a perpendicular orientation to the long axis of the epidermis (Fig. 5.5, e-figs. 5.1–5.10).

Not all investigators have found regression to have a significant survival impact.[72,81–83] In the study of Barnhill et al.,[58] regression, when not assessed quantitatively or semiquantitatively, did not emerge as a significant variable. Regression of over 75% of a given tumor may be the critical volume that portends metastasis.[19,84] One case-control study confirmed that extensive regression was present in 42% of melanomas <1 mm in thickness that metastasized, versus only 5% of thin melanomas that did not.[85]

MICROSCOPIC SATELLITES. Microscopic satellites, characterized by reticular dermal and/or subcuticular nodules of tumor greater than 0.05 mm in width separated from the main vertical growth phase component (Fig. 5.6), are associated with lymph node metastasis and with decreased disease-free and overall survival.[10,53,86–89] Clark et al.[10] found a reduction of actuarial 8-year survival from 75% to 40% when satellites were identified. It has

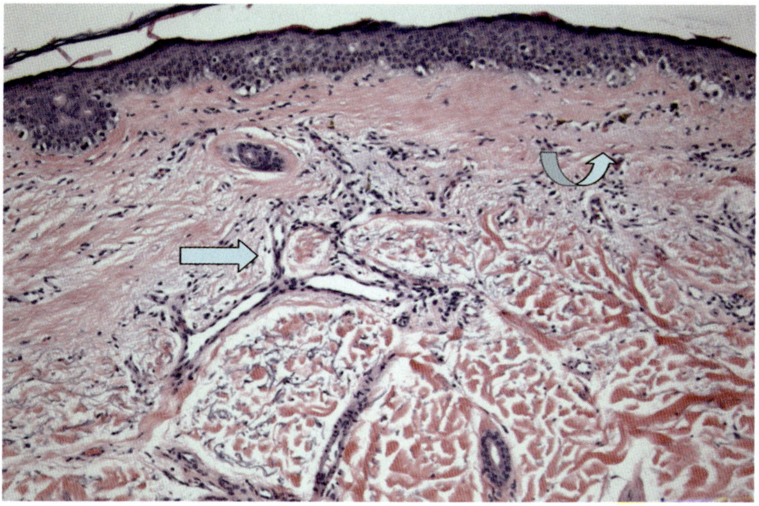

FIGURE 5.5 **Regression.** Regression of over 75% of the tumor volume of a melanoma is considered a bad prognostic sign. Regression is characterized by haphazard, patternless fibrosis, accompanied by vertically oriented, ectatic blood vessels (*straight arrow*), melanophages (*curved arrow*), and patchy lymphocytic infiltration of the stroma. In complete, as opposed to partial regression, there is a total absence of neoplastic melanocytes in the dermis and in the overlying epidermis.

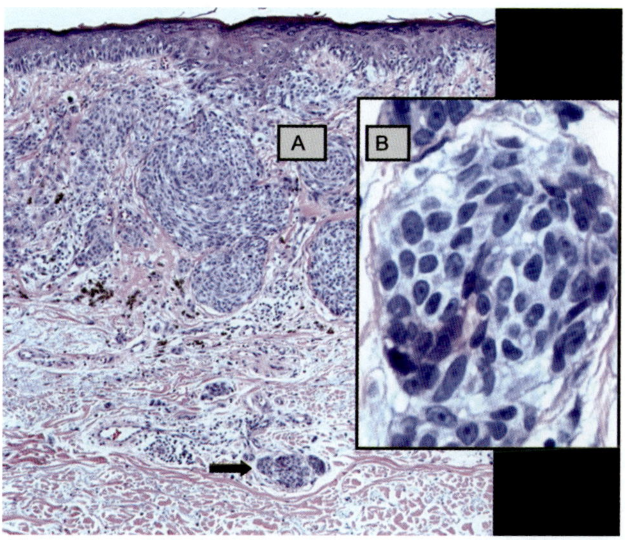

FIGURE 5.6 **Microscopic Satellites.** Microscopic satellites, in the most recent AJCC Classification scheme, are considered equivalent to an N1 lymph node metastatic station **(A)**. The satellite is characterized by a group of neoplastic melanocytes greater than 0.05 mm in diameter, typically located at Clark level 3, 4, or 5. This neoplastic group is discontinuous (*arrow*) from the overlying vertical growth phase component demonstrated in the papillary and superficial and reticular dermis. To qualify as a microscopic satellite, the melanocytes must have a malignant cytomorphology **(B)**.

been suggested that this is a difficult criterion to assess, as tumor tongues radiating from the main vertical growth phase nodule may mimic satellites due to artifacts of sectioning.[73]

BLOOD VESSEL AND LYMPHATIC INVASION. The presence or absence of blood vessel and lymphatic invasion should be reported (Fig. 5.7). Some studies have correlated the frequency of angiolymphatic invasion with increasing depth and level of tumor invasion,[59] while others have shown vascular invasion to be a significant predictor of metastasis[90] or of reduced survival.[11] It is perhaps the low frequency of this finding that prevented its emergence as an independent prognostic variable in many earlier series, but more recent data has shown a reduced survivorship of some 40% over 8 years when angioinvasion is demonstrated in primary tumors in vertical growth phase.[10] In modern multivariate analytic systems, angioinvasion is equivalent in prognostic import to ulceration, and second only to thickness, as a measure of survival probability.[91] Angioinvasion is focal within any given tumor, generating potential difficulties with respect to false negative studies in a single or few paraffin sections. Immunostaining with antibodies such those against endothelial antigenic targets CD31 and CD34 can prove beneficial in the avoidance of false positive diagnoses, as stromal retraction artifact around tumor nests can be easily misinterpreted as angioinvasion.

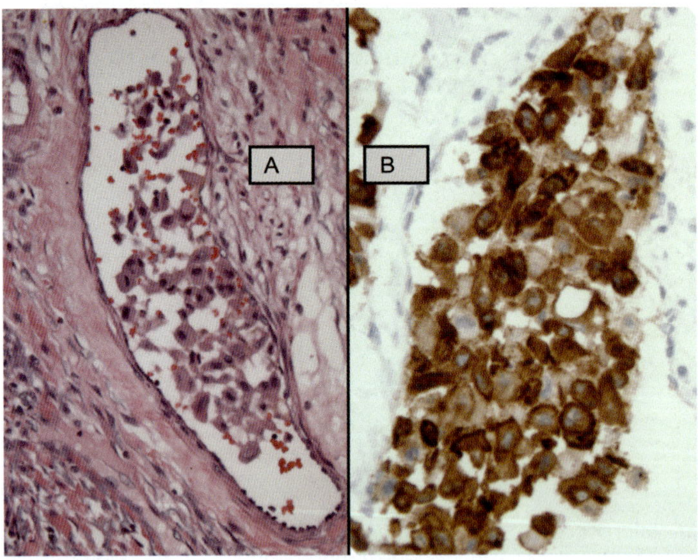

FIGURE 5.7 **Angioinvasion.** Although vascular invasion emerges as a powerful negative prognostic variable only in larger sample sizes, its presence is nonetheless an ominous sign and should be reported. Neoplastic epithelioid melanocytes are present within the lumen of a venule **(A)**. Their melanocytic character is confirmed by immunohistochemistry with a Melan-A antibody **(B)**.

ANATOMIC SITE. Melanomas of the head and neck area, upper back, axial skeleton, subungual region, and/or on the palms or soles have a worse prognosis than do extremity-based lesions.[2,53]

SEX. Women have a better prognosis than men in some but not all studies.[10,53] The statistical significance of gender is confounded by anatomic site, as women tend to have more extremity-based neoplasms, with better survivorship as a result.[73]

AGE. Some studies indicate that patients over the age of 60 years have a worse prognosis.[10,53]

Ulceration

Ulceration not attributable to trauma in any melanoma, irrespective of the diameter of the ulcer, represents an adverse independent prognostic factor (Fig. 5.8).[92] The reason that ulceration correlates with substantially increased risk of local recurrence and metastasis likely reflects rapid tumor growth and relative tumor ischemia as a function of rapid growth. By convention, we measure the size of any ulcer.[93] The 5-year survivorship in stage I and stage II melanomas decreased from 80% to 55% in the presence of

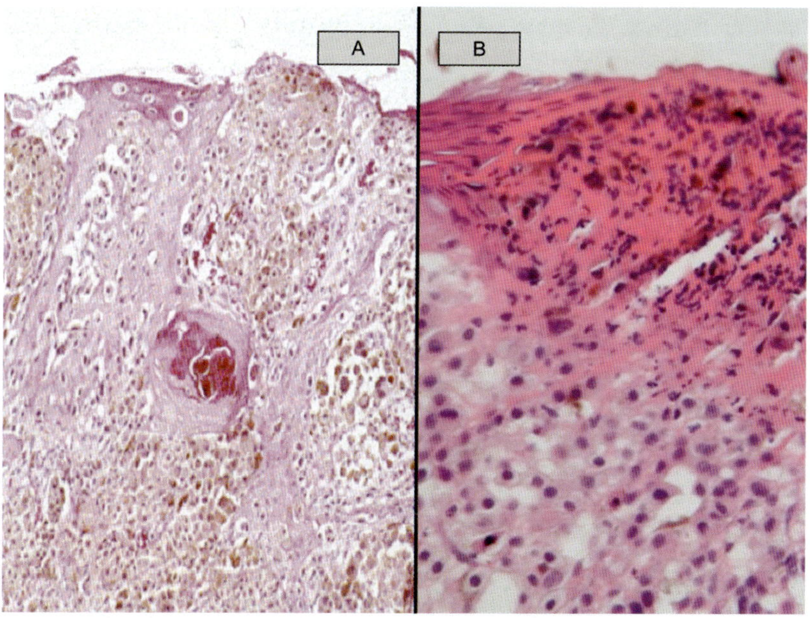

FIGURE 5.8 **Ulceration.** Ulceration emerges as a powerful negative prognostic indicator. It is important not to misinterpret artifactual fragmentation of the epidermal surface **(A)** from ulceration **(B)**. In the former instance, nests of neoplastic cells can be artifactually extruded to the epidermal surface during processing. The absence of an in vivo response as indicated in **(B)**, namely, a fibrinopurulent exudate directly overlying the neoplastic melanocytes and/or papillary dermal stroma, is the clue to a correct interpretation.

ulceration and for stage III melanomas dropped from 53% to 12%. The majority of melanomas greater than 4 mm in thickness are ulcerated. When tumors had an ulcer diameter of greater than 6 mm, the prognosis was even worse. Important changes with respect to the T classification were therefore effected from 1997 to 2002 (Tables 5.1 and 5.2). In particular, the T1 level, formerly 0.75 mm, is now set at less than 1 mm. T2 tumors are

TABLE 5.1 AJCC Melanoma TNM Classification (Revised 2002)

T Classification	Thickness	Ulceration Status
T_1	≤1.0 mm	a: w/o ulceration and level II or III b: with ulceration or level IV or V
T_2	1.01–2.00 mm	a: w/o ulceration b: with ulceration
T_3	2.01–4.0 mm	a: w/o ulceration b: with ulceration
T_4	>4.0 mm	a: w/o ulceration b: with ulceration
N Classification	**Number of Metastatic Nodes**	**Nodal Metastatic Mass**
N_1	1 node	a: micrometastasis[a] b: macrometastasis[b]
N_2	2–3 nodes	a: micrometastasis[a] b: macrometastasis[b] c: in transit met(s)/ satellite(s) without metastatic nodes
N_3	4 or more metastatic nodes, or matted nodes, or in transit met(s)/satellite(s) with metastatic node(s)	
M Classification	**Site**	**Serum LDH**
M_{1a}	Distant skin, subcutaneous or nodal mets	Normal
M_{1b}	Lung metastases	Normal
M_{1c}	All other visceral metastases	Normal
	Any distant metastasis	Elevated

[a]Micrometastases are diagnosed after elective or sentinel lymphadenectomy.

[b]Macrometastases are defined as clinically detectable nodal metastases confirmed by therapeutic lymphadenectomy or when nodal metastasis exhibits gross extracapsular extension.

TABLE 5.2 Stage Groupings For Cutaneous Melanomas

Clinical Staging[a]				Pathologic Staging[b]			
0	Tis	N0	M0	0	Tis	N0	M0
IA	T1a	N0	M0	IA	T1a	N0	M0
IB	T1b	N0	M0	IB	T1b	N0	M0
	T2a	N0	M0		T2a	N0	M0
IIA	T2b	N0	M0	IIA	T2b	N0	M0
	T3a	N0	M0		T3a	N0	M0
IIB	T3b	N0	M0	IIB	T3b	N0	M0
	T4a	N0	M0		T4a	N0	M0
IIC	T4b	N0	M0	IIC	T4b	N0	M0
III	Any T	Any N	M0	IIIA	T1–4a	N1a	M0
					T1–4a	N2a	M0
				IIIB	T1–4b	N1a	M0
					T1–4b	N2a	M0
					T1–4a	N1b	M0
					T1–4a	N2b	M0
					T1–4 a/b	N2c	M0
				IIIC	T1–4b	N1b	M0
					T1–4b	N2b	M0
					T1–4b	N2c	M0
					Any T	N3	M0
IV	Any T	Any N	Any M	IV	Any T	Any N	Any M

[a]Clinical staging includes microstaging of the primary melanoma and clinical/radiologic evaluation for metastases. By convention, it should be used after complete excision of the primary melanoma with clinical assessment for regional and distant metastases.

[b]Pathologic staging includes microstaging of the primary melanoma and pathologic information concerning regional lymph nodes after partial or complete lymphadenectomy. Patients with pathologic stage 0 or stage IA disease are the exception; they do not require pathologic evaluation of their lymph nodes.

1.1 to 2 mm in thickness and T3 tumors 2.1 to 4 mm. A T4 neoplasm is any tumor greater than 4 mm in thickness. The subscript "a" is added for the absence of ulceration and the subscript "b" for the presence of ulceration. Microscopic satellites are considered to represent N3 disease in the 2002 staging classification. In the new classification, a T4b tumor (i.e., >4 mm in thickness with an ulcer present) is associated with roughly 30% 10-year survivorship.[6,94]

DNA Ploidy Status

DNA ploidy status can be assessed in paraffin-embedded tissues using static image-analysis software, or in fresh tissue using flow cytometry. Conflicting data are reported, some showing no prognostic import of DNA analysis.[95,96] Some authors have found, in contrast, a significant association between aneuploidy and diminished survivorship in stage I and stage II melanoma patients.[97] The import of aneuploidy diminishes in multivariate analysis; a majority of melanomas are diploid and thicker tumors tend to be more often aneuploid, diminishing the necessity of ploidy analysis to routine prognostic analysis. The S-phase fraction of a given neoplasm can be similarly expressed; median survival times were 45 months for tumors with an S-phase fraction greater than 5% and 19 months for an S-phase fraction greater than 10%.[98] Mitotic rate and S-phase fraction proved to correlate independently with survivorship in one multivariate anaylsis.[99]

Lymph Node Status

Survival from melanoma drops progressively from 90% at 10 years for stage I to 10% at 10 years for stage IV disease. The major independent variable predicting survivorship in thick (i.e., >4 mm in depth) melanoma is the presence or absence of micrometastatic disease in the SLN.[100,101] The number of involved lymph nodes has been shown to be a powerful prognosticator with a p value of 0.00001.[53] Furthermore, microscopic versus macroscopic metastasis is of major significance; if a lymph node is clinically palpable in a suspicious fashion and is proven histologically to contain tumor, this has more significance than a clinically negative lymph node containing microscopic disease. With respect to survival by a number of positive lymph nodes, the 10-year survivorship drops from 50% with one positive node to 20% with greater than four positive lymph nodes. The number of lymph nodes positive in any definitive resection specimen correlates with the presence of ulceration. With respect to the issue of clinical node positive versus clinical node negative disease, the 10-year survivorship drops from 50% in those microscopically positive nodes held clinically to be negative to 30% in those microscopically positive nodes held clinically to be suspicious for metastatic disease.

Visceral and Other Remote Metastatic Sites

With respect to visceral and other metastatic deposit sites, a high LDH, more than one visceral site involved, male gender, and low serum albumin levels all correlate with short survival times ranging from 3 to 7 months.

Satellites

The presence of microscopic and macroscopic satellites, the former defined by Day et al.[86] as a nest of tumor cells 0.05 mm in diameter that is distinct from the main vertical growth phase tumor mass, has been assigned the significance of a micrometastasis and therefore moved to the *N* stage classification.[5] The macroscopic satellite is defined as a clinical evidence of tumor deposit(s) 2 cm from the primary neoplasm along the line of drainage to the nearest regional lymph node station.

Sentinel Lymph Node Biopsy as a Prognostic Tool

The SLN biopsy status has proven to be a powerful predictor of survivorship.[100,101] The pattern and volume of lymph node involvement are predictive of the likelihood of finding metastatic deposits in other nodes in the drainage basin at time of completion lymphadenectomy (Fig. 5.9). Although some studies have shown significant improvements in survivorship with elective and/or completion lymphadenectomy, most such series have not. In the data of Cherpelis et al.,[102] SLN status and ulceration were the only independent predictive factors of 5-year survival for tumors greater than 3 mm in thickness, while others have shown thickness, ulceration, and mitotic rate all to be independent prognostic factors for patients with thick melanomas.[103] We recommend SLN biopsy as part of the prognostic workup for a patient with a T2 or T3 tumor, or any patient with a T1 tumor in vertical growth phase or with ulceration or significant regression at the primary site, as previously defined next.

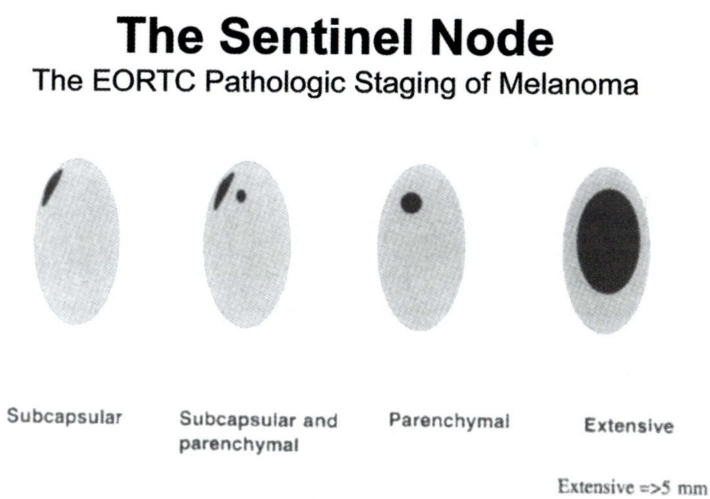

FIGURE 5.9 **The sentinel Lymph Node: Architectural Patterns Indicative of Probable Involvement of Nonsentinel Lymph Nodes.** The restriction of clusters of neoplastic melanocytes to a subcapsular location in a sentinel lymph node is associated with a very low (i.e., <5%) risk of nonsentinel lymph node involvement in the drainage basin. Subcapsular parenchymal deposits or parenchymal deposits of small size in isolation from subcapsular components portend a roughly 10% to 20% incidence of nonsentinel lymph node positivity. Extensive lymph node involvement, defined in the quoted study of Ruiter et al.[109] as deposit or deposits greater than 5 mm in diameter, is associated with an incidence of nonsentinel lymph node involvement of roughly 25%.

UTILITY OF SENTINEL LYMPH NODE BIOPSY TO DIRECT THERAPEUTIC COMPLETION LYMPHADENECTOMY

Compelling data demonstrate a statistically significant survival benefit in those patients with melanomas greater than 1 mm in thickness who have positive SLN biopsies and go on to immediate completion lymphadenectomy in the setting of node-negative disease, as opposed to those who wait for subsequent clinical evidence of further lymph node metastases. Dessureault et al.[104] showed a statistically significant survivorship benefit with a reduction of mortality of 68.5% in such patients. More recent work by Morton et al.[105] has shown survivorship benefit in a trial of 1,269 patients with intermediate thickness melanomas (1.2 to 3.5 mm in depth) who were randomly assigned to immediate SLN biopsy or to delayed lymphadenectomy following observation for clinically detectable lymph nodes in the drainage basin. In the latter group, the finding of a palpable lymph node would prompt a subsequent lymphadenectomy. In the former group, a SLN biopsy showing microscopic metastasis prompted immediate radical lymphadenectomy. This trial demonstrated unequivocally that the SLN biopsy provided immediate important prognostic information and identified those patients with nodal metastases whose survivorship could be prolonged by lymphadenectomy.[106] This trial also demonstrated that clinically occult nodal metastases could be detected through the SLN biopsy technique at a median of 16 months earlier than lymph node metastases could be detected by physical examination alone. Among those patients with nodal metastases, the 5-year survivorship was 72% in the immediate completion lymphadenectomy arm versus 52% in the observation group ($p = 0.004$).[105] Admittedly, there is a dilutional effect of those patients who undergo SLN biopsy and have a negative lymph node status. Overall, the 5-year disease-free survivorship is higher in the biopsy group than in the observation group (78% vs. 73%; $p = 0.009$).[106] As has been pointed out, those 80% of patients with melanoma who have pathologically negative results from SLN biopsy can also be spared some of the cost of subsequent oncology clinic visits, as well as the anxiety of being held in suspense concerning the possibility of metastatic tumor events having gone undetected.

Once a SLN is proven to contain metastatic melanoma, the next step is completion lymphadenectomy. Only 15% to 25% of patients will have any evidence of metastases in the SLN,[107] and it is therefore imperative to predict which patients with a positive SLN will require further surgery in the draining lymph node basin so as to avoid the morbidity which occurs with this operation in patients who do not require it. The contributions of Cochran et al.[108] have provided valuable clues as to which patients with metastatic deposits in the biopsied SLN will be found to have positive non-SLNs at the time of completion lymphadenectomy. The thickness of the primary melanoma, the relative area of tumor in the SLN, and the density of dendritic leukocytes in the paracortex of the lymph node have all been proven to be predictive of the risk of positive non-SLNs at completion lymphadenectomy. Specifically, the mean Breslow thickness of primary melanomas from patients whose non-SLNs were tumor free was 2.3 mm, while the mean Breslow thickness was 4.3 mm in those patients whose non-SLNs were positive. The percentage of SLN area containing melanoma cells was 4.3% in those patients whose non-SLNs were negative versus 30.16% in patients whose non-SLNs were positive. The density of dendritic cells in the SLN paracortex in patients whose non-SLNs were tumor free was 69.34/mm^2 versus 35.65/mm^2 in patients with positive non-SLNs (Fig. 5.10). The p values of significance for these data points ranged from 0.08 to 0.0001.[108]

Data from the European Organisation for the Research and Treatment of Cancer (EORTC) showed that the finding of an extensive lymph node deposit, defined as a deposit greater than 5 mm in diameter, correlates with tumor deposits in the non-SLNs of the draining lymph node basin in over 20% of patients.[109] Data from Toronto indicated that none of 127 patients with positive SLN biopsies, of whom 15.8% had a positive non-SLN in the drainage basin at completion lymphadenectomy, had a positive non-SLN if the SLN deposit was less than or equal to 0.2 mm.[110]

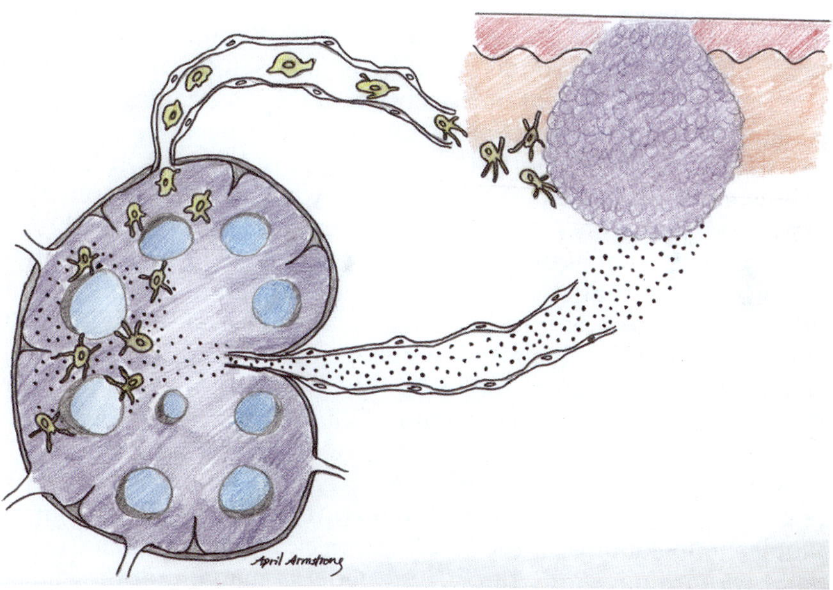

FIGURE 5.10 **Sentinel Lymph Node Involvement and the "veiled" Antigen-presenting Cell.** Dendritic antigen presenting cells migrate from the lymphatic bed of the primary cutaneous melanoma to enter the draining lymph node through afferent lymphatics. While in transit, these dendritic antigen presenting cells lose their dendritic morphology, the phenotypic hallmark of which is loss of CD80 and CD86 expressions. If these antigen presenting cells remain "veiled" (i.e., CD80 and CD86 negative) when in the paracortex of the lymph node, the possibility of nonsentinel lymph node involvement in the drainage basis may be higher. This process is alleged to reflect immune suppression mediated by some cytokine or cytokines elaborated by the melanoma cells.

Of 504 patients in one Colorado series, 31 had SLN deposits greater than 2 mm in size, which correlated with a 5-year survival of 47%. By contrast, among 49 patients whose SLN deposits were at or less than 2 mm in size, the 5-year survival rate of 85% was essentially identical to SLN-negative patients in the study pool.[111] The method of van Akkooi et al.,[112] in a histologic analysis of 262 patients, was to divide deposits into three groups: less than 1.0 mm, 0.1 to 1.0 mm, and greater than 1.0 mm in size. They found that neither the location nor the number of SLN deposits less than 0.1 mm affected survival. The 5-year survival rates for the three groups were 100%, 63%, and 35%, respectively. Patients with deposits less than 0.1 mm would therefore not be expected to benefit from completion lymphadenectomy.

Certain caveats must be applied to the adoption of the SLN biopsy as a standard of care. First, neither the choice of the radioactive label, nor the technique and optimal timing for the injection of the radiocolloid and of the pigmented dye has been strictly defined,[113] nor is it clear how many lymph nodes should be removed at the time of SLN biopsy.[114] In one study, authors found that the metastases in some 5% of patients were confined to nodes that were neither stained blue by the supravital dyes nor those which generated the highest gamma counts.[114] The "ten percent rule" has been applied in some facilities to determine which lymph nodes merit consideration as SLNs; namely, those draining nodes that are removed until the background count by lymphoscintigraphy is less than 10% of the original count at the inception of the surgical procedure.[115,116] The logic behind this approach is that the false negative rate of SLN biopsy rises if only the "hottest" lymph node is sampled. It is also not clear how many drainage basins identified by lymphoscintigraphy should be explored operatively or how many nodes should be removed.[113,114] In 37 prior reports summating over 14,000 patients, the total number of SLNs removed per patient was 2.16, with the mean of the total number ranging from 1.2 to 3.6.[117] In the large data set assembled by the AJCC, the number of positive lymph nodes as well as the clinical status (positive versus negative prior to the histopathologic demonstration of lymph node deposits) impacted survivorship.[5,6] Similarly, the number of negative SLNs has been shown to be predictive of time to recurrence.[117]

In addition to the foregoing, patients with certain melanoma subtypes may not benefit from the SLN biopsy technique. In particular, pure desmoplastic melanoma of the head and neck appears to metastasize to regional lymph nodes only rarely, and patients may die of disseminated metastases without ever first compromising the draining lymph node basin.[118]

CONCLUSION

The essential elements of the pathology report for primary cutaneous melanoma should include all of the statistically proven prognostic variables as discussed earlier. Enclosed is the melanoma diagnostic template used at Regional Medical Laboratory in Tulsa, Oklahoma (Table 5.3). In light of the

TABLE 5.3 Synoptic Report for Primary Cutaneous Melanoma (Regional Medical Laboratory, Tulsa, Oklahoma)

Name: ______________	Case No.: __________
Location: ______________	
Histological type:	
Lentigo maligna	❑
Superficial spreading	❑
Nodular	❑
Acral lentiginous	❑
Not otherwise specified	❑
Clark level:	
I	❑
II	❑
III	❑
IV	❑
V	❑
Thickness (Breslow):	___________ mm
Mitotic index (mitoses/mm^2):	___________
Radial growth phase	Y ❑ N ❑
Vertical growth phase	Y ❑ N ❑
Microscopic satellites	Y ❑ N ❑
Regression	Y ❑ N ❑
Ulceration	Y ❑ N ❑
Diameter___________	
Host immune response	
	Brisk Nonbrisk Absent
Neurotropism	Y ❑ N ❑
Vascular invasion	Y ❑ N ❑
Microscopic satellites	Y ❑ N ❑
Precursor lesion	Y ❑ N ❑
Type	___________
Margin positive	Y ❑ N ❑
Location if positive	___________
Minimum distance from tumor if negative	___________
Lymph nodes involved	Y ❑ N ❑
Number___________	
Sentinel lymph node positive	Y ❑ N ❑ not assessed
Distant metastases	Y ❑ N ❑
Site___________	

This synoptic report is appended to a narrative description of all malignant melanomas except for in situ disease, where the "microstaging" of prognostic risk factors, i.e., ulceration, regression, Breslow depth, etc., is not given.

modern approaches to the assessment of metastatic risk, the old "quick and dirty report," namely "Melanoma, not otherwise specified: Breslow depth 0.4 mm; margin negative" does the patient a disservice. In the modern era, clinicians and oncologists must recognize specific risk factors for metastatic disease so as to guide adjuvant chemotherapy or immunomodulatory therapy and further surgical therapy including sentinel and completion lymphadenectomy when necessary. The most recent data of Morton et al.[105] suggests that the SLN biopsy has emerged as a standard of care for patients with melanoma greater than 1.1 mm in thickness. It is our view that the sentinel lymphadectomy must be considered not only part of the prognostic armamentarium, but also one which leads to potentially beneficial further surgical therapy. We recommend SLN biopsy, therefore, as part of our prognostic workup for a patient with a T2 or T3 tumor or any patient with a T1 tumor in vertical growth phase or whose T1 tumor has ulceration or extensive (i.e., >75%) regression at the primary site. Further, it can be argued that patients with primary cutaneous nevomelanocytic proliferations deemed to be prognostically indeterminate from a histologic perspective, for example, the atypical Spitzoid lesions, ought to undergo SLN biopsy as part of their prognostic microstaging with the proviso that one would have evaluated and treated unequivocal melanoma at the same lesional thickness by a SLN biopsy and completion lymphadenectomy as indicated.[119]

Although the once promising work concerning alpha interferon therapy has not borne fruit, suggesting that no current adjuvant therapy is available to confer increased survival benefits upon patients with metastatic or disseminated disease, evolving adjuvant genetic therapies may soon dramatically impact survivorship. The metastastic potential of any given patient's melanoma therefore needs to be ascertained as precisely and accurately as possible, as in the near future we anticipate that specific gene-based therapy will target the molecular events of melanomagenesis[15,120] and that the subtype of melanoma and its pattern of invasion will illuminate specific molecular therapeutic targets. It is therefore considered essential that patients receiving melanoma diagnoses be provided with the accurate and comprehensive diagnostic assessment upon which these novel therapeutic strategies will be based.

ACKNOWLEDGMENT

We thank April Armstrong for the illustration in Figure 5.10.

REFERENCES

1. Clark WH Jr. A classification of malignant melanoma in man correlated with histogenesis and biological behaviour. In: Montagna W, Hu F, eds. *Advances in the Biology of the Skin*. Vol VIII. New York, NY: Pergamon; 1967:621–647.
2. Clark WH Jr, From L, Bernardino EA, Mihm MC. Histogenesis and biologic behavior of primary human malignant melanomas of the skin. *Cancer Res* 1969;29:705–726.

3. Breslow A. Thickness, cross-sectional areas and depth of invasion in the prognosis of cutaneous melanoma. *Ann Surg* Nov 1970;172(5):902–908.
4. Crowson AN, Barnhill RL, Magro CM, Mihm MC Jr. The pathology of melanoma. In: Balch C, Houghton A, Sober A, et al. eds. *Cutaneous Melanoma*, 4th Ed. St Louis: Quality Medical Publishers Inc.; 2003:171–206.
5. Balch CM, Buzaid AC, Akins MB, et al. A new American Joint Committee on Cancer staging system for cutaneous melanoma. *Cancer* 2000;88:1484–1491.
6. Balch CM, Soong SJ, Gershenwald JE, et al. Prognostic factors analysis of 17,600 melanoma patients: Validation of the American Joint Committee on Cancer melanoma staging system. *J Clin Oncol* 2001;19:3622–3634.
7. Balch CM, Gershenwald JE, Buzaid AC, et al. Staging and classification. In: Balch C, Houghton A, Sober A, et al. eds. *Cutaneous Melanoma*. 4th Ed. St Louis: Quality Medical Publishers Inc, 2003:55–76.
8. Crowson AN, Magro CM, Mihm MC Jr. Malignant melanoma. In: *The Melanocytic Proliferations: A Comprehensive Textbook of Pigmented Lesions*. New York, NY: John Wiley and Sons; 2001:281–397.
9. Clark EH Jr, Elder DE, Guerry D IV, et al. A study of tumor progression: The precursor lesions of superficial spreading and nodular malignant melanoma. *Hum Pathol* Dec 1984;15(12):1147–1165.
10. Clark WH Jr, Elder DE, Guerry D, et al. Model predicting survival in stage I melanoma based on tumor progression. *J Natl Cancer Inst* 1989;81:1893–1904.
11. Barnhill RL, Fine JA, Roush GC, Berwick M. Predicting five-year outcome for patients with cutaneous melanoma in a population-based study. *Cancer* 1996;78:427–432.
12. Day CL, Lew RA, Mihm MC Jr, et al. A multivariate analysis of prognostic factors for melanoma patients with lesions greater than or equal to 3.65 mm in thickness. The importance of revealing alternate Cox models. *Ann Surg* Jan 1982;195(1):44–49.
13. Day CL, Mihm MC Jr, Sober AJ, et al. Prognostic factors for melanoma patients with lesions 0.76–1.69 mm in thickness. An appraisal of "thin" level IV lesions. *Ann Surg* 1982;95(1):30–34.
14. Day CL, Mihm MC Jr, Lew RA, et al. Prognostic factors for clinical stage I melanoma of intermediate thickness (1.51–3.39 mm). A conceptual model for tumor growth and metastasis. *Ann Surg* 1982;195(1):35–43.
15. Crowson AN, Magro C, Mihm MC Jr. The biology of melanoma progression: From melanocyte to metastatic seed. In: Hearing VJ, Leong SPL, eds. *From Melanocytes to Malignant Melanoma*. Totowa, NJ: Humana Press, 2006:365–399.
16. Guerry D IV, Synnestvedt M, Elder DE, et al. Lessons from tumor progression: the invasive radial growth phase of melanoma is common, incapable of metastasis, and indolent. *J Invest Dermatol* 1993;100(3):342S–345S.
17. Taran JM, Heenan PJ. Clinical and histological features of level 2 cutaneous malignant melanoma associated with metastasis. *Cancer* 2001;91:1822–1825.
18. Lefevre M, Vergier B, Balme B, et al. Relevence of vertical growth pattern in thin level II cutaneous superficial spreading melanomas. *Am J Surg Pathol* 2003;27:717–724.
19. Ronan SG, Eng AM, Briele HA, et al. Thin melanomas with regression and metastases. *Arch Dermatol* 1987;123:1326–1330.
20. Ronan SG, Han MC, Das Gupta TK. Histologic prognostic indicators in cutaneous malignant melanoma. *Semin Oncol* 1988;15:558–565.
21. Elder DE, Guerry D IV, Epstein MN, et al. Invasive melanomas lacking competence for metastasis. *Am J Dermatopathol* Summer 1984;6(Suppl. 1):55–61.
22. Kesmodel SB, Karakousis GC, Botbyl JD, et al. Mitotic rate as a predictor of sentinel lymph node positivity in patients with thin melanomas. *Ann Surg Oncol* 2005; 12:449–458.

23. Otto FJ, Goldmann T, Biess B, et al. Prognostic classification of malignant melanomas by combining clinical, histological, and immunohistochemical parameters. *Oncology* 1999;56:208–214.
24. Conley J, Lattes R, Orr W. Desmoplastic malignant melanoma (a rare variant of spindle cell melanoma). *Cancer* 1971;28:914–936.
25. Egbert B, Kempson R, Sagebiel R. Desmoplastic malignant melanoma. A clinicopathologic study of 25 cases. *Cancer* 1988;62:2033–2041.
26. Bruijn JA, Mihm MC Jr, Barnhill RL. Desmoplastic melanoma. *Histopathology* 1992;20: 197–205.
27. Fearns C, Dowdle EB. The desmoplastic response: Induction of collagen synthesis by melanoma cells in vitro. *Int J Cancer* 1992;50:621–627.
28. Carlson JA, Dickersin GR, Sober AJ, Barnhill RL. Desmoplastic neurotropic melanoma. A clinicopathologic analysis of 28 cases. *Cancer* 1995;75:478–494.
29. Gyorki DE, Busam K, Panageas K, et al. Sentinel lymph node biopsy for patients with cutaneous desmoplastic melanoma. *Ann Surg Oncol* 2003;10:403–407.
30. Busam KJ, Zhao H, Coit DG, et al. Distinction of desmoplastic melanoma from non-desmoplastic melanoma by gene expression profiling. *J Invest Dermatol* 2005;124:412–418.
31. Hawkins WG, Busam KJ, Ben-Porat L, et al. Desmoplastic melanoma: a pathologically and clinically distinct form of cutaneous melanoma. *Ann Surg Oncol* 2005;12:197–199.
32. Iwamoto S, Odland PB, Piepkorn M, Bothwell M. Evidence that the p75 neurotrophin receptor mediates perineural spread of desmoplastic melanoma. *J Am Acad Dermatol* 1996;35(5 Pt 1):725–731.
33. Al-Alousi S, Carlson JA, Blessing K, et al. Expression of basic fibroblast growth factor in desmoplastic melanoma. *J Cutan Pathol* 1996;23:118–125.
34. Clark WH, Mihm MC. Lentigo maligna and lentigo maligna melanoma. *Am J Pathol* 1969;55:39–54.
35. Reed RJ. Acral lentiginous melanoma. In: Reed RJ, ed. *New Concepts in Surgical Pathology of the Skin*. New York, NY: Wiley; 1976:89–90.
36. Koh HK, Michalik E, Sober AJ, et al. Lentigo maligna melanoma has no better prognosis than other types of melanoma. *J Clin Oncol* 1984;2:994–1001.
37. Vollmer RT. Malignant melanoma. A multivariate analysis of prognostic factors. *Pathol Annu* 1989;24:383–407.
38. Thorn M, Ponten F, Bergstrom R, et al. Clinical and histopathologic predictors of survival in patients with malignant melanoma: A population-based study in Sweden. *J Natl Cancer Inst* 1994;86:761–769.
39. Weinstock MA, Sober AJ. The risk of progression of lentigo maligna to lentigo maligna melanoma. *Br J Dermatol* 1987;116:303–310.
40. Massi D, Borgognoni L, Franchi A, et al. Thick cutaneous malignant melanoma: A reappraisal of prognostic factors. *Melanoma Res* 2000;10:153–164.
41. Slingluff CL Jr, Vollmer RT, Reintgen DS, Seigler HF. Lethal "thin" malignant melanoma. Identifying patients at risk. *Ann Surg* 1988;208:150–161.
42. Kato T, Suetake T, Kumasaka N, et al. Nodular melanoma in 62 Japanese patients: influence of initial surgical treatment of local recurrence and prognosis. *J Dermatol* 1995;22:723–728.
43. Fidler IJ. Tumor heterogeneity and the biology of cancer invasion and metastasis. *Cancer Res* 1978;38:2651–2660.
44. Cox NH, Aitchison TC, Sirel JM, MacKie RM. Comparison between lentigo maligna melanoma and other histogenetic types of malignant melanoma of the head and neck. Scottish Melanoma Group. *Br J Cancer* 1996;73:940–944.
45. Mehnert JH, Heard JL. Staging of malignant melanoma by depth of invasion. *Am J Surg* 1965;110:168–176.

46. Balch CM, Murad TM, Soong SJ, et al. A multifactorial analysis of melanoma: Prognostic histopathological features comparing Clark's and Breslow's staging methods. *Ann Surg* 1978;188:732–742.

47. Balch CM, Soong SJ, Murad TM, et al. A multifactorial analysis of melanoma. II. Prognostic factors in patients with stage I (localized) melanoma. *Surgery* 1979;86:343–351.

48. Cascinelli N, Morabito A, Bufalino R. Prognosis of stage I melanoma of the skin. *Int J Cancer* 1980;26:733–739.

49. Sondergaard K, Schou G. Survival with primary cutaneous malignant melanoma, evaluated from 2012 cases. A multivariate regression analysis. *Virchows Arch A Pathol Anat Histopathol* 1985;406:179–195.

50. Rigel DS, Friedman RJ, Kopf AW, Silverman MK. Factors influencing survival in melanoma. *Dermatol Clin* 1991;9:631–642.

51. Stidham KR, Johnson JL, Seigler HF. Survival superiority of females with melanoma. A multivariate analysis of 6383 patients exploring the significance of gender in prognostic outcome. *Arch Surg* 1994;129:316–324.

52. Garbe C, Buttner P, Bertz J, et al. Primary cutaneous melanoma. Identification of prognostic groups and estimation of individual prognosis for 5093 patients. *Cancer* 1995;75:2484–2491.

53. Balch CM, Soong S, Ross MI, et al. Long-term results of a multi-institutional randomized trial comparing prognostic factors and surgical results for intermediate thickness melanomas (1.0 to 4.0 mm). Intergroup Melanoma Surgical Trial. *Ann Surg Oncol* Mar 2007;7(2):87–97.

54. Retsas S, Henry K, Mohammed MQ, MacRae K. Prognostic factors of cutaneous melanoma and a new staging system proposed by the American Joint Committee on Cancer (AJCC): validation in a cohort of 1284 patients. *Eur J Cancer* 2002;38:511–516.

55. Vollmer RT, Seigler HF. A model for pretest probability of lymph node metastasis from cutaneous melanoma. *Am J Clin Pathol* 2000;114:875–879.

56. Mihm MC Jr, Googe PB. *Problematic Pigmented Lesions. A Case Method Approach.* Philadelphia, PA: Lea and Febiger; 1990:241–250.

57. Buttner P, Garbe C, Bertz J, et al. Primary cutaneous melanoma. Optimized cutoff points of tumor thickness and importance of Clark's level for prognostic classification. *Cancer* 1995;75:2499–2506.

58. Barnhill RB, Katzen J, Spatz A, et al. The importance of mitotic rate as a prognostic factor for localized cutaneous melanoma. *J Cutan Pathol* 2005;32:268–273.

59. Schmoeckel C, Braun-Falco O. Prognostic index in malignant melanoma. *Arch Dermatol* 1978;114:871–873.

60. Kopf AW, Gross DF, Rogers GS, et al. Prognostic index for malignant melanoma. *Cancer* 1987;59:1236–1241.

61. Scolyer RA, Shaw HM, Thompson JF, et al. Interobserver reproducibility of histopathologic prognostic variables in primary cutaneous melanomas. *Am J Surg Pathol* 2003;27:1571–1576.

62. Azzola MF, Shaw HM, Thompson JF, et al. Tumor mitotic rate is a more powerful prognostic indicator than ulceration in patients with primary cutaneous melanoma: An analysis of 3661 patients from a single center. *Cancer* 2003;97:1488–1498.

63. Gimotty PA, Guerry D, Ming MF. Thin primary cutaneous malignant melanoma: A prognostic tree for 10-year metastasis is more accurate than American Joint Committee on Cancer staging. *J Clin Oncol* 2004;22:3651–3653.

64. Ramsay JA, From L, Iscoe NA, Kahn HJ. MIB-1 proliferative activity is a significant prognostic factor in primary thick cutaneous melanomas. *J Invest Dermatol* 1995;105:22–26.

65. Sparrow LE, English DR, Taran JM, Heenan PJ. Prognostic significance of MIB-1 proliferative activity in thin melanomas and immunohistochemical analysis of MIB-1 proliferative activity in melanocytic tumors. *Am J Dermatopathol* 1998;20:12–16.

66. Penneys N, Seigfried E, Nahass G, Vogler C. Expression of proliferating cell nuclear antigen in Spitz nevus. *J Am Acad Dermatol* 1995;32:964–967.

67. Vecchiato A, Rossi CR, Montesco MC, et al. Proliferating cell nuclear antigen (PCNA) and recurrence in patients with cutaneous melanoma. *Melanoma Res* 1994;4: 207–211.

68. Karlsson M, Boeryd B, Carstensen J, et al. Correlation of Ki-67 and PCNA to DNA ploidy, S-phase fraction and survival in uveal melanoma. *Eur J Cancer* 1996;32A:357–362.

69. Niezabitowski A, Czajecki K, Rys KJ, et al. Prognostic evaluation of cutaneous malignant melanoma: A clinicopathologic and immunohistochemical study. *J Surg Oncol* 1999;70:150–160.

70. Goldmann T, Ribbert D, Suter L, et al. Tumor characteristics involved in the metastatic behaviour as an improvement in primary cutaneous melanoma prognostics. *J Exp Clin Cancer Res* 1998;17:483–489.

71. Reddy VB, Gattuso P, Aranha G, Carson HJ. Cell proliferation markers in predicting metastases in malignant melanoma. *J Cutan Pathol* June 1995;22(3):248–251.

72. Clemente CG, Mihm MC Jr, Bufalino R, et al. Prognostic value of tumor infiltrating lymphocytes in the vertical growth phase of primary cutaneous melanoma. *Cancer* 1996;77:1303–1310.

73. Piepkorn M, Barnhill RL. Prognostic factors in cutaneous melanoma. In: Barnhill RL, Piepkorn M, Busam KJ, eds. *Pathology of Melanocytic Nevi and Malignant Melanoma.* 2nd Ed. New York, NY: Springer, 2004:372–394.

74. Pastorfide GC, Kibbi AG, de Roa AL, et al. Image analysis of stage I melanoma (1.00–2.50mm): Lymphocytic infiltrates related to metastasis and survival. *J Cutan Pathol* 1992;19:390–397.

75. Mascaro JM, Molgo M, Castel T, Castro J. Plasma cells within the infiltrate of primary cutaneous malignant melanoma of the skin. A confirmation of its histoprognostic value. *Am J Dermatopathol* 1987;9:497–499.

76. Brocker EB, Zwaldo G, Suter L, et al. Infiltration of primary and metastatic melanomas with macrophages of the 25F9-positive phenotype. *Cancer Immunol Immunother* 1987;25:81–86.

77. Paladagu RR, Yonemeto RH. Biologic behavior of thin malignant melanomas with regressive changes. *Arch Surg* 1983;118:41–44.

78. Sondergaard K, Hou-Jensen K. Partial regression in thin primary cutaneous malignant melanomas clinical stage I. A study of 486 cases. *Virchows Arch A Pathol Anat Histopathol* 1985;408:241–247.

79. Naruns PL, Nizze JA, Cochran AJ, et al. Recurrence potential of thin primary melanomas. *Cancer* 1986;57:545–548.

80. Blessing K, McLaren KM, McLean A, Davidson P. Thin malignant melanomas (<1.5mm) with metastasis: a histological study and survival analysis. *Histopathology* 1990;17:389–395.

81. Shaw HM, McGovern VJ, Milton GW, et al. Malignant melanoma: Influence of site of lesion and age of patient in the female superiority in survival. *Cancer* 1980;46:2731–2735.

82. Kelly JW, Sagebiel RW, Blois MS. Regression in malignant melanoma. A histologic feature without independent prognostic significance. *Cancer* 1985;56:2287–2291.

83. Vilmer C, Bailly C, Le Doussal V, et al. Thin melanomas with unusual aggressive behaviour: A report on nine cases. Melanoma Groups of French Federation of Cancer Centers. *J Am Acad Dermatol* 1996;34:439–444.

84. Byers HR, Bahwan J. Pathologic parameters in the diagnosis and prognosis of primary cutaneous melanoma. *Hematol Oncol Clin North Am* 1998;12:717–725.

85. Guitart J, Lowe L, Piepkorn M, et al. Identification of histological features associated with metastasizing thin melanomas: A case-control study of 43 cases. *Arch Dermatol* 2002;138:603–608.

86. Day CL, Harrist TJ, Gorstein F, et al. Malignant melanoma. Prognostic significance of "microscopic satellites" in the reticular dermis and subcutaneous fat. *Ann Surg* Jul 1981;194(1):108–112.

87. Harrist TJ, Rigel DS, Day CL Jr, et al. "Microscopic satellites" are more highly associated with regional lymph nodes metastases than is primary melanoma thickness. *Cancer* 1984 May; 53(10):2183–2187.

88. Leon P, Daly JM, Synnestvedt M, et al. The prognostic implications of microscopic satellites in patients with clinical stage I melanoma. *Arch Surg* 1991;126:1461–1468.

89. Rao UN, Ibrahim J, Flaherty LE, et al. Implications of microscopic satellites of the primary and extracapsular lymph node spread in patients with high-risk melanoma: Pathology corollary of Eastern Cooperative Oncology Group Trial E1690. *J Clin Oncol* 2002;20:2053–2057.

90. Mraz-Gernhard S, Sagebiel RW, Kashani-Sabet M, et al. Prediction of sentinel lymph node micrometastasis by histological features in primary cutaneous malignant melanoma. *Arch Dermatol* 1998;134:983–987.

91. Kashani-Sabet M, Sagabiel RW, Ferreira CM, et al. Vascular involvement in the prognosis of primary cutaneous melanoma. *Arch Dermatol* 2001;137:1169–1173.

92. Buzaid AC, Ross MI, Balch CM, et al. Critical analysis of the current American Joint Committee on Cancer staging system for cutaneous melanoma and proposal of a new staging system. *J Clin Oncol* 1997;15:1039–1051.

93. Balch CM, Wilkerson JA, Murad TM, et al. The prognostic significance of ulceration of cutaneous melanoma. *Cancer* 1980;45:3012–3017.

94. Kim SH, Garcia C, Rodriguez J, Coit DG. Prognosis of thick cutaneous melanoma. *J Am Coll Surg* 1999;188:241–247.

95. Herzberg AJ, Kerns BJ, Borowitz MJ, et al. DNA ploidy of malignant melanoma determined by image cytometry of fresh frozen and paraffin-embedded tissue. *J Cutan Pathol* 1991;18:440–448.

96. Skowronek J, Adamska K, Filipiak K, et al. DNA ploidy in malignant melanoma, skin cancer and pigmented nevi. *Neoplasma* 1997;44:282–288.

97. Kheir SM, Bines SD, Vonroenn JH, et al. Prognostic significance of DNA aneuploidy in stage I cutaneous melanoma. *Ann Surg* 1988;207:455–461.

98. Karlsson M, Boeryd B, Carstensen J, et al. DNA ploidy and S-phase in primary malignant melanoma as prognostic factors for stage III disease. *Br J Cancer* 1993;67:134–138.

99. Karjalainen JM, Eskelinen MJ, Nordling S, et al. Mitotic rate and S-phase fraction as a prognostic factor in stage I cutaneous malignant melanoma. *Br J Cancer* 1998;77:1917–1925.

100. Gershenwald JE, Mansfield PF, Lee JE, Ross MI. Role for lymphatic mapping and sentinel lymph node biopsy in patients with thick (> or = 4 mm) primary melanoma. *Ann Surg Oncol* 2000;7:160–165.

101. Zettersten E, Sagebiel RW, Miller JR III, et al. Prognostic factors in patients with thick cutaneous melanoma (>4 mm). *Cancer* 2002;94:1049–1056.

102. Cherpelis BS, Haddad F, Messina J, et al. Sentinel lymph node micrometastasis and other histologic factors that predict outcome in patients with thicker melanomas. *J Am Acad Dermatol* 2001;44:762–766.

103. Massi D, Franchi A, Borgognoni L, et al. Thin cutaneous malignant melanoma (< or = 1.5 mm): Identification of risk factors indicative of progression. *Cancer* 1999; 85:1067–1076.

104. Dessureault S, Soong SJ, Ross MI. Improved staging of node-negative patients with intermediate to thick (>1 mm) with the use of lymphatic mapping and sentinel lymph node biopsy. *Ann Surg Oncol* 2001;8:766–770.

105. Morton DL, Thompson JF, Cochran AL, et al. Sentinel-node biopsy or nodal observation in melanoma. *New Engl J Med* 2006;355:1307–1317.

106. Balch CM, Cascinelli NF. Sentinel-node biopsy in melanoma. *New Engl J Med* 2006;355:1370–1371.
107. Dalal KM, Patel A, Brady MS, et al. Patterns of first-recurrence and post-recurrence survival in patients with primary cutaneous melanoma after sentinel lymph node biopsy. *Ann Surg Oncol* 2007;14(6):1934–1942.
108. Cochran AJ, Wen DR, Huang RR, et al. Prediction of metastatic melanoma in nonsentinel nodes and clinical outcome based on the primary melanoma and the sentinel node. *Mod Pathol* 2004;17:747–755.
109. Ruiter DJ, Spatz A, van den Oord JJ, et al. Pathologic staging of melanoma. *Semin Oncol* 2002;29:370–381.
110. Govindarajan A, Ghazarian DM, McCready DR, Leong WL. Histological features of melanoma sentinel lymph node metastases associated with status of completion lymphadenectomy and rate of subsequent relapse. *Ann Surg Oncol* 2007;14:906–912.
111. Pearlman NW, McCarthy MD, Frank M, et al. Size of sentinel lymph node metastases predicts other nodal disease and survival in malignant melanoma. *Am J Surg* 2006;192:878–881.
112. van Akkooi AC, de Wilt JH, Verhoef C, et al. Clinical evidence of melanoma micrometastases (<0.1 mm) in sentinel lymph nodes: Are these nodes to be considered negative? *Ann Oncol* 2006;17:1578–1585.
113. White DC, Schuler FR, Pruit SK, et al. Timing of sentinel lymph node mapping after lymphoscintigraphy. *Surgery* 1999;126:156–161.
114. Porter GA, Ross MI, Berman RS, et al. How many lymph nodes are enough during sentinel lymphadenectomy for primary melanoma? *Surgery* 2000;128:306–311.
115. Emery RE, Stevens JS, Nance RW, et al. Sentinel lymph node staging of primary melanoma by the "10% rule": Pathology and clinical outcomes. *Am J Surg* 2007;193:618–622.
116. Kroon HM, Lowe L, Wong S, et al. What is a sentinel node? Re-evaluating the 10% rule for sentinel lymph node biopsy in melanoma. *J Surg Oncol* 2007;95:623–628.
117. Stewart LE, Tyler DS, Vollmer RT. The importance of total number of sentinel lymph nodes in patients with stage N0 cutaneous melanoma. *Am J Clin Pathol* 2005;124:77–82.
118. Hawkins WG, Busam KJ, Ben-Porat L, et al. Desmoplastic melanoma: A pathologically and clinically distinct form of cutaneous melanoma. *Ann Surg Oncol* 2005;12:197–199.
119. Gamblin TC, Edington H, Kirkwood JM, Rao UN. Sentinel lymph node biopsy for atypical melanocytic lesions with spitzoid features. *Ann Surg Oncol* 2006;13:1664–1670.
120. Crowson AN, Magro C, Miller A, et al. The molecular basis of melanomagenesis and the metastatic phenotype. *Semin Oncol* 2007;34:476–490.

6

BASAL CELL CARCINOMA: CLINICAL FEATURES, HISTOLOGY, AND BIOLOGY

INTRODUCTION

Basal cell carcinoma (BCC), first described by Jacob in 1827,[1] is the most common malignant neoplasm of humans.[2–4] After a rise in incidence of roughly 20% between 1971 and 1977,[5] by 1998, roughly one million new cases were being diagnosed annually in the United States.[6] In consequence of its high incidence, BCC, although eminently curable when the diagnosis is made promptly and the lesion treated in its early phase, constitutes an enormous financial burden on the healthcare system.

Lesions occur on both sun-protected and sun-exposed skin but often have a different biology and morphology in these locations.[7] Typically, BCCs occur in the fourth decade of life and beyond,[8] although exceptions to this occur, in particular, in the setting of specific genodermatoses or in patients with immune compromise.[9] As sun exposure plays a role in the development and transformation of BCC,[7] patients with light skin phenotypes are particularly predisposed as expected; this includes in the context of blue eyes, red hair, and easy freckling[8] as well as those whose occupational or leisure activities lead them to pronounced and prolonged sun exposure. Additional risk factors for BCC include the exposure to arsenic, coal tar derivatives, and irradiation, although by far, ultraviolet light is the most important factor in lesion development and progression.[5,7,8,10,11] BCC may, like squamous cell carcinoma, arise in the setting of scars, draining sinuses, ulcers, burn sites, and foci of chronic inflammation.[8,10,11] The role of immune compromise in provoking an increased risk of BCC may be due to an impairment of the immune surveillance of oncogenic viruses.[12] The genodermatoses which enhance the risk of BCC include the prototype xeroderma pigmentosa, Rasmussen syndrome, Rombo syndrome, Bazex–Christol–Dupre syndrome, albinism, and Darier disease.[5,11,13] These syndromes variably either decrease epidermal pigmentation and thus increase the risk of ultraviolet light-induced oncogenic transformation[7] or promote genotypic instability in the epidermis.

BCC has been associated with a variety of other lesions and/or neoplasms in the same or a nearby anatomic location. For example, desmoplastic trichilemmoma is said to be associated with coexistent atypical basaloid neoplasms including BCC in up to 19% of cases[14]; the aforementioned study shows the impact of selection bias as it was first based upon the detection of the coincidence of BCC and desmoplastic trichilemmoma followed by a retrospective analysis of all accessioned desmoplastic trichilemmomas over a set time interval. Other lesions associated with coexistent BCCs include acantholytic processes of diverse type (personal observation), warts, porokeratosis, neurofibromata, nevi sebaceus and epidermal nevi, condylomata accuminata, hemangiomas, cysts of hair follicle derivation, pilomatricomas, and a variety of common banal neoplasms such as seborrheic keratoses and melanocytic nevi, which are so common as to make their coexistence with BCC in any given patient a random event in all probability.[8,11,13,14] BCCs have also been reported in collision with a common dermal fibrosing reaction to trauma (i.e., dermatofibroma), but in this setting, the presence of dermal proplastic cytokines could explain the epidermal proliferation. As in nevi sebaceus, the basaloid epidermal proliferation overlying a dermatofibroma often shows a form of follicular stromal induction suggesting a recapitulation of hair follicle growth. Whether a component of a hamartoma or as a response to proplastic cytokines, it is not clear that such basaloid proliferations frequently have a propensity to eventuate in a malignant neoplasm with the capacity for local tissue invasion or destruction or, ultimately, of metastatic events. Before considering the pathogenesis of BCC, it is first necessary to define the clinical characteristics and their corresponding histologic expression.

Clinical Features

The typical BCC is a pearly pink or flesh-colored papule with telangiectasia. Lesions may be translucent or slightly erythematous with a rolled border (Fig. 6.1), occasionally accompanied by bleeding, scaling, or crusting. Aggressive-growth tumors tend to show more frequent ulceration and large, untended neoplasms can be locally destructive of eyes, ears, and nares.[15] The different histomorphologic subgroups have their specific clinical correlates; the aggressive-growth variants such as infiltrative (Fig. 6.2) or morpheaform BCC manifest as a depressed scariform plaque while the superficial variant presents as a reddish plaque with variegated depigmentation and a spreading peripheral margin and/or an atrophic or scarlike peripheral border that raises consideration clinically to Bowen's disease, nummular eczema, and other annular dermatoses such as superficial fungal infections.[11] The presence of a surrounding hypo- or hyperpigmented flare has been designated "halo" BCC,[11] the histologic correlate of which is a heavy bandlike lymphoid infiltrate. Lesions of the superficial variety are frequently multifocal (the so called field fire basal cell cancer).[11]

The linear variant in childhood and adolescence manifests a longitudinal arrangement.[16] Apart from presenting with a papule or nodule typically on sun-exposed skin, patients generally have no other complaints referable to the tumor. On rare occasions, a lesion manifests tenderness or pain, which can be a clue to perineural infiltration in the aggressive-growth varieties.[17] Sensorimotor compromise has been reported particularly in lesions of the preauricular and cheek areas.[17]

Metastases are rare and most are said to more closely correlate to the size and depth and less so to the histologic subtype of the original tumor.[18–20] Lesions which recur after radiotherapy may infiltrate widely prior to becoming clinically apparent; this plus the fact that radiotherapy is often reserved for aggressive-growth tumors ought to enhance the suspicion of perineural infiltration in recurrent BCC post irradiation.[19] The incidence of metastases and/or death is said to correlate to large tumors greater than 3 cm in diameter, in which setting patients are said to have a 1% to 2% risk of metastases that increases to up to 20% to 25% in lesions greater than 5 cm and up to 50% in lesions greater than 10 cm in diameter.[21] A "giant" BCC is designated as one that is greater than 5 cm in diameter and has a significant risk of morbidity and mortality.[19,20] A BCC arising in a young person (i.e., <35 years of age) may have an aggressive clinical course.[19]

NEVOID BASAL CELL CARCINOMA (BASAL CELL NEVUS) SYNDROME

Described originally by Howell and Caro in 1959,[22] the nevoid BCC syndrome is also known as the Gorlin–Goltz's syndrome[23,24] and is inherited as an autosomal dominant trait with some 30% to 50% of cases representing sporadic mutations.[23,24] Typically, the syndrome is expressed in young adulthood but on occasion, children as young as two years of age manifest disease expression characterized by the presence of multiple basal cell cancers and other anomalies as described below. The prevalence is roughly 1 in 56,000.[8] In most cases, the abnormality represents a mutation in the human homologue of the Drosophila patched gene (PTCH).[25] Perturbation of this tumor suppressor gene on chromosome 9 q22-q31[26,27] results in upregulated cell proliferation. The biology of sporadic BCC and of tumors arising in the setting of nevoid BCC syndrome is discussed in greater detail below.

Clinical Features

The clinical manifestations of nevoid BCC syndrome include the presence of numerous (up to thousands) BCCs (Fig. 6.3),[24] in essence similar to those which occur sporadically in the population but with an emphasis on nodular, superficial, and, in our experience, infundibulocystic types. Patients also manifest cysts of the skin and of the jaws, the latter showing a corrugated eosinophilic internal cuticular lining cognate to odontogenic

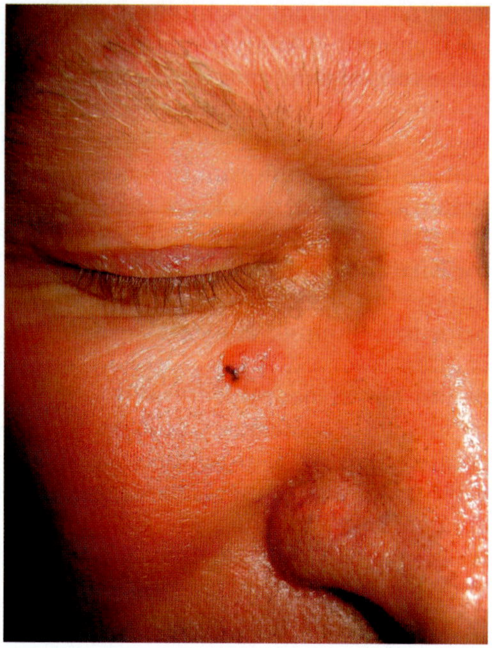

FIGURE 6.1 **Nodular Basal Cell Carcinoma—Clinical Morphology.** This pearly, nodular lesion shows telangiectasia on its surface and a sharp contour with a smooth margin. An incisional biopsy has been performed. (Case courtesy of Dr George Monks, Tulsa, OK.)

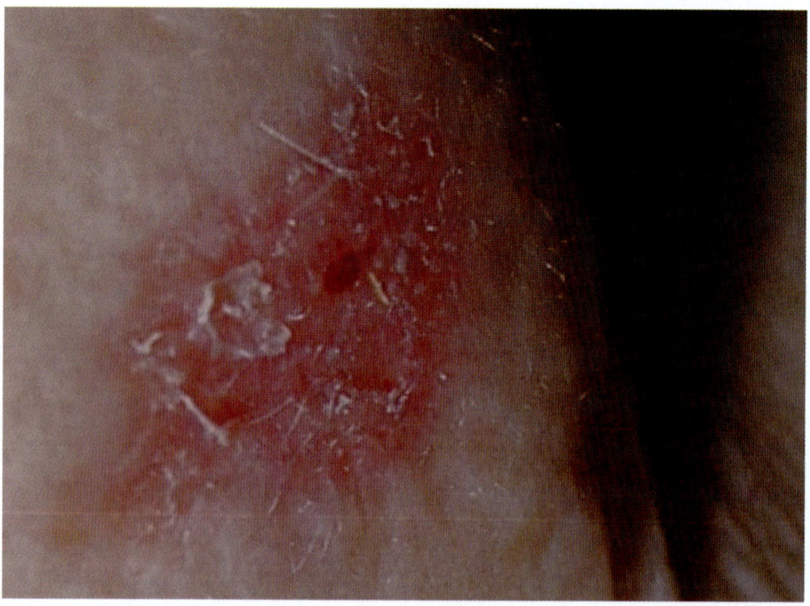

FIGURE 6.2 **Infiltrative Growth Basal Cell Carcinoma, Clinical Morphology.** The infiltrative growth BCC has a scaly surface, a pink to reddish color, and an irregular, ill-defined margin. This is a plaque lesion which can be either slightly elevated or depressed with palpable induration at the tissue edges. (Case courtesy of Dr Michael Wilkerson, Galveston, TX.)

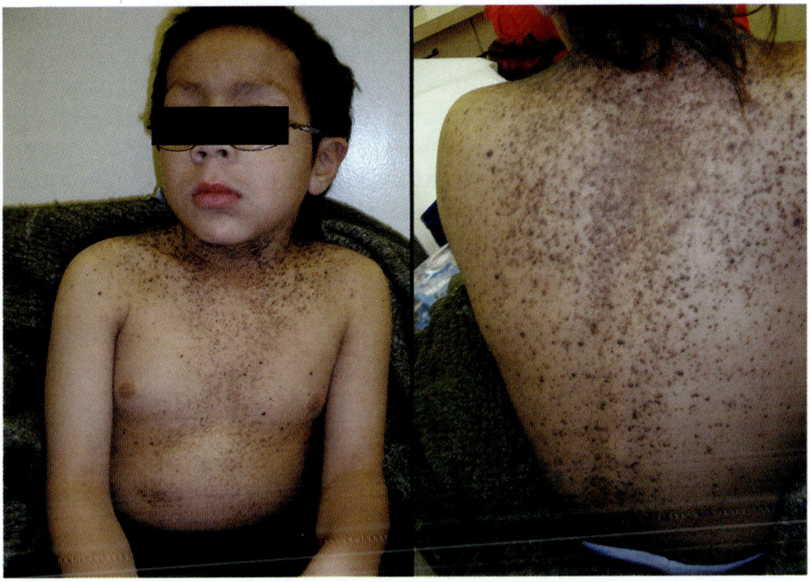

FIGURE 6.3 **Basal Cell Nevus Syndrome: Clinical Morphology.** This 9-year-old boy with basal cell nevus syndrome has thousands of pigmented papules and skin tag-like lesions on his trunk, which correspond histologically to infundibulocystic BCC; the histology of one of these lesions is represented in Figure 6.12. (Case courtesy of Dr David Adelson, Department of Dermatology, University of Oklahoma.)

keratocysts[24] and the former showing a similar eosinophilic internal cuticle as is seen in steatocystomas.[28] Also present are skeletal anomalies including spinal and rib deformities, excessive ossification with bossing of the frontal skull, and bridging of the sella turcica. Calcification of the falx cerebri is another manifestation.[10,24] Palmoplantar pits typically 1 to 3 mm in depth and 2 to 3 mm in diameter appear during the second decade of life.[29] Neuropsychiatric impacts include schizophrenia, abnormal electroencephalograms, mental retardation, and cerebellar degeneration.[30] Some patients manifest tumors and other anomalies of the reproductive system.

Histopathology

The histologies of most BCCs encountered in the nevoid BCC syndrome are, as mentioned, typically not dissimilar from those seen in sporadic BCCs. The epidermal cysts are usually derived from the follicular infundibula with a pronounced keratohyalin granular layer in the internal squamous epithelial lining, while in some cases, the histology is more cognate to steatocystomata but differs by the absence of sebaceous glands.[28]

Differential Diagnosis

Although generally one cannot tell from a single biopsy that a patient does or does not have basal cell nevus syndrome, the astute pathologist will suspect the diagnosis when an individual in the second or third decade of life has a BCC in a biopsy submitted with no clinical information. Multiple tumor syndromes which can produce basaloid adnexal neoplasms include Muir–Torre's syndrome and Cowden's syndrome, but these produce neoplasms with sebaceous and trichilemmal differentiation, respectively. The cystic structures will resemble steatocystoma multiplex congenita while dermoid cysts show pilosebaceous differentiation, sometimes with eccrine or apocrine glands and frequently with true follicular differentiation including in the context of hair shaft production. The cutaneous pits of pitted keratolysis manifest Gram positive filamentous or rounded bacteria in the cornified layer.

Histopathology

Traditionally, BCCs have been classified as solid (or undifferentiated) versus those tumors that manifest specific differentiation features (i.e., to eccrine, sebaceous, or other cell lines). However, the only proven histologic prognosticator of biologic behavior, and therefore a major determinant of what constitutes an appropriate therapeutic approach, is the architectural growth pattern. Thus, the architecture is a critical issue, while the differentiation patterns need to be considered only insofar as they must be recognized as part of the histologic spectrum of BCC and as they impact differential diagnosis. Their misidentification as Merkel cell carcinoma or as sebaceous, eccrine, or follicular neoplasia is a diagnostic pitfall that carries with it a risk of over- or undertreatment.

One needs to be aware that shave and punch biopsy specimens have an intrinsic error rate, due to the nature of the tissue sample, of roughly 20% in predicting classification of BCC subtypes when compared to completion excisions at the same anatomic location.[31] The reason for this may be explained by the fact that biological transformation of BCC tends to occur at the base and edges of the growing neoplasm.

UNDIFFERENTIATED BASAL CELL CARCINOMAS

We classify BCCs as belonging to indolent-growth or aggressive-growth subsets. The indolent-growth variants include superficial and nodular BCC. The aggressive-growth tumors are infiltrative BCC, metatypical BCC, and morpheiform or sclerosing BCC.[7] In one large retrospective series of 1,039 consecutive neoplasms, and using a slightly dissimilar classification scheme, 21% were nodular, 17.4% were superficial, 14.5% were micronodular, 7.4% were infiltrative, and 1.1% were morpheiform.[32] Roughly one-third of all tumors showed an admixture of patterns.[32]

Superficial Basal Cell Carcinoma

Superficial BCC is characterized by a proliferation of atypical basaloid cells, which form an axis parallel to the epidermal surface, and demonstrates slitlike retraction of the palisaded basal cells from the subjacent stroma (Fig. 6.4, e-figs. 6.1–6.3).[7] The resulting cleftlike spaces often contain alcian blue-positive mesenchymal mucoid material, a presumed product of

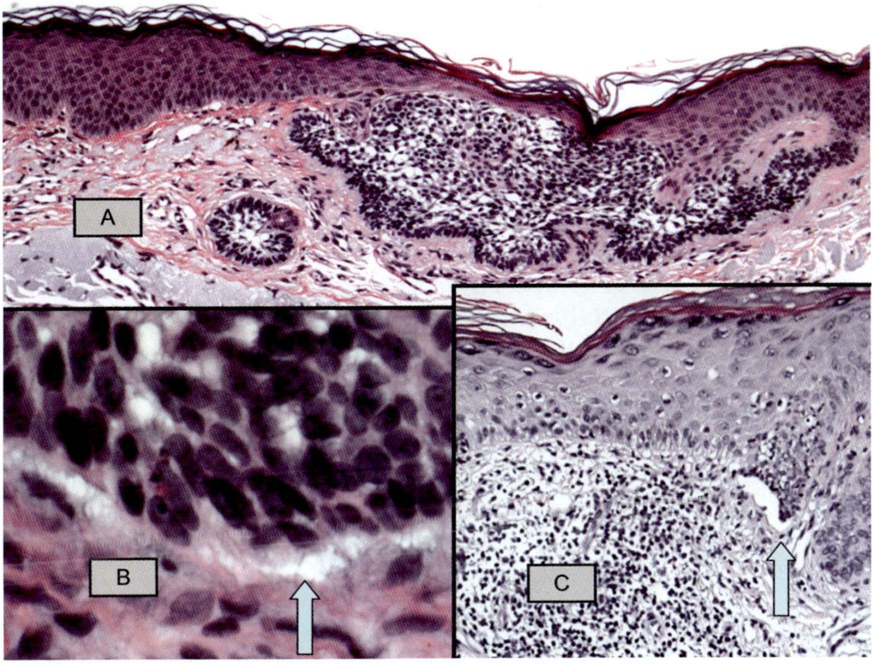

FIGURE 6.4 **Superficial Basal Cell Carcinoma: Histomorphology. (A)** Proliferation of basaloid cells parallel to the long axis of the epidermis. Serial sectioning showed the small nest at left to connect to the remainder of the tumor which is in continuity with the undersurface of the epidermis **(A)**. **(B)** Slitlike stromal retraction (*arrow*) with mucin deposition in the papillary dermis. **(C)** Bandlike lymphoid infiltrate in apposition to the basaloid nests (*arrow*) and the undersurface of the epidermis. If only the bandlike lymphoid infiltrate is present in a biopsy intended to confirm the presence of BCC, serial deeper step sections through the tissue block are advised.

the stromal cells. Tumor cells may colonize the hair follicle and rarely the eccrine adnexal structures and, as mentioned above, often take origin from the follicular bulges. Mitoses are infrequent and apoptotic cells rare in the atypical basaloid buds for reasons reflecting their biologic derivation as described above. Some cases manifest melanin pigmentation of the epithelium and in the histiocytes in the subjacent stroma; of pigmented BCCs, most are held to reflect superficial tumors in some series,[32] although in our experience, nodular BCCs constitute the most frequent form of pigmented BCC. A bandlike, often heavy, lymphoid infiltrate may be present. When seen in the setting of a biopsy for suspect superficial or superficial multifocal BCC, a bandlike lymphoid infiltrate should prompt a careful search through multiple levels looking for foci of superficial BCC.

Nodular Basal Cell Carcinoma

Nodular BCC represents the most common form of the neoplasm in our experience. Nodular BCC is also referred to as nodulocystic BCC by some observers, although this term is not employed by us. This is the type of BCC that clinically shows a translucent pearly papule or nodule with a rolled border and telangectasia (Fig. 6.1). The nodular form of BCC is characterized by discrete large and/or small nests of basaloid cells in either the papillary or reticular dermis accompanied by slitlike retraction from a stroma in which the fibroblasts do not appear to be plump or proplastic (Fig. 6.5, e-figs. 6.4–6.6). Any of the differentiated elements (eccrine, sebaceous, etc.) may be seen in nodular tumors and roughly one-third of cases will show a coexistent superficial component. As both superficial and nodular BCC can be seen in sun-exposed or sun-protected skin, the dermis may show solar elastosis and this may be pronounced. The surrounding stroma shows myxoid change, is rarely fibrotic, and may show calcification in discrete islands of tumor or in adjacent stroma. Mitoses and individual cell necrosis are uncommon. The presence of abundant slitlike retraction may cause tumor nests to drop out from the stroma during processing yielding empty spaces with a rounded contour in the mid or deep dermis (Fig. 6.6, e-fig. 6.7). This is an important clue to the diagnosis in the setting of the nodular and/or infiltrative growth patterns.[33] A significant proportion of

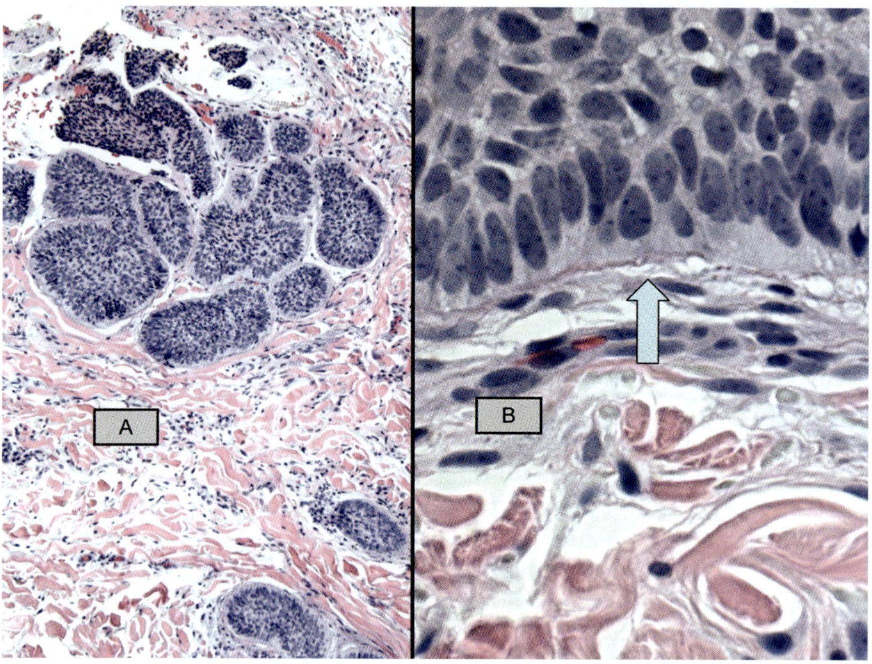

FIGURE 6.5 **Nodular Basal Cell Carcinoma: Histomorphology.** Nodular BCC manifests multiple variably sized and rounded nodules with a pushing contour in apposition to a stroma that shows no significant fibroplasias **(A)**. The nodules of tumor show a peripheral palisade of basaloid cells and, at their interface with the stroma, slitlike retraction is seen (*arrow*) **(B)**. Note also the eosinophilic condensation of basement membrane material adherent to the cytoplasms of the palisading basaloid cells **(B)**.

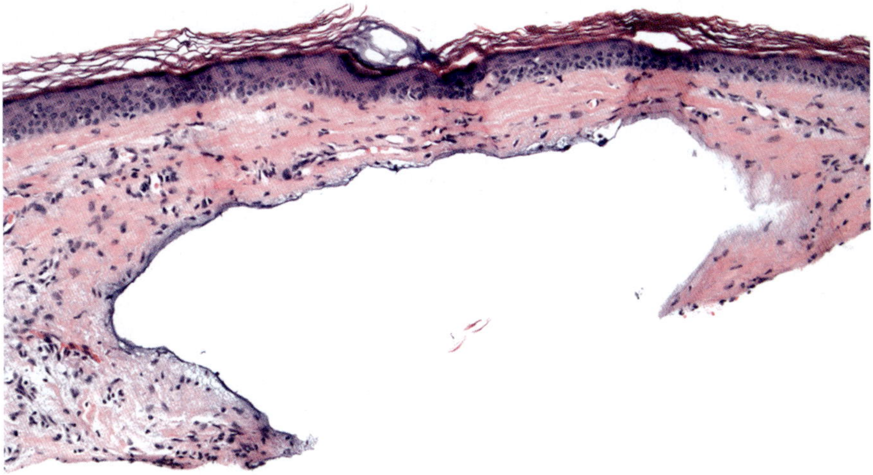

FIGURE 6.6 **Nodular Basal Cell Carcinoma: Histomorphology.** The slitlike retraction with mucin deposition in the adjacent stroma causes the nests of BCC to be only loosely adherent to the collagen. Thus, during processing, the tumor cell nests can drop out of the tissue sample, leaving nothing but an empty space, an important clue to BCC.

BCCs with a nodular component manifests a variable admixture of superficial and/or micronodular morphologies.[32]

Melanin pigmentation of tumor cells and adjacent stromal histiocytes may be seen. Transition to micronodular and other aggressive-growth forms of BCC may be seen (e-figs. 6.8–6.10).

Micronodular Basal Cell Carcinoma

Micronodular BCC manifests a plaquelike indurated lesion with a poorly demarcated contour.[34] As mentioned above, lesions may be difficult to remove, and so they have an increased incidence of recurrence.[32,35] Micronodular BCC manifests tumor nests with roughly the same shape and contour as nodular BCC, but which are nonetheless smaller and widely dispersed in an often asymmetric distribution extending deeper into the dermis and/or subcutis (Fig. 6.7, e-figs. 6.11–6.14). These monotonous, small, round tumor nests are accompanied by stromal proliferation cognate to that seen in infiltrative growth BCC. Retraction spaces are not common and the surrounding stroma shows either a myxoid or a collagenized morphology suggesting that these lesions may be an intermediate step between nodular and aggressive-growth subtypes.[7,32,34] The micronodular BCC has been reported to have a higher incidence of local recurrence[32,34] and may penetrate more deeply into the reticular dermis and/or subcutis.

Aggressive-Growth Basal Cell Carcinoma

The aggressive-growth BCCs include the prototypic morpheaform BCC, infiltrative growth BCC, and metatypical BCC.

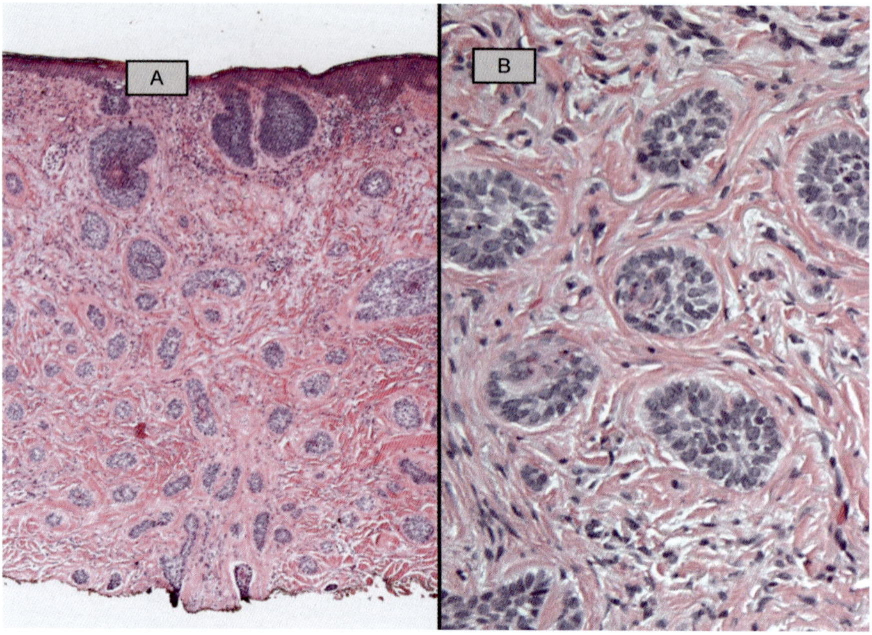

FIGURE 6.7 **Micronodular Basal Cell Carcinoma: Histomorphology.** Micronodular BCC manifests uniformly small nests of neoplastic basal cells with rounded peripheral contours extending widely throughout the sampled dermis **(A)**. The adjacent stroma shows fibroplasia **(B)** indicating a transition step in evolution from nodular to aggressive-growth BCC.

Morpheaform Basal Cell Carcinoma

Morpheaform or sclerosing BCC is characterized by columns of basaloid cells one to two cells thick enmeshed in a densely collagenized stroma containing proplastic fibroblasts (Fig. 6.8, e-figs. 6.15 and 6.16). Individual cell necrosis and mitotic activity are brisk considering the relative tumor volume and the neoplasms themselves are poorly demarcated, showing widespread invasion of the reticular dermis and penetration into the subcutaneous tissue. Slitlike retraction from stroma is less common for morpheaform BCC than for the nodular and superficial variants but is still often demonstrable. These neoplasms may coexist with other aggressive- and/or indeolent-growth morphologic variants. Morpheaform BCCs represent roughly 1% to 5% of all BCCs and clinically present as white or yellow depressed fibrotic scars that rarely ulcerate or bleed.[8] In our experience, these cancers occur mainly in a sun-exposed distribution.[7] Although typically one to two cells in thickness, cords up to five cells in thickness may be present; the architecture comprises sharp angulation of such cords. Pronounced stromal fibroplasia or fibrosis surrounds the tumor tongues. By electron microscopy, it has been determined that a basal lamina is absent.[36]

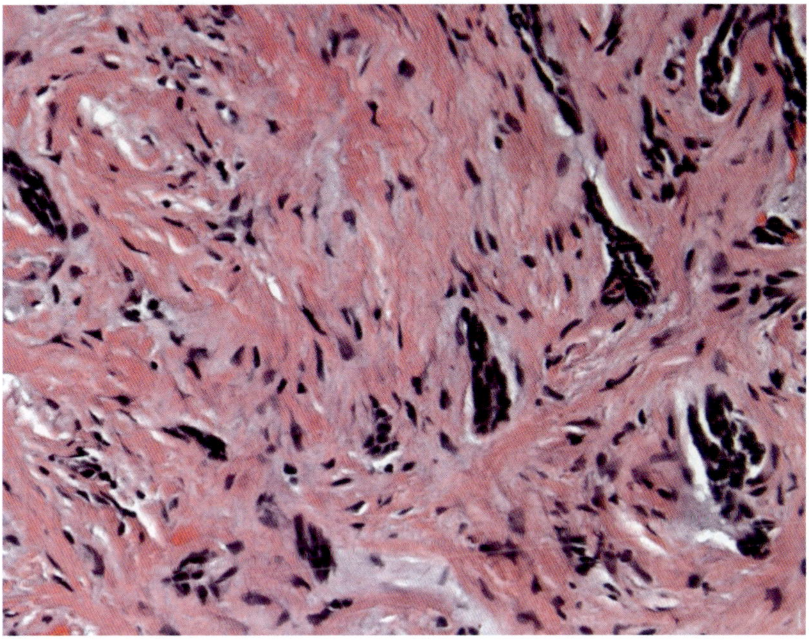

FIGURE 6.8 **Morpheaform (Sclerosing) Basal Cell Carcinoma: Histomorphology.** In a densely proplastic and heavily collagenized stroma, small irregular (sharply angulated) tongues of neoplastic basaloid cells, often one to four cells thick, are embedded in the collagen table. Slitlike retraction may be much less conspicuous than that seen in this particular example.

Infiltrative Growth Basal Cell Carcinoma/ Basosquamous Carcinoma

Infiltrative growth BCC comprises, at the light microscopic level, irregularly sized and shaped nests of tumor cells; the nests show sharp angulation of their peripheral contours, occasional foci of slitlike retraction, and frequent mitotic activity and individual cell necrosis of the neoplastic cells (Fig. 6.9, e-figs. 6.17–6.19). The stroma is frequently fibrotic with plump proplastic stromal fibroblasts. The nests are variable in size and shape with jagged contours.[14,32,37]. Typically, the elongated tumor cell strands of the infiltrative growth component are five to eight cells in thickness. Roughly one-third of such cases show an admixed nodular component from which the lesions are held to derive following ultraviolet irradiation (Fig. 6.10, e-figs. 6.20–6.21).[38] Like the morpheaform variant, these tumors are poorly circumscribed and may show invasion of subcutis and adjacent muscular and other structures. Perineural infiltration is a distinct risk in this variant as in the morpheaform BCC, and, like the morpheaform variant, the clinical correlate is a depressed yellowish or fibrotic plaque that typically lacks a rolled border or an elevated pearly nodule unless a nodular BCC component coexists.

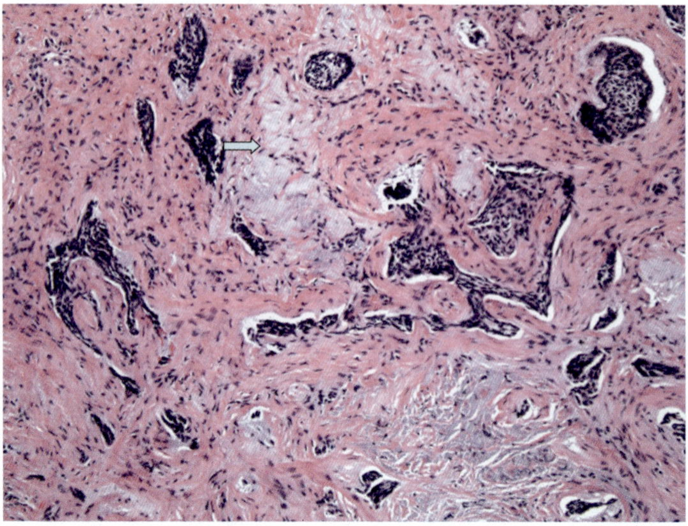

FIGURE 6.9 **Infiltrative Growth Basal Cell Carcinoma: Histomorphology.** Like morpheaform BCC, the infiltrative growth BCC shows heavy stromal collagenization and proplasia of stromal fibroblasts. However, the tumor tongues manifest an admixture of rounded nodules, large nodules with irregular contours, and small irregular tongues of tumor cells embedded in the fibrous stroma. These lesions almost invariably arise in sun-damaged skin, the morphologic evidence of which is solar elastosis (*arrow*).

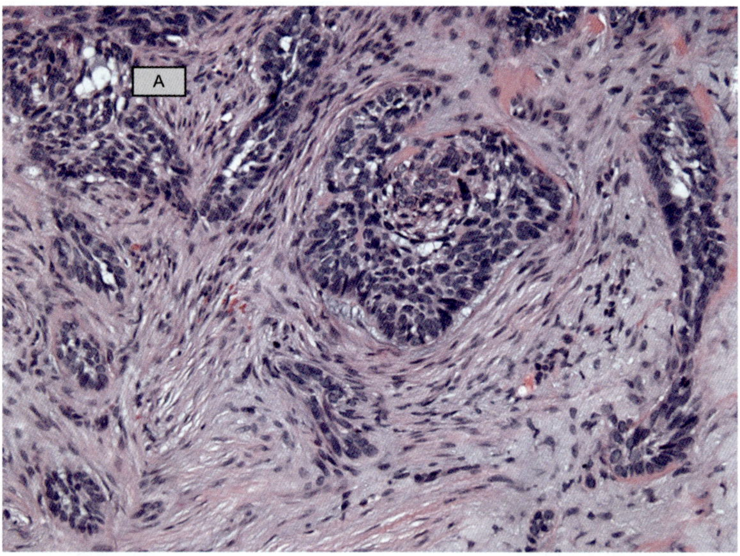

FIGURE 6.10 **Mixed Nodular and Infiltrative Growth Basal Cell Carcinoma.** There is an admixture of rounded and irregularly contoured tumor cell nests imbedded in a fibrous stroma. In our experience, this is a very common histologic form of BCC **(A)**. **(B)** High power microscopy shows the presence of mitotic figures (*arrow*) and apoptotic nuclear debris (*curved arrow*), which characterizes the aggressive-growth BCCs.

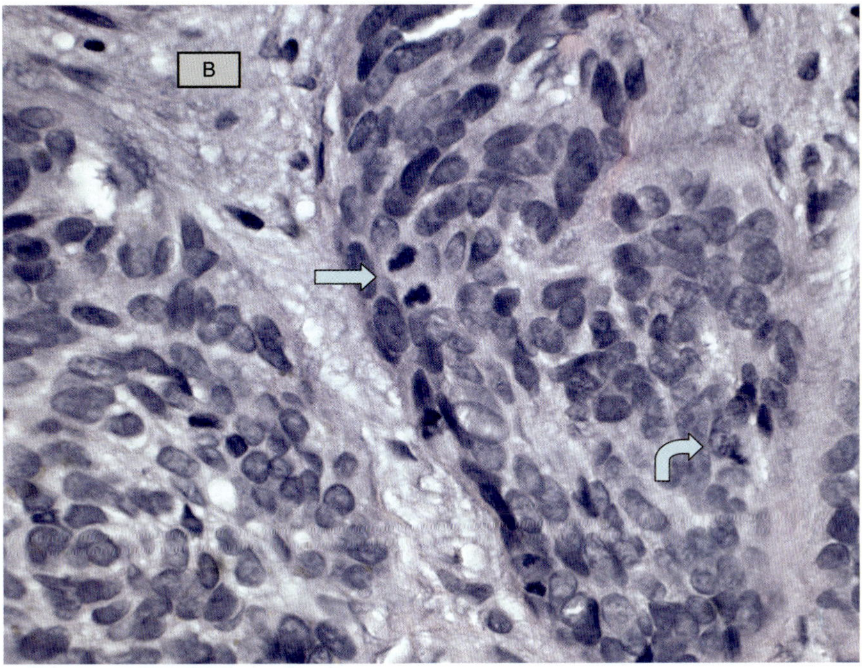

FIGURE 6.10 Cont'd.

Metatypical Basal Cell Carcinoma

The metatypical BCC (equated by some authors with "basosquamous carcinoma"[39]) is, in our view, a form of aggressive-growth BCC with infiltrating jagged tongues of tumor cells, some of which manifest an abortive peripheral palisade and clear-cut basaloid morphology, admixed with other areas that show intercellular bridge formation and/or cytoplasmic keratinization (Fig. 6.11, e-figs. 6.22–6.24). Clinching the diagnosis is the presence of a coexistent classic nodular or superficial component. We distinguish these neoplasms from keratotic BCC, which is most often a nodular BCC with central squamous differentiation, and from the mixed basal cell–squamous cell carcinomas that represent a collision between two clonally distinctive and geographically separate neoplasms in the same biopsy or excision specimen. Metatypical BCC is the subtype of BCC that can be confused with squamous cell carcinoma and that promotes controversy considering its precise histomorphologic classification,[39,40,41,42] as it shows both basal cell and squamous cell carcinoma differentiation in a continuous fashion.[15,43] One must recognize that use of the terms "metatypical BCC" and "basosquamous carcinoma" delineates a largely semantic distinction with the proviso that the clinician recognizes what the pathologist is referring to and also that the diagnosis has a specific clinical implication. In summation, in our hands, "metatypical" and "basosquamous" carcinomas are used synonymously.

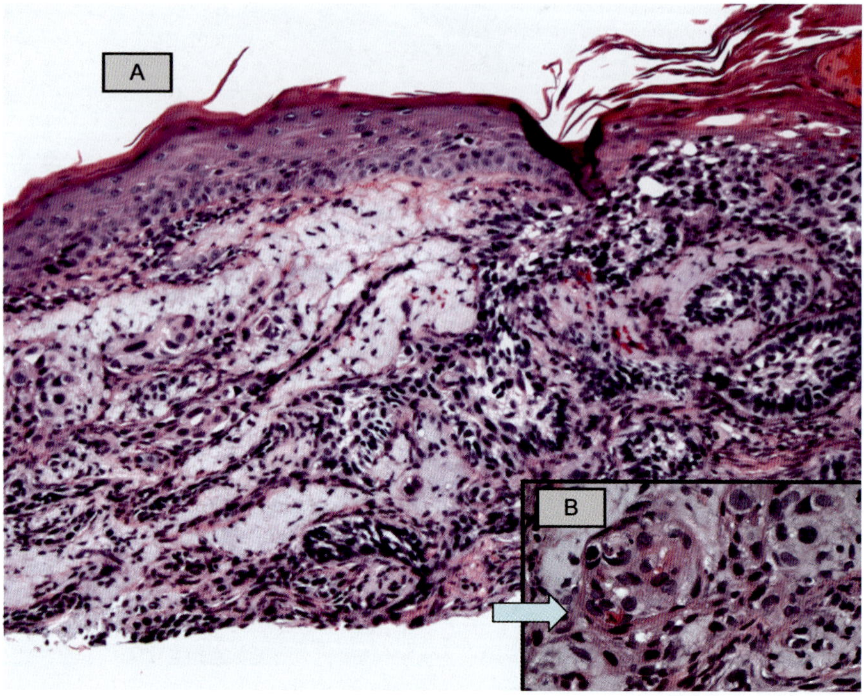

FIGURE 6.11 **Metatypical Basal Cell Carcinoma: Histomorphology.** The metatypical BCC is an aggressive-growth neoplasm arising in sun-damaged skin and showing irregular tongues of tumor and/or an admixed nodular BCC component **(A)**. High power microscopy shows cytoplasmic keratinization and/or intercellular bridges in the squamous areas (*arrow*) **(B)**.

DIFFERENTIATED BASAL CELL CARCINOMAS

BCCs may show a variety of specific cell lineage differentiation features which do not impact prognosis. These include, but are not restricted to, keratotic BCC,[39] infundibulocystic BCC (Fig. 6.12),[44,45] follicular BCC,[46–49] which shows collision features with pilomatricoma, pleomorphic BCC (Fig. 6.13),[50,51] BCC with eccrine differentiation,[52,53] BCC with sebaceous differentiation, the fibroepithelioma of Pinkus (Fig. 6.14),[54] and the BCC with myoepithelial differentiation.[55]

Keratotic Basal Cell Carcinoma

Also known as pilar BCC, as it appears to differentiate along pilosebaceous lines, the keratotic BCC manifests large basaloid tumor nests which are rounded and show central keratinization and degeneration. We deem these to represent a variant of nodular BCC. The central cysts typically lack a granular cell layer and are filled with keratin and parakeratotic debris (e-figs. 6.25 and 6.26); a granular cell layer is present in some cases and the cysts may show central calcification surrounded by the basaloid

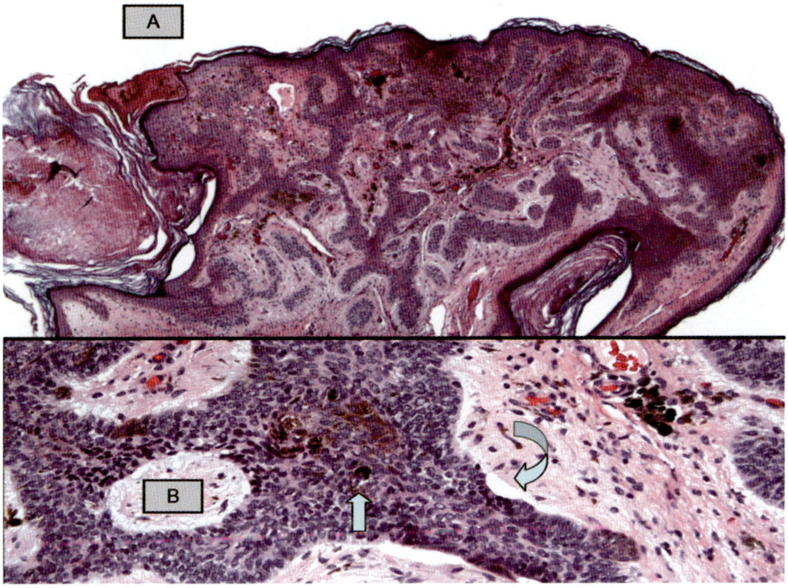

FIGURE 6.12 **Infundibulocystic Basal Cell Carcinoma: Histomorphology.** In a skin taglike growth removed from the young patient illustrated in Figure 6.3, a polypoid surface contour is noted **(A)**; basaloid tumor tongues are in continuity with the undersurface of the epidermis at multiple points. The individual tumor nests show cytoplasmic melanization **(B)**, an important criterion separating BCC from trichoepithelioma and trichofolliculoma. Classic slitlike stromal retraction is seen (*curved arrow*).

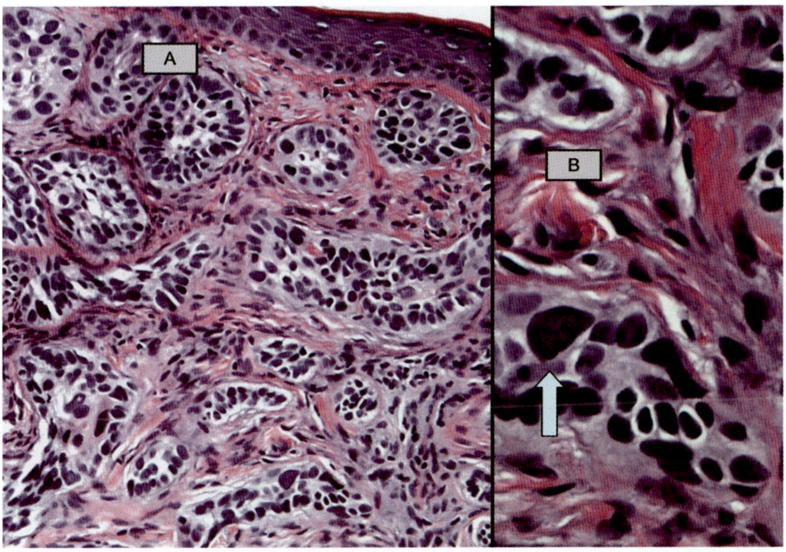

FIGURE 6.13 **Pleomorphic Basal Cell Carcinoma: Histomorphology.** In pleomorphic BCC, the tumor nests have a similar architectural pattern to nodular or mixed nodular and infiltrative growth BCC **(A)**. However, the tumors under high power microscopy show pleomorphic nuclei with large diameters (monster cells) (*arrow*) **(B)**.

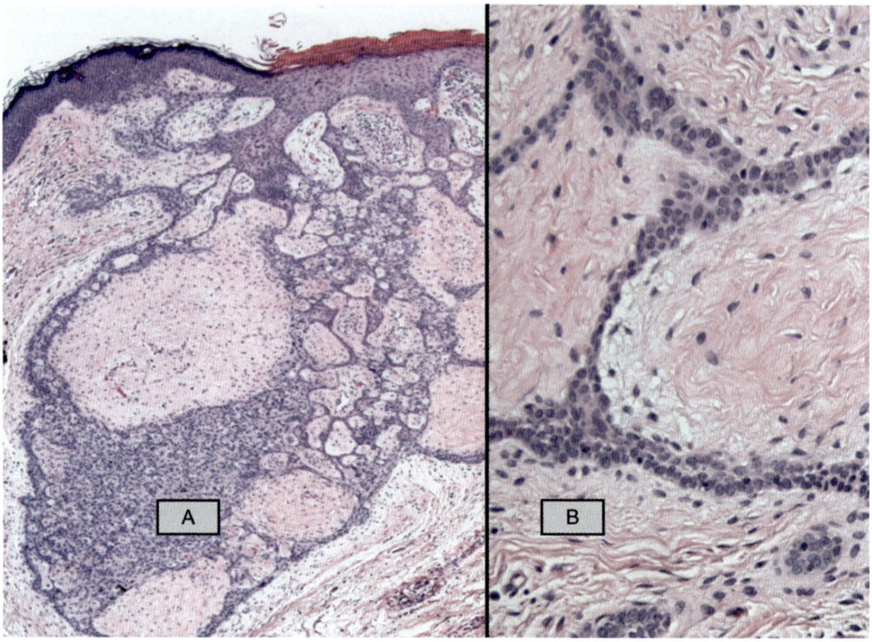

FIGURE 6.14 **Fibroepithelioma of Pinkus: Histomorphology.** The fibroepithelioma of Pinkus manifests atypical basaloid cells which grow in thin lacy strands radiating down from points of continuity with the overlying epidermis **(A)**. The stroma is often myxoid or shows plump stromal cells with collagen deposited around the basaloid tumor tongues **(B)**.

tumor cells. As with other nodular BCCs, the stroma is neither proplastic nor highly collagenized, and mitotic activity is minimal as is the presence of individual cell necrosis.[39] True hair production is absent.

Infundibulocystic Basal Cell Carcinoma

In the infundibulocystic BCC, proliferating basaloid cells, typically in continuity with the overlying epidermis, proliferate as oblong and rounded nests surrounding keratin filled structures lined by a stratified epithelium that shows a granular cell layer. The cells which line these keratin-filled cysts manifest progressive squamoid differentiation with an outer basaloid rim (e-figs. 6.27–6.30). Follicular bulbs, dermal papillae, and papillary mesenchymal bodies typical of true follicular differentiation, and often seen in trichoepitheliomata, are typically absent. Hair shaft production is not seen. Although the surrounding stroma contains plump cells of presumed fibroblastic lineage and shows minimal myxoid change,[44] the circumscribed, well-demarcated and differentiated stroma of a trichoepithelioma is not present, nor is there a desmoplastic stromal reaction as typifies the infiltrative growth BCC, which is one differential diagnostic consideration. The other differential diagnostic possibility is a basaloid follicular hamartoma. The basaloid follicular hamartoma manifests abortive hair papillae, is typically centered around a folliclelike structure in continuity with the epidermis, and is typically smaller than the infundibulocystic BCC. The infundibulocystic BCC is a tumor held to show differentiation toward the hair follicle infundibulum. A sebaceous component is usually absent. This morphology is seen in lesions associated with a familial pattern of inheritance. We have also seen infundibulocystic BCC in the setting of skin taglike polypoid growths in patients with nevoid BCC syndrome of Gorlin and Goltz (Fig. 6.3).

Follicular Basal Cell Carcinoma

On occasion, a BCC will show matrical differentiation whereby shadow cells adjacent to islands of proliferating basaloid cells are present, and so mimic a pilomatricoma.[46–49] The shadow cells have an anucleate morphology and eosinophilic cytoplasms often accompanied by zones of calcification.[47] Mitoses, apoptic cells, and high-grade nuclear atypia are absent.[46] The term "follicular squamous cell carcinoma" has been used to describe squamous cell carcinoma arising in the wall of an epidermal cyst; BCC arising in this setting is a rare event but is not unique to our experience (personal observation).

Pleomorphic Basal Cell Carcinoma

Some BCCs, particularly of nodular architecture, show strikingly enlarged giant hyperchromatic nuclei with amorphous nucleoplasms. These are termed as pleomorphic BCCs or "basal cell epithelioma with monster cells".[50] Typically, these misshapen giant nuclei are either scattered individually through tumor lobules or show clustering suggesting that they are components of a similar clone (Fig. 6.13, e-figs. 6.31 and 6.32). All cases evaluated by static image analysis cytometry have proven to be aneuploid[51] but paradoxically, mitoses, although present in roughly the same frequency as seen in typical nodular BCCs, are not often atypical.[50,51] As these pleomorphic monster cells impart no prognostic significance from the standpoint of enhanced biologic aggressiveness, we speculate that this represents a form of senescent atypia.

Basal Cell Carcinoma with Sweat Duct Differentiation

Typically seen in nodular BCC in some 1% of cases in our experience is otherwise typical eccrine, and sometimes apocrine, differentiation (see e-figs. 6.39–6.42)[52,53] whereby tubules lined by cuboidal epithelium with an internal eosinophilic cuticle are centrally disposed in otherwise typical basaloid tumor cell aggregates. The internal eosinophilic cuticle decorates with immunohistochemical stains for carcinoembryonic antigen (CEA) and epithelial membrane antigen (EMA).[44,52]

Basal Cell Carcinoma with Sebaceous Differentiation

The BCC with sebaceous differentiation is differentiated from sebaceous adenoma by having a germinative cell component which occupies greater than 50% of the transverse diameter of tumor lobules that typically manifest a rounded morphology with areas of slitlike retraction accompanied by mitoses and apoptotic debris (e-figs. 6.33–6.35). Unlike sebaceous carcinoma, there is no pagetoid spread in the overlying epidermis, no haphazard infiltrative growth morphology, no desmoplastic stromal reaction, and no invasion of adjacent structures. Sebaceous adenoma, in contrast, is characterized by a lining of germinative cells less than 50% of the diameter of the neoplastic lobule while sebaceous hyperplasia typically has a peripherally disposed layer of germinative cells one to two cells thick. In contrast is the sebaceoma (see e-figs. 6.43–6.45), a tumor that manifests a haphazard array of germinative epithelium admixed with sebocytes and structures that recapitulate sebaceous ducts. Particularly problematic are the sebaceous neoplasms of Muir–Torre's syndrome, which sometimes defy precise classification by the foregoing scheme.

Fibroepithelioma of Pinkus

Described by Pinkus in 1953,[54] the fibroepithelioma typically arises above the natal cleft or on the lower trunk as a pink or flesh-colored nodule with a constricted inferior margin suggesting a seborrheic keratosis.[56] In this tumor, elongated basaloid epithelial strands manifesting slitlike retraction from stroma are enmeshed in a myxoid matrix or a background of proliferating spindle cells with abundant collagen (Fig. 6.14, e-figs. 6.36–6.38). If a lesion is completely excised, a well-demarcated, pushing inferior and lateral margin is noted; the tumor frequently connects to the overlying epidermis at multiple points. A cystic variant is described.[56] The important differential diagnostic consideration is the eccrine syringofibroadenoma of Mascaro, characterized by a typical acral disposition and comprising elongated basaloid strands containing central eccrine ductal cells and a well-defined cuticle; these connect to the undersurface of the overlying epidermis in the fashion of eccrine straight ducts. Deeper levels through the paraffin block will show the basaloid strands of the eccrine syringofibroadenoma to have a central eccrine ductal differentiation and cuticle, unlike the solid undifferentiated basaloid epithelial columns of fibroepithelioma.[57] Some observers regard the fibroepithelioma as a form of "fenestrated" trichoblastoma, a lesion held to be a benign analog of BCC that shares many morphologic features of BCC but has not, to date, been shown to manifest PTCH mutations and dominantly affects sun-protected skin.[58]

Recurrent Basal Cell Carcinoma

In approximately 10% of BCCs treated by conventional management, either surgical excision or curettage followed by fulguration of the lesional base, recurrent tumors appear at some future point (Fig. 6.15).[2,3] The recurrence rate reflects margin positivity after attempted surgical excision and varies by histologic type, being highest for the aggressive-growth variants (for example, 26.5% for infiltrative BCCs) and lowest in the indolent-growth variants (for example, 6.4% and 3.6% for nodular and superficial BCCs,

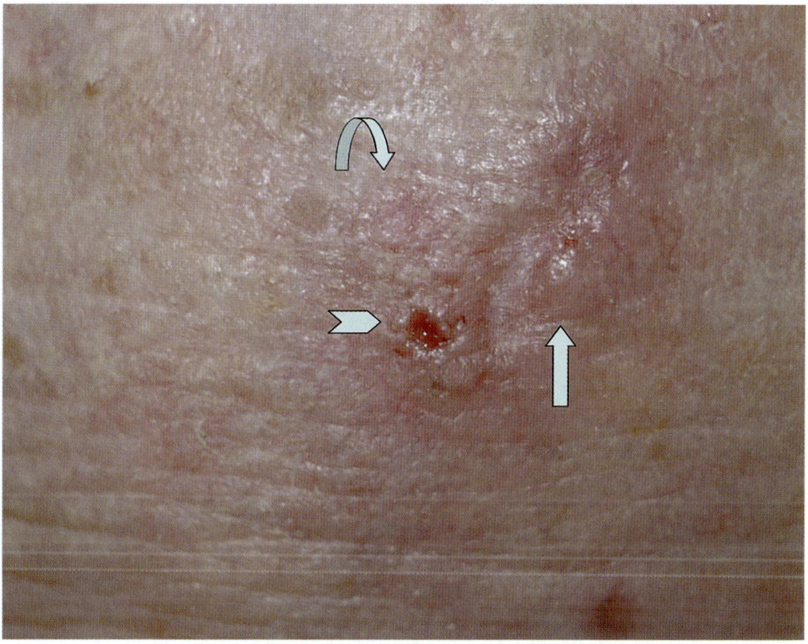

FIGURE 6.15 **Recurrent Basal Cell Carcinoma: Clinical Morphology.** In this tumor, a scariform plaque is present at the site of a previous biopsy. There is a rolled edge along one side of the tumor representing a nodular growth component (*straight arrow*) while the infiltrative growth component is recognizable only by pink discoloration of the skin (*curved arrow*) and has a poorly demarcated border. The *arrowhead* marks a recent biopsy site. (Case courtesy of Dr Michael Wilkerson, Galveston, TX.)

respectively).[32] Following Mohs micrographic surgery, the recurrence rate is said to be in the 1% range.[2,3] The recurrence rates may also differ based upon the anatomic site, particularly as regards lesions of the nose and ears,[2,3,20] where higher recurrence rates may reflect peculiarities of the anatomy or a natural hesitancy on the part of clinicians to perform mutilating surgical procedures in these locations. While most recurrences are seen within 3 years following the original operative procedure, some 20% of the recurrences manifest themselves between 6 and 10 years after the original surgery.[20] Any subsequently managed recurrent lesion has a further enhanced risk of recurrence, which is said to be in the 40% range.[15] This, too, reflects the difficult anatomic locations and the disruption of pre-existing architecture by scarring.[8] Recurrent BCC is characterized clinically by areas of induration, erythema, ulceration, or bleeding at a prior operative site for known BCC (Fig. 6.16). The histomorphology of recurrent BCC reflects, therefore, the character of the neoplasm, which is more often an aggressive-growth variant than an indolent-growth variant,[2,3,32,59] the presence of scar formation that disrupts the pre-existing native anatomy, and the depth of

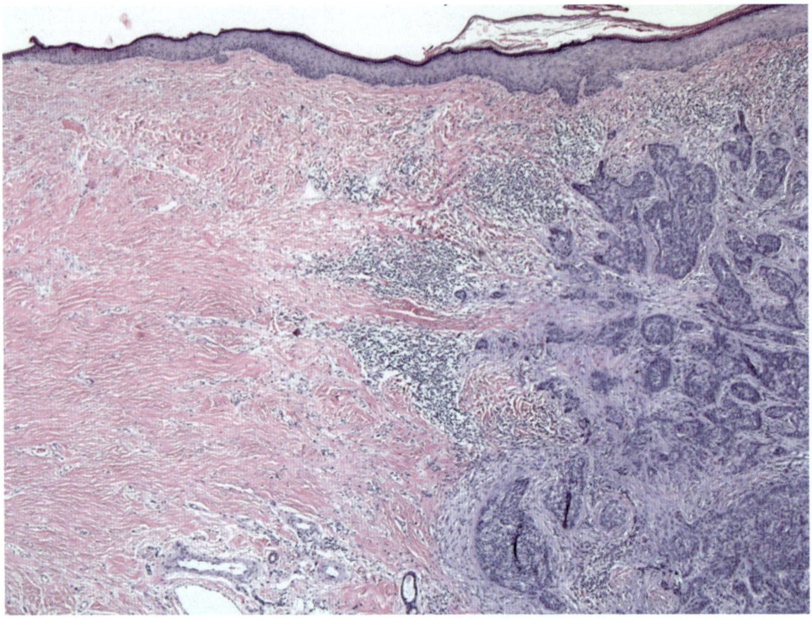

FIGURE 6.16 **Recurrent Basal Cell Carcinoma: Histomorphology.** In the same lesion illustrated in Figure 6.15, a biopsy showed a mature fibrous scar in continuity with areas of recurrent BCC of mixed nodular and infiltrative growth types.

infiltration, whereby recurrent lesions tend to have, at least in so far as the aggressive-growth variants are concerned, no connection to the overlying epidermis or to the pre-existing follicular structures (Fig. 6.16, e-figs. 6.46–6.48). There is an apparent correlation between the measured distance of the tumor to the nearest lesional edge and the recurrence rate.[6]

PATHOGENESIS

BCC is held to derive from basaloid epithelia located in the follicular bulges, in the anagen hair bulbs and the follicular matrix cells, and in specific basaloid cells of the interfollicular epidermis.[7,8,37,60] The cells of origin are held to be pluripotent progenitor epithelia in adults or epithelial germ cells in the case of those neoplasms arising in childhood (i.e., linear basal cell nevi). BCCs manifest a keratin profile similar to that of the lower part of the hair follicle[61] and that is therefore distinct from that of the adjacent epidermal basal layer epithelia.[61] In particular, and held to reflect their derivation from basaloid epithelia, BCCs express keratins type 5, 6[62], and 14[63] and also $\alpha 2$ and $\beta 1$ integrins[64] in a fashion that does not correlate well to tumor subtype. The expression of CD10 supports derivation from the folliculosebaceous unit.[65] Key to our understanding of the pathogenesis of BCC has been the unraveling of the molecular basis of the nevoid BCC syndrome.

Nevoid Basal Cell Carcinoma

The nevoid BCC syndrome, or Gorlin–Goltz's syndrome,[23,24] is inherited as an autosomal dominant trait with a minority of cases representing sporadic mutations.[23,24] Typically expressed in young adulthood, the syndrome comprises multiple basal cell cancers and other anomalies as described below. It is now recognized that for most patients, the abnormality represents a mutation in the human homolog of the Drosophila patched gene (PTCH).[25] A tumor suppressor gene, PTCH is sited on chromosome 9 q22-q31[26] results. The PTCH gene product functions as a transmembrane receptor for the Sonic hedgehog (SHH) protein; when binding of the wild-type protein occurs, the inhibition by PTCH of a second seven-span transmembrane protein termed smoothened (SMO) is downregulated. The inhibition of SMO is held to be relieved by mutations of PTCH or SMO that eventuate in cell proliferation (Fig. 6.17)[66]; PTCH gene mutations produce truncated proteins incapable of binding to and inactivating SMO.[67] Perturbations of the SHH pathway can occur through mutations or deletions of PTCH, SMO, and presumably of the zinc-finger glioma transcription factor (Gli)-1 that is normally expressed in the human hair follicle.[68] Upregulation of Gli proteins (Figs. 6.18 and 6.19) has been shown by quantitative reverse transcriptase polymerase chain reaction assay in BCC[69,70] and may play

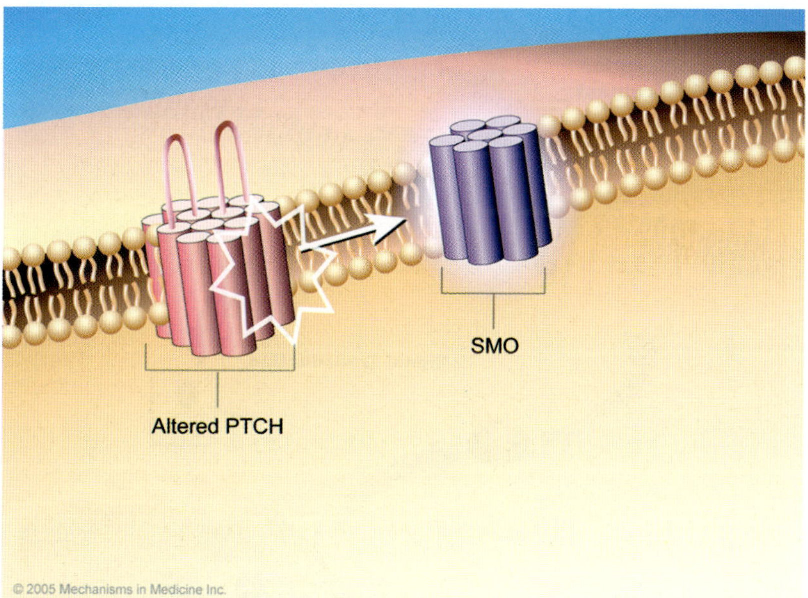

FIGURE 6.17 The patched (PTCH) gene product resides in the phospholipid bilayer of the plasma membrane. Its normal function is to bind smoothened (SMO), which is released after binding of the Sonic hedgehog (SHH) signaling protein. Mutations which cause truncation of the PTCH protein result in a situation where SMO expression is constitutively upregulated in the absence of the binding of SHH protein.

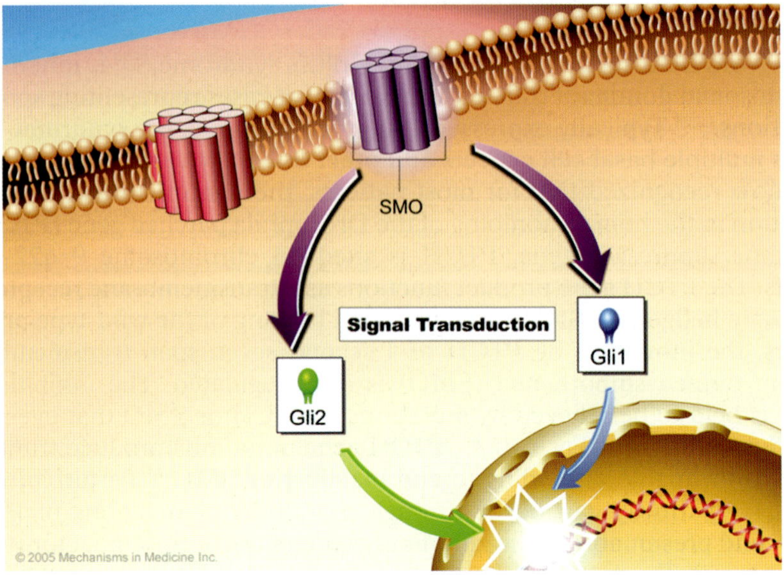

FIGURE 6.18 The SMO protein, when unbound by PTCH, acts as a signal transducer upregulating the expression of glioblastoma (Gli)-1 and Gli-2 signaling proteins.

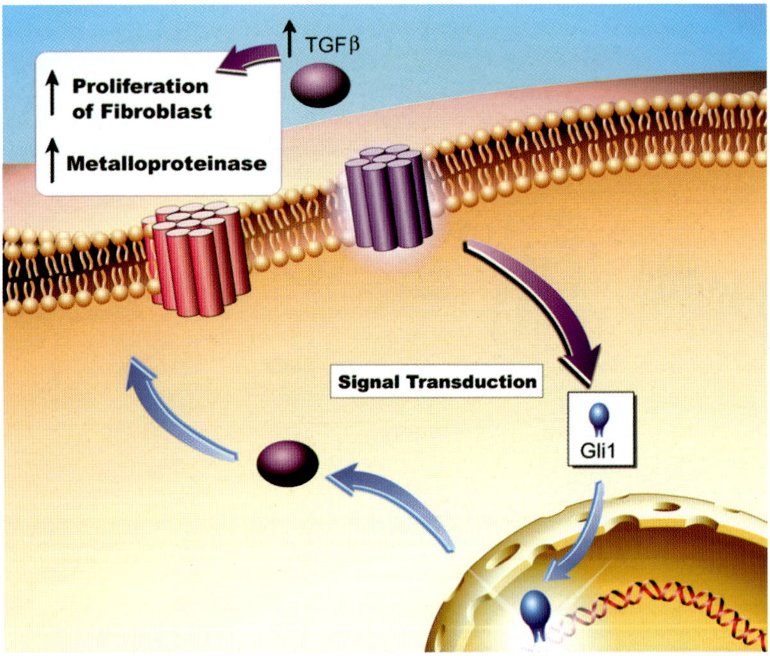

FIGURE 6.19 The Gli-1 protein binds to DNA to cause upregulation of the expression of transforming growth factor beta (TGF-β). TGF-β then migrates through holes in the nuclear envelope into the extracellular space to cause proliferation of fibroblasts and upregulated expression of metalloproteinases that cause dissolution of basement membrane material.

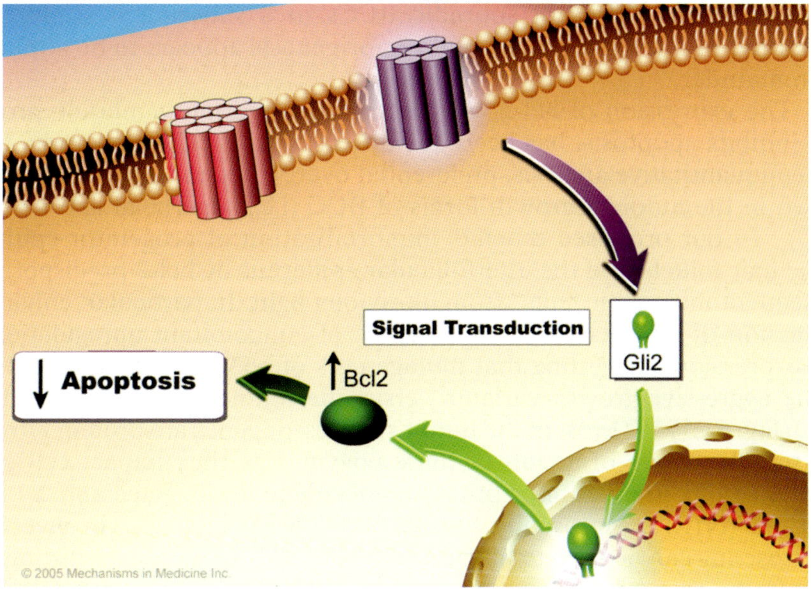

FIGURE 6.20 The Gli-2 protein product binds to chromosome 18 to cause upregulated expression of bcl-2 protein. The bcl-2 protein is believed to then migrate through the nuclear envelope. Its function along the internal cristae of mitochondria appears to impact oxygen consumption and ATP utilization. Bcl-2 is an antiapoptotic protein which helps to increase cell longevity. Normally functional in the operation of the hair follicle in a fashion that appears to prevent conversion from anagen through to the catagen phase of the hair cycle, bcl-2 may be the common pathway where those sporadic BCCs not impacted by PTCH mutations acquire similar properties to those neoplasms that are seen in basal cell nevus syndrome and in the setting of those sporadic mutations that impact the PTCH/SMO system.

an important role in the initiation of BCC through the activation of the bcl-2 gene (Fig. 6.20).[71] Gli proteins are also downstream regulators of the SHH signaling pathway, leading to increased tRNA expression through the basonuclin gene system[72] and possibly as well through the forkhead/winged-helix domain transcription factor FOXE-1.[73] Increased FOXM-1 levels, upregulated through SHH signaling via Gli-1, may be specific for sporadic BCC.[74] Gli-2 is able to induce G1-S phase progression in contact-inhibited keratinocytes, apparently through the transcription factor E2F1.[75] Antagonists of the SHH/SMO signaling pathway, such as the steroidal alkaloid cyclopamine, can selectively induce differentiation and apoptosis of tumor cells in vivo and may emerge as a potential therapeutic modality in the future.[76]

Sporadic Basal Cell Carcinoma

Perturbation of the SHH pathway, which is the rule in heredofamilial BCC, appears to be frequently operative in the sporadic BCC as well. Mutations of SMO or PTCH were detected in 12 of 31 sporadic BCCs in one study[77]; the same group of researchers showed mutations in this pathway in two-thirds of sporadic BCCs in a subsequent study.[78] An additional or alternate pathway of tumorigenesis appears to be at play in the remainder.

The expression of bcl-2, an inner mitochondrial membrane protein that inhibits apoptosis, has been demonstrated in BCCs of sporadic type. By semiquantitative analysis, preferential overexpression of bcl-2 has been shown in the indolent-growth forms of BCC (i.e., superficial and nodular BCC).[7] In our proposed scheme, immortalization of progenitor epithelia of the hair follicle and the interfollicular epidermis by bcl-2 predisposes to subsequent mutagenic "hits" from ultraviolet light. In particular, enhanced expression of p53 occurs in the absence of concomitant upregulation of p21 expression, suggesting that mutagenesis of p53 appears preferentially in the aggressive-growth variants versus the indolent-growth variants of BCC (Fig. 6.21).[38,79] Most of the tumor suppressor genes are protein tyrosine kinases; the mode of action of these enzymes as they impact cell cycle activity results in alterations of tissue phosphate levels detectable by near infra-red (NIR) spectroscopy.[80–82] By noninvasive methods, in vivo NIR spectroscopy can be used to map the extent of BCCs and also to distinguish them from other cutaneous tumors with a high degree of accuracy.[80–84]

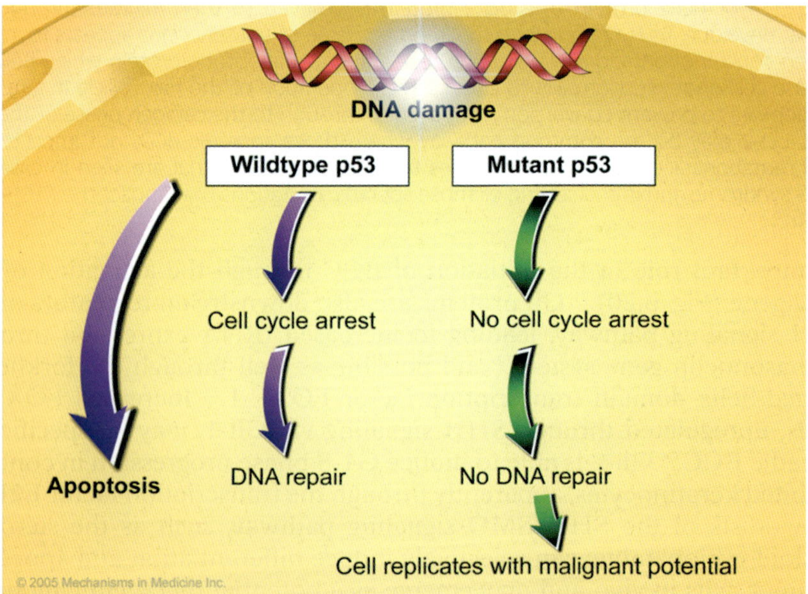

FIGURE 6.21 Ultraviolet light-induced damage causes conversion from wild type to mutant p53. Wild-type p53 causes cell cycle arrest through the p21/retinoblastoma gene product pathway in order to enable the repair of DNA in cells subjected to sublethal genotoxic injury. It also promotes apoptosis of irreparably damaged cells through the bcl-2/bax system. Mutant p53, in contrast, does not effect cell cycle arrest. As a consequence, DNA repair does not take place and cells are not driven down the apoptotic pathway, enabling them to then replicate and to acquire further genomic instabilities leading to an enhanced malignant potential.

That the two proposed mechanisms of tumorigenesis are complementary is suggested by the fact that SHH-expressing cells also manifest increased expression of bcl-2,[85] likely through the activation of the Gli proteins, which are expressed in the outer root sheath of the normal hair follicle and in BCCs[66]; Gli-2 in particular appears to play an important role in the activation of the bcl-2 gene.[71]

Ultraviolet Light-Induced Mutagenesis and Biologic Transformation

BCCs express p53 protein and do so in a preferential fashion in aggressive-growth variants.[79,86,87] Mutations of p53 have been documented in up to 40% of studied BCCs;[78] 72% of the mutations bear the signature of UV light induction. The aggressive-growth variants of sporadic BCC are associated with stromal fibroplasia and overexpression of what is likely a mutant p53.[38,79] It is this stromal response to tumor which makes the aggressive-growth BCC less amenable to local therapy and control.[32] The interaction between tumor and stroma, as demonstrated in many neoplastic systems, is critical to lesional pathogenesis. Loss of basement membrane material around individual tumor cell nests occurs with progression from indolent to aggressive-growth neoplasms.[36] The working hypothesis is that activation of matrix metalloproteinases in the process of transformation results in the digestion of basal lamina around tumor nests, promoting the elaboration and/or release of proplastic cytokines and their subsequent availability to the rapidly proliferating aggressive-growth neoplasms. Perhaps corroborating this hypothesis is the fact that the aggressive-growth BCCs have been shown to selectively express syndecan-1 in the adjacent stroma, but not in the tumor cells.[88] Syndecan-1 is a member of the syndecan glycoprotein family, held to play an important role in inhibiting tumor growth and invasion through its role as a receptor for growth factors in the extracellular matrix.

In our hands, the indolent-growth variants are found widely distributed on both sun-exposed and sun-protected skin, whereas the aggressive-growth variants such as infiltrative and morpheaform BCC are more frequent in sun-exposed skin.[7] Australian observers have confirmed these findings in a large series using conventional histology.[89] Men and women are affected in roughly equal proportions with the majority of tumors occurring in the head and neck region.[2,3,20] In our experience, men tend to manifest more frequent localization to the left side of the face, which may reflect the fact that many of our patients were driving vehicles in North America prior to the advent of sun screens. Roughly one-quarter of cases occur on the nose, the most frequently involved site.[2–6] Overall, it is less prevalent in more darkly pigmented races; the histologic types of BCC seen in Africans and Hispanics have a similar histomorphology.[90]

Other Risk Factors for Sporadic Basal Cell Carcinoma

The incidence of BCC is much more common in individuals who have received a solid organ transplant[91,92] in whom herpes virus-like DNA sequences have been demonstrated[91,92] and in whom tumors appear to have an increased tendency for recurrence and metastasis.[93] In concert with this more aggressive behavior, the histologic types are different in patients with immune suppression in whom infiltrative growth BCC is more common than nodular and/or superficial variants.[12] In contrast, superficial BCC predominates in individuals with renal failure, diabetes mellitus, and human immunodeficiency virus infection.[12]

Host Response to Neoplasm and Tumor–Stromal Interactions

Most inflammatory cells in the stroma of a BCC are lymphocytes of T-helper phenotype,[94] while T-cytotoxic/suppressor cells and B-lymphocytes are uncommon[8] and plasma cells, when present, are generally held to reflect coexisting ulceration. Patients with immune suppression have reduced numbers of T-lymphocytes around their tumor nests and tongues. Histiocytes are often present in significant numbers, most expressing HLA-DR antigens[8,81] and some representing Langerhans cells.[8] The apposition of human lymphocyte antigen (HLA) DR-expressing lymphocytes appears to be associated with upregulation of HLA-DR antigens on the surface of some tumor cells.[94] Mast cells are often present in increased numbers around the periphery of tumor islands[8,95] and may play a role, through release of their cytosolic products, in provocation of fibrosis around the tumor tongues of aggressive-growth neoplasms. An amyloidlike substance held to derive from degenerating epithelia is present in and around some indolent-growth BCCs (e-fig. 6.49)[96,97] but mucin deposition is a far more common finding. The mesenchymal mucins, likely products of stromal cells, represent hyaluronic acid and dermatan sulfate.[96,97] Cylinderlike inclusions of hyalin material resembling those seen in cylindroma are demonstrated in some nests of nodular BCCs[98] and appear to comprise intermediate filaments vimentin, keratin, and myosin.[98] In rare cases, needle-shaped fibers comprising collagenous crystalloids are identified[99] and contain types I and III collagen, held to reflect degeneration of extracellular matrix components.

Ultrastructural examination gives some clues to the pathogenesis and transformation characteristics of BCC. Both the superficial and nodular variants of BCC[36,100,101] are surrounded by a continuous basement membrane zone comprising collagens type IV and V admixed with laminin (Fig. 6.22). The aggressive-growth variants (i.e., morpheaform, metatypical, and infiltrative growth subtypes) manifest an absent basement membrane (Fig. 6.23).[36,101] Although formerly held to constitute a barrier to invasion,[100] the basement membrane zone may first be secreted by and later dissolved by neoplastic cell systems, such as in the case of upregulated transmembrane metalloproteinase activity in vertical growth phase melanoma-derived cell lines in vitro,[102] a biologic function which has specific implications. In particular, we speculate that the basement membrane material may act as a trap for proplastic cytokines derived from tumor cells, stromal cells, and inflammatory cells. These proplastic cytokines, when liberated by a transmembrane or other matrix metalloproteinase, may then be bioavailable to

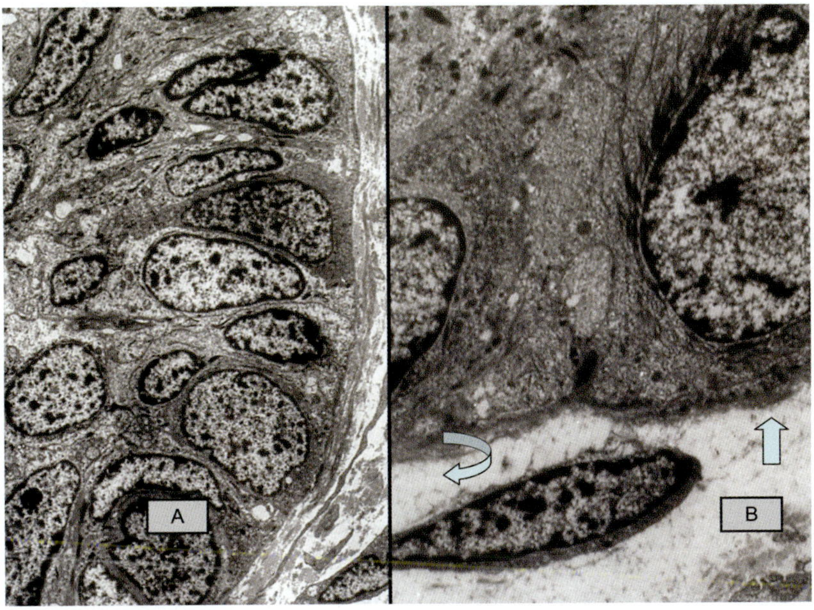

FIGURE 6.22 **Nodular Basal Cell Carcinoma: Ultrastructural Features.** The nodular BCC is characterized by rounded nests of neoplastic basaloid cells **(A)** which are delineated by an almost continuous basal lamina **(B**, *straight arrow***)**. Note the presence of numerous hemidesmosomes at the interface between the plasma membrane of the neoplastic basal cells and the adjacent delimiting basal lamina (*straight arrow*), and the absence of anchoring fibrils (*curved arrow*), which helps to explain the slitlike stromal retraction so characteristic of BCC at the light microscopic level.

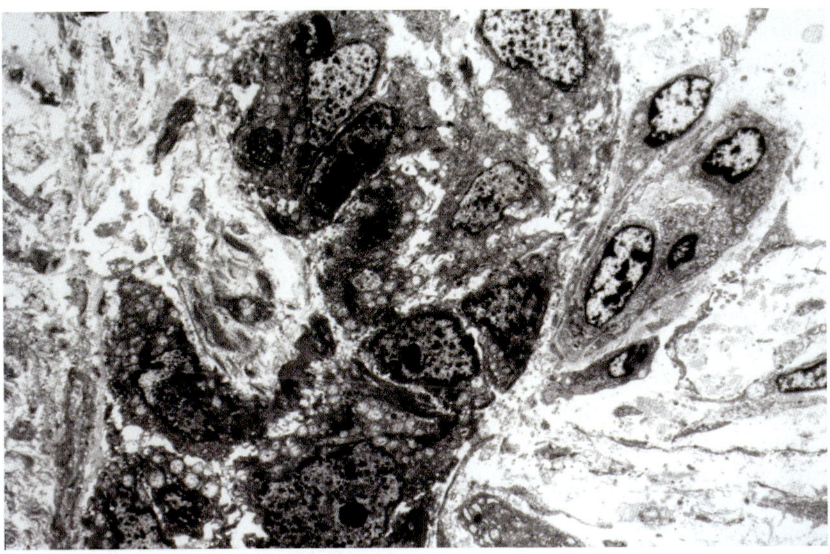

FIGURE 6.23 **Infiltrative Growth Basal Cell Carcinoma: Ultrastructural Characteristics.** In this infiltrative growth BCC, the tumor tongues have irregular contours. There is no delimiting zone of basement membrane material.

promote tumor growth.[102] In any event, the interaction between tumor and stroma plays a key role in basal cell cancer biology. The aggressive-growth variants, manifesting pronounced stromal desmoplasia, are not easily treatable by simple curettage and fulguration. The clinician can, with reasonable accuracy, predict when he or she is dealing with an aggressive-growth variant as the curette loop will strike the tumor and its fibrotic matrix to produce a "gritty" sensation quite unlike the nongritty character of superficial and nodular BCCs. It is the percolation of cells through stroma and their protection from the curette loop by the desmoplastic collagen table which necessitates an alternative approach, typically a surgical one, to the aggressive-growth tumors. Other ultrastructural features which find expression at the light microscopic level include the presence of hemidesmosomes along the margin of a nodular or superficial BCC in decreased numbers versus normal adjacent epidermis. This reduction in hemidesmosome concentration in concert with the absence of type VII collagen anchoring fibrils is held to be a potential explanation for the retraction spaces seen at the light microscopic level between the nodules of tumor cells and the adjacent stroma. Cytoskeletal microfilaments uncommon in normal epithelia are present in BCC, particularly in the invasive subtypes,[103] and could, in part, explain enhanced tumor mobility through stroma. Actin protein expression is upregulated in BCCs versus adjacent normal tissue via a series of specific protein kinases (unpublished data of Crowson and Garcia, 2005); differential expression of actin filaments and their attachment plaques has also been implicated as a significant event in the evolution of melanoma.[104,105]

Differential Diagnosis

The different forms of BCC carry with them a different set of differential diagnostic possibilities. Superficial BCC, by showing oftentimes sharply demarcated clones of basaloid cells, calls to mind Bowen's disease and sometimes other clonal proliferations such as clonal seborrheic keratosis or even intraepidermal eccrine porocarcinoma in situ. Essential to the distinction is the identification of a peripheral palisade along the base of the lesion at the dermal–epidermal junction in concert with slitlike retraction of the stroma. Eccrine cancers often have true lumenal margins or intracytoplasmic lumina reflecting glandular differentiation. Bowen's disease shows pronounced intercellular bridge formation and cytoplasmic keratinization and has frequent and atypical mitotic figures, which are uncommon in superficial BCC. Seborrheic keratoses can cause surprising difficulty in distinction from both superficial and early nodular BCCs, but generally the seborrheic keratosis manifests a plaquelike architecture whereby a straight line drawn between the native epidermides at the shoulders of the lesion lies beneath the plane of the proliferation. Seborrheic keratoses comprise basaloid epithelia, usually without atypia or mitotic activity, accompanied by pseudohorn cyst formation and a pigmented reticulated, a solid acanthotic, or a papillomatous architecture. Actinic keratoses occasionally mimic BCCs as well. In particular, some actinic keratoses manifest downward buds of atypical basaloid cells in sun-damaged skin but these are surmounted by parakeratosis and typically lack slitlike retraction from the subjacent stroma I or mucin deposition.

Nodular BCC raises consideration to a nodular intradermal eccrine proliferation such as clear cell hidradenoma or eccrine spiradenoma, the latter showing intertwined dark basaloid and lighter cuboidal lumenal cells reflecting eccrine differentiation. These neoplasms frequently have few mitoses and often do not connect to the overlying epidermis. Peripheral palisading, stroma mucinosis, or individual cell necrosis is unusual in the tumor nests of benign eccrine adnexal neoplasia. The trichoepithelioma manifests abortive hair papilla formation with papillary mesenchymal bodies in basaloid nests, which are in turn encompassed by a distinctive stroma populated by plump stromal cells that is sharply demarcated from the adjacent native dermis. Trichoepitheliomas do not manifest mitotic activity and individual cell necrosis and only infrequently have melanin pigment within tumor nests. Trichoepitheliomas also frequently radiate around central keratin-filled cystic structures. It is the more differentiated BCCs, such as the BCC with abortive hair papilla formation, and the infundibulocystic BCC which can cause confusion with respect to trichoepithelioma.[106] Immunostains can be helpful, such as CD34 that is expressed in the stroma of trichoepitheliomas but not that of BCCs[46,107] and bcl-2 that is expressed diffusely in the indolent-growth BCC but only around the periphery of a trichoepithelioma.[108] Trichofolliculoma, on the other hand, manifests a central keratin-filled pore containing hair shaft material, from which radiate squamoid bands that in turn connect to basaloid islands recapitulating follicular differentiation. The differentiated forms of nodular BCC such as BCC with sebaceous or eccrine adnexal differentiation can be distinguished in the former instance by criteria already listed above and in the latter by the presence of slitlike retraction, individual cell necrosis, and mitotic activity. As well, the eccrine components of BCC, when present, are only a minor contribution to the overall volume of tumor. We do not consider distinction of the "adenoid" form of BCC from digital papillary adenocarcinoma and other malignant eccrine neoplasms to be a significant or realistic concern in the vast majority of cases.

Some BCCs show clear cell differentiation comprising intracytoplasmic glycogen accumulation and apparently recapitulating outer root sheath (trichilemmal) differentiation. In this setting, sebaceous carcinoma enters the differential diagnosis. Sebaceous carcinomas decorate with antibodies to low molecular weight keratins (i.e., CAM 5.2) and strongly with antibodies to EMA in our hands. Others describe absent EMA expression in the poorly differentiated areas of sebaceous carcinoma.[109] Basal and squamous cell carcinomas express EMA only faintly and are typically negative for CAM 5.2. The Thompsen–Freidenreich (T) antigen is expressed in sebaceous neoplasms but not by most basal and squamous cell carcinomas, and has been held to be a useful diagnostic tool.[110] Some authors have found the marker to be less helpful.[111] Androgen receptor expression in sebaceous neoplasms, including in the seboblasts as well as the differentiated sebocytes, has been proposed as a diagnostic adjunct.[112] Androgen receptor expression was reported in 78% of BCCs but no trichogeneic neoplasms in one study[112]; by implication, the utility of this marker in differentiating sebaceous neoplasms from BCC must be considered dubious. The distinction of these clear cell tumors from sebaceous carcinoma and sebaceous epithelioma rests on the demonstration of cytoplasmic glycogen (using an alcian blue-Periodic acid-Schiff (PAS) and PAS-diastase staining combination) and by the expression of CEA. Recognition of sebaceous differentiation in a BCC would not alter the biologic potential of the tumor, but sebaceous carcinomas tend to have more stubborn local aggression and also a metastatic capability, which is likely more significant than for BCC. The presence of balloon cell change in a melanocytic proliferation can mimic clear cell and sebaceous differentiation in BCCs; appropriate immunohistochemical decoration with antibodies to S-100 protein, A103 (Melan-A), and gp100 protein (HMB-45) makes these distinctions possible.[113] Metastatic renal cell cancers and thyroid cancers can have a clear cell morphology. The former are glycogen rich and can therefore cause diagnostic concern but typically have a highly vascular stroma associated with abundant hemorrhage. Renal cell carcinomas express CD10, CD15, AMCAR, specific renal cell antigens recognizable with commercial antibodies, PAX-2, and keratins. Thyroid carcinomas decorate with antibodies to thyroid transcription factor and/or thyroglobulin (if follicular differentiation is present), enabling distinction. On occasion, Merkel cell carcinoma comes into consideration of a solid undifferentiated form of BCC. The Merkel cell carcinoma expresses cytokeratin 20, typically as droplike aggregates in a perinuclear disposition representing Golgi complex accentuation, in concert with neuroendocrine markers, namely, synaptophysin and chromogranin.[114]

With respect to the aggressive-growth BCCs, the morpheaform BCC must be distinguished from other desmoplastic adnexal tumors including desmoplastic trichoepithelioma and microcystic adnexal carcinoma. Some desmoplastic trichoepitheliomas manifest an epidermal "dell," a downward indentation of the epidermal surface, accompanied by proliferating basaloid cells, keratin cysts, and only a very rare mitosis in the tumor cell population. Dermal mucin production and apoptosis are absent, although calcification may be seen. In the microcystic adnexal carcinoma, a widely invasive tumor is seen which goes to all edges of a punch biopsy specimen most typically and comprises columns of vertically oriented atypical cells manifesting individual cell necrosis and mitotic activity surmounted by keratin-containing cystic structures lined by differentiated squamous epithelium. Microcystic adnexal carcinoma is a neoplasm of the mid face typically of middle-aged or elderly woman and can manifest stubborn local recurrence with disfigurement. Its correct diagnosis and appropriate extirpative surgical therapy are therefore necessary.[115]

CONCLUSION

Advances in the biology of BCC have led us to understand the pathways of lesional evolution and have induced clinicians to demand precision as well as accuracy in morphologic classification. The impact upon therapy of the accurate classification of BCC is such that all practicing surgical pathologists should be aware of the histologic criteria for diagnosis and subclassification of this most common human cancer.

ACKNOWLEDGMENTS

Much of the original work on BCC described in this chapter, was funded by the Misericordia General Hospital Research Foundation, Winnipeg, Canada. Funding for the illustrations of tumor biology was provided by the Arthur Curtis Foundation of the University of Oklahoma and by Pathology Laboratory Associates, Tulsa, Oklahoma. I am indebted to my colleagues Drs Thomas Hayakawa, Marshall Kadin, Cynthia Magro, Dragana Pilavdzic, and Mirek Stranc who participated in the original works. The illustrations of patched and smoothened signaling were created in concert with David and Nic Searle and their colleagues at Mechanisms in Medicine, Inc, Toronto, Ontario, Canada.

REFERENCES

1. Jacob A. Observations respecting an ulcer of peculiar character, which attacks the eyelids and other parts of the face. *Dublin Hosp Rep Commun Med Surg* 1827;4:232–239.
2. Miller SJ. Biology of basal cell carcinoma (Part I). *J Am Acad Dermatol* 1991;24:1–13.
3. Miller SJ. Biology of basal cell carcinoma (Part II). *J Am Acad Dermatol* 1991;24: 161–175.
4. Lacour JP. Carcinogenesis of basal cell carcinomas: Genetics and molecular mechansisms. *Br J Dermatol* 2002;146 (Suppls 61):17–19.
5. Carter DM, Lin AN. Basal cell carcinoma, In: Fitzpatrick TM, Eisen AZ, Wolff K, et al., eds. *Dermatology in General Medicine*, 4th Ed. New York: McGraw-Hill, 1993:840–847.
6. Miller DL, Weinstock MA. Nonmelanoma skin cancer in the United States: Incidence. *J Am Acad Dermatol* 1994;30:774–778.
7. Crowson AN, Magro CM, Kadin M, Stranc M. Differential expression of bcl-2 oncogene in human basal cell carcinoma. *Hum Pathol* 1996;27:355–359.
8. Goldberg LH. Basal cell carcinoma. *Lancet* 1996;347:663–667.
9. Price MA, Goldberg LH, Levy ML. Juvenile basal cell carcinoma. *Ped Dermatol* 1994;11:176–177.
10. Goldstein AM, Bale SJ, Peck GL, et al. Sun exposure and basal cell carcinoma in the nevoid basal cell carcinoma syndrome. *J Am Acad Dermatol* 1993;29:34–41.
11. Johnson TM, Tschen J, Ho C, et al. Unusual basal cell carcinomas. *Cutis* 1994;54:85–92.
12. Oram Y, Orengo I, Griego RD, et al. Histologic Patterns of basal cell carcinoma based upon patient immunostatus. *Dermatol Surg* 1995;21:611–614.
13. Rao BK, Freeman RG, Poulos EG, et al. The relationship between basal cell epithelioma and seborrheic keratosis. *J Dermatol Surg Oncol* 1994;20:761–764.

14. Crowson AN, Magro CM. Desmoplastic trichilemmoma and its association with basal cell carcinoma. *Am J Dermatopathol* 1996;18:43–48.
15. Boyd AS. Tumors of the epidermis. In: Barnhill R, Crowson AN, eds. *Textbook of Dermatopathology*. 2nd Ed. New York: McGraw-Hill Co., 2004:575–634.
16. Peschen M, Lo JS, Snow SN, et al. Linear basal cell carcinoma. *Cutis* 1993;51: 287–289.
17. Niazi ZBM, Lamberty BGH. Perineural infiltration in basal cell carcinomas. *Br J Plast Surg* 1993;6:156–157.
18. Lo JS, Snow SN, Reizner GT, et al. Metastatic basal cell carcinoma: Report of twelve cases with a review of the literature. *J Am Acad Dermatol* 1991;24:715–719.
19. Sahl WJ. Basal cell carcinoma: Influence of tumor size on mortality and morbidity. *Int J Dermatol* 1995;34:319–321.
20. Randle HW. Basal cell carcinoma: Identification and treatment of the high-risk patient. *Dermatol Surg* 1996;22:255–261.
21. Snow SN, Sahl WJ, Lo J, et al. Metastatic basal cell carcinoma: Report of 5 cases. *Cancer* 1994;73:328–335.
22. Howell JB, Caro MR. The basal cell nevus. *Arch Dermatol* 1959;79:67–80.
23. Bale AE, Gailani MR, Leffell DJ. Nevoid basal cell carcinoma syndrome. *J Invest Dermatol* 1994;103:126S–130S.
24. Gorlin RJ. Nevoid basal cell carcinoma syndrome. *Derm Clin N Am* 1995;13:113–125.
25. Nagao K, Fujii K, Yamada M, Miyashita T. Identification of a novel polymorphism involving a CGG repeat in the PTCH gene and a genome-wide screening of CGG-containing genes. *J Hum Genet* 2004;49:97–101.
26. Kim MY, Park HJ, Baek SC, et al. Mutations of the p53 and PTCH gene in basal cell carcinomas: UV mutation signature and strand bias. *J Dermatol Sci* 2002;29:1–9.
27. Bale AE. The nevoid basal cell carcinoma syndrome: Genetics and mechanisms of carcinogenesis. *Cancer Invest* 1997;15:180–186.
28. Barr RJ, Headley JL, Jensen JL, et al. Cutaneous keratocysts of nevoid basal cell carcinoma syndrome. *J Am Acad Dermatol* 1986;14:572–576.
29. Howell JB, Mehregan AH. Pursuit of the pits in nevoid basal cell carcinoma syndrome. *Arch Dermatol* 1970;102:586–597.
30. Pratt MD, Jackson R. Nevoid basal cell carcinoma syndrome. *J Am Acad Dermatol* 1987;16:964–970.
31. Russell EB, Carrington PR, Smoller BR. Basal cell carcinoma: A comparison of shave biopsy versus punch biopsy techniques in subtype diagnosis. *J Am Acad Dermatol* 1999;41:69–71.
32. Sexton M, Jones DB, Maloney ME. Histologic pattern analysis of basal cell carcinoma. *J Am Acad Dermatol* 1990;23:1118–1126.
33. Ackerman AB, Jacobson M, Vitale P. *Clues to Diagnosis in Dermatopathology*. Chicago, IL: ASCP Press, 1991:245–248.
34. Hendrix JD, Parlette HL. Micronodular basal cell carcinoma: A deceptive histologic subtype with frequent clinically undetected tumor extension. *Arch Dermatol* 1996;295–298.
35. Boyd AS, Rapini RP. Cutaneous collision tumors. *Am J Dermatopathol* 1994; 16:253–257.
36. Hayakawa TJ, Pilavdzic D, Magro CM, et al. The ultrastructure of aggressive-versus indolent-growth basal cell carcinoma: A comparative study [abstract]. *Lab Invest* 1998; 78:50A.
37. Siegle RJ, MacMillan J, Pollack SV. Infiltrative basal cell carcinoma: A nonsclerosing subtype. *J Dermatol Surg Oncol* 1986;12:830–836.

38. Crowson AN, Magro CM, Pilavdzic D, et al. Differential stromal p53 expression in human basal cell carcinoma [abstract]. *Lab Invest* 1997;76:43A.

39. de Faria JL. Basal cell carcinoma of the skin with areas of squamous cell carcinoma: A basosquamous cell carcinoma. *J Clin Pathol* 1985;38:1273–1277.

40. Wick MR. Malignant tumors of the epidermis. In: Farmer ER, Hood AF, eds. *Pathology of the Skin*, 2nd Ed. New York: McGraw-Hill, 2000:969–1006.

41. Garcia C, Poletti E, Crowson AN. Basosquamous carcinoma. *J Am Acad Dermatol* 2009 Jan;60(1):137–143. Review.

42. Crowson AN. Basal cell carcinoma: biology, morphology and clinical implications. *Mod Pathol* 2006;19:S127–S147.

43. Lever WF, Shamberg-Lever G. *Histopathology of the Skin*, 7th Ed. Philadelphia, PA: Lippincott, 1989.

44. Kato N, Ueno H. Infundibulocystic basal cell carcinoma. *Am J Dermatopathol* 1993;15:265–267.

45. Walsh N, Ackerman AB. Infundibulocystic basal cell carcinoma: A newly described variant. *Mod Pathol* 1990;3:599–608.

46. Aloi FG, Molinero A, Pippione M. Basal cell carcinoma with matrical differentiation. *Am J Dermatopathol* 1988;10:509–513.

47. Ambrojo P, Aguilar A, Simon P, et al. Basal cell carcinoma with matrical differentiation. *Am J Dermatopathol* 1992;14:293–297.

48. Haskel HD, Maynes HA, McKee PH, et al. Basal cell carcinoma with matrical differentiation: A case study with analysis of beta-catenin. *J Cutan Pathol* 2005;32:245–250.

49. Ali F, Brown A, Gottwald L, Thomas J. Basal cell carcinoma with matrical differentiation in a transplant patient: A case report and review of the literature. *J Cutan Pathol* 2005;32:445–448.

50. Elston DM, Bergfeld WF, Petroff N. Basal cell carcinoma with monster cells. *J Cutan Pathol* 1993;20:70–73.

51. Garcia JA, Cohen PR, Herzberg AJ, et al. Pleomorphic basal cell carcinoma. *J Am Acad Dermatol* 1995;32:740–746.

52. Hanke CW, Temofeew RK. Basal cell carcinoma with eccrine differentiation (eccrine epithelioma). *J Dermatol Surg Oncol* 1986;12:820–824.

53. Misago N, Satoh T, Narisawa Y. Basal cell carcinoma with ductal and glandular differentiation: A clinicopathological and immunohistochemical study of 10 cases. *Eur J Dermatol* 2004;14:383–387.

54. Pinkus H. Premalignant fibroepithelial tumors of the skin. *Arch Dermatol* 1953;67:598–603.

55. Suster S, Cajal SR. Myoepithelial differentiation in basal cell carcinoma. *Am J Dermatopathol* 1991;13:350–357.

56. Jones CC, Ansari SJ, Tschen JA. Cystic fibroepithelioma of Pinkus. *J Cutan Pathol* 1991;18:220–222.

57. Spoonemore K, Crowson AN. Eccrine syringofibroadenoma in a patient with chronic graft-versus-host disease [abstract]. *J Cutan Pathol* 2004;1:128–129.

58. Bowen AR, LeBoit PE. Fibroepithelioma of Pinkus is a fenestrated trichoblastoma. *Am J Dermatopathol* 2005;27:149–154.

59. Lang PG, Maize JC. Histologic evolution of recurrent basal cell carcinoma and treatment implications. *J Am Acad Dermatol* 1986;14:186–196.

60. Kore-eda S, Horiguchi Y, Ueda M, et al. Basal cell carcinoma cells resemble follicular matrix cells rather than follicular bulge cells: Immunohistochemical and ultrastructural studies. *Am J Dermatopathol* 1998;20:362–369.

61. Shimizu N, Ito M, Tazawa T, et al. Immunohistochemical study on keratin expression in certain cutaneous epithelial neoplasms. *Am J Dermatopathol* 1989;11:534–540.

62. Plumb SJ, Argenyi ZB, Stone MS, De Young HR. Cytokeratin 5/6 immunostaining in cutaneous adnexal neoplasms and metastatic adenocarcinoma. *Am J Dermatopathol* 2004;26:447–451.
63. Bigelow RL, Jen EY, Delehedde M, et al. Sonic hedgehog induces epidermal growth factor dependent matrix infiltration in HaCaT keratinocytes. *J Invest Dermatol* 2005;124:457–465.
64. Pentel M, Helm KF, Maloney MM. Cell surface molecules in basal cell carcinomas. *Dermatol Surg* 1995;21:858–861.
65. Yada K, Kashima K, Daa T, et al. Expression of CD10 in basal cell carcinoma. *Am J Dermatopathol* 2004;26:463–471.
66. Xie J, Murone M, Luoh SM, et al. Activating Smoothened mutations in sporadic basal-cell carcinoma. *Nature* 1998;391:90–92.
67. Barnes EA, Heidtman KJ, Donoghue DJ. Constitutive activation of the shh-ptc1 pathway by a patched1 mutation identified in BCC. *Oncogene* 2005;24:902–915.
68. Dahmane N, Lee J, Robins P, et al. Activation of the transcription factor Gli1 and the Sonic hedgehog signaling pathway in skin tumours. *Nature* 1997;389:876–881.
69. Tojo M, Kiyosawa H, Iwatsuki K, et al. Expression of the GLI2 oncogene and its isoforms in human basal cell carcinoma. *Br J Dermatol* 2003;148:892–897.
70. Hatta N, Hirano T, Kimura T, et al. Molecular diagnosis of basal cell carcinoma and other basaloid cell neoplasms of the skin by the quantification of Gli1 transcript levels. *J Cutan Pathol* 2005;32:131–136.
71. Regl G, Kasper M, Schnidar H et al. Activation of the BCL2 promoter in response to hedgehog/GLI1 signal transduction is predominantly mediated by GLI2. *Cancer Res* 2004;64:7724–7731.
72. Cui C, Elsam T, Tian Q, et al. Gli proteins up-regulate the expression of basonuclin in basal cell carcinoma. *Cancer Res* 2004;64:5651–5658.
73. Eichberger T, Regl G, Ikram MS. FOXE1, a new transcription target of GLI2 is expressed in human epidermis and basal cell carcinoma. *J Invest Dermatol* 2004;122:1180–1187.
74. The MT, Wong ST, Neill GW, et al. FOXM1 is a downstream target of Gli1 in basal cell carcinomas. *Cancer Res* 2002;62:4773–4780.
75. Regl G, Kasper M, Schnidar H, et al. The zinc-finger transcription factor GLI2 antagonizes contact inhibition and differentiation of human epidermal cells. *Oncogene* 2004;23:1263–1274.
76. Tas S, Avci O. Induction of the differentiation and apoptosis of tumor cells in vivo with efficiency and selectivity. *Eur J Dermatol* 2004;14:96–102.
77. Reifenberger J, Wolter M. Weber RG, et al. Missense mutations in SMOH in sporadic basal cell carcinomas of the skin and primitive neuroectodermal tumors of the central nervous system. *Cancer Res* 1998;58:1798–1803.
78. Reifenberger J, Wolter M, Knobbe SB, et al. Somatic mutations in the PTCH, SMOH, SUFUH and TP53 genes in sporadic basal cell carcinomas. *Br J Dermatol* 2005;152:43–51.
79. Crowson AN, Pilavdzic D, Stranc M, Magro CM. Expression of p21$^{WAF1/CIP1}$ in aggressive-versus non-aggressive-growth basal cell carcinoma: A comparative study [abstract]. *Lab Invest* 1999;79:56A.
80. McIntosh LM, Jackson M, Mantsch HH, et al. Chemical analysis of basal cell carcinomas by infrared microscopy: Possible diagnostic applications [abstract]. *Lab Invest* 1999;79:60A.
81. McIntosh LM, Mansfield JR, Crowson AN, et al. Pathological diagnosis of basal cell carcinoma by infrared spectroscopy [abstract]. *Proc Society for Invest Dermatol 60th Annual Meeting*, Chicago, IL, May 5–9, 1999:643A.
82. McIntosh LM, Jackson M, Mantsch HH, et al. Infrared spectra of basal cell carcinomas are distinct from non-tumor-bearing skin components. *J Invest Dermatol* 1999;112:951–956.

83. McIntosh LM, Summers R, Jackson M, et al. Non-invasive diagnosis of skin tumors by near infrared spectroscopy [abstract]. *J Invest Dermatol* 2000;112:670.
84. McIntosh LM, Summers R, Jackson M, et al. Towards non-invasive screening of skin lesions by near-infrared spectroscopy. *J Invest Dermatol* 2001;116:175–181.
85. Fan H, Oro AE, Scott MP, Khavani PA. Induction of basal cell carcinoma features in transgenic human skin expressing Sonic Hedgehog. *Nat Med* 1997;3:788–792.
86. Shea CR, McNutt NS, Volkenandt M, et al. Overexpression of p53 protein in basal cell carcinomas of human skin. *Am J Pathol* 1992;141:25–29.
87. De Rosa G, Saibano S, Barra E, et al. p53 protein in aggressive and non-aggressive basal cell carcinoma. *J Cutan Pathol* 1993;20:429–434.
88. Bayer-Garner IB, Dilday B, Sanderson RD, Smoller BR. Syndecan-1 expression is decreased with increasing aggressiveness of basal cell carcinoma. *Am J Dermatopathol* 2000;22:119–122.
89. McCormack CJ, Kelly JW, Dorevitch AP. Differences in age and body site distribution of the histological subtypes of basal cell carcinoma. A possible indicator of different causes. *Arch Dermatol* 1997;133:593–596.
90. Woods SG. Basal cell carcinoma in the black population. *Int J Dermatol* 1995;34:517–518.
91. Bavinck JNB, de Boer A, Vermeer BJ, et al. Sunlight, keratotic skin lesions and skin cancer in renal transplant recipients. *Br J Dermatol* 1993;129:242–249.
92. Rady RL, Yen A, Rollefson JL, et al. Herpes virus-like DNA sequences in non-Kaposi's sarcoma skin lesions of transplant patients. *Lancet* 1995;345:1339–1340.
93. Sitz KV, Keppen M, Johnson DF. Metastatic basal cell carcinoma in acquired immunodeficiency syndrome-related complex. *JAMA* 1987;257:340–343.
94. Kohchiyama A, Oka D, Ueki H. Expression of human lymphocyte antigen (HLA)–DR on tumor cells in basal cell carcinoma. *J Am Acad Dermatol* 1987;16:833–838.
95. Cohen MS, Rogers GS. The significance of mast cells in basal cell carcinoma. *J Am Acad Dermatol* 1995;33:514–517.
96. Satti MB, Azzopardi JG. Amyloid deposits in basal cell carcinoma of the skin. *J Am Acad Dermatol* 1990;22:1082–1087.
97. Olsen KE, Westermark P. Amyloid in basal cell carcinoma and seborrheic keratosis. *Acta Derm Venereol (Stockh)* 1994;74: 273–275.
98. Sahin AA, Ro JY, Grignon DJ, et al. Basal cell carcinoma with hyaline inclusions. *Arch Pathol Lab Med* 1989;113:1015–1018.
99. Zamecnik M, Skalova A, Michal M. Basal cell carcinoma with collagenous crystalloids. *Arch Pathol Lab Med* 1996;120:581–582.
100. Kallioinen M, Autio-Harmainen A, Dammert K, et al. Discontinuity of the basement membrane in fibrosing basocellular carcinomas and basosquamous carcinomas of the skin: An immunohistochemical study with human laminin and type IV collagen antibodies. *J Invest Dermatol* 1984;82:248–251.
101. Barsky SH, Grossman DA, Bhuta S. Desmoplastic basal cell carcinomas possess unique basement membrane-degrading properties. *J Invest Dermatol* 1987;88:324–329.
102. Iida J, Wilhelmson KL, Price MA, et al. Membrane type-I matrix metalloproteinase promotes human melanoma invasion and growth. *J Invest Dermatol* 2004;122:167–176.
103. Jones JCR, Steinman HK, Goldsmith BA. Hemidesmosomes, collagen VII, and intermediate filaments in basal cell carcinoma. *J Invest Dermatol* 1989;93:662–671.
104. Bouffard D, Duncan LM, Howard CA, et al. Actin-binding protein expression in benign and malignant melanocytic proliferations. *Hum Pathol* 1994;25:709–714.
105. Duncan LM, Bouffard D, Howard C, et al. In situ distribution of alpha 2 beta 1 and alpha-actinin in melanocytic proliferations. *Mod Pathol* 1996;9:938–943.
106. Brooke JD, Fitzpatrick JE, Golitz LE. Papillary mesenchymal bodies: A histologic finding useful in differentiating trichoepitheliomas from basal cell carcinomas. *J Am Acad Dermatol* 1989;21:523–528.

107. Kirchmann TT, Prieto VG, Smoller BR. CD34 staining pattern distinguishes basal cell carcinoma from trichoepithelioma. *Arch Dermatol* 1994;130:589–592.
108. Smoller BR, van de Rijn M, Lebrun D, Warnke RA. Bcl-2 expression reliably distinguishes trichoeplthelioma from basal cell carcinomas. *Br J Dermatol* 1994;13:28–31.
109. Bayer-Garner IB, Givens V, Smoller BR. Immunohistochemical staining for androgen receptors: A sensitive marker of sebaceous differentiation. *Am J Dermatopathol* 1999;21:426–431.
110. Hassanein AM. Sebaceous carcinoma and the T-antigen. *Semin Cutan Med Surg* 2004;23:62–72.
111. Ansai S, Mitsuhashi Y, Kondo S, Manabe M. Immunohistochemical differentiation of extra-ocular sebaceous carcinoma from other skin cancers. *J Dermatol* 2004;31: 998–1008.
112. Izikson L, Bhan A, Zembowicz A. Androgen receptor expression helps to differentiate basal cell carcinoma from benign trichoblastic tumors. *Am J Dermatopathol* 2005;27: 91–5.
113. Crowson AN, Magro CM, Mihm MC Jr. *The Melanocytic Proliferations: A Comprehensive Textbook of Pigmented Lesions*. New York: John Wiley and Sons, 2001.
114. Mott RT, Smoller BR, Morgan MB. Merkel cell carcinoma: A clinicopathological study with prognostic implication. *J Cutan Pathol* 2004;31:217–223.
115. Sebastien TS, Nelson BR, Lowe L, et al. Microcystic adnexal carcinoma. *J Am Acad Dermatol* 1993;29:840–845.

7

SQUAMOUS CELL CARCINOMA AND ITS PRECURSORS

Nonmelanoma skin cancer is increasing in incidence worldwide but at varying rates with estimates ranging from 3% to 8% per year since the 1960s.[1] Although the term "nonmelanoma skin cancer" refers to many different types of malignancy with different prognoses, the most common of these are basal cell carcinoma followed by squamous cell carcinoma. The latter represents 20% of all skin cancers and is the most common cutaneous malignancy in the African-American population.[2] Even though most of the cutaneous squamous cell cancers are diagnosed early, the tumor still accounts for approximately 20% of all deaths from skin cancer.[3] Sun exposure is by far the most important risk factor, but others include exposure to carcinogenic agents such as arsenic, chewing tobacco and beetle gum, or aromatic hydrocarbons. Infection with human papilloma virus type 16 is another important causative association. The genodermatosis xeroderma pigmentosum is associated with numerous carcinomas, including squamous cell carcinoma, appearing at an early age.[4,5] There is also a risk associated with chronic inflammation and scarring such as in the setting of burn wounds, non-healing ulcer sites, and persistent draining sinuses as one finds in chronic osteomyelitis.

Certain chronic dermatoses are also associated with development of squamous cell carcinoma, especially lichen planus of the mouth and vulva, lichen sclerosus, lupus erythematosus, and porokeratosis. Indeed the nevus sebaceus and the epidermal nevus have been associated with malignant degeneration, resulting in squamous cell carcinoma. Of the bullous disorders, epidermolysis bullosa dystrophica is often associated with squamous cell carcinoma, which can be fatal in affected individuals. Finally, some of the chronic infective diseases such as granuloma inguinale and lymphogranuloma venereum and deep fungal infections such as chromoblastomycosis have also been associated with squamous cell carcinoma.[2,6]

We address the subtypes of squamous cell carcinoma in light of a classification offered by Cassarino et al.,[3] which groups the lesions into low-risk (<2% risk of metastasis), intermediate-risk (3% to 10% risk of metastasis), and high-risk (>10% risk of metastasis) squamous cell carcinomas. Some lesions that comprise the indeterminate behavior group are rare and are so classified despite insufficient data to reliably impute prognosis. This classification is a synthesis of extensive studies of the metastatic potential and aggressiveness of each squamous cell carcinoma type. We consider that this represents a valid attempt to better understand these entities and to obtain a true clinicopathological view of lesions that were for a long time considered to constitute a homogeneous group[3] and is a complementary tool to be used along with the well-established attributes utilized to assess these lesions such as the histological grade of differentiation (Broders' classification), perineural invasion, and depth of invasion. We will also discuss some prognostic factors under consideration by the American Joint Committee on Cancer (AJCC) for cutaneous squamous cell carcinomas, for inclusion in a new staging system. A table of immunohistochemical stains that may be employed to dissect the differential diagnosis of squamous cell carcinoma is offered. Finally, some molecular findings in squamous cell carcinoma and the role of chronic inflammation in causation of the tumor will be reviewed.

LOW-RISK TUMORS

Squamous Cell Carcinoma Arising in Actinic Keratoses

This type of squamous cell carcinoma occurs most commonly in sun-exposed areas of the body where there is usually clinical evidence of sun damage, or "dermatoheliosis". The precursor lesion, the actinic keratosis, presents mainly on the face, arms, and dorsum of the hands, on the superior aspect of the ear, and on the scalp, particularly in bald men. These lesions are usually slightly erythematous, are sometimes flesh-colored, and usually have a scale that is whitish and densely adherent to the skin. Some are markedly hyperkeratotic and resemble seborrheic keratoses or verruca vulgaris. There is a type that is rather flat and variably pigmented that gradually expands, termed the superficial pigmented actinic keratosis (SPAK). A squamous cell carcinoma that arises in actinic keratosis is first identifiable as an area of thickening of the precursor lesion. This thickening with some increase in erythema can lead to a hyperkeratotic lesion that has a densely adherent crust initially. As the lesion progresses the thickened area may give rise to a nodule or may become ulcerated, manifesting a central crust. These lesions are often associated with a history of bleeding after trauma, especially after washing and abrading the area with a wash cloth or towel. In the presence of a SPAK, the lesion may be pigmented and may resemble a melanoma. In some instances, the ulcerated lesion may have an irregularly raised border with telangiectasia, resembling a basal cell carcinoma. Squamous cell carcinoma on the lip is associated with actinic cheilitis characterized by fissuring and thinning of the lip mucosa and scaling. In such instances the carcinoma can appear as a superimposed thickened area or a nodule or plaque with ulceration. Squamous cell carcinoma is usually asymptomatic other than for the scaling, but sometimes it manifests with itching and intermittent bleeding. Large lesions, greater than

2 cm, can be associated with perineural invasion and then will present with anesthesia, dysesthesia, or even tic douloureux.[7]

The pathogenesis of squamous cell carcinoma arising in sun-exposed skin of elderly individuals reflects ultraviolet light induced mutations of p53 and other tumor suppressor genes in which a specific CC→TT "fingerprint" mutation is demonstrated[8]; p53 acts through $p21^{WAF1/CIP1}$ to arrest the cell cycle through the retinoblastoma gene product. When p53 mutation occurs, the overexpression of mutant type p53 in the absence of corresponding upregulation of p21 can be seen in paraffin-embedded tissue.[9]

HISTOLOGY. The lesion of squamous cell carcinoma arising in actinic keratosis (Figs. 7.1–7.3) usually begins as an in situ carcinoma in which there is hyperplasia of the skin with atypia affecting all layers. Thus, the basal layer is abnormal with keratinocytes showing large, hyperchromatic, and crowded nuclei with dyskeratosis (e-figs. 7.1–7.8). The remainder of the epidermis shows irregular shape and size of the keratinocyte nuclei with no evidence of maturation. Finally, there is either a very abnormal granular cell layer with large cells, scattered granules, and atypical nuclei or there is no granular cell layer with the cells abruptly forming a parakeratotic scale. The nuclei are often hyperchromatic and large in the scale, a finding we term "dysplastic parakeratosis" (e-figs. 7.9 and 7.10). Early invasion is associated with tongues of atypical cells that in some foci infiltrate the dermis (e-figs. 7.11 and 7.12). As the lesion progresses, the tumor is organized into

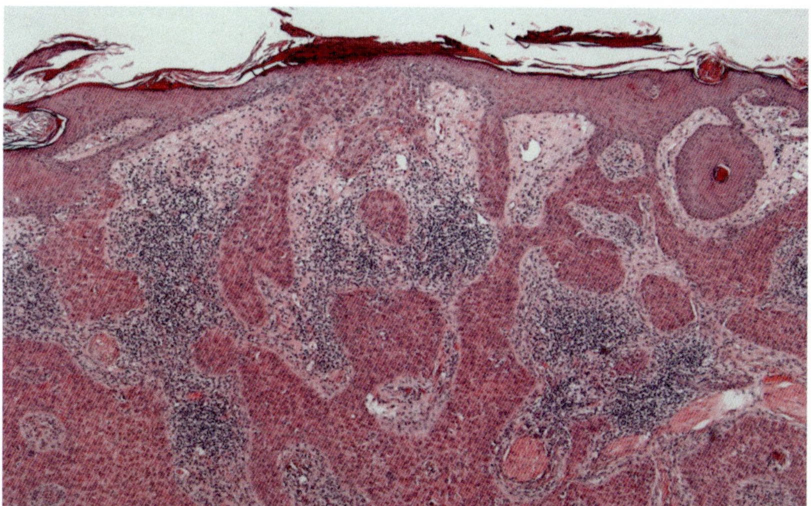

FIGURE 7.1 **Squamous Cell Carcinoma Arising in an Actinic Keratosis.** The actinic keratosis manifests basal layer atypia and crowding, parakeratosis, and solar elastosis of the collagen table. This is associated with an adjacent well-differentiated squamous cell carcinoma. Note, to the left of the biopsy, the sparing of the acrosyringium by the hyperplastic actinic keratosis.

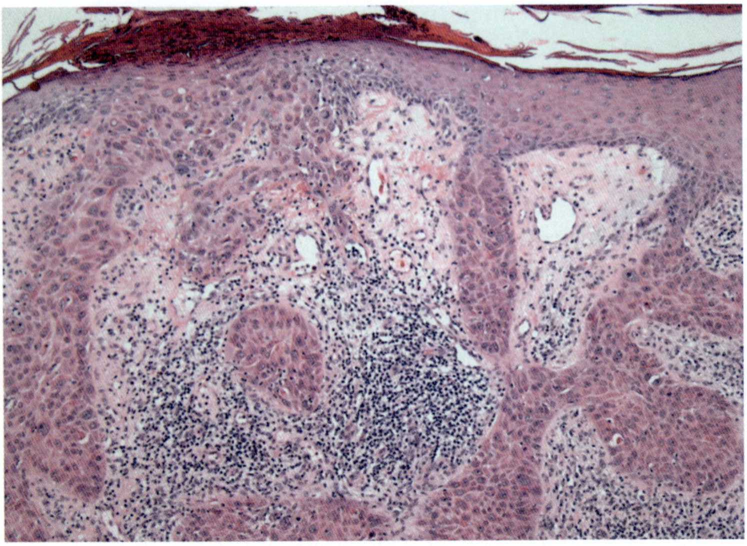

FIGURE 7.2 **Squamous Cell Carcinoma Arising in an Actinic Keratosis.** The actinic keratosis exhibits marked basaloid atypia and then extends as invasive tongues of squamous cell carcinoma into the dermis.

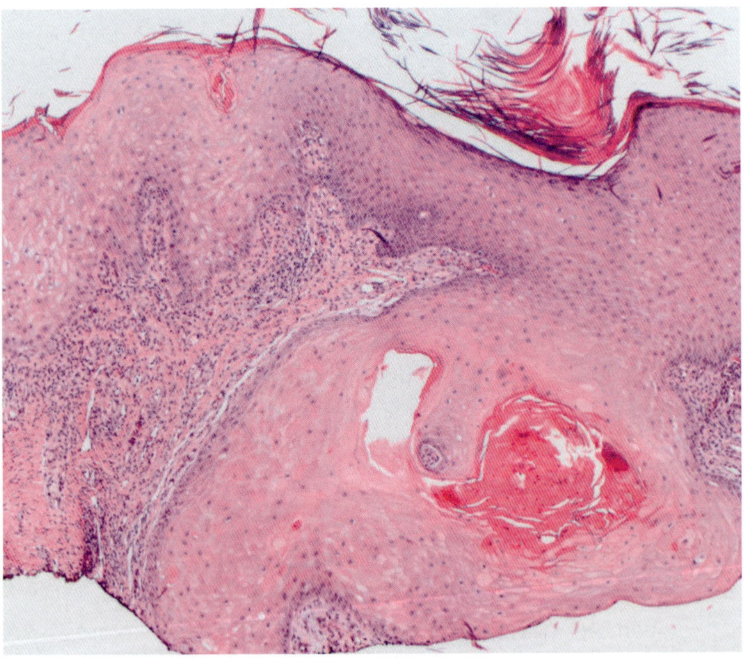

FIGURE 7.3 **The Squamous Cell Carcinoma Extends as an Expansile Nodule into the Dermis.** Note the well-differentiated cellular appearance and the areas of single cell dyskeratosis.

expansile nodules that extend into the dermis and are associated typically with a desmoplastic host response of fibroblast proliferation with a collagenized stroma containing inflammatory cells (e-figs. 7.13 and 7.14). The malignant squamous cells will show foci of individual cell dyskeratosis in the midst of the infiltrating tumor. In some cases, one will see dyskeratotic keratin abutting the stroma (e-figs. 7.15 and 7.16), a finding characteristic of squamous cell carcinoma. The cells usually are epithelioid in type. As nodules extend into the reticular dermis, deformation and destruction of appendages can be observed. In general, but not always, the squamous cell carcinoma will share characteristics of the precursor lesion, at least in the early steps of invasion of the tumor. Other types of carcinomatous cells can be identified including spindle cells (e-figs. 7.17–7.20), acantholytic cells (e-figs. 7.21–7.25), and sarcomatous variants among others. The prognosis varies depending on a variety of factors that are to be discussed.

Verrucous Carcinoma and Human Papillomavirus (HPV)-related Low-risk Squamous Cell Carcinoma

SQUAMOUS CELL CARCINOMA. Verrucous carcinoma is an uncommon lesion that is found in squamous mucosae, such as the mouth or larynx, in the anogenital region, and on the plantar surfaces. Different names have been given to these lesions in different sites, for example, in the oral cavity the lesion is named oral florid papillomatosis or Ackerman's tumor, and on the plantar surface, it is called epithelioma cuniculatum.[10,11] On the sole of the foot, the lesion usually begins as a "wart," gradually increases in size, and becomes markedly exophytic. The etiology is considered to be either chronic trauma or infection with HPV types 6 and 11.[12] This variant has been reported on the penis as well.[13] The anogenital cancer is a highly exophytic lesion that has been noted to occur predominantly on the uncircumcised glans penis in middle aged men.[12,14] Lesions in the oral cavity present as a focus of leukoplakia that continues to grow and eventually become quite warty and papillomatous. These lesions have also been reported to be closely related to HPV infection, especially with types 16 and 18 and are a form of verrucous carcinoma that occurs in the larynx.[15]

Another important entity related to HPV is epidermodysplasia verruciformis. In this disorder, patients exhibit numerous flat warts, superimposed upon which squamous cell carcinoma appears in 30% to 50% of cases.[16] There are sporadic and inherited forms. The latter has both a benign and malignant presentation. In the benign presentation, there are multiple flat warts scattered over the body. In the malignant presentation, the lesions can go on into invasive squamous cell carcinoma in 30% of cases, with patients occasionally dying of the disease. The benign and malignant forms have different HPV types associated with their lesions.[16,17]

Squamous cell carcinoma caused by HPV type 16 involves dysregulation of cell cycle control through the inactivation of the retinoblastoma gene product (pRB) through binding of a specific protein product of HPV (HPV-E6) to an internal pocket on pRB.

HISTOLOGY. All the various types of verrucous carcinoma have a similar picture which includes an endophytic pattern of growth with an exophytic component (Figs. 7.4–7.6, e-figs. 7.26–7.30). The lesion characteristically shows a papillomatous growth caused by broad, bulbous rete ridges that at their base have a blunted appearance. The area between the rete ridges is associated with minimal stroma and vascularity. There is no evidence of dermal invasion by single cells or tongues. There is a dense inflammatory infiltrate which is rich in plasma cells in most cases (e-figs. 7.31 and 7.32). The presence of dyskeratosis and significant nuclear atypia in the elongated rete ridges signifies a well-differentiated squamous cell carcinoma rather than a verrucous carcinoma.[18]

The genital warty carcinoma has been reported as a more aggressive type of carcinoma than verrucous carcinoma (Fig. 7.7). The important differences between the two lesions include a striking papillomatous appearance with often very prominent koilocytic atypia as well as squamous cell atypia. Frequent mitotic figures also occur, and the lesion has a more truly infiltrative pattern.[14] This type of tumor has been described in the penis and vulva and will be further discussed under high-risk lesions.

Although in most instances verrucous carcinoma manifests an indolent clinical course, an aggressive course occasionally manifests itself as metastasis to lymph nodes and viscera. The initial presentation of this lesion is similar to the less aggressive type. Local radiotherapy has been

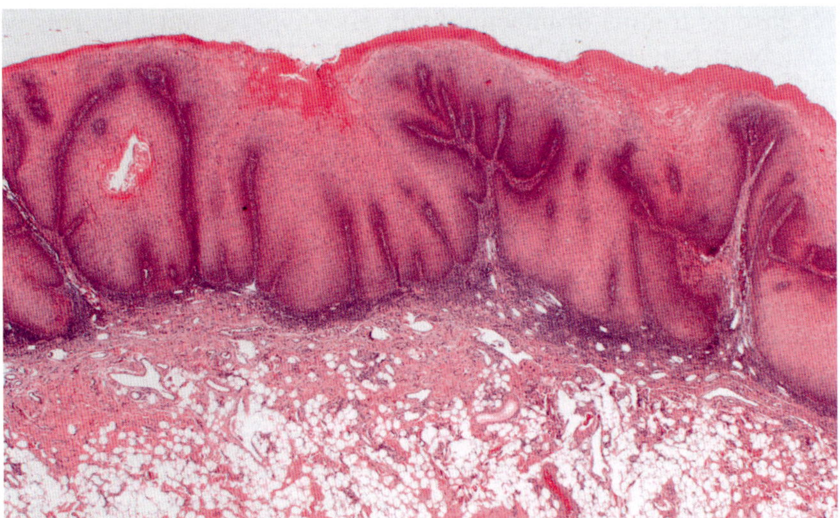

FIGURE 7.4 **Verrucous Squamous Cell Carcinoma.** On low-power a plaque of hyperplastic epidermis is associated with bulbous rete ridges with minimal connective tissue separating the epithelial projections. Note the striking uniformity of the extent of the tumor projections highlighted by an inflammatory infiltrate.

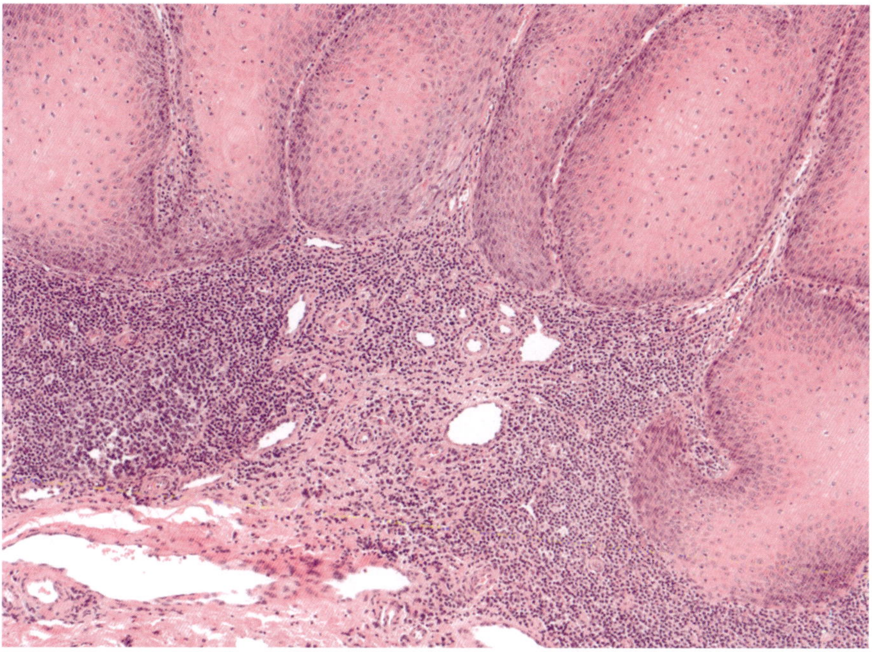

FIGURE 7.5 **Verrucous Squamous Cell Carcinoma.** The hyperplastic epidermis exhibits uniform squamous cells without any individual cell dyskeratosis with elongated tongues showing a basaloid peripheral proliferation.

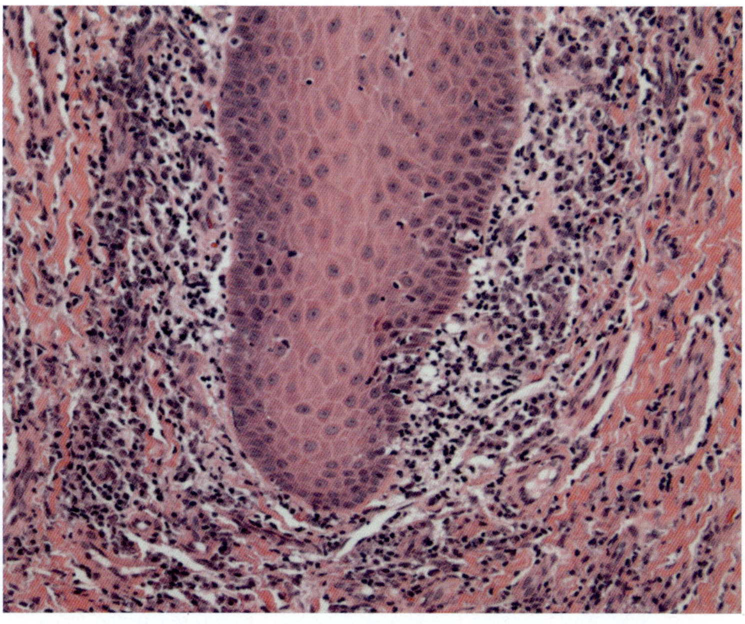

FIGURE 7.6 **Verrucous Squamous Cell Carcinoma.** High power reveals the characteristic "pushing border" with some stromal condensation and a dense inflammatory infiltrate.

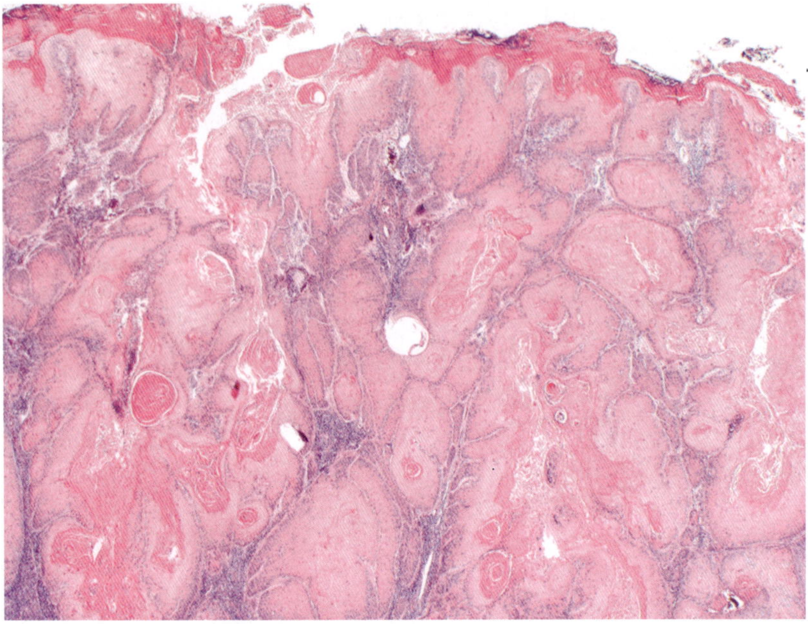

FIGURE 7.7 **Warty Squamous Cell Carcinoma.** The warty squamous cell carcinoma shows a highly arborescent epidermal hyperplasia producing a condylomatous appearance with prominent parakeratosis and with keratin forming a striking component of the invasive tongues. This type of squamous cell carcinoma is associated with higher risk of regional node metastasis. (Courtesy of Dr Antonio L. Cubilla.)

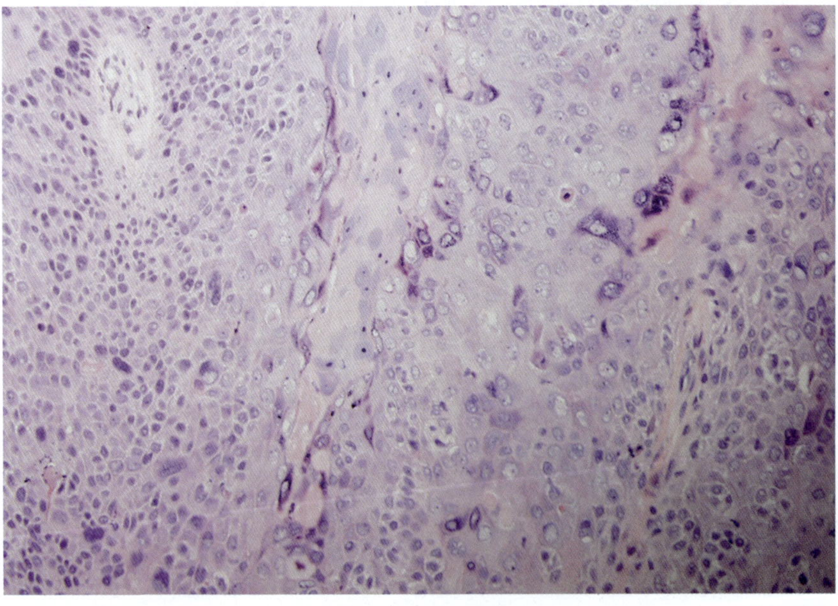

FIGURE 7.8 **Squamous Cell Carcinoma In Situ Arising in Epidermodysplasia Verruciformis.** This carcinoma exhibits the marked dysplasia associated with such tumors, while the adjacent epidermal keratinocytes have basophilic cytoplasms.

said anecdotally to be associated with a transformation to an aggressive disease process.

The histology of epidermodysplasia verruciformis includes viral cytopathic changes in the upper granular cell layer (e-figs. 7.33 and 7.34), comprising prominent basophilic cytoplasms. As the lesions transform into malignancy, there is first in situ change and then invasion (Fig. 7.8).

Low-risk Spindle Cell Squamous Cell Carcinoma

Spindle cell squamous cell carcinoma presents as a nodule or exophytic tumor that is often ulcerated and/or bleeding. It occurs typically in areas of heavy sun exposure, especially in the head and neck region. These lesions have a more indolent course in contrast to those spindle cell squamous cell carcinomas that occur in areas of prior radiation therapy. The parameters that are most useful in predicting behavior will be reviewed.

HISTOLOGY. The tumor has a highly variable presentation. It is usually composed of spindle cells, but with some evidence of typical squamous cell carcinoma being evident (Figs. 7.9 and 7.10). There may be an adjacent actinic keratosis. On low-power examination, the lesion appears as a cellular nodule with infiltration of single cells into the adjacent stroma in the periphery. Pleomorphic cells are often present, sometimes including giant cells, and there may be other elements including mucin deposition and in some cases fibrosis. Mitotic figures are usually easily observable. These

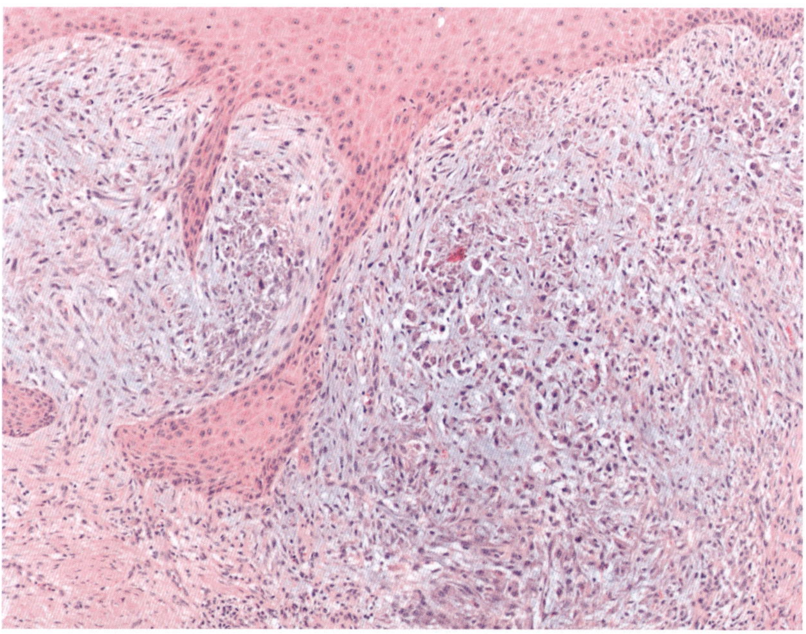

FIGURE 7.9 **Spindle Cell Squamous Cell Carcinoma.** Beneath this hyperplastic squamous cell carcinoma, a plaque of infiltrative spindle-shaped tumor cells extends into the deep reticular dermis.

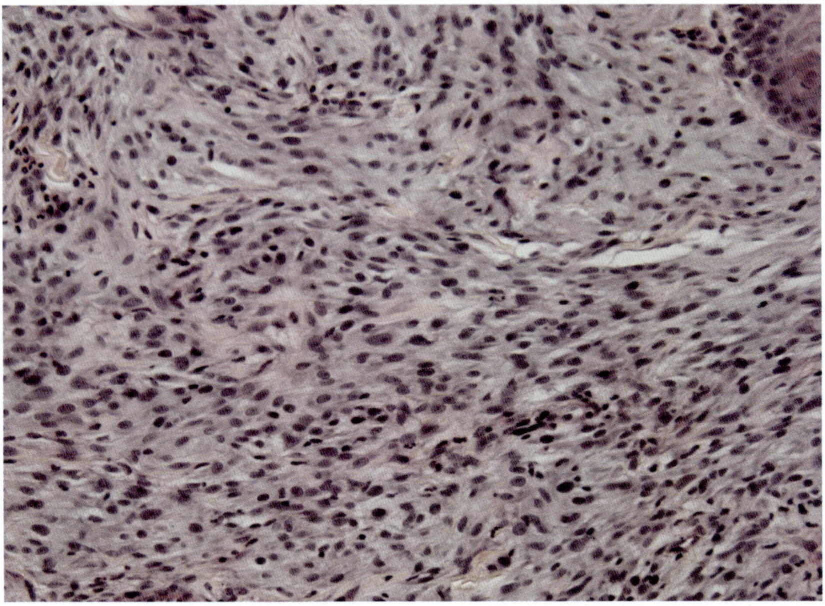

FIGURE 7.10 **Spindle Cell Squamous Cell Carcinoma.** The histogenesis of the malignant spindle cells is often inapparent without the use of immunohistochemistry.

lesions can infiltrate deeply, even into muscle. In those lesions in which there is no evidence of squamous differentiation, one must consider the differential diagnosis of spindle cell melanoma, atypical fibroxanthoma, and leiomyosarcoma. In such cases, immunohistochemical stains will usually result in successful identification of the tumor as a squamous cell carcinoma. The immunochemical picture includes decoration with antibodies to cytokeratins and epithelial membrane antigen (EMA). Antibodies to CK5/6, 34BE12, and p63 are the most reliable to identify the nature of the spindle cells (e-fig. 7.35).[19–21]

INTERMEDIATE-RISK TUMORS

Adenoid (Acantholytic) Squamous Cell Carcinoma

This tumor is most commonly observed in sun-exposed areas in men of advanced age. As do virtually all squamous cell carcinomas, it appears as a nodule that can be pink, red, or occasionally flesh-colored. It has also been noted to occur in other sites of the body, even in genitalia.[22] The prognosis of this particular lesion is probably not different from other types of squamous cell carcinoma, but there have been reports of mortality as high as 19%.[3,23]

HISTOLOGY. On low-power, one observes an expansile nodule descending from the epidermis into the dermis, often with small nests of cells palisading around a central nodule. The overlying stratum corneum shows hyperkeratosis and parakeratosis. The striking feature of the tumor is the extensive dyscohesion of the cells or acantholysis. The acantholytic cells may be focally present or may occupy 90% of the tumor area. They form tubulelike structures in the midst of the acantholysis where the cells coalesce. The acantholytic cells have varying degrees of dyskeratosis (Figs. 7.11 and 7.12). The differential diagnosis includes a basal cell carcinoma with acantholysis, metastatic adenocarcinoma, or some type of poorly differentiated eccrine carcinoma.[24]

Lymphoepitheliomalike Carcinoma of the Skin

This lesion is rare and occurs mainly in the head and neck regions. There is no sex predilection, and like many tumor in the skin, it presents as a nodule.[25] The lesion may ulcerate.

HISTOLOGY. On low power, one observes a large, usually lymphoid-appearing nodule in the dermis. Scattered throughout the lesion are rather pale cells that have either an amphophilic or eosinophilic coloration. The cells are present in small aggregates or may appear to be in a syncytial array (Figs. 7.13–7.15, e-figs. 7.36–7.40). These epithelioid islands lie in the midst of a dense lymphoid background. They have large nuclei with vesicular nucleoplasm and large nucleoli. These cell aggregates are sometimes mistaken for sarcoidal granulomas, but their large polyhedral cell shape, nuclear atypia and nucleolation, as well as the variation in cytoplasmic color and lack of organization help one to arrive at the correct diagnosis. The

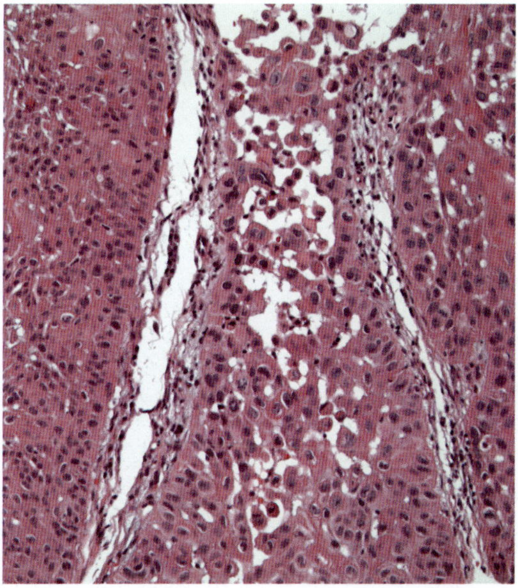

FIGURE 7.11 **Acantholytic Squamous Cell Carcinoma.** Numerous rounded "acantholytic" keratinocytes lie in an apparent cavity formed by the dyscohesion of the cells. Note the varying degrees of acantholysis present in the invasive tumor tongues.

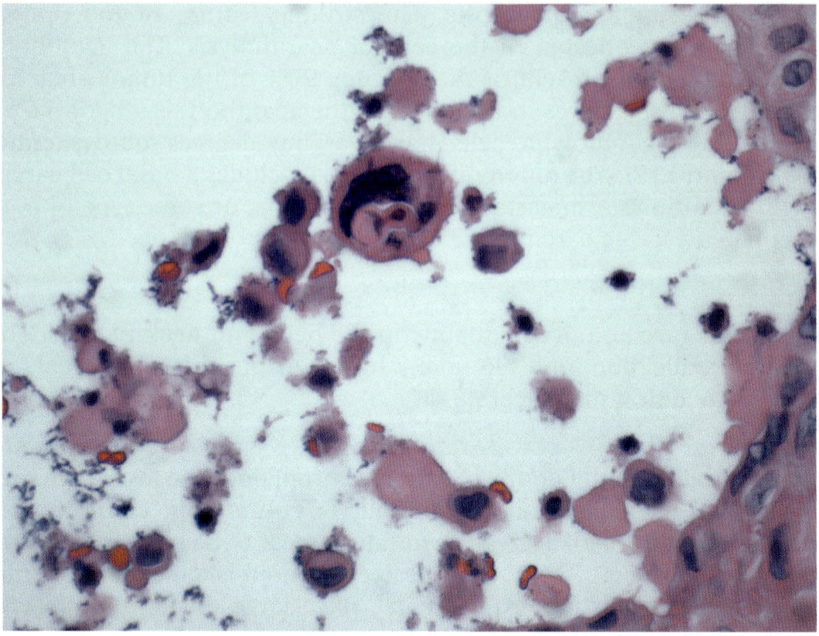

FIGURE 7.12 **Acantholytic Squamous Cell Carcinoma.** High power reveals quite numerous mitoses, varying degrees of dyskeratosis, including *corp rond*-like structures.

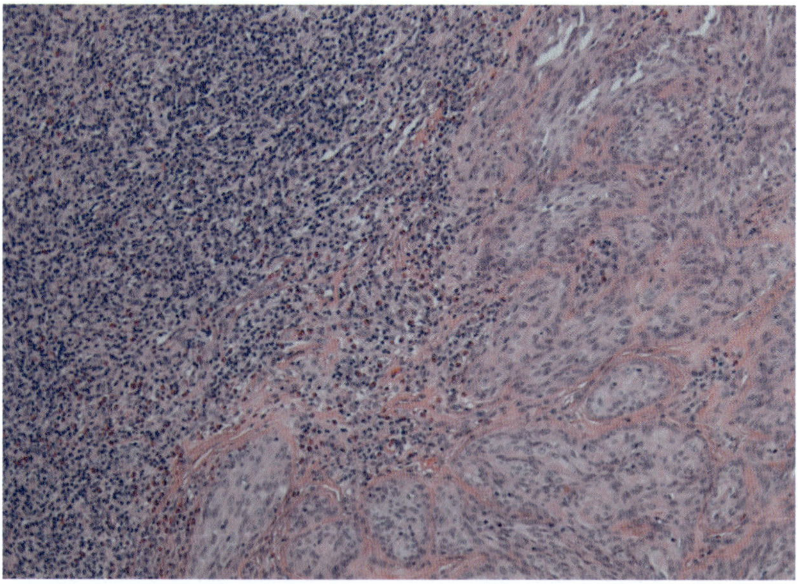

FIGURE 7.13 **Lymphoepithelial Carcinoma.** Nests of neoplastic epithelia are present surrounded by a sheetlike inflammatory infiltrate, in this case comprising lymphocytes and eosinophils.

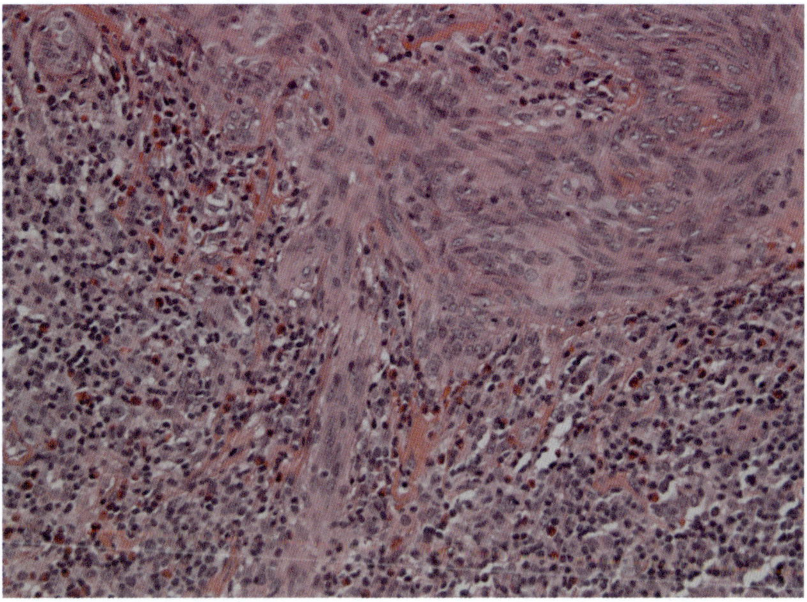

FIGURE 7.14 **Lymphoepithelial Carcinoma.** The neoplastic epithelia have atypical nuclear features and are mitotically active.

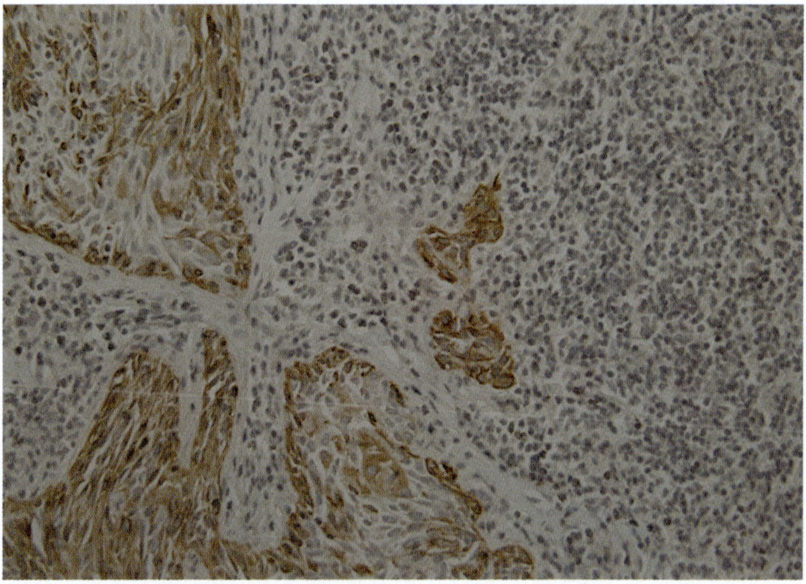

FIGURE 7.15 **Lymphoepithelial Carcinoma.** A pan-cytokeratin immunostain shows the epithelial character of the neoplastic cells.

lymphoid infiltrate varies from sparse to dense. Immunohistochemically, the tumor cells stain for cytokeratins (e-fig. 7.41), EMA, and sometimes carcinoembryonic antigen (CEA). The lymphocytes are all T cells with virtually no B cells (e-figs. 7.42 and 7.43).[25]

The principal differential diagnosis is a metastasis from a lymphoepithelioma of the nasopharynx. However, this tumor, when of skin primary derivation rarely metastasizes. Among other differential diagnosis considerations are squamous cell carcinoma metastatic from other sites. Rarely, the Merkel cell carcinoma can have a similar appearance. Atypical lymphoid infiltrates including lymphomas can be differentiated principally by immunohistochemistry. In some of the low-grade malignant B cell lymphomas, there are monocytoid B cells, but these cells do not form aggregates such as nests or syncytia. The immunoperoxidase stains again help to resolve the diagnostic problem. Metastatic melanoma with prominent epithelioid cells and lymphoid infiltrate can be differentiated on the basis of S100 and Mart-1 positivity of the tumor.[26,27]

Intraepidermal Epithelioma/Borst–Jadassohn

Cassarino et al.[3] considered this lesion to be a squamous cell carcinoma in situ or a special type of clonal cellular proliferation that can go on to invade and metastasize. The Borst-Jadassohn phenomenon has come to be recognized as a pattern reflective of intraepithelial clonality that may represent a clonal seborrheic keratosis, clonal actinic keratosis, clonal Bowen's disease, porocarcinoma in situ, or even the benign intraepidermal poroma termed hidroacanthoma simplex.[28,29] The lesion clinically is a flat or slightly raised tan plaque with scaling. The lesion occurs predominantly on extremities, but can occur elsewhere. The presence of invasion in these tumors is usually highlighted by the appearance of a raised area or by erythema.

HISTOLOGY. These lesions manifest as a multifocal intraepidermal proliferation of cells in discrete nests. When they represent a malignant lesion, they show characteristic hyperchromatic nuclei with mitoses and dyskeratosis. A purely intraepidermal lesion is not associated with inflammation in most cases, except in the irritated seborrheic keratosis. When invasion, however, appears in a malignant intraepidermal epithelioma, then inflammation would often accompany the invasive dermal component. The differential diagnosis of the lesion is successfully handled by high-power microscopic examination of the cell types in the intraepidermal nests.[29]

HIGH-RISK TUMORS

Invasive Squamous Cell Carcinoma Arising in Bowen's Disease

Bowen's disease is the name given to a distinct presentation of squamous cell carcinoma in situ that occurs predominantly in chronically sun-exposed skin of a patient, most often a male, in mid- to late life. The lesions occur commonly on the head and neck but also can occur on the trunk and extremities. In the first half of the 20th century, Bowen's disease frequently occurred in association with arsenical exposure and had a wider distribution in the skin. The lesion classically presents as a beefy-red, well-defined plaque with scaling and sometimes crusting. Changes on the lesion such as ulceration or thickening may herald invasion.[30] Recent studies have shown that invasion was found in 5% of Bowen's disease cases. Metastasis developed in up to 13% to 20% of the latter patients. In a small series of black patients, the lesion exhibited invasion in 20% with subsequent metastatic spread in 60% of the patients with invasive carcinomas.[31,32]

HISTOLOGY. In the classic lesion, there is a hyperkeratosis and parakeratosis that overlies cells with cytologically malignant characteristics, including marked hyperchromasia and irregularly-thickened and -contoured nuclear rims, associated with dyskeratosis, atypical mitoses, and loss of polarity (Figs. 7.16–7.18). Usually, the basal layer is comparatively spared in contrast to squamous cell carcinoma arising in an actinic keratosis where the abnormality initiates in the basal layer of the epidermis (e-figs. 7.44–7.48). Also, Bowen's disease will manifest malignant transformation of the hair follicular lining epithelium in contrast to actinic keratosis that only affects the upper follicle at the junction with the epidermis.

Adenosquamous Carcinoma

This rare variant of squamous cell carcinoma occurs principally in elderly patients, and again tends to involve the head and neck.[33] The lower trunk and penis are also affected. This tumor is one in which there is a true glandular

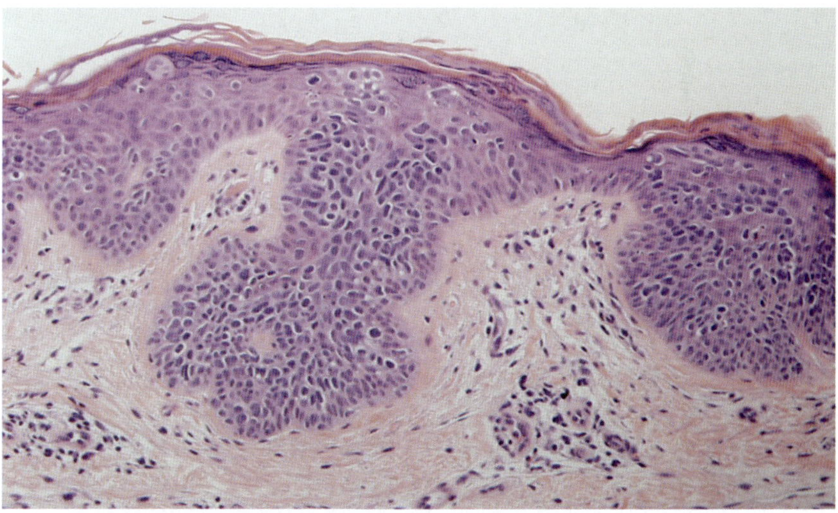

FIGURE 7.16 **Bowen's Disease.** This form of squamous cell carcinoma in situ exhibits a characteristic of sharply demarcated border at its junction with the normal epidermis.

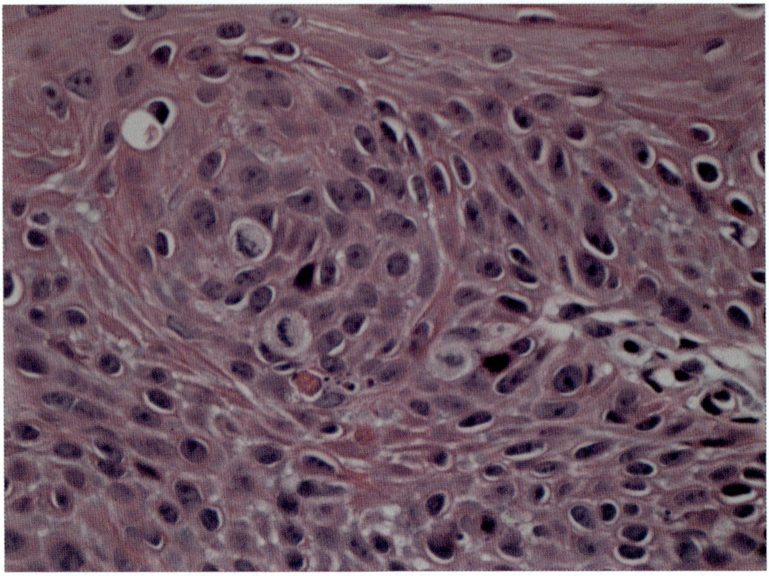

FIGURE 7.17 **Bowen's Disease.** The proliferative nature of this tumor is clearly evidenced by the markedly increased cellularity and prominent mitoses. A preserved basal layer present in Bowen's disease helps to differentiate it from squamous cell carcinoma in situ arising in actinic keratosis.

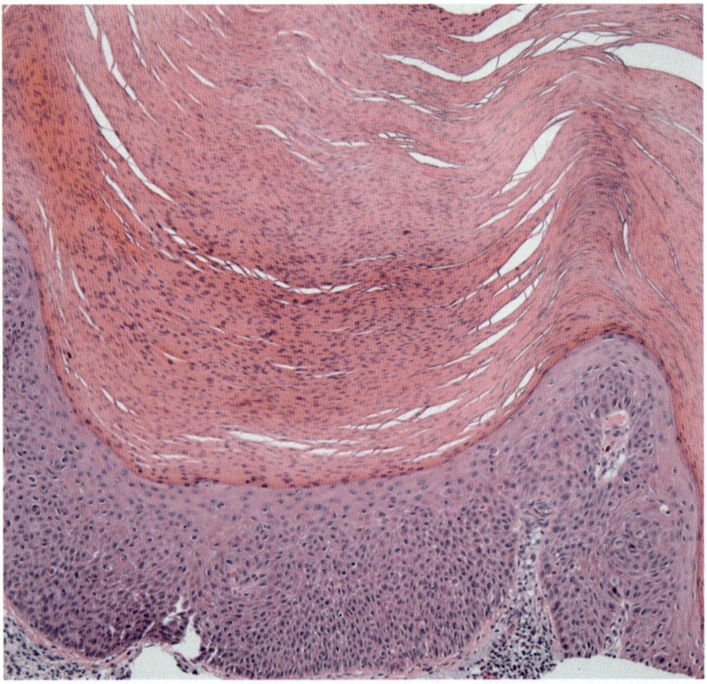

FIGURE 7.18 **Bowen's with Cutaneous Horn.** Bowen's disease in this instance is associated with marked hyperkeratosis resulting in a cutaneous horn.

differentiation and is usually aggressive in its course. The prognosis of the patient is poor, and in one series of 10 patients mortality was 50%.[34]

HISTOLOGY. The tumor on low-power exhibits nests and cords of poorly differentiated squamous cells that focally interconnect and form keratocysts. There is usually at least one clear area of origin in the epidermis, although multiple foci of origin have been described.[34] The glands may appear in a disposition which is focal or quite extensive. The deeper, more invasive component is the usual site of the glandular differentiation (e-figs. 7.49–7.52). The glands lie between squamous nests and small cystlike areas. The cysts focally exhibit a lining that shows a columnar epithelium. There is an inspissated intraluminal material that is often positive with alcian blue at pH 2.5, the staining pattern of sialomucin (e-figs. 7.53 and 7.54). The differential diagnosis includes metastatic mucoepidermoid carcinoma that does not show any evidence of epidermal connection. The acantholytic squamous cell carcinoma can be differentiated by the absence of lesion of glands with mucin.

Squamous Cell Carcinoma Arising in Association with Proliferating Pilar Proliferating Tumor/Cysts and Epidermal Cysts

Proliferating pilar tumors occur more frequently in women. The average age of a person with this tumor is 60 years. The lesions present as nodules in the scalp with multiple cystlike structures that occasionally ulcerate. The proliferating epidermal cyst is more frequent in men and more commonly occurs in the anogenital area. They may also occur on the scalp and extremities. The characteristic behavior of these lesions when associated with malignant degeneration is usually the rapid growth of a previously indolent mass. A second presentation is the rapid recurrence within weeks to months of a tumor after a resection of a pilar or epidermal cyst.

HISTOLOGY. While most proliferating pilar tumors are considered benign, malignancy has been reported in as many as 10 of 63 cases in one series.[35] Likewise, in 7 out of 33 proliferating epidermal cysts, carcinoma was found.[36] The great majority of carcinomas that arise in proliferating pilar tumors are well differentiated and are identifiable as tongues and cords of atypical squamous cells that have marked cytological atypia, easily visible mitoses and characteristic invasion associated with stromal desmoplasia around aggressive tongues of tumor, which usually occur toward the edges of the original lesion. In some instances, one can find epidermal continuity as well (Figs. 7.19–7.21).[35] In the proliferating epidermal cyst, there is also a proliferation of nests and nodules of cells undergoing progression from well-differentiated carcinoma close to the edge of the lesion to more poorly differentiated carcinoma with many mitoses and invasive tongues at the periphery where they infiltrate the adjacent stroma. The most important finding in these lesions is the evidence of invasion into stroma, with attendant desmoplasia, well away from the central area

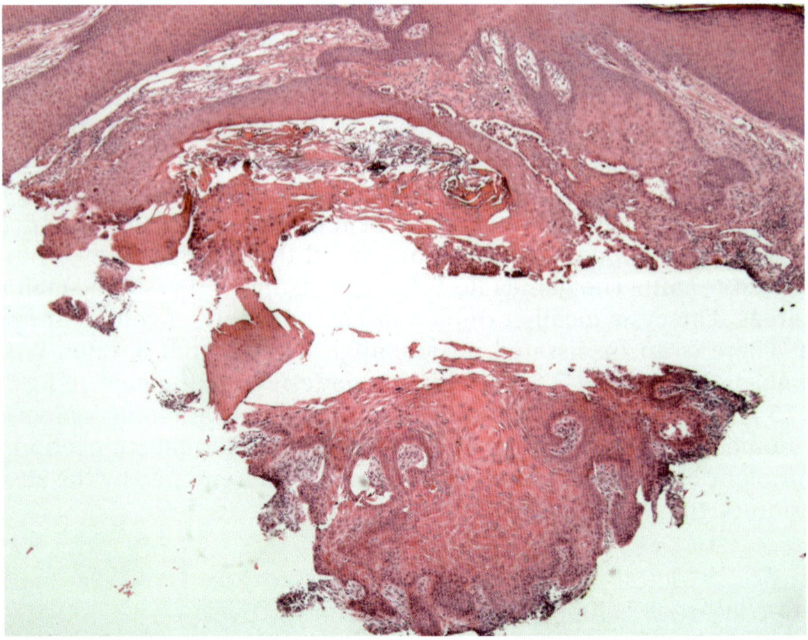

FIGURE 7.19 **Squamous Cell Carcinoma Arising in an Epidermal Cyst.** To one edge of a typical infundibular cyst, which shows normal keratinization in the cyst cavity, an infiltrating well-differentiated carcinoma arises and invades the adjacent dermis.

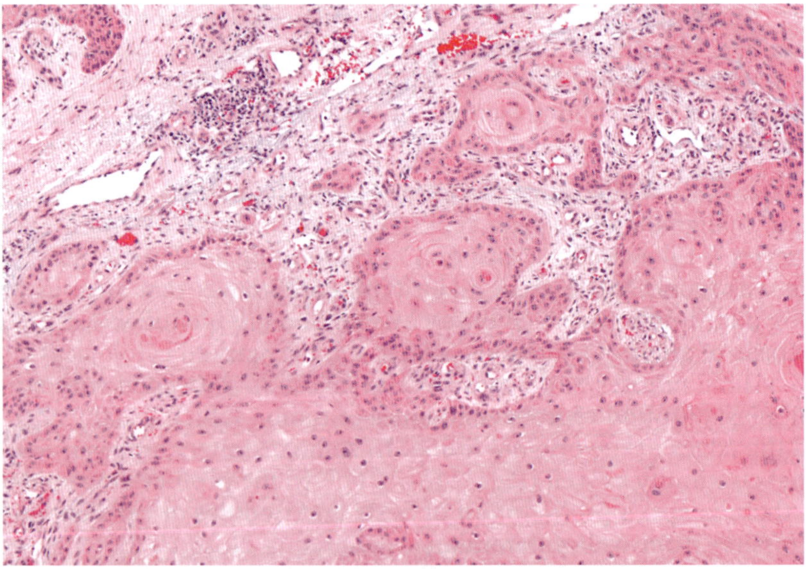

FIGURE 7.20 **Squamous Cell Carcinoma Arising in an Epidermal Cyst.** High power reveals the highly infiltrative and atypical nature of this carcinoma with small invasive nests and single-cell dyskeratosis, highlighting the malignant cells.

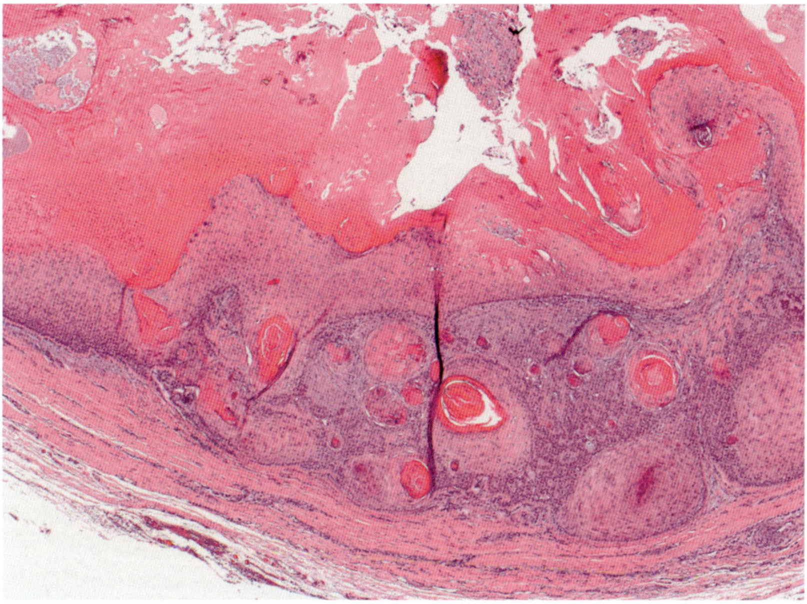

FIGURE 7.21 **Squamous Cell Carcinoma Arising in Proliferating Pilar Tumor.** Adjacent to the proliferating pilar tumor, the squamous cell carcinoma invades the adjacent stroma both as large and small nests. Note that the dyskeratotic keratin abuts the stroma, a characteristic of carcinoma.

of the cyst.[37] One important observation is that mitotic activity in benign proliferating pilar tumors is usually found only in the basal layer, whereas the malignant lesions exhibit proliferative activity throughout the entire epithelium.[38]

De Novo Squamous Cell Carcinoma

This tumor arises in either normal non-sun-exposed skin or in sun-damaged skin, typically with no evidence of a precursor lesion. These tumors are singled out because they show an aggressive behavior with one series indicating 8% to 14% regional or disseminated metastasis.[39] The presentation is as nodules or plaques with crusting and even ulceration in some cases. The tumors range from 1.2 to 5 cm in size.[39]

HISTOLOGY. On low power, one observes a hyperplastic epidermis with progressive atypia from which cords and tongues of squamous cell carcinoma emanate. Toward the center of the lesion, there is often ulceration or an area of atrophy overlying the tumor. In the overwhelming majority of cases, in addition to the absence of an actinic keratosis precursor, not even an actinic lentigo is identified (Figs. 7.22–7.24).[40]

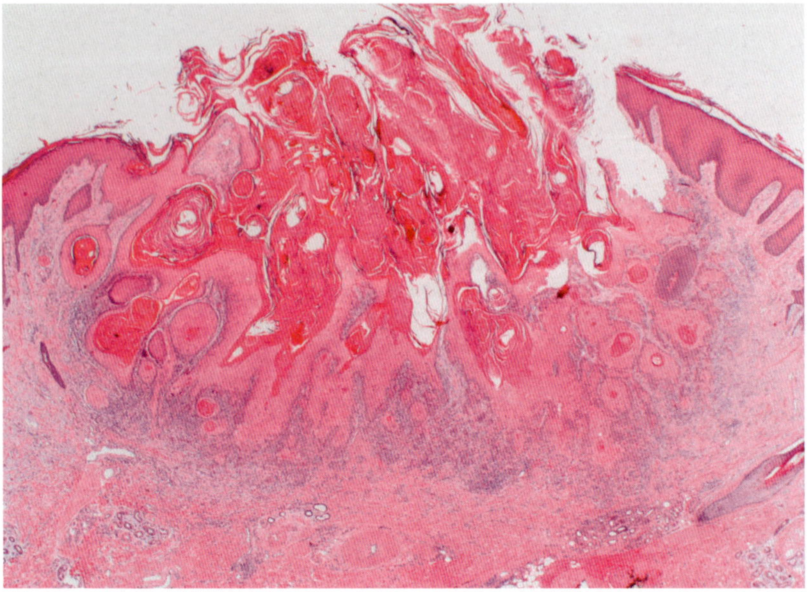

FIGURE 7.22 **De Novo Squamous Cell Carcinoma.** An invaginated epidermal hyperplasia exhibits marked hyperkeratosis and parakeratosis arising form an hyperplastic tumor, forming the base of the lesion. To one side, there is a progressive change from the normal epidermis to an atypical eosinophilic proliferation leading then to invasion.

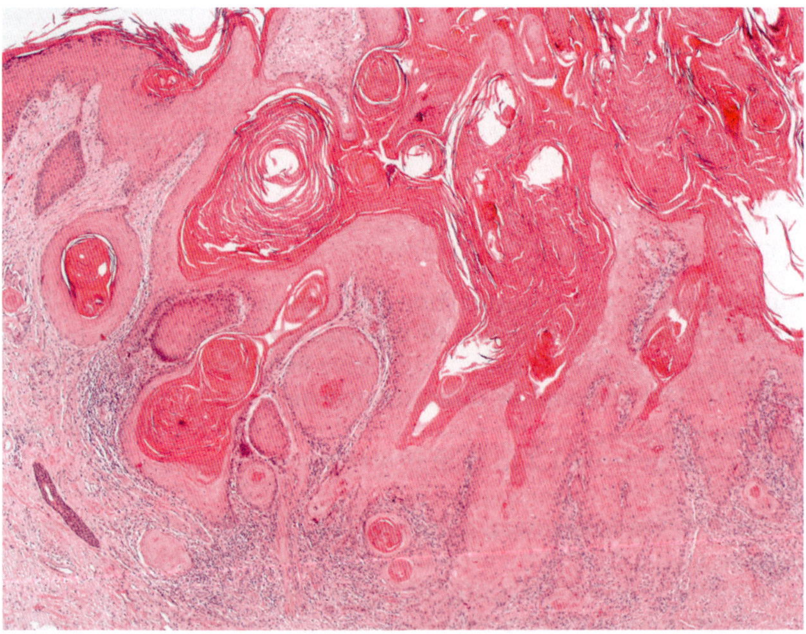

FIGURE 7.23 **De Novo Squamous Cell Carcinoma.** Note the highly infiltrative tongues and nests of tumor associated with a prominent inflammatory infiltrate and some stromal hyperplasia.

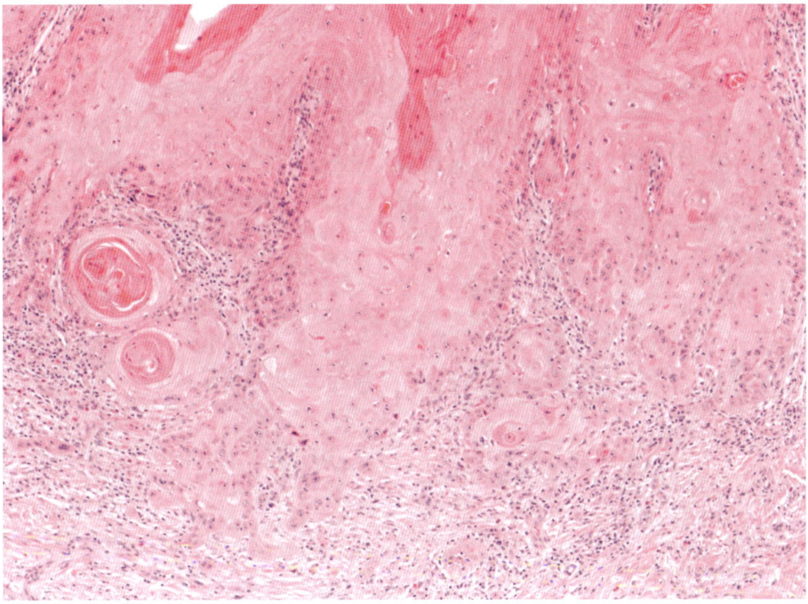

FIGURE 7.24 **De Novo Squamous Cell Carcinoma.** The tumor infiltrates as small cords and nests with single cell dyskeratosis. There is no basal layer around the infiltrative tongues, so that the eosinophilic dyskeratotic cells in nests abut directly on the inflamed stroma.

Basaloid squamous cell carcinoma

This uncommon squamous cell carcinoma variant typically occurs on the penis and is associated with HPV type 16 infection. The lesion presents as a mass on the glans, especially in the perimeatal area. In a study done by Cubilla et al., 10 of 17 patients died of the disease at an average time of 34 months from the time of diagnosis. This unusual carcinoma is an example of a high-grade malignancy invoked by HPV infection, in contrast to the low-grade tumors already discussed.[41]

HISTOLOGY. These neoplasms, which range in size from 2 to 10 cm, manifest a downward proliferation of large tumor nests separated by minimal intervening fibrous or hyalinized stroma with prominent inflammation and prominent central necrosis. The individual cells are basophilic, uniform, and small, but with large nuclear to cytoplasmic ratios (Figs. 7.25–7.27). Usually, a space or cleft caused by artifact of separation is present around the nodules. Numerous mitoses are characteristic, with as many as 120 per HPF in some areas. There is a "starry sky" appearance in some cases, caused by individual cell necrosis. In some areas, typical squamous cell differentiation, pseudoglandular change, and anaplasia are noted among the otherwise basaloid tumor. Perineural and vascular invasion was noted in almost all cases in the quoted series. The differential diagnosis includes urethral transitional cell, basal cell, small cell neuroendocrine, and metastatic carcinoma.[41]

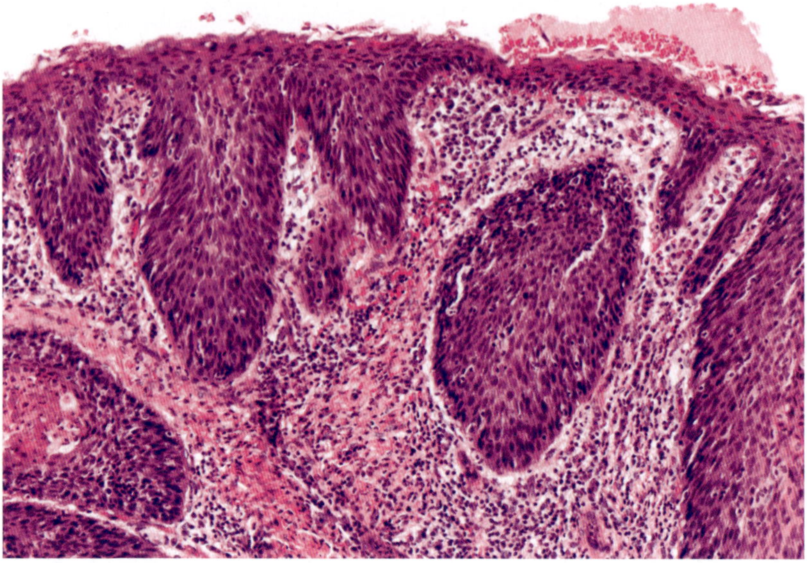

FIGURE 7.25 **Basaloid Squamous Cell Carcinoma.** Prominent basaloid cells form the in situ component of the tumor and then invade as large tongues of cells with basaloid features. The tongues infiltrate irregularly into the stroma and are associated with chronic inflammation. (Courtesy of Dr Antonio L. Cubilla.)

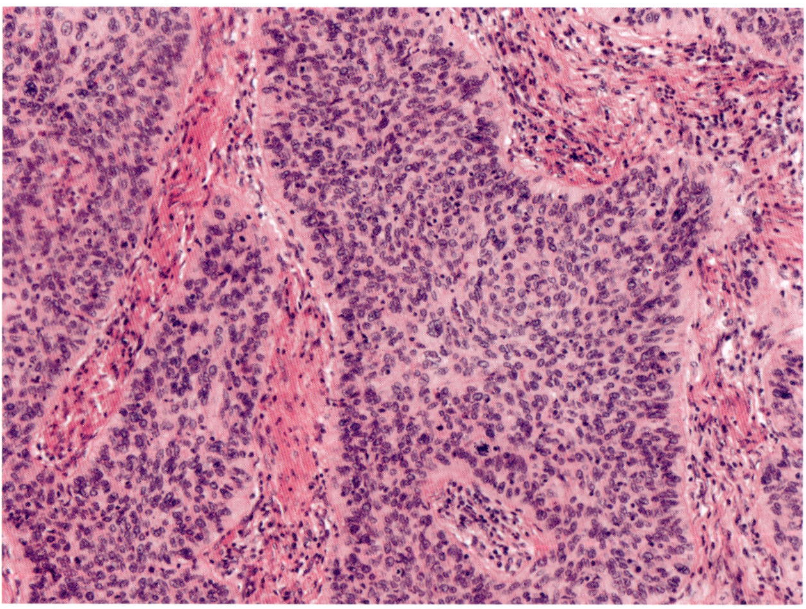

FIGURE 7.26 **Basaloid Squamous Cell Carcinoma.** The intraepidermal in situ component of the tumor is composed of strikingly atypical basaloid cells that give rise to the invasive tumor. (Courtesy of Dr Antonio L. Cubilla.)

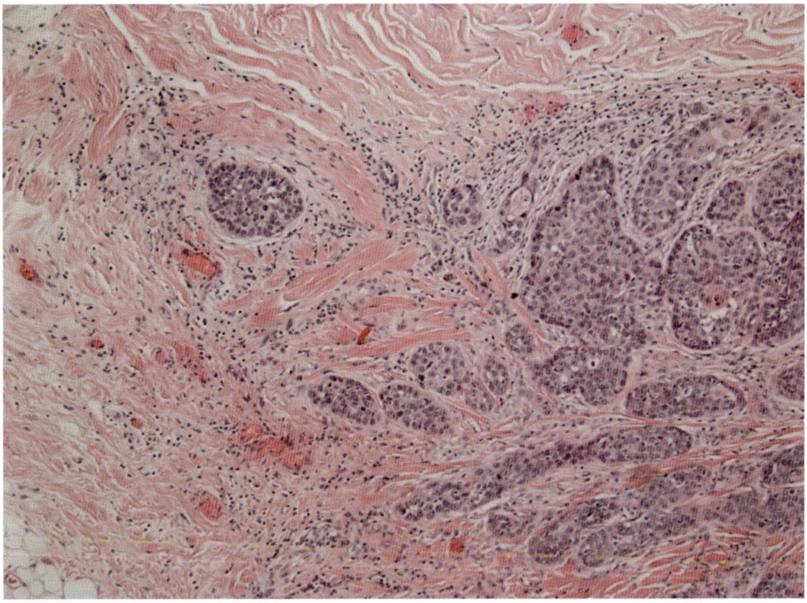

FIGURE 7.27 **Basaloid Squamous Cell Carcinoma.** The invasive component maintains the basaloid appearance of the tumor with poorly differentiated areas exhibiting numerous mitoses, as evidence of the highly aggressive nature of this lesion. (Courtesy of Dr Antonio L. Cubilla.)

Squamous Cell Carcinoma Arising in Association with Radiation and in Disorders with Chronic Inflammation

The pathogenesis of radiation dermatitis is associated with DNA mutations, the effect of which may express itself in squamous cell carcinoma anywhere from 1 to 64 years later, with an average of 20 to 23 years, after exposure to ionizing radiation.[42,43] On the other hand, the mechanisms of induction of squamous cell carcinoma in chronic conditions involving chronic inflammation and burn scars are related to several mechanisms involving the inflammatory chemokine system[44] as well as possible toxins secreted by burn tissue.[45,46] Squamous cell carcinomas arising in chronic lesions such as lichen sclerosis, lichen planus, and dystrophic epidermolysis bullosa may invoke neoplasia by an alternate mechanism. For example, upregulation of bcl-2 expression as a result of the inflammatory cytokine interleukin-2 elaborated by Th-1 lymphoid cells has been proposed in sites of chronic inflammation,[47] immortalizing squamous epithelia in a fashion similar to that proposed for sporadic basal cell cancer. There is a putative risk of subsequent mutagenic "hits" by ultraviolet light or other factors as is postulated for basal cell carcinoma.[47] This particular mechanism might be involved in the Marjolin's ulcer, and in squamous cell carcinoma developing in a chronic draining fistula, sinus tract, ulcer, or other chronic inflammatory site[5]; these lesions have a 30% risk of metastatic disease (Figs. 7.28 and 7.29).

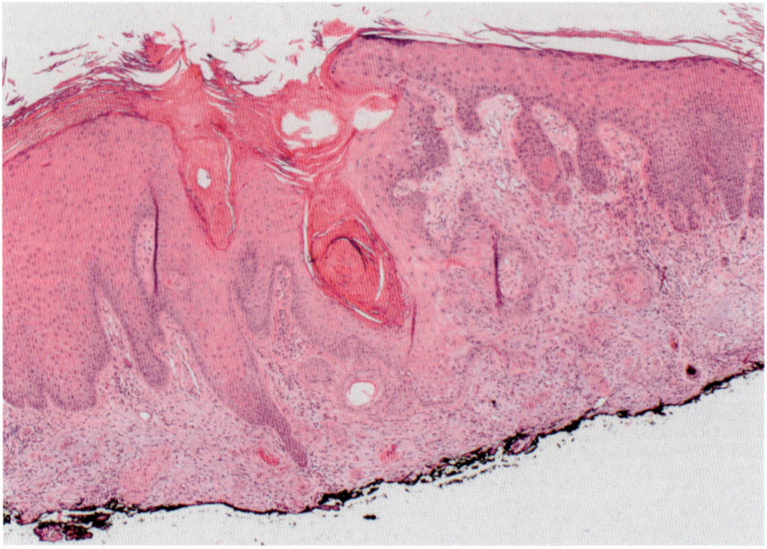

FIGURE 7.28 **Squamous Cell Carcinoma Arising in Lichen Simplex Chronicus.** In the midst of an epidermis showing psoriasiform hyperplasia, hypergranulosis and hyperkeratosis arise as a well-differentiated squamous cell carcinoma that is superficially invasive.

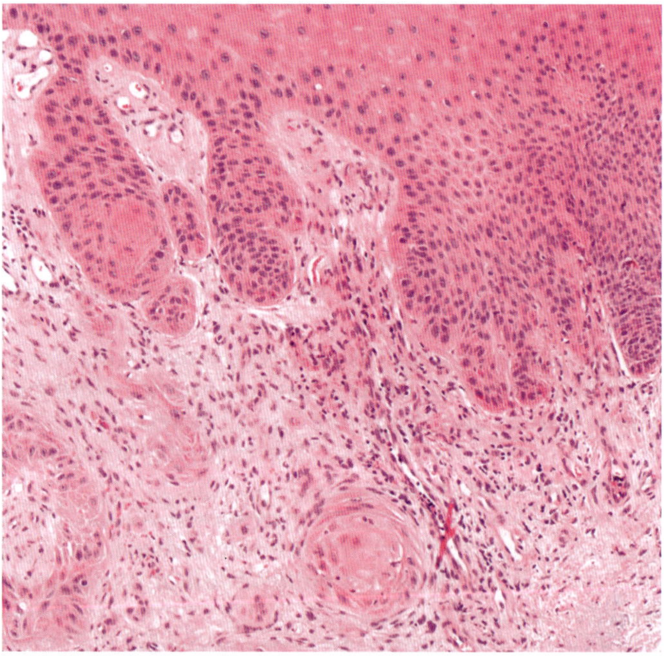

FIGURE 7.29 **Squamous Cell Carcinoma Arising in Lichen Simplex Chronicus.** There is infiltration of small nests of squamous cell carcinoma showing individual cell dyskeratosis in a reactive stroma.

HISTOLOGY. The lesions associated with chronic inflammation and burns are usually moderately or well differentiated. Likewise the radiation induced carcinoma usually appears to be moderately differentiated, but in this particular setting a spindle cell carcinoma can also be observed. In both of these settings, while the carcinomas appear similar to other carcinomas arising, for example, in a sun-damaged skin, including a spindle cell squamous cell carcinoma, they behave in a much more aggressive fashion.[3,46,48]

INDETERMINATE RISK TUMORS

Clear Cell Squamous Cell Carcinoma

Clear cell carcinomas of the skin represent tumors of several cell lineages; in this discussion, we restrict our focus to those of squamous epithelial derivation, which typically occur in older men in the head and neck region. The tumors have been classified into three types,[49] all characterized by cells with very clear cytoplasm with varying degree of nuclear pleomorphism (Fig. 7.30, e-figs. 7.55–7.58). The first two types had evidence of cells with bubbled or finely reticulated cytoplasm. The third type exhibited very

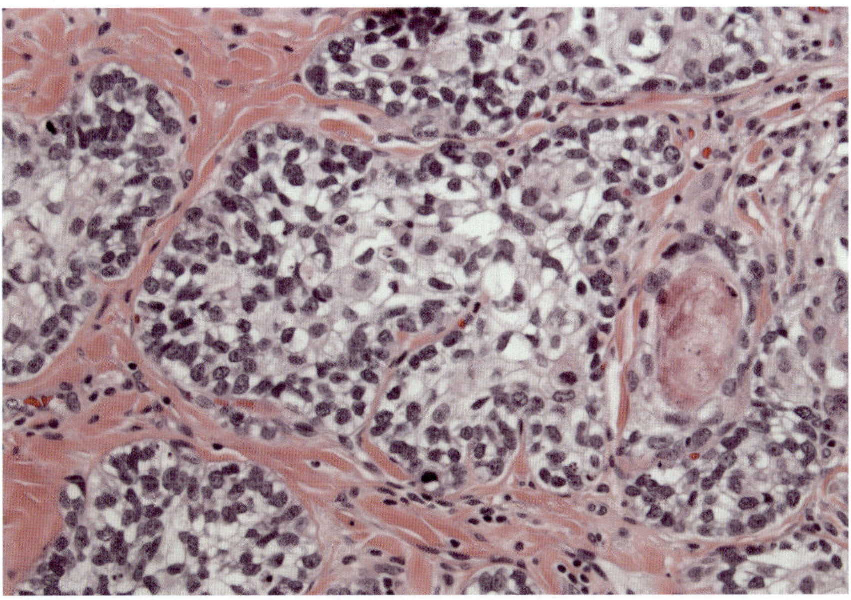

FIGURE 7.30 **Clear Cell Squamous Cell Carcinoma.** There is a spectrum of clear cell differentiation; some cells appear to have little cytoplasm while in others there is a reticulated appearance. Indentation and scalloping of nuclei as one sees in neoplastic sebocytes is not conspicuous.

prominent nuclear pleomorphism, acantholysis, and even individual cell necrosis. Perineural and vascular invasion were extensive. No evidence of mucin is demonstrable in these tumors. In our estimation, these reflect an abortive form of outer root sheath differentiation that does not connect to the hair follicle. The differential diagnosis includes clear cell acanthoma, clear cell hidradenoma, and trichilemmal carcinoma, all of which are glycogen-rich, sebaceous carcinoma[49,50], balloon cell melanocytic lesions, and metastatic renal cell carcinoma.[51] Careful histology and the use of immunohistochemical stains allow for definitive diagnosis. Sebaceous carcinoma, metastatic renal cell carcinoma and balloon cell melanoma are discussed elsewhere.

Follicular Squamous Cell Carcinoma

While most squamous cell carcinoma clearly arise from the epidermis, a minority take origin in the follicle in which case this tumor may appear as a squamous cell carcinoma or a clear cell trichilemmal-type carcinoma or a carcinoma with sebaceous differentiation.[3] These lesions most commonly appear on the face in persons of advanced age. They present as nodules that are not ulcerated but often have a central indentation. This picture is most commonly mistaken for an epidermal-derived squamous cell carcinoma or as a metastasis when the hair follicle origin is not visualized in the biopsy, but there is little or no dysplasia of the overlying native epidermis.[52,53]

HISTOLOGY. The infundibulum or upper part of the hair follicle is the most common site of origin for these lesions. The tumor usually exhibits an in situ component that replaces the follicular keratinocytes and then extends into the dermis (Figs. 7.31 and 7.32, e-figs. 7.59–7.64). Most cases will show definite squamous differentiation with large cytoplasms and prominent nuclei but also show dyskeratosis with single cell penetration of the collagen table. Less common is a clear cell carcinoma resembling trichilemmal carcinoma, with prominent pale cells replacing the follicular lumen and extending into the dermis.[54]

Other Indeterminate Risk Tumors

There are other squamous cell carcinoma variants including squamous cell carcinoma arising form benign cysts of sweat gland derication, pigmented squamous cell carcinoma, and squamoid eccrine ductal carcinoma that are sufficiently rare in our opinion as to not need a separate discussion. The reader is referred to Cassarino et al.[3] for a review of these entities.

Prognostic Factors

Prognosis in squamous cell carcinoma has been one of the more difficult features of the tumor to define with confidence. Various breakpoints have been proposed. In the following, we will present the results of a preliminary study of the AJCC staging system for cutaneous squamous cell carcinoma.

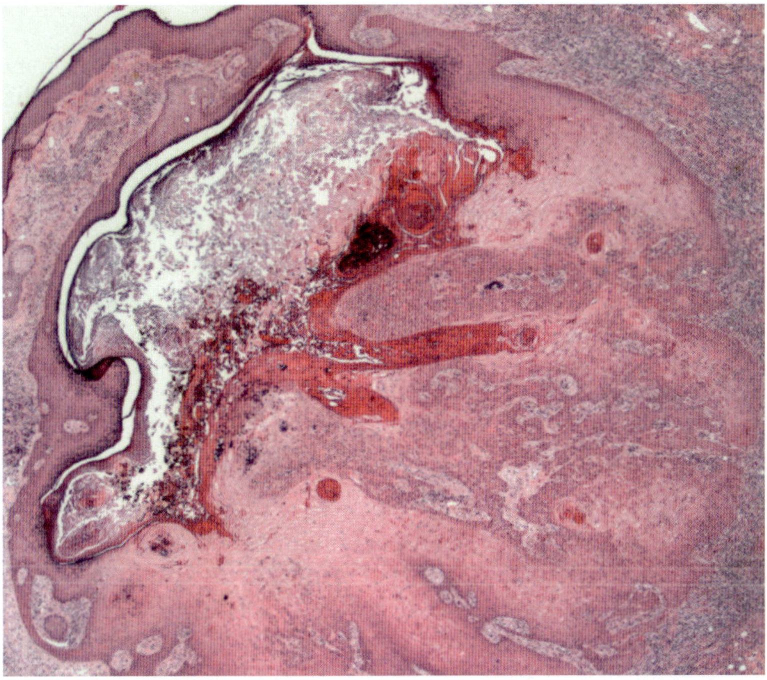

FIGURE 7.31 **Follicular Squamous Cell Carcinoma.** Low power examination reveals follicular involvement by neoplastic cells arising in continuity with a pre-existing benign epidermal cyst.

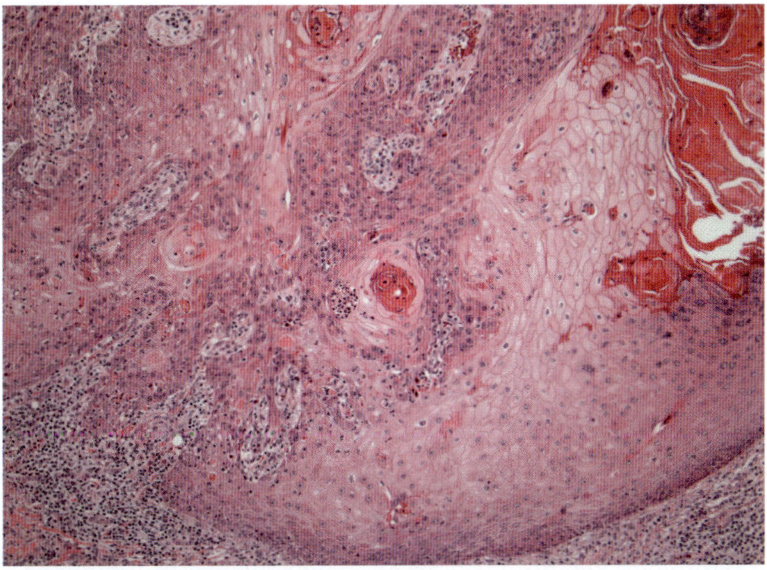

FIGURE 7.32 **Follicular Squamous Cell Carcinoma.** High power examination reveals complete replacement of the cyst wall by malignant squamous epithelia that radiate in an invasive manner into the adjacent dermal stroma.

Tumor Diameter

A review of the literature on prognosis of squamous cell carcinoma on the skin and lip since 1940 showed that tumors that exceeded 2 cm in diameter had double the local recurrence rate and triple the metastatic rate. The tumor diameter has been adopted by the AJCC task force as a significant factor.[55]

Depth of the Tumor

For depth, two parameters are recommended. Tumors greater than 4 mm in measured depth are considered to have high risk as are tumors invasive to Clark level IV or higher. Invasion into bone and invasion directly into a nerve or in perineural spaces are considered to be high-risk independent prognostic factors.[55–57]

Perineural and Vascular Invasion

Perineural (e-figs. 7.65 and 7.67) and vascular (e-fig. 7.68) invasion are both cited as significant prognostic factors. Perineural invasion has been shown to be associated with an increased risk of both cervical lymphadenopathy and distant metastasis.[58,59] Lymphovascular invasion, while significant, has not been shown to have the same effect on prognosis as perineural invasion.

Tumor Grading

Histological grade has definitely shown to be associated with risk of recurrence. Tumors graded as poorly differentiated appear to be the only ones in which high risk for metastasis occurs.[60,61] We utilize a system loosely based on that of Broders, which includes well to moderate to poorly differentiated tumors. Well-differentiated tumors show undifferentiated cells (i.e., those lacking cytoplasmic keratinization or intercellular bridge formation) to represent less than 25% (e-figs. 7.69 and 7.70) of the tumor population, while such cells represent greater than 75% (e-figs. 7.71 and 7.72) of the tumor in poorly differentiated squamous cell carcinoma. A moderately differentiated tumor in this system shows 25% to 75% of the cells to manifest cytoplasmic keratinization or intercellular bridge formation (e-figs. 7.73 and 7.74).[60]

Immunohistochemical Studies

Table 7.1 represents the immunohistochemical findings that help to confirm the diagnosis of squamous cell carcinoma and to distinguish such a lesion from a malignant adnexal tumor. This is one of the salient problems in skin pathology. We do not offer an exhaustive list of lesions or studies but rather a table that will help one to resolve the more common problems in cutaneous tumor pathology.[62–66]

TABLE 7.1 Immunohistochemical Differentiation of Cutaneous Carcinomas

	BCC	SCC	SEB CA	EC CA	MAC	Tricho-epithelioma
Androgen Receptor	+		+			–
Anti-bcl-2	+ (diffuse)	– (25% focally +)			+ (focal)	+ (peripheral cells only)
BerEP4	+ (diffuse)	– (+ in mets)			–	+ (60%)
CK 5/6	+	+	+	–		+
CK 7	(focal weak)	(focal weak)	+	+	–	–
CK15	–	–	+		+	+ (focal)
CK17	+			+		
CK20	–	–	–	–		+ (focal)
CK903 (HMWCK)	+	+			+	+
CAM 5.2 (LMWCK)		–	+	–		
CD10	+ (60%)	–				+ (stromal cells)
CD34	–				–	+ (spindle cells around nests)
c-Erb-B2	–				–	–
CEA	–	–	– (+ in ducts)	+	–	–
EMA	–	+	+	+	±	±
HMFG-1	–		+	–		
Ki-67 prolif index	20% to 40%				5%	<1%
PAS/D				+		
P53	+		–	+	–	–
P63	+	+	+	+	+	+
SMA	±	–		+		

BCC, basal cell carcinoma; EC CA, eccrine carcinoma; MAC, microcystic adnexal carcinoma; Rec, receptor; mets, metastases; HMW, high molecular weight; LMW, low molecular weight; SCC, squamous cell carcinoma; SEB CA, sebaceous carcinoma; SMA, smooth muscle actin; +, positive expression; –, no expression.

Molecular Aspects of the Genesis and Progression of Squamous Cell Carcinomas

RAS AND P53 MUTATIONS. Mutations in *ras* genes are found in 10% to 30% of squamous cell carcinomas. These mutations occur predominantly in H-*ras* and K-*ras*, the latter being the most prevalent. The mutations are related with the UV radiation-triggered formation of pyrimidine dimers.[67,68]

On the other hand, the *p53* gene is mutated in more than 50% of human cutaneous squamous cell carcinomas. Most of these alterations are missense mutations that result in the change of a single amino acid, yielding an altered *p53* protein. This is produced also by the influence of UV radiation to induce the thymidine dimer switch of TT to CC.[69] The resultant *p53* mutations can be grouped in loss-of-function mutations (loss of *p53*) or gain-of-function mutations (overexpression of *p53*). Both mutations play a part in tumoral progression. However, the gain-of-function mutations are thought to be associated with poorer prognosis.[70]

One can find *p53* missense mutations in normal keratinocytes in sun-exposed skin.[71,72] However, skin tumors rarely arise from the cells harboring these mutations, suggesting that additional alterations are necessary to give rise to malignant neoplasia. It appears that ras mutations play an important role in initiation of the tumors, while p53 mutations, especially gain-of-function mutations, are associated with later stages of the malignant progression.[73] The ras and p53 mutations act in synergy to initiate skin cancer.[74]

Role of Chronic Inflammation

The link between skin malignancies and chronic inflammation is well documented. In the 19th century, Marjolin described an ulcer arising in burn scars; later, in that same century, Virchow found evidence through microscopy that cancers have a close relationship with inflammatory processes. In this chapter, we discussed earlier the role of Th-1 cytokine products in immortalizing keratinocytes. At the present time, tremendous efforts are being carried out to unravel the intricate clockwork mechanisms of the inflammatory phenomenon and its relationship with cancer. There are several cellular and humoral elements playing different roles in the "pathologic inflammation" that occurs in most of the epithelial malignant proliferations.[75] Recently, it has been found that a specific type of chemokine receptor expressed in lymphatics, the D6 receptor plays an important role in limiting the chronic inflammatory process by acting as a "deceptor," sequestering pro-inflammatory chemokines and inactivating them.[76] The absence of this receptor in knock-out mice leads to the development of a psoriasiform skin pathology, after application of irritant chemicals on the skin.[44] The understating of these rather intimate mechanisms in SCC carcinogenesis may offer helpful leads to combat SCC in humans in the future (Fig. 7.33).

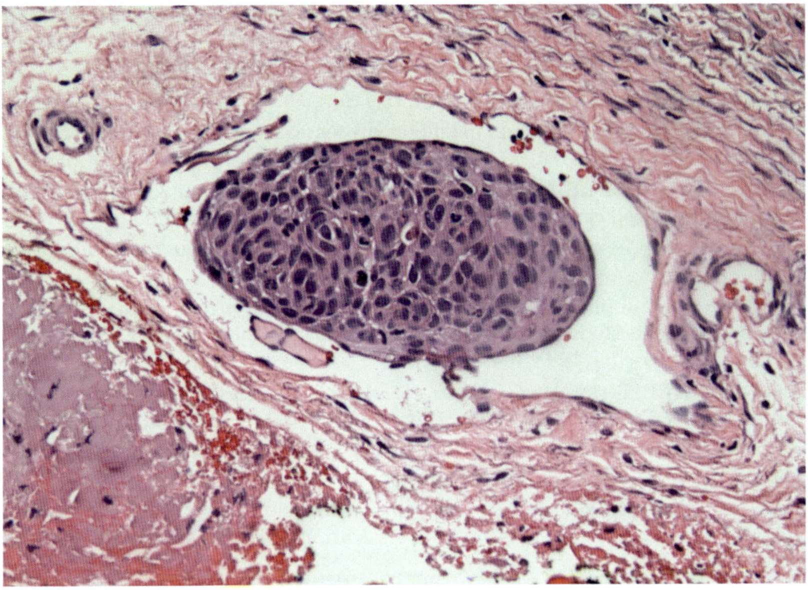

FIGURE 7.33 **Lymphatic Invasion in Squamous Cell Carcinoma.** This perianal SCC exhibited lymphatic invasion, evidence of its aggressive nature.

ACKNOWLEDGMENT

We thank Dr Rosalynn Nazarian for her work in assembling the data in Table 7.1.

REFERENCES

1. Kirkham N. Tumors and cysts of the epidermis In: Elder D, ed. *Lever's Histopathology of the Skin,* 10th Ed. Philadelphia, PA: Lippincott Williams & Wilkins, 2009;791–850.
2. Johnson TM, Tschen J, Ho C, et al: Unusual basal cell carcinomas. *Cutis* 1994;54:85–92.
3. Cassarino DS, DeRienzo DP, Barr RJ. Cutaneous squamous cell carcinoma: A comprehensive clinicopathologic classification. Part One. *J Cutan Pathol* 2006;33:191–206.
4. Kwa RE, Campana K, Moy RL. Biology of cutaneous squamous cell carcinoma. *J Am Acad Dermatol* 1992;26:1–16.
5. Berstein SC, Lim KK, Brodland DG, et al. The many faces of squamous cell carcinoma. *Dermatol Surg* 1996;22(3):243–254.
6. Horan TA, Urschel J, MacEachern NA, et al. Esophageal perforation in recessive dystrophic epidermolysis bullosa. *Ann Thorac Surg* 1994;57:1027–1029.
7. Ampil FL, Hardin JC, Peskind SP, et al. Perineural invasion in skin cancer of the head and neck: A review of nine cases. *J Oral Maxillofac Surg* 1995;53:34–38.
8. Crowson AN. Basal cell carcinoma: Biology, morphology and clinical implications. *Mod Pathol* 2006;19:S127–S147.
9. Crowson AN, Pilavdzic D, Stranc M, Magro CM. Expression of $p21^{WAF1/CIP1}$ in aggressive- versus non-aggressive-growth basal cell carcinoma: A comparative study [abstract]. *Lab Invest* 1999;79:56A.

10. Ackerman LV, Hermann P. Verrucous cancer of the oral cavity. *Proc Int Acad Oral Pathol* 1969:7–13.
11. Aird I, Johnson HD, Lennox B, Stansfeld AG. Epithelioma cuniculatum: A variety of squamous carcinoma peculiar to the foot. *Br J Surg* 1954;42(173):245–250.
12. Harwood CA, Prody CM. Human papillomaviruses and non-melanoma skin cancer. *Curr Opin Infect Dis* 2002;15:101–114.
13. Barreto JE, Velazquez EF, Ayala E, et al. Carcinoma cuniculatum: A distinctive variant of penile squamous cell carcinoma: Report of 7 cases. *Am J Surg Pathol* 2007;31(1):71–75.
14. Cubilla AL, Velazques EF, Reuter VE, et al. Warty (condylomatous) squamous cell carcinoma of the penis. *Am J Surg Pathol* 2000;24:505–512.
15. Fliss DM, Noble-Topham SE, McLachlin M, et al. Laryngeal verrucous carcinoma: A clinicopathologic study and detection of human papillomavirus using polymerase chain reaction. *Laryngoscope* 1994;104:146–152.
16. de Oliveira WRP, Festa Neto C, Rady PL, et al. Clinical aspects of epidermodysplasia verruciformis. *J Euro Acad Dermatol Venereol* 2003;17(4):394–398.
17. Androphy EJ, Dvoretzky I, Lowy DR. X-linked inheritance of epidermodysplasia verruciformis. *Arch Dermatol* 1985;121:864–868.
18. Kao GF, Graham JH, Helwig EB. Carcinoma cuniculatum (verrucous carcinoma of the skin): A clinicopathologic study of 46 cases with unltrastructural observations. *Cancer* 1982;49:2395–2403.
19. Sigel JE, Skacel M, Bergfeld WF, et al. The utility of cytokeratin 5/6 in the recognition of cutaneous spindle cell squamous cell carcinoma. *J Cutan Pathol* 2001;28(10):520–524.
20. Heintz PW, White CR. Diagnosis: Atypical fibroxanthoma or not? Evaluating spindle cell malignancies on sun damaged skin: A practical approach. *Semin Cutan Med Surg* 1999;18:78–83.
21. Dotto JE, Glusac EJ. p63 is a useful marker for cutaneous spindle cell squamous cell carcinoma. *J Cutan Pathol* 2006;33(6):413–417.
22. Lasser A, Corong JL, Morris JM. Adenoid squamous cell carcinoma of the vulva. *Cancer* 1974;33:224–227.
23. Nappi O, Pettinato G, Wick MR. Adenoid (acantholytic) squamous cell carcinoma of the skin. *J Cutan Pathol* 1989;16:114–121.
24. Johnson WC, Helwig EB. Adenoid squamous cell carcinoma (adenoacanthoma). A clinicopathologic study of 155 patients. *Cancer* 1966;19:1639–1650.
25. Swanson SA, Cooper PH, Mills SE, Wick MR. Lymphoepithelioma-like carcinoma of the skin. *Mod Pathol* 1988;1(5):359–365.
26. Okamura JM, Barr RJ. Cutaneous lymphoepithelial neoplasms. *Adv Dermatol* 1997; 12:277–294.
27. Lind AC, Breer WA, Wick MR. Lymphoepithelioma-like carcinoma of the skin with apparent origin in the epidermis-a pattern or an entity? *Cancer* 1999;85:884–890.
28. Hodge SJ, Turner JE. Histologic concepts of intraepithelial epithelioma. *Int J Dermatol* 1986;25:372–375.
29. Cook MG, Ridgeway HA. The intra-epidermal epithelioma of Jadassohn: A distinct entity. *Br J Dermatol* 1979;101:659–667.
30. Kossard S, Rosen R. Cutaneous Bowen's disease. An analysis of 1001 cases according to age, sex, and site. *J Am Acad Dermatol* 1992;27(3):406–410.
31. Kao G. Carcinoma arising in Bowen's disease. *Arch Dermatol* 1986;122(10):1124–1126.
32. Mora RG, Perniciaro C, Lee B. Cancer of the skin in blacks III. A review of nineteen black patients with Bowen's disease. *J Am Acad Dermatol* 1984;11(4 Pt 1):557–562.
33. Weidner N, Foucar E. Adenosquamous carcinoma of the skin. An aggressive mucin-and gland-forming squamous carcinoma. *Arch Dermatol* 1985;121:775–779.

34. Banks ER, Cooper PH. Adenosquamous carcinoma of the skin: A report of 10 cases. *J Cutan Pathol* 1991;18:227–234.
35. Sau P, Graham JH, Helwig EB. Proliferating epithelial cysts. *J Cutan Pathol* 1995; 22:394–406.
36. Lopez-Rios F, Rodriguez-Peralto J, Aguilar A, et al. Proliferating trichilemmal cyst with focal invasion. *Am J Dermatopathol* 2000;22:183–187.
37. Takata M, Rehman I, Rees JL. A trichilemmal carcinoma arising from a proliferating trichilemmal cyst: Loss of the wild-type p53 is a critical event in malignant transformation. *Hum Pathol* 1998;29:193–195.
38. Rutty GN, Richman PI, Laing JH. Malignant change in trichilemmal cysts: A study of cell proliferation and DNA content. *Histopathology* 1992;21:465–468.
39. Graham JH, Helwig EB. Premalignant cutaneous and mucocutaneous diseases. In: Graham JH, Johnson WC, Helwig EB, eds. *Dermal Pathology*. Hagerstown, MD: Harper & Row, 1972:561.
40. Graham JH. Selected precancerous skin and mucocutaneous lesions. In: Clark RL, ed. *Proceedings of the Annual Clinical Conference on Cancer by the University of Texas M.D. Anderson Hospital and Tumor Institute; Neoplasms of the Skin and Malignant Melanoma*. Chicago, IL: Year Book Medical Publishers, 1976:82.
41. Cubilla AL, Reuter VE, Gregoire L, et al. Basaloid squamous cell carcinoma: A distinctive human papilloma virus-related penile neoplasm: A report of 20 cases. *Am J Surg Pathol* 1998;22(6):755–761.
42. Goldschmidt H, Breneman JC, Breneman DL. Ionizing radiation therapy in dermatology. *J Am Acad Dermatol* 1994;30:157–182.
43. Ron E, Modan B, Preston D, et al. Radiation-induced skin carcinomas of the head and neck. *Radiat Res* 1991;125:318–325.
44. Nibbs RJ, Gilchrist DS, King V, et al. The atypical chemokine receptor D6 suppresses the development of chemically induced skin tumors. *J Clin Invest* 2007;117:1884–1892.
45. Dupree MT, Boyer JD, Cobb MW. Marjolin's ulcer arising in a burn scar. *Cutis* 1998; 62:49–51.
46. Trent JT, Kirsner RS. Wounds and malignancy. *Adv Skin Wound Care* 2003;16:31–34.
47. Crowson AN, Magro CM, Kadin M, Stranc M. Differential expression of bcl-2 oncogene in human basal cell carcinoma. *Hum Pathol* 1996;27:355–359.
48. Bartle EJ, Sun JH, Wang XW, Schneider BK. Cancers arising from burn scars: A literature review and report of twenty-one cases. *J Burn Care Rehabil* 1990;11:46–49.
49. Kuo T. Clear cell carcinoma of the skin. A variant of squamous cell carcinoma that simulates sebaceous carcinoma. *Am J Surg Pathol* 1980;4:573–583.
50. Rulon DB, Helwig EB. Cutaneous sebaceous neoplasms. *Cancer* 1974;33:82–102.
51. Wong TY, Suster S. Tricholemmal carcinoma. *Am J Dermatopathol* 1994;16:463–473.
52. Diaz-Cascajo C, Borghi S, Weyers W, Bastid-Inarrea J. Follicular squamous cell carcinoma of the skin: A poorly recognized neoplasm arising from the wall of hair follicles. *J Cutan Pathol* 2004;31(1):19–25.
53. Shendrik I, Crowson AN, Magro CM. Follicular cutaneous squamous cell carcinoma: An under-recognized neoplasm arising from hair appendage structures [abstract]. *Lab Invest* 2007;20(Suppl. 2):98A.
54. Yamamoto O, Asahi M, Horie A, et al. Medusa head-like granules in squamous cell carcinoma with differentiation toward a hair follicle structure. *J Cutan Pathol* 1991; 18(4):298–302.
55. Rowe DE, Carroll RJ, Day CL Jr. Prognostic factors for local recurrence, metastasis, and survival rates in squamous cell carcinoma of the skin, ear, and lip. Implications for treatment modality selection. *J Am Acad Dermatol* 1992;26(6):976–990.

56. Dinehart SM, Pollack SV. Metastases from squamous cell carcinoma of the skin and lip. An analysis of twenty-seven cases. *J Am Acad Dermatol* 1989;21(2 Pt 1):241–248.
57. Friedman HI, Cooper PH, Wanebo HJ. Prognostic and therapeutic use of microstaging of cutaneous squamous cell carcinoma of the trunk and extremities. *Cancer* 1985; 56(5):1099–1105.
58. Goepfert H, Dichtel WJ, Medina JE, et al. Perineural invasion in squamous cell skin carcinoma of the head and neck. *Am J Surg* 1984;48(4):542–547.
59. Fagan JJ, Collins B, Barnes L, et al. Perineural invasion in squamous cell carcinoma of the head and neck. *Arch Otolaryngol Head Neck Surg* 1998;124(6):637–640.
60. Broders AC. Squamous cell epithelioma of the skin. *Ann Surg* 1921;73:141–160.
61. Mohs FE. Chemosurgery: Microscopically controlled surgery for skin cancer. *J Dermatol Surg Oncol* 1978;4(1):41–54.
62. Alsaad KO, Obaidat NA, Ghazarian D. Skin adnexal neoplasms–part 1: An approach to tumours of the pilosebaceous unit. *J Clin Pathol* 2007;60(2):129–144. Epub 1 Aug 2006.
63. Hoang MP, Dresser KA, Kapur P, et al. Microcystic adnexal carcinoma: An immunohistochemical reappraisal. *Mod Pathol* 2008;(2):178–185. Epub 7 Dec 2007.
64. Obaidat NA, Alsaad KO, Ghazarian D. Skin adnexal neoplasms–part 2: An approach to tumours of cutaneous sweat glands. *J Clin Pathol* 2007;60:145–159. Epub 1 Aug 2006.
65. Fan YS, Carr RA, Sanders DS, et al. Characteristic Ber-EP4 and EMA expression in sebaceoma is immunohistochemically distinct from basal cell carcinoma. *Histopathology* 2007;51(1):80–86.
66. Smith KJ, Williams J, Corbett D, Skelton H. Microcystic adnexal carcinoma: An immunohistochemical study including markers of proliferation and apoptosis. *Am J Surg Path* 2001;25(4):464–471.
67. Pierceall WE, Goldberg LH, Tainsky MA, et al. Ras gene mutation and amplification in human nonmelanoma skin cancers. *Mol Carcinog* 1991;4(3):196–202.
68. Spencer JM, Kahn SM, Jiang W, et al. Activated ras genes occur in human actinic keratoses, premalignant precursors to squamous cell carcinomas. *Arch Dermatol* 1995;131(7):796–800.
69. Brash DE, Rudolph JA, Simon JA, et al. A role for sunlight in skin cancer: UV-induced p53 mutations in squamous cell carcinoma. *Proc Natl Acad Sci USA* 1991; 88(22):10124–10128.
70. Cadwell C, Zambetti GP. The effects of wild-type p53 tumor suppressor activity and mutant p53 gain-of-function on cell growth. *Gene* 2001;277(1–2):15–30.
71. Nakazawa H, English D, Randell PL, et al. UV and skin cancer: Specific p53 gene mutation in normal skin as a biologically relevant exposure measurement. *Proc Natl Acad Sci USA* 1994;91(1):360–364.
72. Jonason AS, Kunala S, Price GJ, et al. Frequent clones of p53-mutated keratinocytes in normal human skin. *Proc Natl Acad Sci USA* 1996;93(24):14025–14029.
73. Kemp CJ, Donehower LA, Bradley A, et al. Reduction of p53 gene dosage does not increase initiation or promotion but enhances malignant progression of chemically induced skin tumors. *Cell* 1993;74(5):813–822.
74. Caulin C, Nguyen T, Lang GA, et al. An inducible mouse model for skin cancer reveals distinct roles for gain- and loss-of-function p53 mutations. *J Clin Invest* 2007;117(7): 1893–1901.
75. Mueller MM. Inflammation in epithelial skin tumours: Old stories and new ideas. *Eur J Cancer* 2006;42(6):735–744. Epub 9 Mar 2006.
76. Jamieson T, Cook DN, Nibbs RJ, et al. The chemokine receptor D6 limits the inflammatory response in vivo. *Nat Immunol* 2005;6(4):403–411. Epub 6 Mar 2005.

8

BENIGN ADNEXAL NEOPLASMS

Benign and malignant neoplasms may arise in the apocrine and eccrine sweat glands of humans. As the histologic expression of both eccrine and apocrine neoplasms is extremely wide, and as the tumors can be seen in combination with complex hamartomas and/or can exhibit divergent differentiation, an overwhelming and confusing lexicon of diagnostic appellations has been applied to eccrine and apocrine neoplasia. In this chapter, we discuss the best recognized diagnostic entities for which specific nomenclature should logically be applied.

CYLINDROMA

These neoplasms present as nodules on the face, neck, and scalp. A multifocal variant is seen in the Ancell–Spiegler's ("turban tumor") syndrome[1–5] that links to chromosome 16q12–13 and the CYLD1 gene at that location. Patients manifest red or violaceous, sometimes tender nodules often covering the entire scalp and sometimes extending to involve the face and the upper trunk, typically first presenting in the 20 to 40 year age group. Women are more commonly affected. Some are seen in association with trichoepithelioma of the midface (i.e., Brooke syndrome) or with a coexistent eccrine spiradenoma.

Histopathology

There is a characteristic histomorphology comprising sharply demarcated nests of cuboidal cells with banal round to oval nuclei in the 8 to 15 μm size range which are associated with abundant quantities of lightly granular eosinophilic cytoplasm, sharply defined plasma membranes, and cohesive, compact nests surrounded by a thick eosinophilic mantle of basement membranelike material (Fig. 8.1, e-figs. 8.1–8.3). The tumor derives its name from eosinophilic "cylinders" located within the islands of eccrine epithelia, reflecting laminin 5 produced by the tumor cells.[6] Extension into the subcutaneous fat can occur (Fig. 8.2). Angioinvasion, necrosis, and invasion of adjacent structures are not seen. A rare example of a cylindroma will show significant mitotic activity that does not impart a capacity for aggressive biologic behavior.

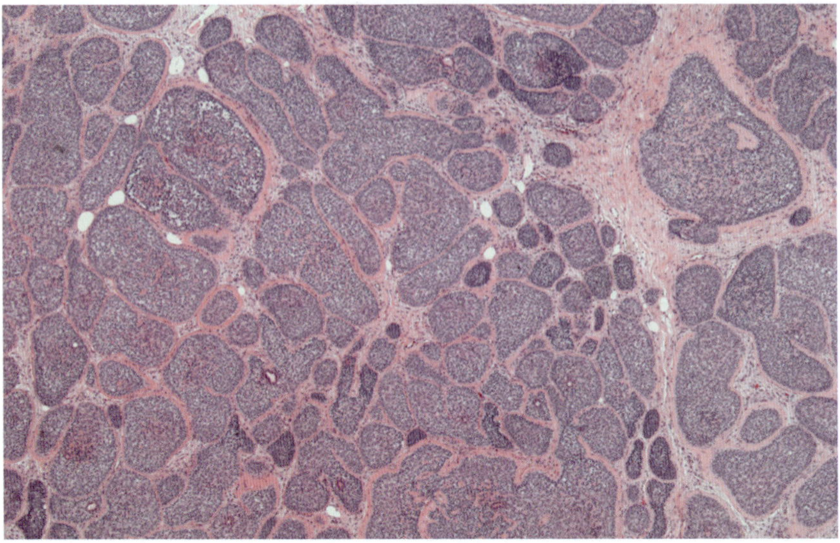

FIGURE 8.1 The cylindroma manifests a characteristic low power morphology comprising sharply demarcated nests of cuboidal cells associated with abundant quantities of lightly granular eosinophilic cytoplasm, sharply defined plasma membranes, in cohesive, compact nests surrounded by a thick eosinophilic mantle of basement membrane-like material.

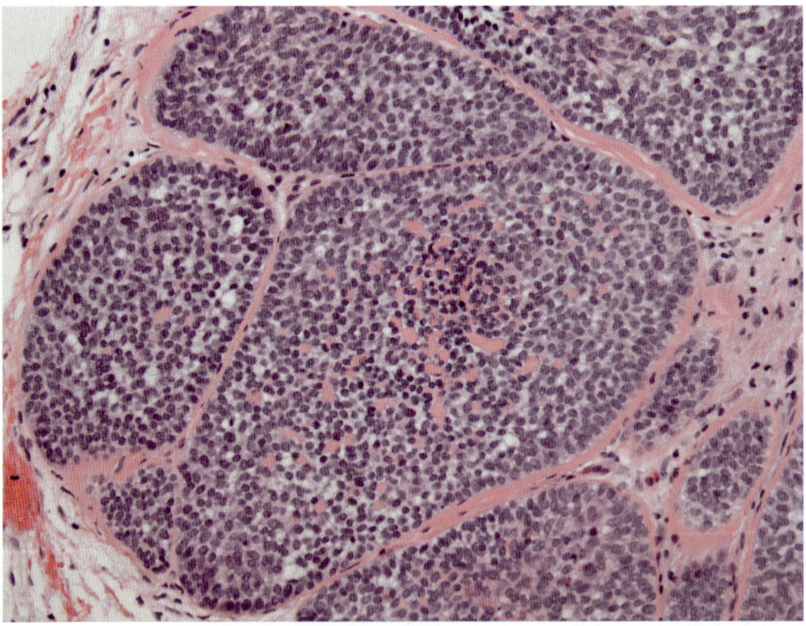

FIGURE 8.2 The tumor derives its name from eosinophilic "cylinders" located within the islands of eccrine epithelia, reflecting laminin 5 produced by the tumor cells.

ECCRINE SPIRADENOMA

Presenting in young adults as a painful solitary bluish or skin-colored nodule 5 mm to 5 cm size range, these lesions occur typically on the ventral aspect of the upper trunk but can be multiple and in that setting, exhibit a grouped, linear or whorled configuration.

Histopathology

Generally lacking the jigsaw or mosaic pattern of a cylindroma, the spiradenoma has two cell populations arranged as intertwining cords and bands of cells, an internal eosinophilic cuboidal cell lining a glandlike space, and a peripheral small hyperchromatic cell with scant cytoplasm (Fig. 8.3, e-figs. 8.4–8.6). These intertwining bands of "dark and light cells" are disposed in one or a few large lobules in the reticular dermis, often surrounded by an eosinophilic mantle of basement membranelike material. The neoplasms may be highly vascular and in this context, the blood vessels may be strikingly dilated to fashion the so-called *giant vascular spiradenoma*[7] potentially mimicking vascular neoplasms.[8–11]. The spiradenoma

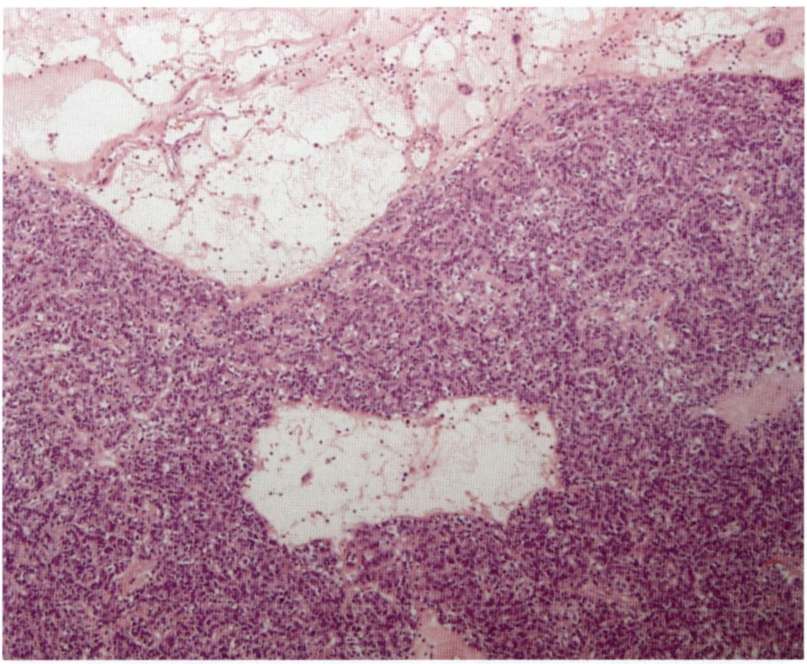

FIGURE 8.3 Generally lacking the jigsaw or mosaic pattern of a cylindroma, the spiradenoma has two cell populations arranged as intertwining cords and bands of cells: an internal eosinophilic cuboidal cell lining a glandlike space and a peripheral small hyperchromatic cell with scant cytoplasm. Cystification can be seen as shown here. The intertwining bands of "dark and light cells" are disposed in one or a few large lobules in the reticular dermis, often surrounded by an eosinophilic mantle of basement membranelike material.

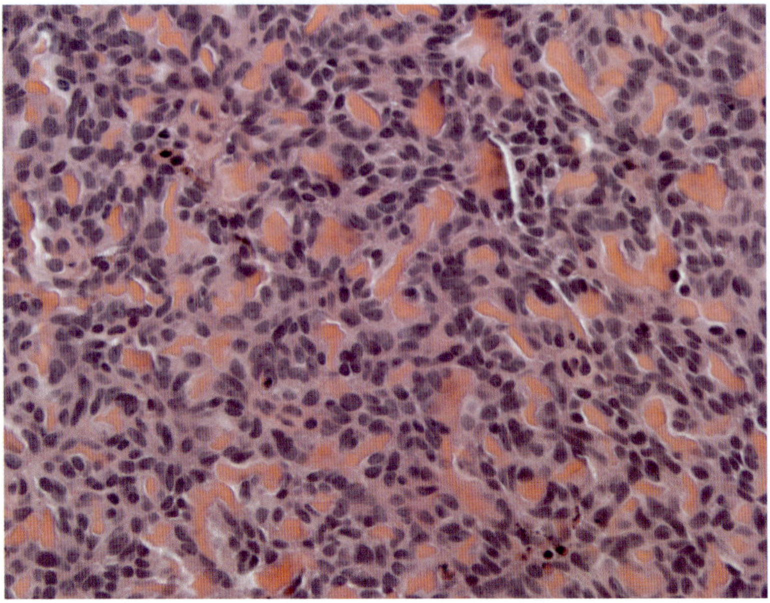

FIGURE 8.4 Cylinders comprising basement membrane material may be present within the neoplasms, thus causing considerable overlap with cylindroma.

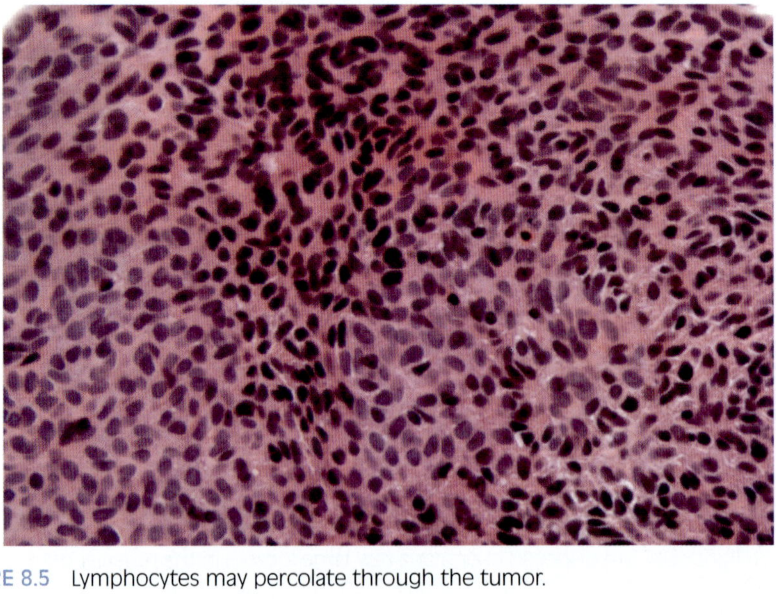

FIGURE 8.5 Lymphocytes may percolate through the tumor.

may penetrate to the level of the subcutis[12] and may have an infiltrative peripheral margin.[12] Cylinders comprising basement membrane material may be present within the neoplasms, thus causing considerable overlap with cylindroma. Patients with the Ancell–Spiegler's syndrome may have multifocal spiradenomas.[5,8,9] Lymphocytes may percolate through the tumor and cystification can occur (Figs. 8.4 and 8.5).

SYRINGOMA

The syringoma typically presents as a multifocal or agminate cluster of papules largely restricted to the skin of the face, in particular the eyelids, and less commonly the genitalia, the scalp, or acral sites. Solitary lesions are also not uncommon. Some observers view this as a form of eccrine ductal hamartoma as opposed to a true neoplasm.[13-22] The typical morphology of the individual lesion is that of a yellow-, a tan-, or a white-colored 1 to 4 mm papule; localization of the lower eyelid is prototypic.[15] Lesions may be plaquelike, linear, milialike, eruptive or disseminated. A rare form resembles the confluent and reticulated papillomatosis of Gougerot and Carteaud.[16]

Histopathology

Classical is a cluster of tubular structures with central concretions of mucin-like material. The tubules have a commalike architecture and are typically lined by a central cuboidal layer with a peripheral myoepithelial mantle embedded in a fibrotic stroma (Fig. 8.6, e-figs. 8.7–8.9). The lining cells are polygonal or flattened with eosinophilic or clear cytoplasms.[13,15,21,22] Nuclei are small and banal, lacking hyperchromasia, nucleoli, mitoses, or necrosis. While sharply circumscribed lesions may penetrate the immediately adjacent stroma, that stroma in turn is well demarcated from the native dermis. Due to their association with a collagenized stroma, an infiltrative growth pattern with a desmoplastic stromal response may be mimicked in small biopsy samples, raising concern with respect to microcystic adnexal carcinoma. Excisional biopsies are therefore prudent but not mandated from a therapeutic perspective. Cytologic variants of the syringoma include a clear cell form, whereby the cuboidal epithelium manifests abundant quantities of glycogen in part or all of the sampled neoplasm (Fig. 8.7).

ECCRINE POROMA

Derived from the acrosyrinx and from the eccrine straight duct, eccrine poroma can manifest as a benign neoplasm with a purely intraepidermal disposition, a mixed dermal and epidermal one, or as a purely intradermal proliferation.[23-28] Typically arising in older woman as a slightly elevated papule or nodule, or sometimes as a brown macule, the intraepidermal form of eccrine poroma is termed *hidroacanthoma simplex*.[29] It may have a verruciform surface. Those with a dermal component form a nodule most

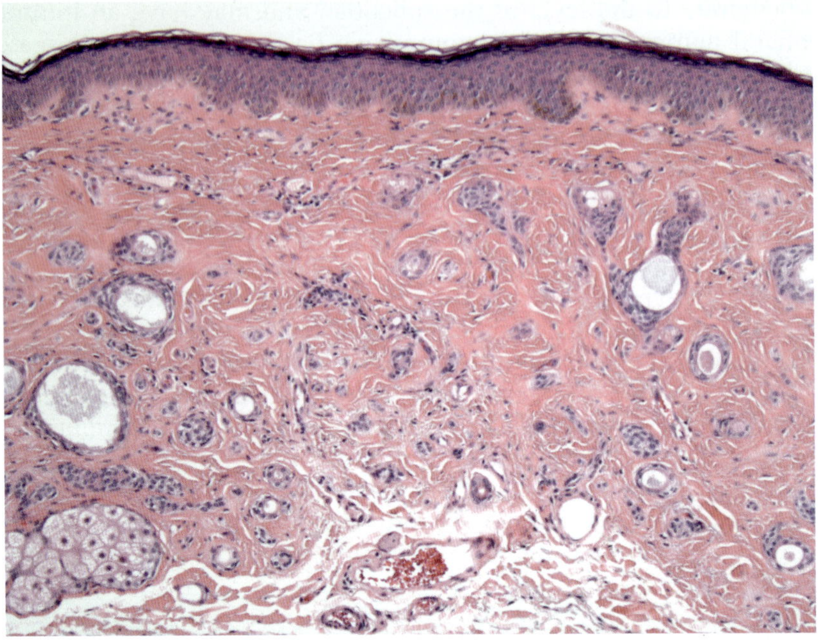

FIGURE 8.6 The syringoma manifests classically as a cluster of tubular structures containing central concretions of mucinlike material. The tubules have a commalike architecture and are typically lined by a central cuboidal layer with a peripheral myoepithelial mantle. These are embedded in a densely fibrotic stroma.

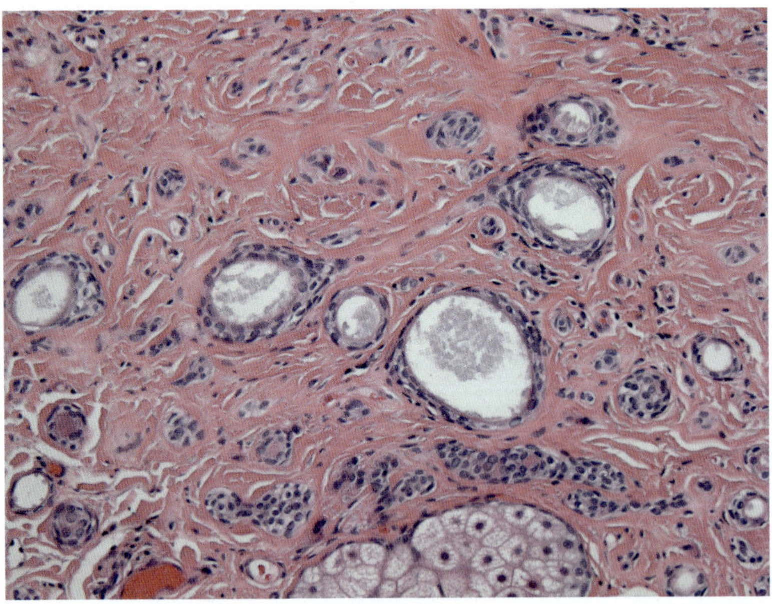

FIGURE 8.7 The lining cells are polygonal or flattened with eosinophilic or clear cytoplasms. Nuclei are small and banal, lacking hyperchromasia, nucleoli, mitoses, or necrosis.

commonly on the palms and soles reflecting the high concentration of sweat ducts and glands in this area. As with the hidroacanthoma simplex, the surface may be verruciform, hence resembling a seborrheic keratosis or verruca. The purely intradermal form of eccrine poroma, the *dermal duct tumor*,[30,31] manifests as a papule or nodule which is skin-colored or tan and raises consideration to an amelanotic melanoma or any one of a variety of benign dermal-based lesions.

Histopathology

The critical cells have round to oval nuclei with eosinophilic glassy, clear or granular cytoplasms and may show intracytoplasmic lumens and/or be arranged into duct structures (Fig. 8.8, e-figs. 8.10–8.12). Some degree of nuclear size and shape variation can be seen and could denote supervening dysplasia. The hidroacanthoma simplex manifests discrete nests of cells sharply demarcated from the adjacent epidermis to form the *Borst–Jadassohn phenomenon* (e-figs. 8.13 and 8.14). The eccrine poroma seen most commonly has both epidermal and dermal components, the latter comprising broad sheets and anastomosing bands of cells that take their origin from the epidermis and extend to the reticular dermis. The junction with the native epidermis is sharply defined (Fig. 8.9). There, stroma is often highly vascular with tortuous and ectatic capillaries embedded in hyalinized or edematous collagen (Fig. 8.10). The dermal duct tumor manifests as one or a few nodules within the dermis showing no connection to the overlying epidermis. Morphological variants include those that show extensive squamous metaplasia, melanin pigment, glandular, sebaceous, apocrine, or follicular differentiation (Fig. 8.11, e-figs. 8.15 and 8.16).[32] Some examples of eccrine poroma have marked epidermal hyperplasia associated with them, for which the term syringoacanthoma has been applied.[33] As mentioned earlier, eccrine poromas can exhibit varying degrees of atypia and are recognized precursor lesions to porocarcinomas (Fig. 8.12). In our experience, it is not uncommon to see some degree of atypia including in the context of scattered atypical mitoses. All lesions of eccrine poroma should be excised completely if cosmetic and/or functional considerations permit.

ECCRINE SYRINGOFIBROADENOMA

The eccrine syringofibroadenoma was first described by Mascaro in 1963.[34] The precise character of the eccrine syringofibroadenoma is a subject of open debate. The presence of solitary acral lesions has led some authorities to consider it a neoplasm, while eruptive variants or those that manifest as agminate plaques have prompted some to consider it a form of hamartoma. We have seen an eccrine syringofibroadenoma in the setting of persistent sclerodermoid graft versus host disease and have postulated that abnormalities of immune function may lead to relative cell immortalization in a fashion cognate to that proposed for basal cell carcinoma.[35,36] We have also encountered malignant variants suggesting its true categorization as a neoplasm.

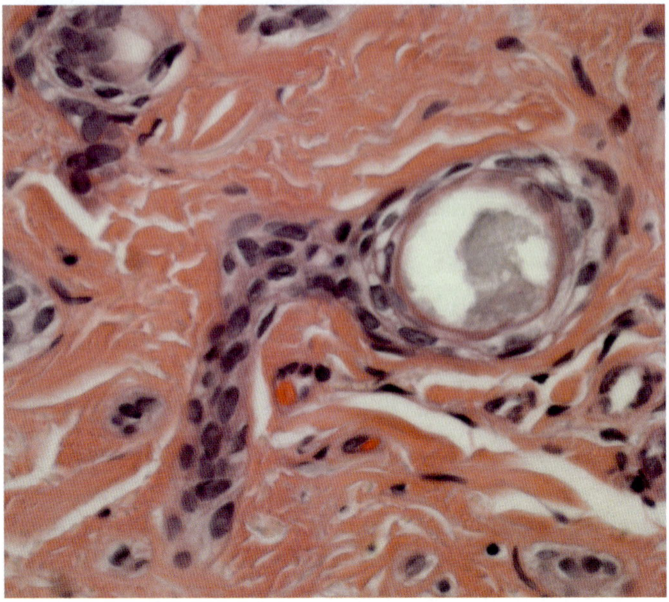

FIGURE 8.8 The critical cells have round to oval nuclei with eosinophilic glassy, clear, or granular cytoplasms and may show intracytoplasmic lumens and/or be arranged into duct structures.

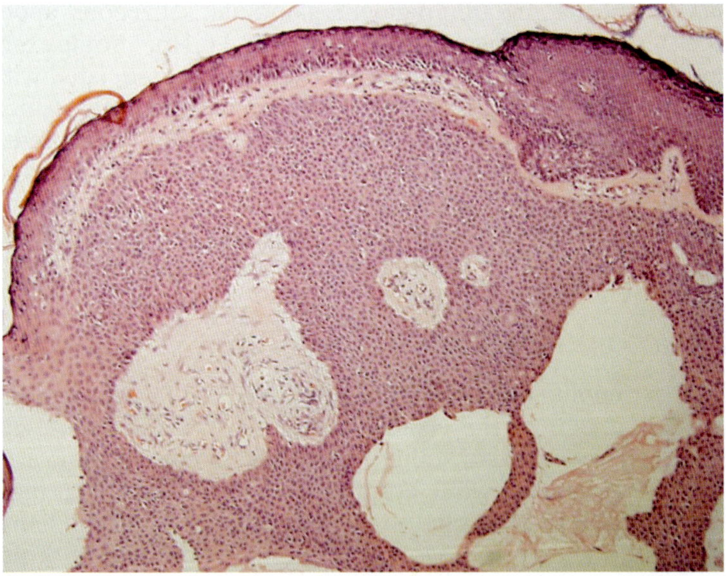

FIGURE 8.9 The classic eccrine poroma seen most commonly in routine practice has both epidermal and dermal components. The latter comprises broad sheets of cells and anastomosing bands which take their origin from the epidermal compartment and extend down to the level of the reticular dermis.

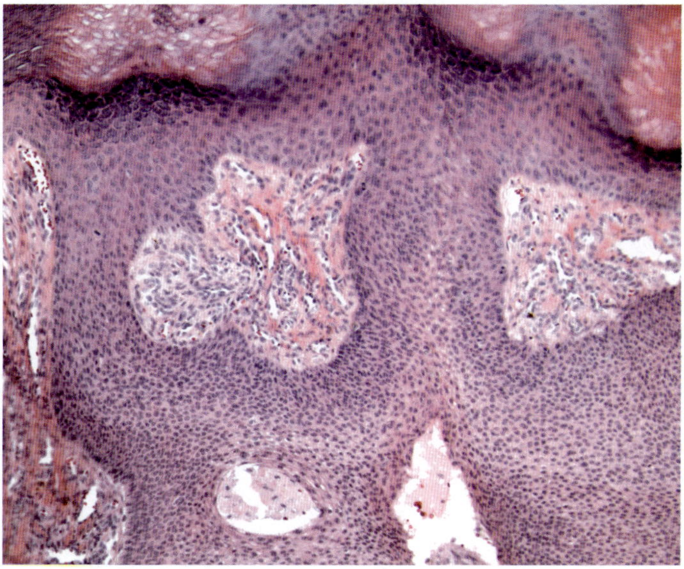

FIGURE 8.10 The classic eccrine poroma manifests a highly vascular dermal stroma with tortuous and ectatic capillaries embedded in a hyalinized or edematous stroma. Note the distinct intraepidermal epithelioma growth pattern in the epidermis.

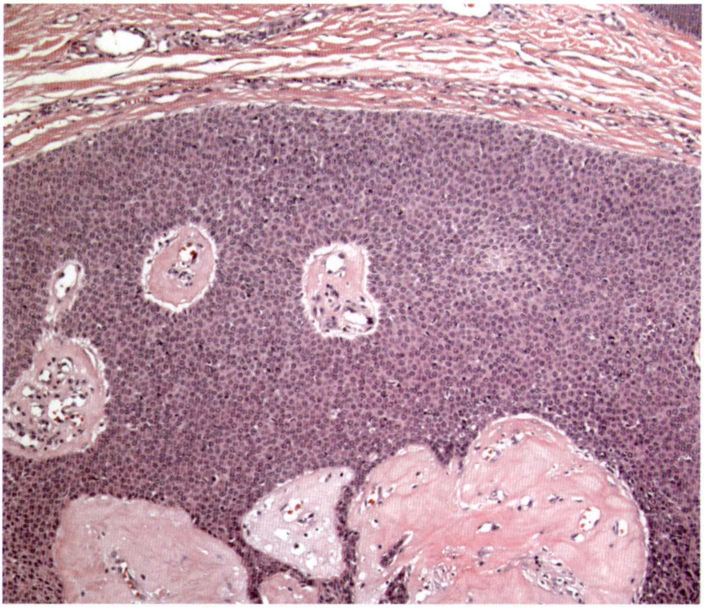

FIGURE 8.11 The dermal duct tumor manifests as one or a few nodules within the dermis showing no connection to the overlying epidermis. Morphological variants include those which show extensive squamous metaplasia, melanin pigment, glandular, sebaceous, apocrine, or follicular differentiation.

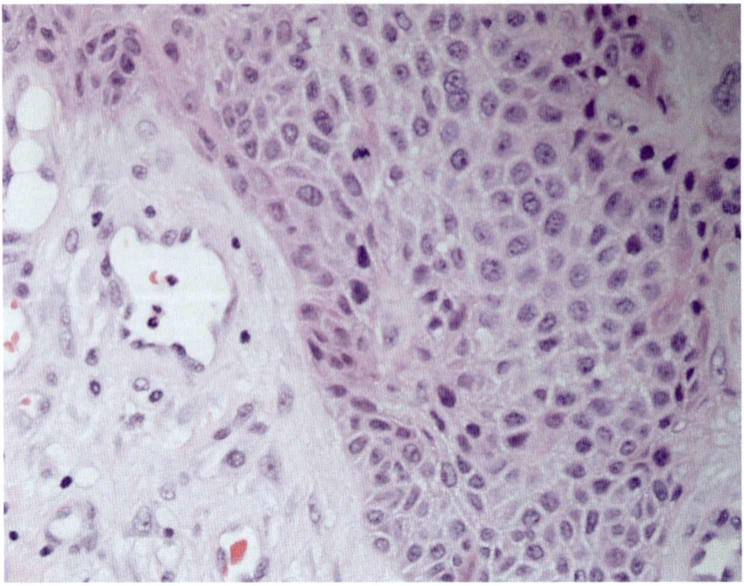

FIGURE 8.12 Eccrine poromas can exhibit varying degrees of atypia and are recognized precursor lesions to porocarcinomas. In our experience, it is not uncommon to see some degree of atypia including in the context of scattered atypical mitoses.

Clinical Features

This lesion can manifest as a solitary nodule or papule, typically on the plantar or palmar surface, as an agminate plaque that may extend progressively over the ventral and/or dorsal surfaces of the distal upper or lower extremities, or as a rare disseminated or eruptive variant. Reflecting confusion over the pathogenetic basis, some observers have suggested the appellation *acrosyringeal nevus*,[37] while others consider it a malformation of the terminal eccrine duct.[38]

Histopathology

The histology is diagnostic. Arising from the undersurface of a thickened epidermis and coursing through a fibrotic or edematous stroma are columns of basaloid cells reminiscent of those seen in the fibroepithelioma of Pinkus, but distinctive by virtue of their showing, in multiple step sections, demonstrable lumina lined by cuboidal cells of evident eccrine derivation with a lining cuticle (e-figs. 8.17–8.20).[39,40]

PAPILLARY ECCRINE ADENOMA

Known also as tubulopapillary eccrine hidradenoma, this lesion presents as a 1 cm nodule on the extremities of middle-aged or elderly patients.[41–47] Distinction of this benign neoplasm from digital papillary adenocarcinoma is difficult, and any lesion showing cytologic atypia when occurring on the digits is best treated as the latter. It is clear, however, that benign papillary and papillary–tubular sweat duct neoplasms manifesting eccrine and/or apocrine cytologic features do exist.[48,49] Those showing eccrine differentiation are said to be more common.

Histopathology

Papillary eccrine hidradenoma manifests uniform polygonal cells with small round to oval nuclei containing discrete nucleoli arranged into multilayered discrete structures separated by a fine fibrous stroma. These structures have rounded external profiles and show multilayered papillary proliferations internally. The formation of intradermal tubulopapillary complexes and microcysts has prompted some authorities to designate this tumor as *tubulopapillary hidradenoma*,[48] and when apocrine differentiation dominates, as tubular or papillary tubular apocrine adenoma (Figs. 8.13 and 8.14).[49] The truly benign form of this process may recur but does not metastasize. Its aggressive counterpart, low grade papillary adenocarcinoma, has a capacity to metastasize.

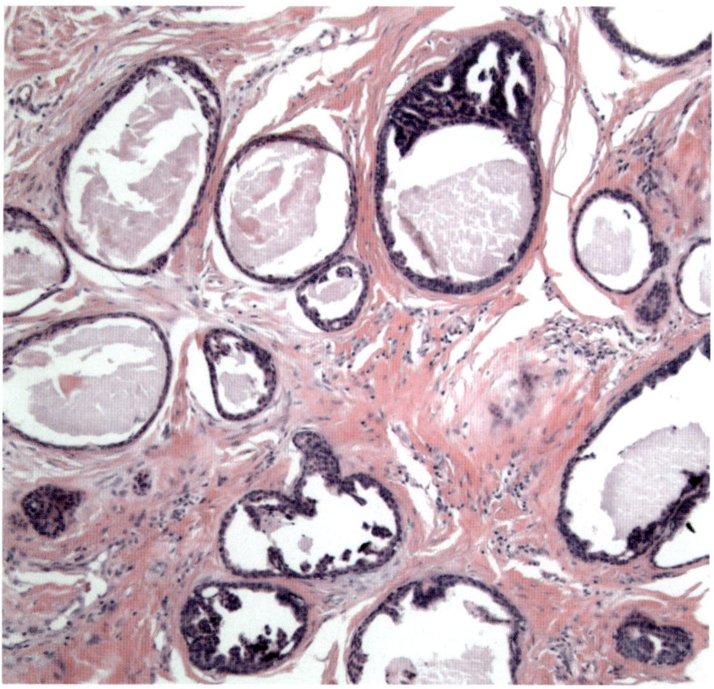

FIGURE 8.13 The papillary eccrine or tubulopapillary eccrine hidradenoma is arranged in rounded multilayered structures of varying sizes. In an acral location, this lesion would be classified as a low grade papillary digital adenocarcinoma. Prediciting the biologic behavior by histologic grounds is notoriously problematic. Our approach is to excise all such lesions completely and comment on the risk of metastatic disease.

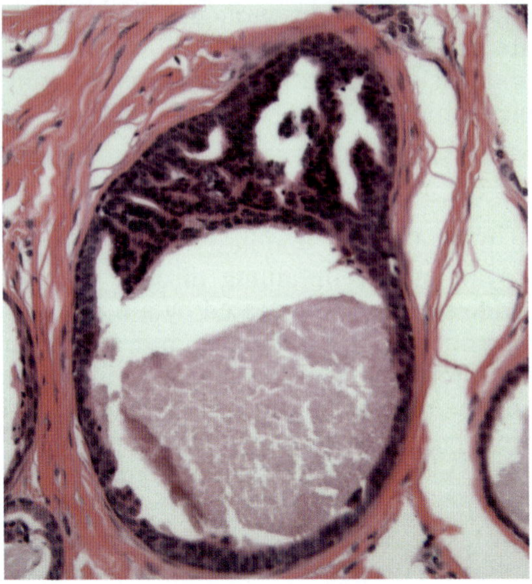

FIGURE 8.14 The cells lining the rounded luminal structures show multilayered papillations. In an acral location, this lesion would be classified as a low grade papillary digital adenocarcinoma. Prediciting the biologic behavior by histologic grounds is notoriously problematic.

ECCRINE ACROSPIROMA

The eccrine acrospiroma goes by a variety of synonyms including clear cell hidradenoma, cystic and solid hidradenoma, nodular eccrine hidradenoma, and clear cell myoepithelioma. These names can be used interchangeably and in some instances, we prefer to issue a diagnosis of "benign eccrine adnexal neoplasm, not otherwise specified" which is a perfectly acceptable alternative to subclassification.

Clinical Features

Typically, these present as a solitary 1 to 2 cm solid and/or cystic lesion in either sex and at any anatomical location. Through neglect, a lesion may reach a size of up to 6 cm in diameter.

Histopathology

Typical is a solid nodule or multiple coalescing smaller nodules comprising a monomorphous population of cuboidal cells with round, regular nuclei in the 8 to 12 μm size range associated with modest quantities of eosinophilic granular cytoplasm showing polygonal external contours and often associated with the formation of discrete ductal lumina, either via common lumenal margins formed by adjacent cells or in the context of intracytoplasmic lumina with a discrete cuticle (Fig. 8.15).[50,51] Microcyst formation is variable; when it is prominent, the term *cystic and solid hidradenoma* has been applied (e-figs. 8.21–8.24). Like most benign eccrine adnexal tumors, the eccrine acrospiroma has a pushing contour at its peripheral margins where it compresses the adjacent stroma. There may be a modest band of basement membrane-like material cognate to that seen in the cylindroma, separating the peripheral aspects of tumor nests from the adjacent stroma. When the peripheral margin manifests a tonguelike pattern of growth with associated stromal desmoplasia, the risk of recurrence is higher, albeit difficult to define. Some authorities view neoplasms with an infiltrative border as low grade hidradenocarcinomas. Squamous metaplasia is seen in eccrine acrospiroma as in all other forms of eccrine neoplasia and has no specific biological import. Some observers hold high grade cytologic atypia affecting the majority of cells in an individual neoplasm, as opposed to just scattered cells, tumor necrosis, and/or tumor giant cells as being indicators of potentially aggressive biologic behavior. The same has been said of neoplasms showing extensive clear cell change, although this has not been our experience (Fig. 8.16). Mitoses may be conspicuous but do not necessarily import adverse prognostic significance.[52] In roughly half of cases, the eccrine acrospiromas show connection to the overlying epidermis in a fashion cognate to that of eccrine poromas; this distinguishes the entity from eccrine spiradenoma which does not connect to the epidermis

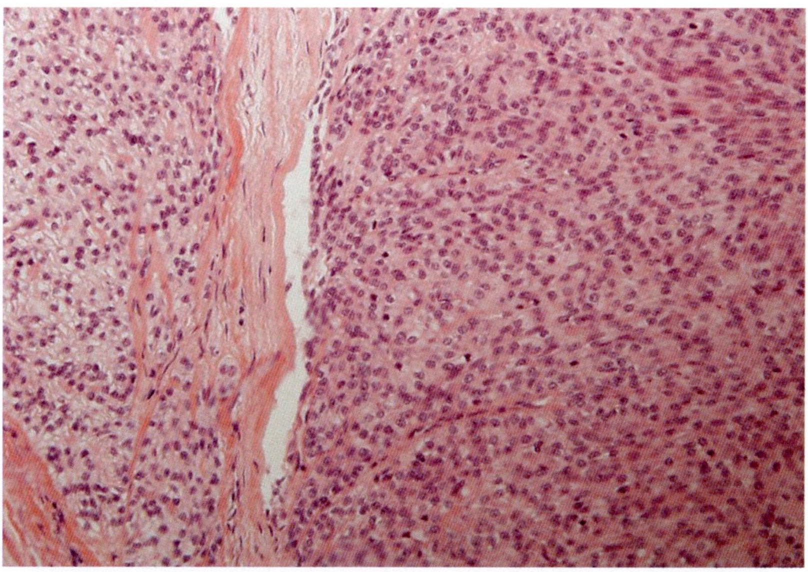

FIGURE 8.15 This eccrine acrospiroma manifests a solid nodule comprising a monomorphous population of cuboidal cells with round, regular nuclei in the 8 to 12 μm size range associated with modest quantities of eosinophilic granular cytoplasm showing polygonal external contours and often associated with the formation of discrete ductal lumens, either via common lumenal margins formed by adjacent cells or in the context of intracytoplasmic lumena with a discrete lining cuticle.

(Fig. 8.17).[53] On occasion, the intraepidermal component associated with an eccrine acrospiroma mimics the hidroacanthoma simplex and in some instances, a clear-cut eccrine acrospiroma is present with no connection to an overlying epidermis in which such changes are identified.

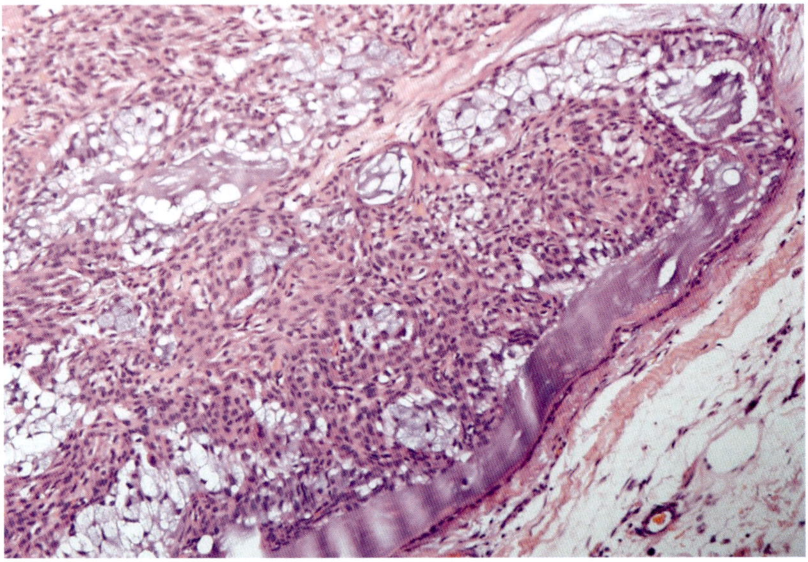

FIGURE 8.16 Clear cell change can be observed.

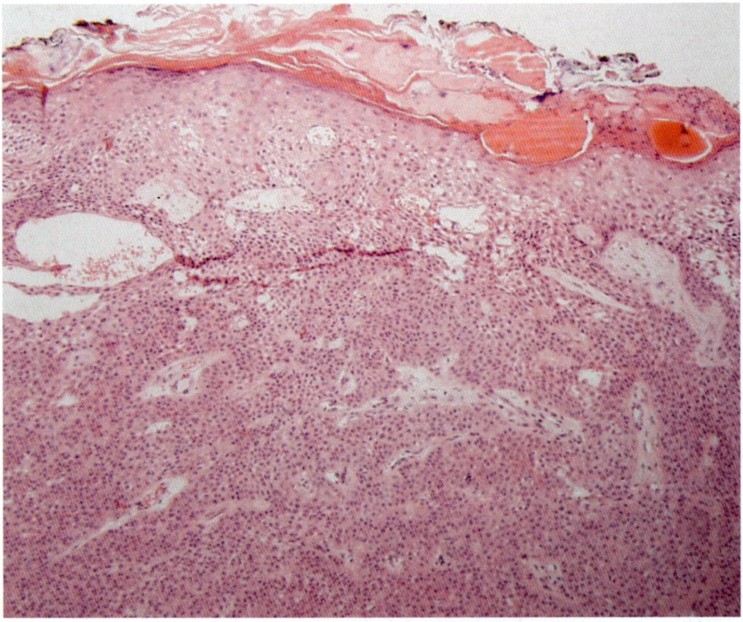

FIGURE 8.17 In roughly half of the cases, the eccrine acrospiromas connect to the overlying epidermis in a fashion cognate to that of the eccrine poroma.

APOCRINE NEOPLASMS

The apocrine sweat apparatus enters the hair follicle structure through a duct that terminates in the follicular bulge. As the distribution of apocrine neoplasms closely correlates to the distribution of hair appendage structures, they are concentrated in the head and neck, axillae, groins, and perineal region where hair follicle structures and apocrine glands are numerous.

SYRINGOCYSTADENOMA PAPILLIFERUM

A typically solitary neoplasm which principally affects the scalp, the syringocystadenoma papilliferum is one of the neoplasms seen arising in the nevus sebaceus of Jadassohn which is a form of complex hamartoma with a prominent folliculosebaceous component. The syringocystadenoma papilliferum occurs sporadically in other anatomic locations in the absence of an underlying nevus sebaceus.

Histopathology

The lesion has a typical and diagnostic morphology. Papillary structures comprising multilayered cuboidal epithelia surmounted by a layer showing apocrine decapitation secretion are typical (Figs. 8.18 and 8.19, e-figs. 8.25–8.27). The fibrovascular cores of these papillary structures contain sheets and nodules of plasma cells (Fig. 8.20). The papillary

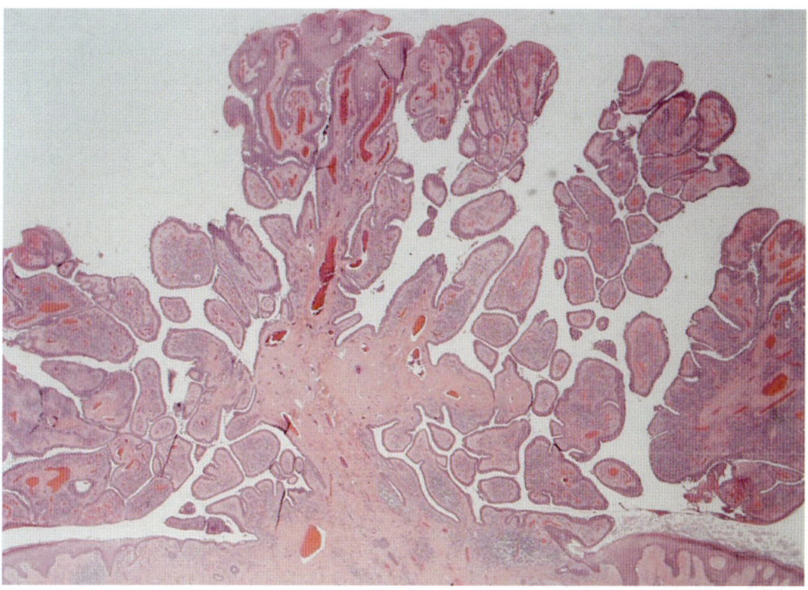

FIGURE 8.18 Papillary structures comprising multilayered cuboidal epithelia surmounted by a layer showing apocrine decapitation secretion are typical of the syringocystadenoma papilliferum.

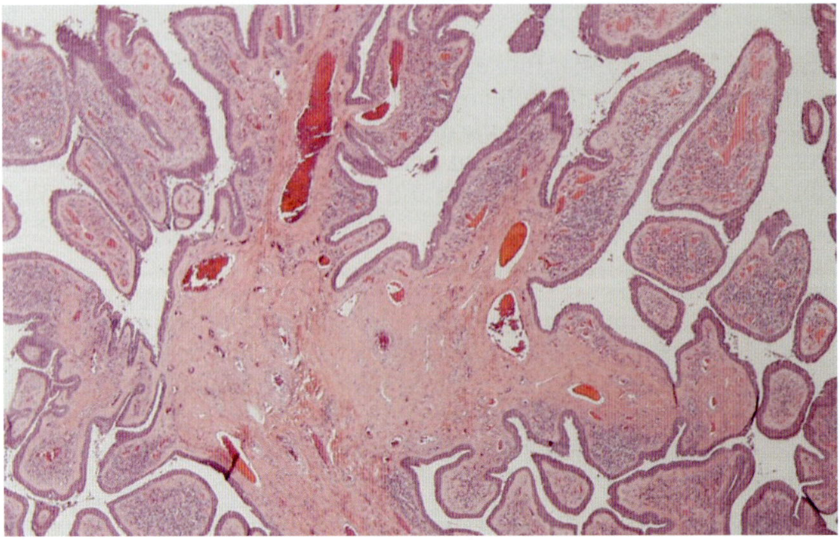

FIGURE 8.19 Papillary structures comprising multilayered cuboidal epithelia surmounted by a layer showing apocrine decapitation secretion are typical.

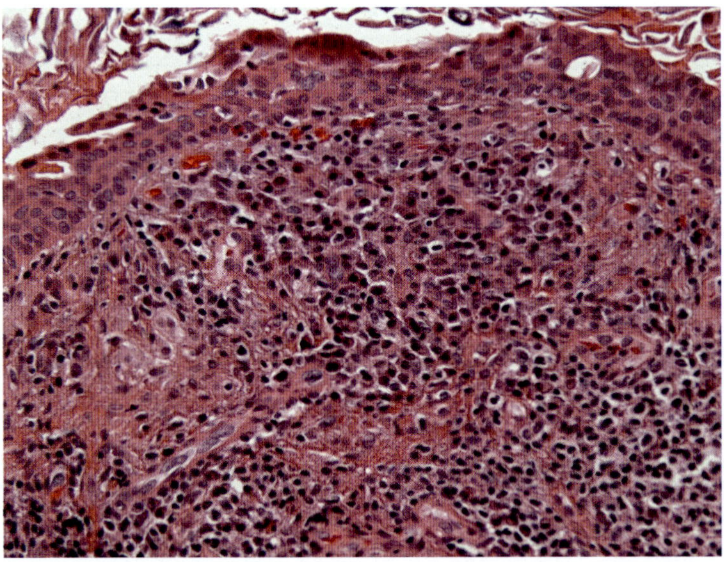

FIGURE 8.20 The fibrovascular cores of these papillary structures contain sheets and nodules of plasma cells. The papillary component typically lies in a central disposition connecting to an overlying epidermis which is centrally deficient, and there is a clinically and histologically demonstrable dell or pit at the epidermal surface.

component typically lies in a central disposition connecting to an overlying epidermis that is centrally deficient, and there is a clinically and histologically demonstrable dell or pit at the epidermal surface (Fig. 8.20). The base of the lesion has a nodular or pushing contour with tubuloalveolar structures admixed with papillary elements. Both components may be randomly disposed or may grow as columns into the underlying dermis, but nonetheless the lesion appears circumscribed at scanning magnification. Mitoses and individual cell necrosis may be seen as bizarre hyperchromatic misshapen nuclei attributed by some authorities to trauma. These lesions are benign with no well-documented examples in the literature having shown a metastatic potential. A striking squamous epithelial proliferative response reminiscent of keratoacanthoma can be seen.

HIDRADENOMA PAPILLIFERUM

The hidradenoma papilliferum typically occurs in the vulva and perineum and, therefore, is most common in woman.[54–56] As the apocrine glandular anlage is more widely dispersed as described earlier, tumors can occur in other locations as well[57] and are also seen in males.

Histopathology

The papillary hidradenoma has some morphological overlap with syringocystadenoma papilliferum, but comprises a homogenous population of apocrine epithelia, has a more pronounced tubuloalveolar and solid pattern of growth, and frequently does not open to the epidermal surface. Lesions may show individual cell atypia and mitotic activity, a finding that may prompt concern with respect to malignancy and in some instances, overdiagnosis (e-figs. 8.28–8.30).[58] Exceptional cases show coexistent extramammary Paget's disease, probably merely reflecting serendipity.

TUBULAR APOCRINE ADENOMA

The tubular or tubulopapillary apocrine adenoma is the apocrine analog of the papillary eccrine adenoma described earlier (e-figs. 8.31 and 8.32).[49,59–61]

MIXED LINEAGE SWEAT GLAND NEOPLASMS

Chondroid Syringoma (Benign Mixed Tumor of Skin)

Typically arising as a solitary nodule of the head and neck area,[62] some authors prefer the designation *benign mixed tumor* for this lesion whose tubular eccrine component, in concert with its clinical morphology, has little resemblance to the syringoma. In a fashion analogous to that of the major salivary gland tumor with a similar histomorphology, the benign mixed tumor reflects the multipotent capabilities of human cell lines.[63] Recognizing divergent differentiation in this neoplasm is the key to diagnosis. The stromal cells are of myoepithelial derivation and so have the capacity to produce cartilage, osteoid, and other matrix glycosaminoglycans as well as skeletal muscle, smooth muscle, and other mesenchymal lines.[64,65]

Histopathology

The chondroid syringoma manifests as a dermal-based myxoid and/or cartilaginous nodule with a well-circumscribed, pushing, lobular peripheral contour (Fig. 8.21, e-figs. 8.33–8.36). Embedded in the cartilaginous or myxoid matrix are tubuloalveolar branching structures comprising banal ductal epithelia of eccrine type with an internal cuticle (Fig. 8.22). A peripheral investiture of myoepithelial cells surrounds these tubules and branches at right angles from them into the stroma as attenuated spindle cells enmeshed in the myxoid matrix. This single cell myoepithelial component may become very prominent and lead to a misdiagnosis of malignant chondroid syringoma. Eccrine, apocrine, sebaceous, pilar, glandular, and squamous differentiation may be seen. These components are admixed in a stroma that variably shows myxoid, cartilaginous, osseous, or myoid features,[66,67] sometimes with nests of mature adipose tissue. All elements are banal with round to oval regular nuclei in the 10 to 15 μm size range showing evenly dispersed chromatin, small discrete nucleoli, and absent mitotic activity (Fig. 8.23). In a fashion analogous to the benign mixed tumor of major salivary glands, areas of solid sheetlike growth of epithelia

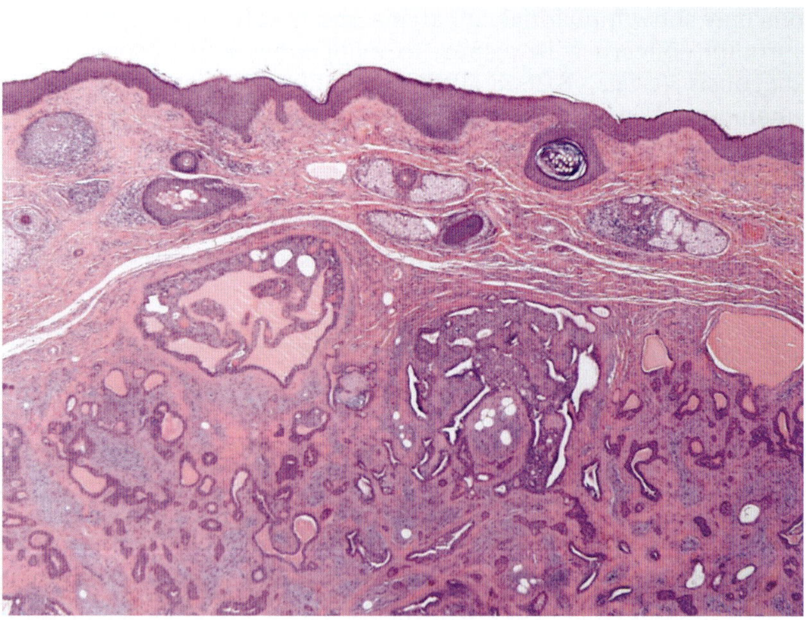

FIGURE 8.21 The chondroid syringoma manifests as a dermal-based myxoid and/or cartilaginous nodule with a well-circumscribed, pushing, lobular peripheral contour.

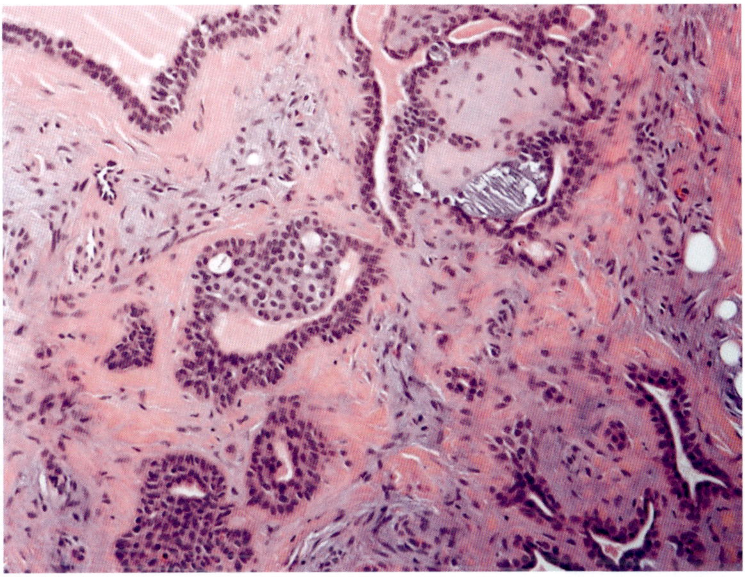

FIGURE 8.22 Embedded in the cartilaginous or myxoid matrix are tubuloalveolar branching structures comprising banal ductal epithelial cells of eccrine type with an internal cuticle. A peripheral investiture of myoepithelial cells surrounds these tubules and branches at right angles from them into the stroma as attenuated spindle and epithelioid cells enmeshed in the myxoid matrix.

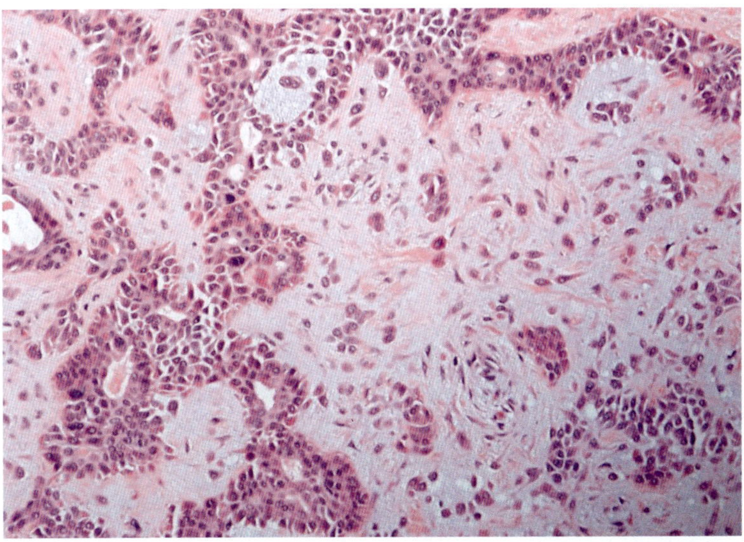

FIGURE 8.23 This single cell myoepithelial component may become prominent and lead to a misdiagnosis of a malignant chondroid syringoma. However, the glandular and myoepithelial elements are banal with round to oval regular nuclei in the 10 to 15 μm size range showing evenly dispersed chromatin, small discrete nucleoli, and absent mitotic activity.

or of the spindle cell component can be seen, and rarely one sees a confluent tubular proliferation with basement membrane material mimicking the adenoid cystic carcinoma of salivary gland type but lacking perineural invasion. Foci of necrosis and clear cell change complete the picture in some cases.[68,69]

Other Adnexal Neoplasms with Divergent Differentiation

Adnexal neoplasms of the skin can show differentiation patterns of bewildering complexity. Typically, these are mature cell lines whose terminal differentiation attests to a benign process. *Inter alia,* these components include those of sebaceous, pilar, admixed eccrine and apocrine, and a variety of mesenchymal cell lines. These lesions prompt an ever expanding plethora of appellations.[70] Some authorities recommend the use of a generic label, i.e., *mixed sweat gland adenoma* or *adnexal adenoma with divergent differentiation*[71]; we apply the terms *benign* or *malignant adnexal neoplasm with divergent differentiation* to those of clearly neoplastic nature and *complex primordial hamartoma* when appropriate.

BENIGN TUMORS OF THE PILOSEBACEOUS APPARATUS

Tumors of the pilosebaceous unit can occur in isolation or in combination with complex proliferations showing multilineal differentiation patterns encompassing those of sweat ducts, epidermis, and stroma with its varied components. We will first turn toward the sebaceous neoplasms and nonneoplastic sebaceous epithelial proliferations.

SEBACEOUS HYPERPLASIA

Sebaceous hyperplasia is a common lesion typically seen in the elderly and occurring most often in the midface including the eyelids.[72–79] Uncommonly, sebaceous hyperplasia is seen in the areolae mammae or in the skin of the genital region where confluent pebblelike plaques can occur.[80,81] When seen in the facial skin of the elderly, the most common differential diagnosis is that of a basal cell carcinoma. Sebaceous hyperplasia may form one of the lesions seen in the sebaceous neoplasia syndrome described by Muir and Torre. Other manifestations include an occasional zosteriform eruption of linear papules with a yellowish hue or occasional giant solitary nodules or plaques with a tendency toward confluence.[72,75,76] A rare autosomal dominantly inherited syndrome predisposes individuals to sebaceous hyperplasia in the second to fourth decades of life.[76,77]

Histology

Wick et al.[82] have attempted to define sebaceous hyperplasia as the presence of greater than three sebaceous lobules attached to the infundibulum of a pilosebaceous structure, but this is merely one form of sebaceous hyperplasia (Fig. 8.24, e-figs. 8.37 and 8.38). The other form comprises the presence

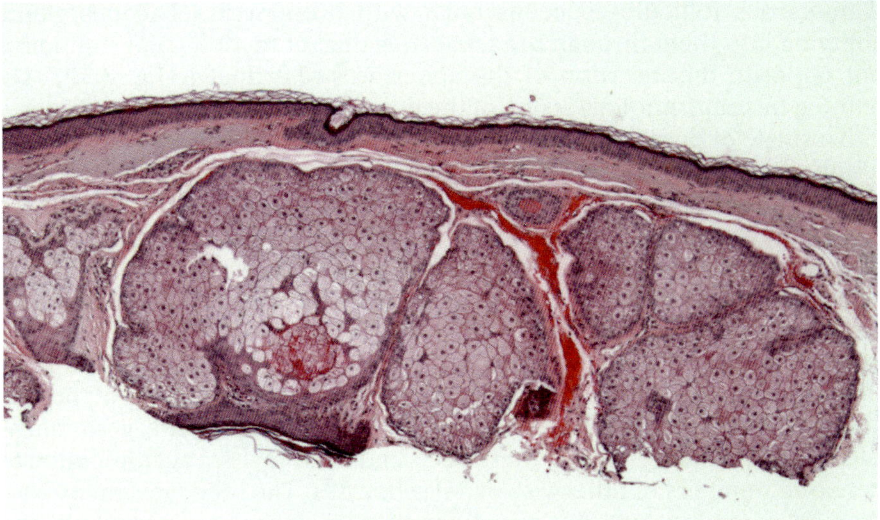

FIGURE 8.24 Wick et al.[82] defined sebaceous hyperplasia as the presence of greater than three sebaceous lobules attached to the infundibulum of a pilosebaceous structure.

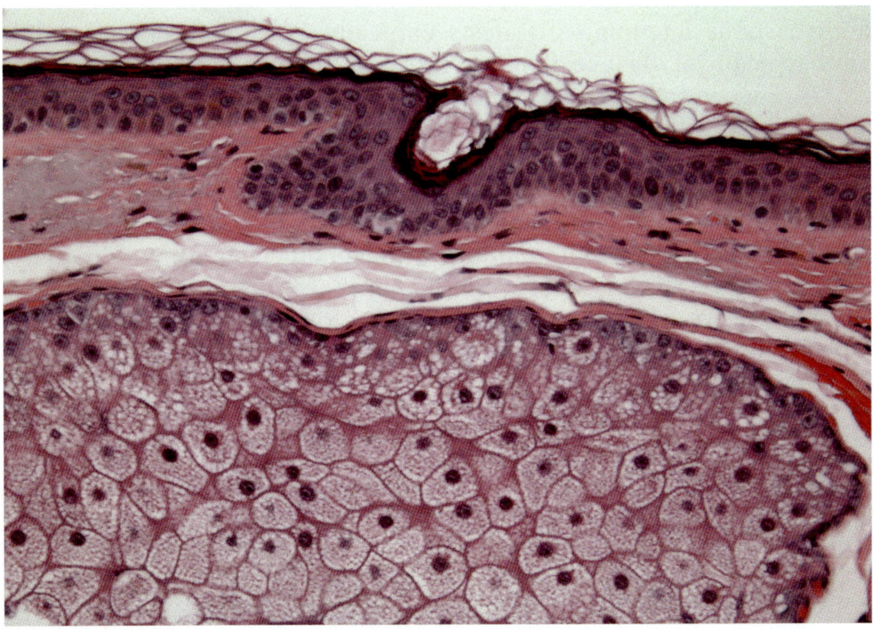

FIGURE 8.25 Irrespective of whether the sebaceous hyperplasia takes the former or the latter form, the defining histomorphology is one of mature sebocytes centrally disposed with a single or occasionally a double layer of germinative epithelium at the periphery of the lobule.

of numerous folliculosebaceous units with prominent sebaceous glands emptying into them through the sebaceous duct at the follicular infundibulum opposite the insertion of the apocrine sweat duct (e-fig. 8.39). The defining histomorphology is one of the mature sebocytes centrally disposed with a single or occasionally a double layer of germinative epithelium at the periphery of the lobule (Fig. 8.25). On occasion, one sees colonization of the follicular infundibulum by mites of *Demodex folliculorum*, particularly in the midfacial lesions of elderly males encompassing the condition termed "rhinophyma" and attributed in some instances to alcohol-based liver disease with impaired estrogen metabolism; this is considered a form of rosacea. A perifollicular lymphoid infiltrate is part of this histomorphology and may contribute to the hyperplasia by the elaboration of cytokines such as interleukin-2 by T helper lymphocytes of the Th1 phenotype; this leukotriene upregulates bcl-2 expression, immortalizing the germinative cells[83] and in theory could, therefore, lead to the slow accumulation of increased numbers of otherwise banal sebocytes. The sebocytes themselves are recognized by abundant quantities of clear vacuolated cytoplasm that often indents the nucleus. The overlying epidermis can be atrophic, thickened, or normal depending upon the presence of exogenous insults such as persistent rubbing.

SEBACEOUS ADENOMA

The sebaceous adenoma manifests clinically as a pale yellow nodular lesion, typically of the face, that expresses itself clinically after the age of 50. Tumors range in size from less than 1 to greater than 5 cm.[84–89] These lesions are associated with the Muir–Torre syndrome, comprising the coexpression of cutaneous neoplasms including those of sebaceous type with well-differentiated squamous epithelial neoplasms and visceral malignancies including carcinomas of breast, ovary, gastrointestinal tract, and larynx.[90–95] An occasional patient may manifest a malignant lymphoma of nodal or extranodal type.[94] Sebaceous neoplasms in the setting of Muir–Torre syndrome are often difficult to classify, showing overlap features between all of the prototypic forms of sebaceous neoplasm ranging from hyperplasia to carcinoma.[95]

Histology

The prototypic sebaceous adenoma manifests 1 to 2 layers of germinative cells that mature to form central sebocytes and have an architecture comprising a sharply circumscribed sebaceous lobule surrounded by a compressed pseudocapsule of dermal stroma. There is no connection to the hair follicle, and the germinative component occupies 30% to 50% of the entire cell population of the sebaceous lobule. The overlying epidermis may be attenuated but sometimes forms a collarette around the peripheral aspect of the neoplasm (Figs. 8.26 and 8.27, e-figs. 8.40 and 8.41). Unlike sebaceous hyperplasia, occasional mitoses may be seen in the lobules

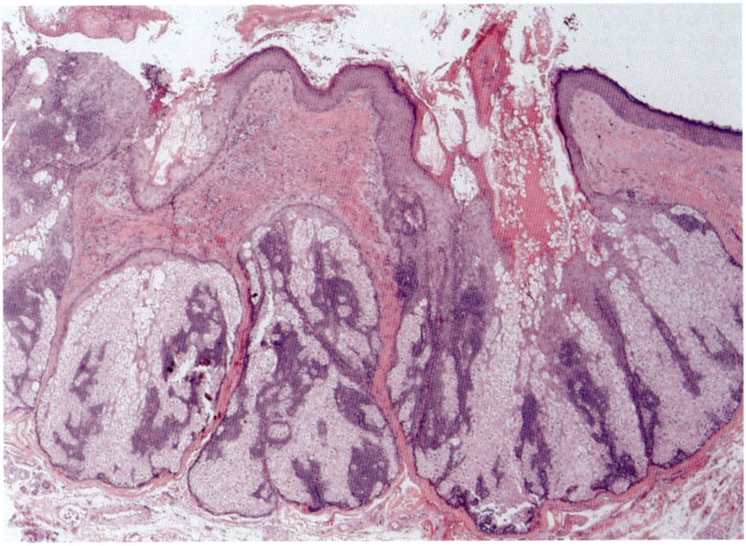

FIGURE 8.26 Sebaceous lobules in the prototypic sebaceous adenoma are contiguous with the epidermis but not in the context of their origin from follicular structures.

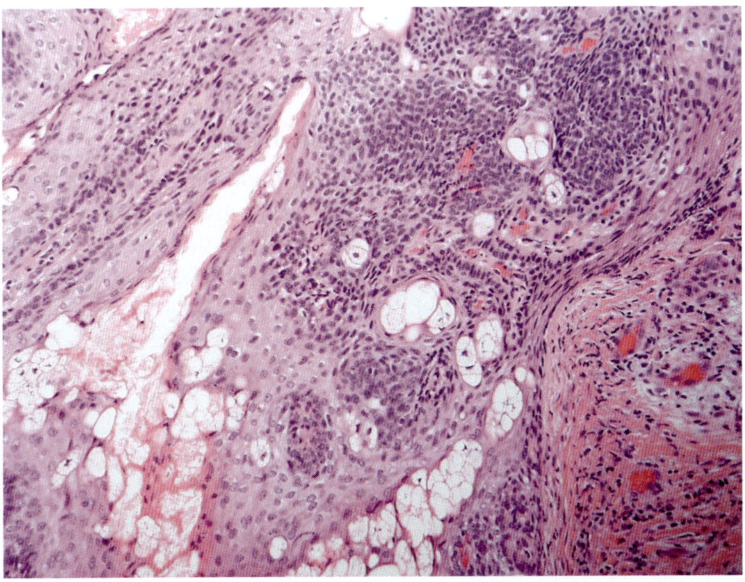

FIGURE 8.27 The lobules are defined by a germinative cell populace which exceeds that encountered in sebaceous gland hyperplasia, typically defining 30% to 50% of the entire cell population with centrally located mature sebocytes.

of a sebaceous adenoma and in concert with this, the nucleoli may be somewhat prominent but pleomorphism, hyperchromasia, and individual cell necrosis of the sebaceous epithelioma are not apparent. Dysplastic epithelial changes may signify an association with Muir–Torre syndrome.

SUPERFICIAL EPITHELIOMA WITH SEBACEOUS DIFFERENTIATION

The superficial epithelioma with sebaceous differentiation appears to represent a slow growing smooth surfaced papule or keratotic nodule on the face, trunk, or thigh.[96]

Histopathology

The lesions mimic a tumor of follicular infundibulum or superficial basal cell carcinoma by virtue of anastomosing cells that connect broadly to the basal layer of epidermis and have an orientation parallel to the epidermal surface. Some examples show peripheral palisading, leading one of us (ANC) to suggest that this represents a form of superficial basal cell carcinoma with sebaceous differentiation cognate to the sebaceous epithelioma,[97] while other examples show squamous differentiation.

SEBACEOUS EPITHELIOMA

This tumor is another benign adnexal neoplasm of sebaceous gland origin, whereby the dominant proliferating cell is a germinative one that typically exceeds 50% of the entire neoplastic cell population. This tumor can be seen in association with Muir–Torre's syndrome.

Histology

The classic tumor is contiguous with the epidermis and exhibits a downward lobulated growth pattern comprising basaloid appearing cells with central foci of sebaceous differentiation. The mature sebocyte component typically defines less than 50% of the entire cell population. Neither necrosis is present, nor is there a significant cytologic atypia or retraction artefact. Dysplastic epithelial changes should prompt consideration of Muir–Torre syndrome (Figs. 8.28 and 8.29, e-figs. 8.42 and 8.43). One of us (ANC) feels that these lesions are best considered part of the spectrum of indolent growth basal cell epithelioma.

NEVUS SEBACEUS

Nevi sebaceus are often present at birth or in young life, but in practical terms, patients may be unaware of these lesions until their adulthood. Thus, even patients in the fourth to sixth decades of life occasionally have a lesion biopsied to exclude a carcinoma or keratosis which is in fact a nevus sebaceus. On the scalp, a nevus sebaceus may produce localized alopecia or manifest as a tan-colored plaque with a rough surface, the latter representing the epidermal component. Prior to puberty, these lesions have no significant sebaceous component, thus the tan or a brown coloration. In and around puberty, sebaceous glands become prominent, the coloration of the plaque changes from tan-brown to yellowish, and the sebaceous component contributes to the verruciform surface. Rare cases are associated with systemic abnormalities such as seizures, mental retardation, or defects in visual fields.[98–103]

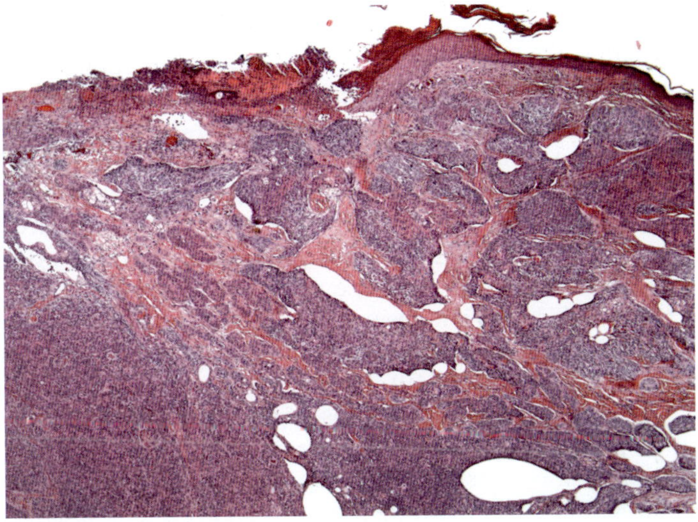

FIGURE 8.28 The tumor is contiguous with the epidermis and exhibits a downward lobulated growth pattern comprising basaloid appearing cells with central foci of sebaceous differentiation.

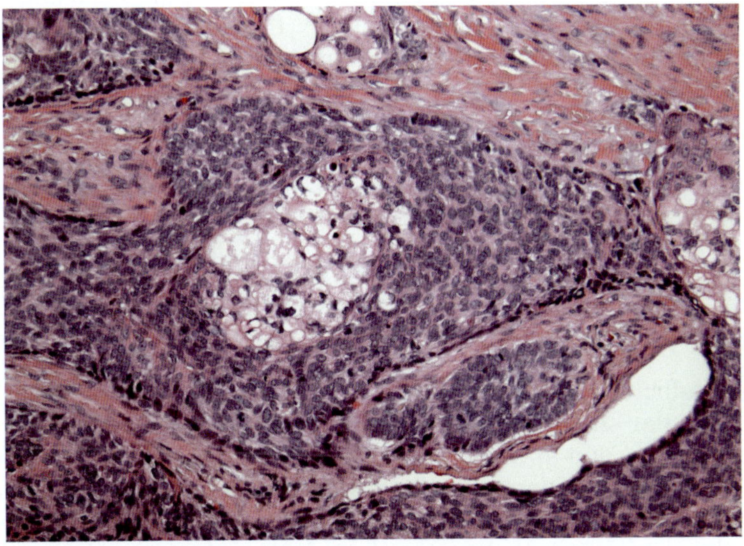

FIGURE 8.29 The mature sebocyte component typically defines more than 50% of the entire cell population. Neither necrosis is present nor is there significant cytologic atypia or retraction artefact.

Histopathology

The nevus sebaceus is a hamartoma with contributions from epidermis, adnexal structures, and mesenchymal elements, the varying proportions of which depend in part upon whether the patient is prepubertal or postpubertal. Prior to puberty, in part the nevus sebaceus may have no recognizable sebaceous elements and is typified by a verruciform epidermal hyperplasia with prominence of adnexal structures including ectopic apocrine glands. Near or after puberty, sebaceous glands become prominent. These are abortive hamartomatous glands that do not connect in the normal fashion through the sebaceous duct to the necks of the follicular bulges. Rather, these miniaturized sebaceous glands open directly to the epidermal surface (e-figs. 8.44–8.47). The lack of association with a mature pilosebaceous unit is associated in turn with a lack of polarizable terminal or vellus hairs, and in consequence one can use polarized light microscopy to delineate the transverse edge of the lesion; where mature hair shafts are identified, the histomorphology represents normal pilosebaceous structures of the native scalp (e-figs. 8.48 and 8.49). Like the sebaceous glands, the apocrine component is typically not conspicuous prior to puberty. A variety of additional lesions may be seen in the setting of nevus sebaceus[104] that are, at least at their inception, possibly hamartomatous in character. These include basal cell epithelioma, proliferating pilar tumor, syringocystadenoma papilliferum, trichilemmoma, apocrine adenoma, sebaceous adenoma, and piloleiomyoma. Although these proliferations may initially be hamartomata, there is no question that neoplastic transformation can occur. In a fashion cognate to that described in the transformation from superficial and nodular to infiltrative growth basal cell carcinoma,[105] the elaboration of cytokines by T-helper lymphocytes may immortalize basaloid epithelia. Subsequent mutagenic "hits" might then lead to an aggressive basal cell carcinoma. Other undisputed malignant neoplasms shown in continuity with nevus sebaceus include squamous cell carcinoma and ductal apocrine adenocarcinoma.[106] The desmoplastic trichilemmoma has also been associated with the nevus sebaceus (Figs. 8.30–8.32, e-figs. 8.50 and 8.51).[105]

BENIGN TUMORS OF THE HAIR FOLLICLE APPARATUS

Tumors of the Outer Root Sheath and Hair Follicle Infundibulum

The hair follicle infundibulum includes the hair pore and that segment of the follicular structure above the follicular bulge (the insertion points of the sebaceous and apocrine ducts). In the infundibulum, keratinization mimics that of the epidermal surface with an internal squamous epithelial lining manifesting keratohyalin granule formation. Deep to the insertion sites of the apocrine and sebaceous ducts is the isthmic portion of the hair follicle where the so-called abrupt or trichilemmal keratinization occurs. In this form of keratinization, the epithelium shows no keratohyalin granule formation separating it from the follicular contents.

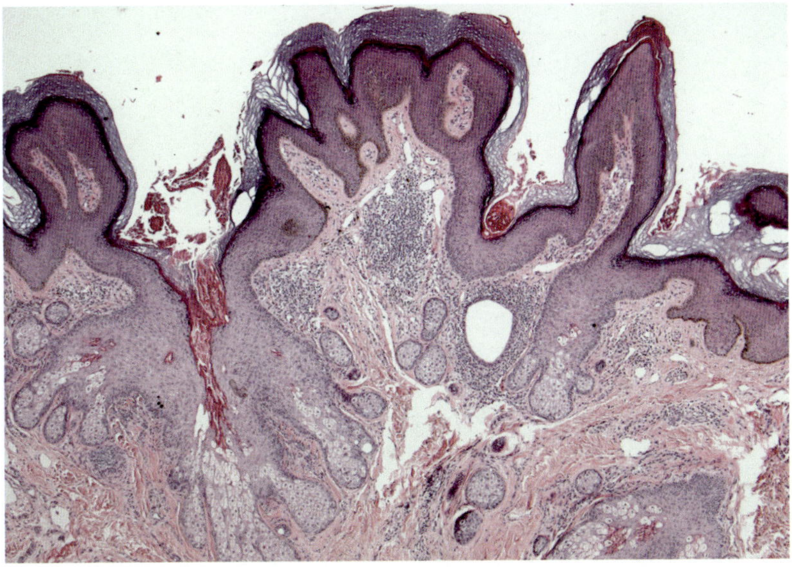

FIGURE 8.30 In nevus sebaceus the surface assumes a verrucous undulating architecture reminiscent of an epidermal nevus. However, there are foci of follicular hamartomatous proliferations contiguous with the epidermis. All components of the hair unit may be present, however, there is no hair shaft production.

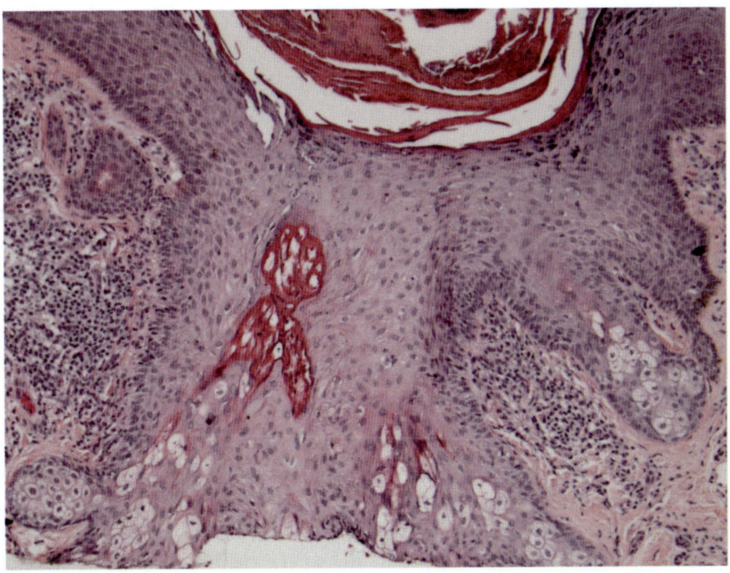

FIGURE 8.31 This hamartomatous follicular structure shows follicular infundibular and germinative epithelium. There is no hair shaft.

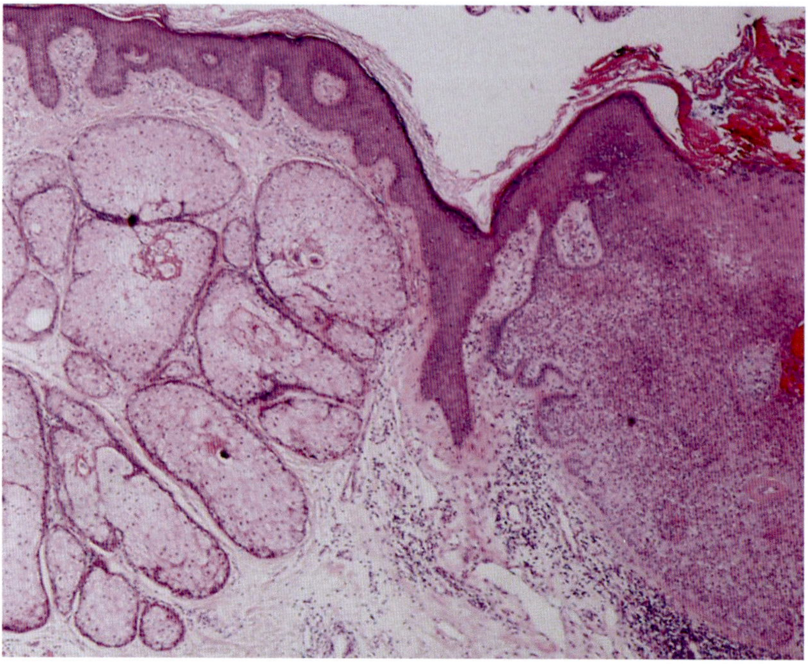

FIGURE 8.32 Neoplasms can arise in lesions of nevus sebaceus. This particular lesion showed an area of trichilemmoma (right half of panel).

Tumor of the Follicular Infundibulum

The tumor of follicular infundibulum is a rare lesion that appears in middle-aged or elderly women as a solitary papule or nodule on the upper lip. Although this is the classic distribution, other sites such as shoulders, head, and neck may be seen. Multiple lesions are extremely uncommon but have been reported arising in a nevus sebaceus or in the setting of Cowden syndrome.[107–111] These lesions are held to represent a superficial variant of trichilemmoma by most. It is our contention that these lesions in fact are an intraepidermal variant of trichilemmoma that lacks the down-growing endophytic growth pattern of the classic example. The histomorphology comprises a platelike horizontal extension of epithelium of presumed follicular infundibular derivation that grows as radiating arrays indented by a prominent stroma. Along its peripheral margins, the epithelia may show nuclear palisading and clear cell change due to high glycogen content held to reflect the outer root sheath derivation (Fig. 8.33, e-figs. 8.52 and 8.53). A corresponding wrinkled eosinophilic external cuticle of the basement membranelike material often surrounds the horizontally disposed cell cords. The cells themselves are banal with neither mitotic activity nor apoptotic debris identifiable. These neoplasms or hamartomata lack hair bulb formation and in consequence, hair shaft material is not seen.[112] The

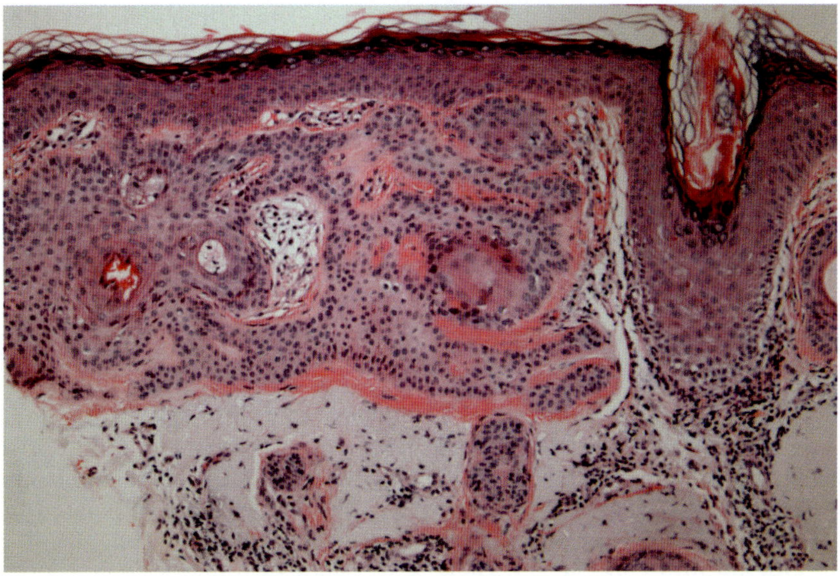

FIGURE 8.33 The tumor of the follicular infundibulum is a superficial variant of a trichilemmoma. It originates in the epidermis; the epithelium can be pale due to intracytoplasmic glycogen accumulation. A horizontal interanastomosing pattern with stromal indentation in a platelike fashion is characteristic.

differential diagnosis includes superficial basal cell carcinoma, seborrheic keratosis, and inverted follicular keratosis. Superficial basal cell carcinomas manifest slitlike retraction of stroma with mucinotic material, while seborrheic keratoses typically have an exophytic component comprising basaloid cells with a mammillated surface even if pseudohorn cysts are not evident. The trichilemmoma may merit consideration, but this is typically a lobular growth pattern of clear cells with a peripheral palisade as opposed to a horizontal platelike epithelial proliferation oriented perpendicular to the epidermal surface. Unlike basal cell carcinoma, the tumor of follicular infundibulum does not decorate with the Ber-EP4 antibody.[113]

Pilar Sheath Acanthoma and Dilated Pore of Winer

The pilar sheath acanthoma classically manifests in middle-aged or elderly patients as a single pink-tan papule of the upper lip or central face, often with a small central keratotic plug.[114–116] The dilated pore of Winer has a rather similar histomorphology but can be seen anywhere on hair bearing skin. Both lesions likely represent a form of hyperplasia of the infundibular component of the pilosebaceous apparatus.

HISTOPATHOLOGY. Both lesions show a keratin-filled central infundibular proliferation that opens to the epidermal surface and has an acanthotic lining with radiating lobules of cells extending into the adjacent dermis. The cells are banal with pale or clear cytoplasms containing glycogen and often manifest a peripheral palisading basaloid rim. These cells have banal nuclei, absent mitoses, and no individual cell necrosis (Fig. 8.34). While the pilar sheath acanthoma is rare, the dilated pore of Winer is common. Typically, the dilated pore has a larger epidermal opening to the skin surface in the fashion of an open comedo and it may have small sebaceous glands or vellus hairs in its base (Fig. 8.35, e-figs. 8.54 and 8.55). The degree of epithelial proliferation is typically less. In that sense, the dilated pore of Winer is an exaggerated comedo with slight acanthosis of the follicular wall.

Trichoadenoma

The trichoadenoma is an uncommon neoplasm of the head and neck and occasionally of the trunk that manifests as a solitary nodule less than 1 cm in diameter.[117–120]

HISTOPATHOLOGY. The trichoadenoma manifests microcysts comprising epithelium showing a pilar keratinization pattern; the cells form grouped and clustered small nodules within the dermal stroma unassociated with desmoplasia or with an epidermal connection. The nuclei are banal, and mitoses and apoptosis are absent (Figs. 8.36 and 8.37, e-figs. 8.56 and 8.57).

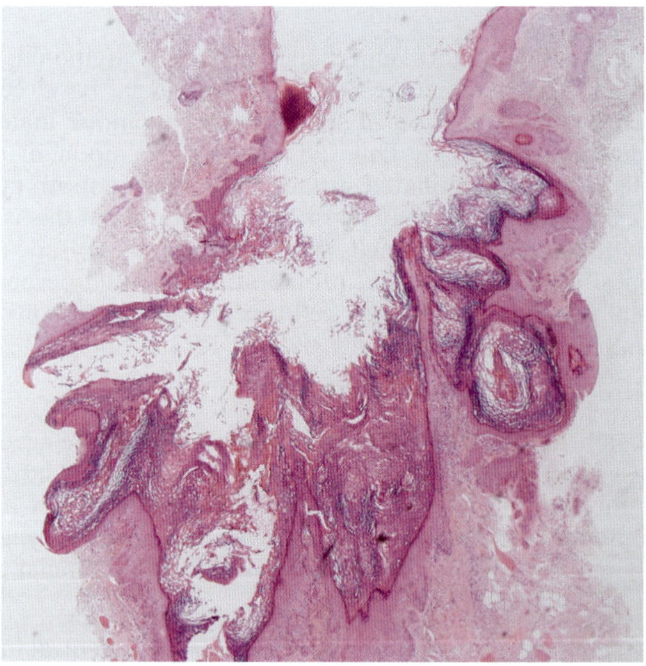

FIGURE 8.34 Both lesions show a keratin-filled central infundibular proliferation that opens to the epidermal surface and has an acanthotic lining with radiating lobules of cells extending into the adjacent dermis.

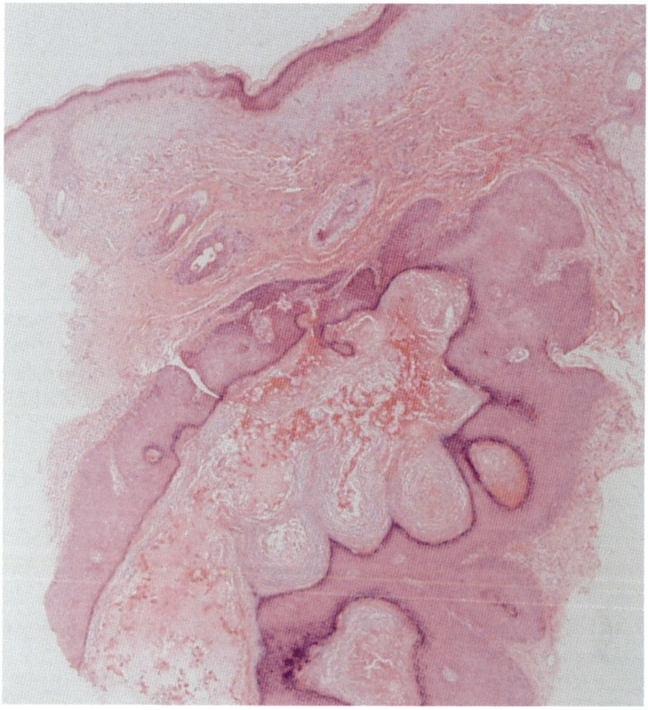

FIGURE 8.35 Typically, the dilated pore has a larger epidermal opening to the skin surface in the fashion of an open comedo and it may have small sebaceous glands or vellus hairs in its base.

Trichilemmoma

Although there is controversy regarding Bernard Ackerman's hypothesis that trichilemmoma is in fact a regressing verruca showing trichilemmal differentiation,[121] we appreciate his observation, as the combination of a verruciform or digitate surface architecture surmounted by columns of parakeratosis with lobular acanthosis in its base encapsulates the morphology well. Different observers have variably shown either the presence or the absence[122] of HPV DNA in trichilemmomas by molecular methodologies. Trichilemmomas comprise glycogen rich cells with a peripheral palisade at their margin and a frequent sharp demarcation from the uninvolved adjacent epidermis. These lesions are typically encountered in the midface or neck and may be seen throughout life, but are most commonly encountered in adults,[123-125] some of whom have multiple lesions in the context of Cowden syndrome.[126-128] Cowden syndrome is a disorder of autosomal dominant inheritance comprising hamartomatous polyps of the intestines with an increased risk of breast, thyroid, and other visceral malignancy and cutaneous tumors[129] including collagenomas and hamartomas of adnexal structures. Cowden syndrome is caused by a mutation of the PTEN gene

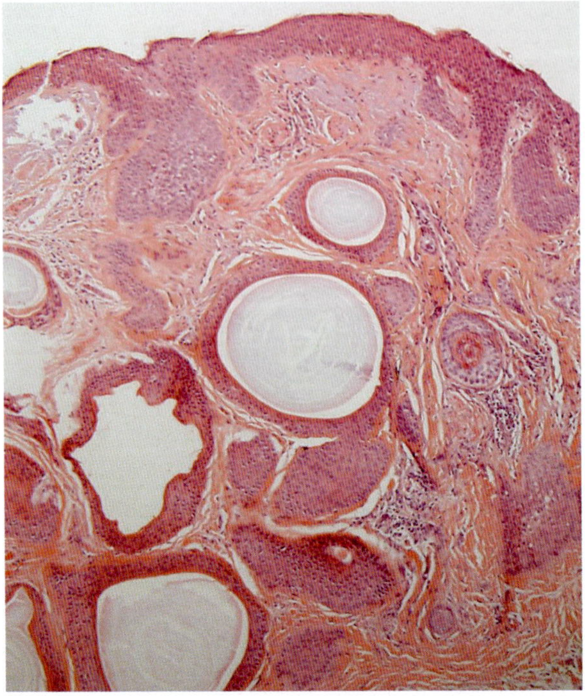

FIGURE 8.36 The trichoadenoma manifests microcysts comprising epithelium showing a pilar keratinization pattern most often.

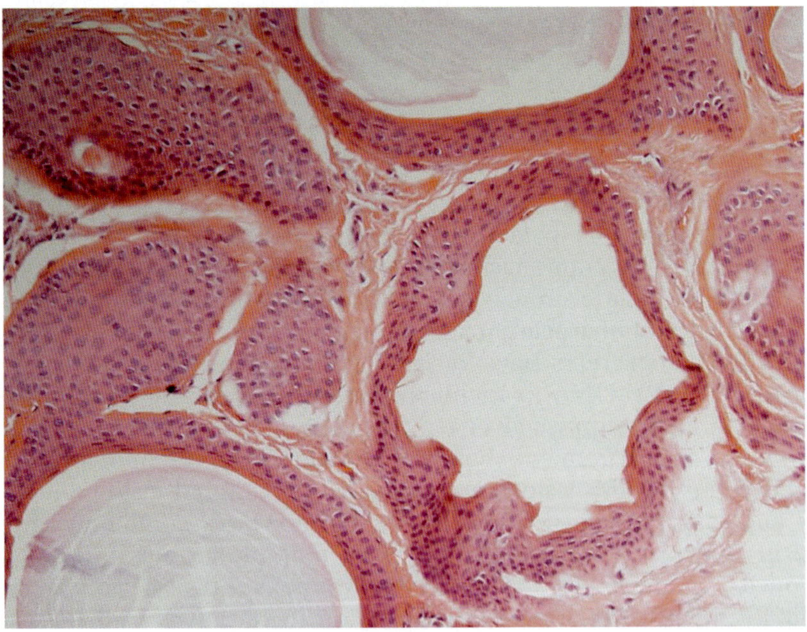

FIGURE 8.37 The cells form grouped and clustered small nodules within the dermal stroma unassociated with desmoplasia or with an epidermal connection. The nuclei are banal, and mitoses and apoptosis are absent.

on chromosome 10q23 that encodes a lipid phosphatase that acts through the phosphoinositol-3-kinase/Akt pathway to promote G1 cell cycle arrest and apoptosis.[130]

HISTOPATHOLOGY. As mentioned, the trichilemmoma combines features of a regressing wart with a glycogen-rich basaloid proliferation showing peripheral palisading but lacking the slitlike retraction of a basal cell carcinoma. Cells are banal cytologically, lack mitosis or individual cell necrosis, and contain abundant quantities of glycogen within their cytoplasms. There is often an underlying eosinophilic cuticle or mantle of basement membranelike material mimicking the outer root sheath of the hair follicle infundibulum (Figs. 8.38 and 8.39, e-figs. 8.58–8.60). An important variant of trichilemmoma is the desmoplastic trichilemmoma.[105,131,132] In this lesion, although the overlying verruciform epidermal architecture and the areas of classic basaloid proliferation with clear cell change seen in the trichilemmoma are frequently identified, in the center growing deep into the thickened basement membrane mantle are tongues of squamoid cells enmeshed in a densely collagenized stroma (Figs. 8.40 and 8.41). These lesions may be misinterpreted as trichilemmal carcinoma with serious consequences for the patients. In some cases, atypical basaloid proliferations including in the context of basal cell carcinoma are present lateral to or in

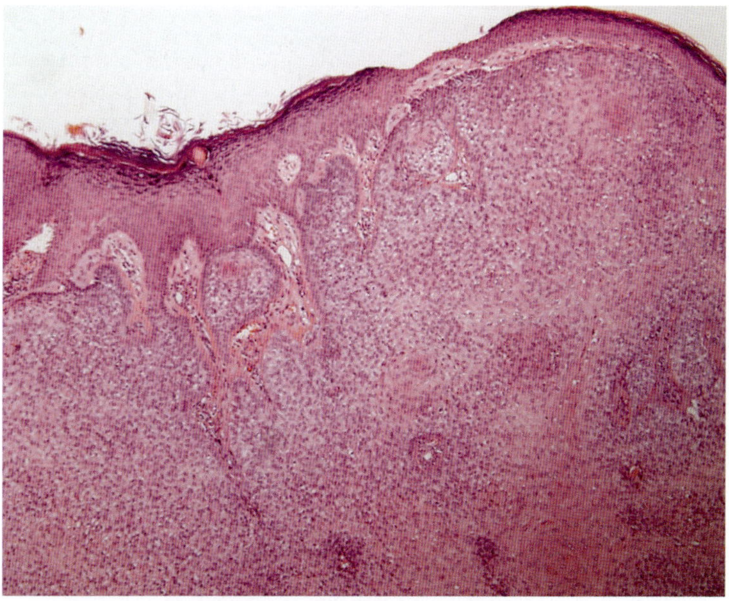

FIGURE 8.38 The trichilemmoma combines features of a regressing wart with a glycogen-rich basaloid proliferation showing peripheral palisading but lacking the slit-like retraction of a basal cell carcinoma. Cells are banal cytologically, lack mitosis or individual cell necrosis, and contain abundant quantities of glycogen within their cytoplasms.

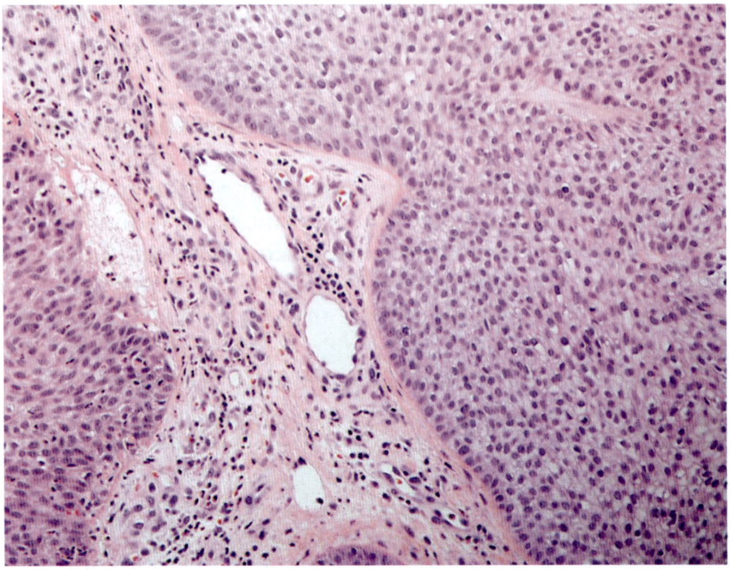

FIGURE 8.39 There is often an underlying eosinophilic cuticle or mantle of basement membrane-like material mimicking the outer root sheath of the hair follicle infundibulum.

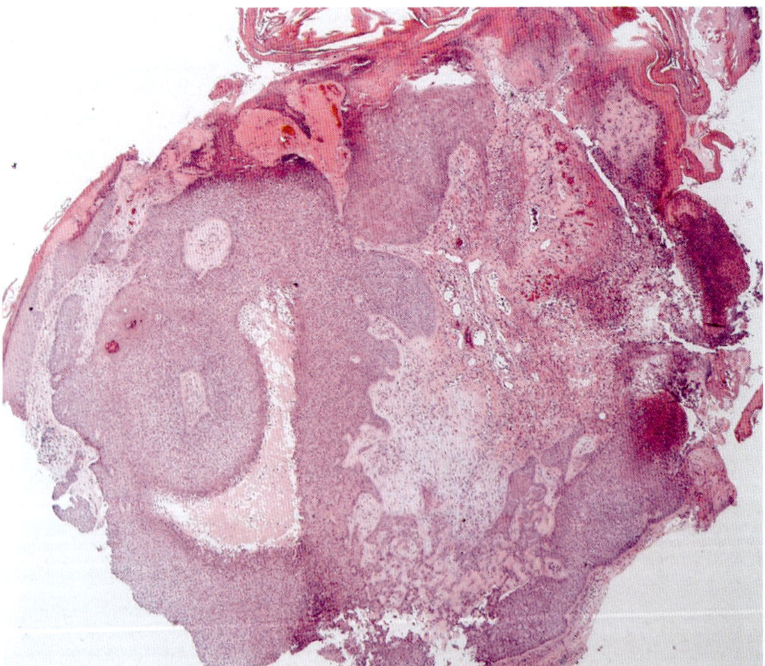

FIGURE 8.40 An important variant is the desmoplastic trichilemmoma. In this lesion, the overlying verruciform epidermal architecture and the areas of classic basaloid proliferation with clear cell change seen in the trichilemmoma are identified.

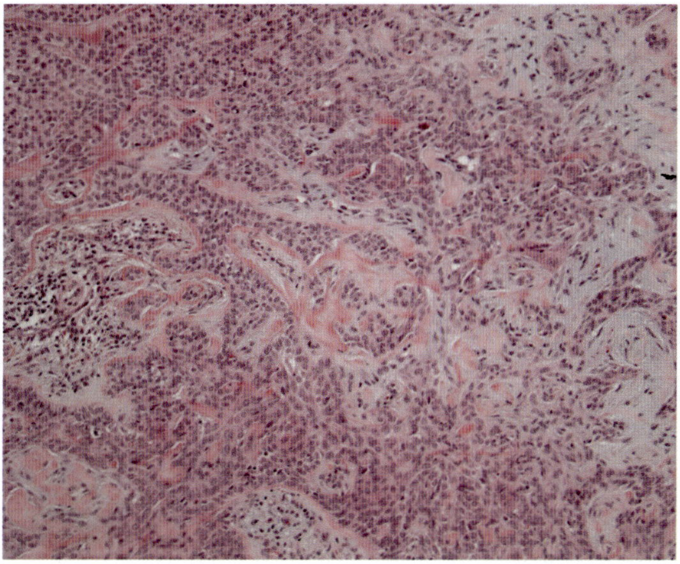

FIGURE 8.41 In the center of the lesions deep into the thickened basement membrane mantle are tongues of squamoid cells enmeshed in a densely collagenized stroma.

continuity with the desmoplastic trichilemmoma.[105] In our experience, this happens in up to 20% of lesions and in consequence, we advise complete excision of all desmoplastic trichilemmoma that we encounter in practice.[105] Unlike trichilemmal carcinoma, which is in our view, a trichilemmal form of squamous cell carcinoma, the desmoplastic trichilemmoma lacks significant mitotic activity or significant nuclear atypia. The best defense against overdiagnosis of trichilemmal carcinoma is knowledge of the entity and recognition of the underlying features of concomitant, otherwise prototypic, trichilemmoma nearby.

Proliferating Pilar Tumor (Proliferating Trichilemmal Cyst)

The proliferating pilar tumor is a benign tumor with a strong predilection for the scalp for elderly women.[133–138] It may occur in other anatomical locations such as the extremities or trunk. The lesion is slow growing and has typically been present for years prior to its being brought to clinical attention due to erosion of the surface.

HISTOPATHOLOGY. The proliferating pilar tumor comprises a sharply circumscribed lesion characterized by an enfolded architecture of thickened bands of squamous epithelia showing pilar-type (i.e., trichilemmal) keratinization, often with an abundant quantity of eosinophilic homogenous intracystic material. The neoplastic cells are large polygonal cells of isthmic hair follicle derivation that lack nuclear atypia or mitotic activity in the prototypic benign neoplasm. Anastomosing fascicles surround a central cystic area; frequently, the eosinophilic polygonal cells are admixed with those having clear cytoplasms rich in glycogen and often surrounded by a thickened wrinkled mantle of basement membranelike material (e-figs. 8.61–8.63). Cytologically, these are proplastic cells with somewhat larger, spherical or oval nuclei than other benign pilosebaceous neoplasms and frequently show prominent nucleoli. When nuclear pleomorphism and mitotic activity supervene, the lesions can have a worrisome morphology suggestive of a malignant proliferating pilar tumor (see next section). Even in benign examples, up to ten mitoses are seen in ten 40× high power fields.[82] Despite the sometimes worrisome cytology and brisk mitotic activity, these lesions are sharply circumscribed with a pushing as opposed to an infiltrative margin.

TUMORS OF THE GERMINATIVE FOLLICULAR ANLAGE

Neoplasms that arise from the germinative components of the hair follicle generate a bewildering array of morphologies cognate to the hair differentiation seen in embryonic and adult human skin. These germinative components of the normal hair follicle are the matrical cells, cells of the cortex, and cells of the inner root sheath. The hallmark of matrical differentiation is the so-called shadow cell that typifies the pilomatrixoma and other matrical neoplasms.[139] We will consider trichoblastomas and trichodysgerminomas, which are in fact derived from the follicular hair germ in the section on tumors with significant follicular mesenchymal stromal participation.

Trichofolliculoma

The trichofolliculoma is a tumor of the head and neck that typically manifests as a small flesh-colored nodule on the nose or midface of an adult, who presents with a dome-shaped lesion having a central keratotic plug from which protrude vellus hair shafts (e-fig. 8.64).[140,141]

HISTOPATHOLOGY. Manifesting a central keratin-filled dilated follicular infundibulum containing the vellus hair material and being in continuity with the epidermal surface when identified in a vertical section, the trichofolliculoma manifests radiating bands or ribbons of squamous epithelial cells that connect to germinative follicular epithelia and form anagen hair bulb structures (Figs. 8.42 and 8.43, e-figs. 8.65–8.67). There is a dense collagenous stroma which indents these radiating squamous epithelial bands, the latter showing isthmic or infundibular differentiation and keratinization. Some cell bands will show outer root sheath differentiation with clear cytoplasms rich in glycogen and peripheral palisading, while others will have matrical morphology. The so-called sebaceous trichofolliculoma is one in which sebaceous differentiation is seen in an otherwise prototypic trichofolliculoma, suggesting that in fact these are hamartomatous lesions.[142] The so-called folliculosebaceous cystic hamartoma is, in our view, closely related to the so-called sebaceous trichofolliculoma if it does not in fact represent the same lesion.[143–146]

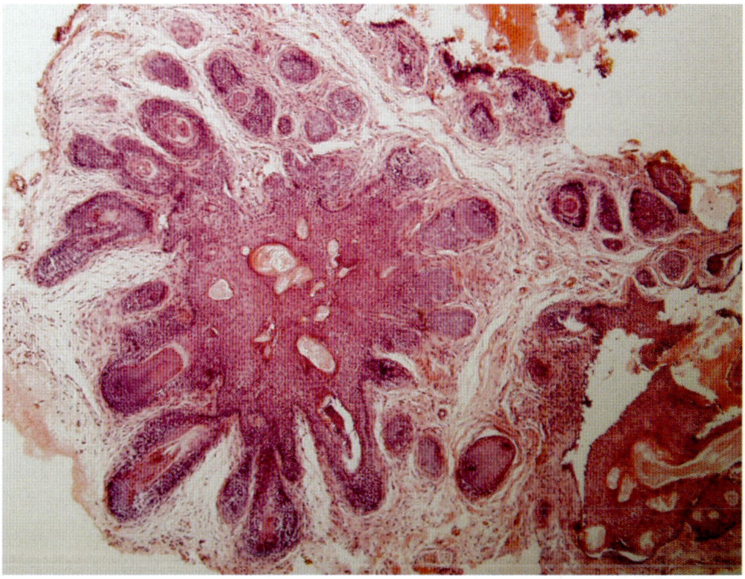

FIGURE 8.42 Manifesting a central keratin-filled dilated follicular infundibulum containing vellus hair material and being in continuity with the epidermal surface when identified in a vertical section, the trichofolliculoma manifests radiating bands or ribbons of squamous epithelial cells which connect to germinative follicular epithelia and form anagen hair bulb structures from which emanate vellus hairs. Each hair unit is complete.

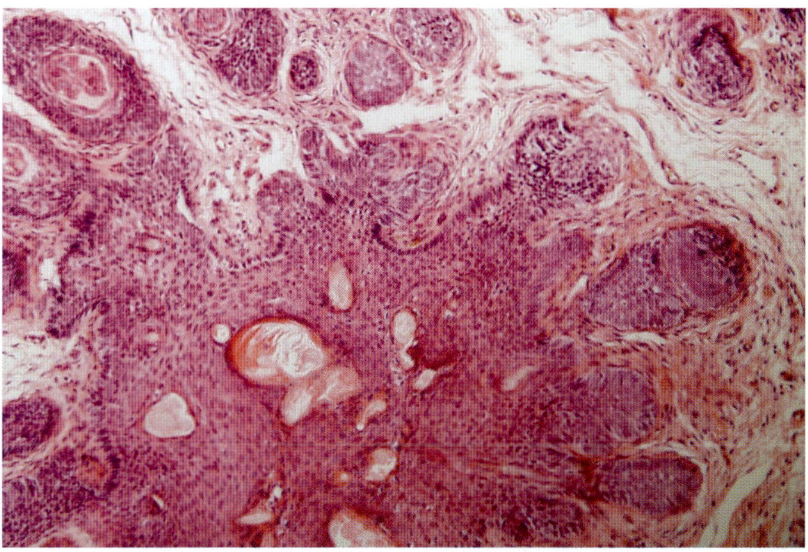

FIGURE 8.43 The trichofolliculoma manifests radiating bands or ribbons of squamous epithelial cells which connect to germinative follicular epithelia and form anagen hair bulb structures from which emanate vellus hairs. Papillary mesenchymal bodies and features of stromal induction are evident.

Trichoepithelioma

Typically arising as a solitary flesh colored papule of the face presenting in childhood or adult life,[147–149] the trichoepithelioma raises consideration to a basal cell epithelioma at the clinical level. Multiple lesions of trichoepithelioma may be seen in the Brooke–Fordyce syndrome transmitted as an autosomal dominant disease complex of multiple trichoepitheliomas up to 1 cm in diameter, involving the face in a sometimes confluent fashion with occasional extrafacial lesions, cylindromas, spiradenomas, tricholemmomas, or basal cell epitheliomas,[150–152] and sometimes with extracutaneous genodermatoses. The latter include the Rombo's syndrome of milia, atrophoderma, hypotrichosis, and vasodilatation; some patients with multiple trichoepitheliomas show an association with systemic connective tissue diseases such as lupus erythematosus and myasthenia gravis.[153,154]

HISTOPATHOLOGY. The trichoepithelioma has a stereotypic morphology irrespective of whether a patient has one or multiple lesions. It comprises uniform basaloid cells arranged in discrete nests associated with the specialized mesenchymal stroma described earlier. The combination of epithelia and stroma together forms a complex that is well circumscribed and sharply demarcated from the adjacent native dermal stroma (e-figs. 8.68–8.70). Depending upon the plane of section examined, the basaloid lobules may connect to each other. Keratin-containing microcysts, typically lined by cells showing infundibular differentiation with the so-called epidermal keratinization and concomitant keratohyaline granules or, less frequently, isthmic differentiation with abrupt trichilemmal keratinization, are dispersed through the lesions. These keratinous microcysts frequently rupture with an associated foreign body giant cell reaction. Reflecting the presence of the germinative hair papillae generated in the trichoepithelioma are papillary mesenchymal bodies that represent protrusions of modified stroma into the clawlike extension of the basaloid epithelia as it recapitulates the anagen bulb (Figs. 8.44 and 8.45). The absence of hair shaft production is a key observation.

Desmoplastic Trichoepithelioma

The tumor that bears the name *desmoplastic trichoepithelioma* may not in fact be of the same histogenetic basis as the conventional trichoepithelioma[82,155,156] The desmoplastic trichoepithelioma is almost always a solitary lesion and is not associated with any specific genodermatosis syndrome. It presents as an umbilicated nodule in the midface of a young or middle-aged woman.

HISTOPATHOLOGY. As the name implies, this is a sclerosing adnexal neoplasm comprising columns of rather banal basaloid epithelia enmeshed in a dense collagenized stroma and unassociated with slitlike stromal retraction, apoptosis, or mitotic activity. Typically, the upper half of the lesion is associated with keratinous microcysts as one associates with conventional trichoepithelioma and in many such cases a foreign body granulomatous reaction to extravasated keratin is identified admixed

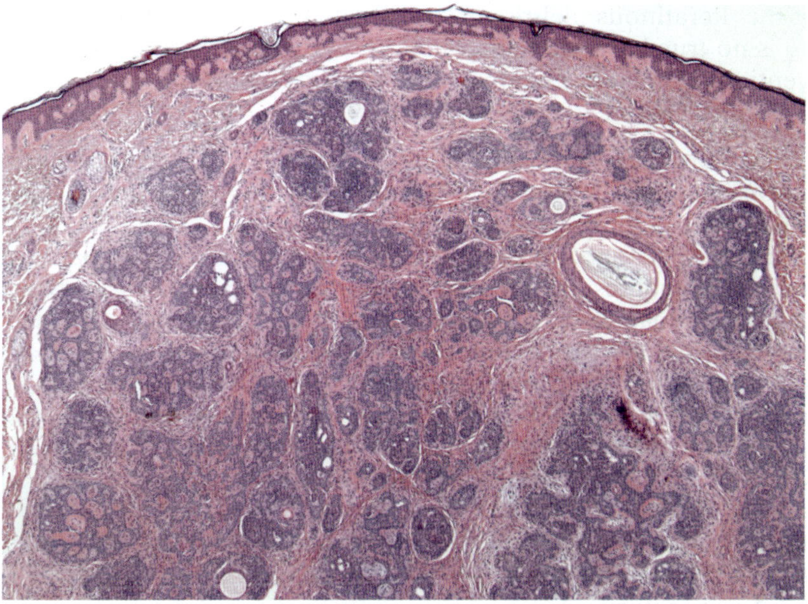

FIGURE 8.44 The trichoepithelioma has a stereotypic morphology irrespective of whether a patient has one or multiple lesions. It comprises uniform basaloid cells arranged in discrete nests associated with the specialized stroma described earlier. The combination of epithelia and stroma together forms a complex that is well circumscribed and sharply demarcated from the adjacent native dermal stroma.

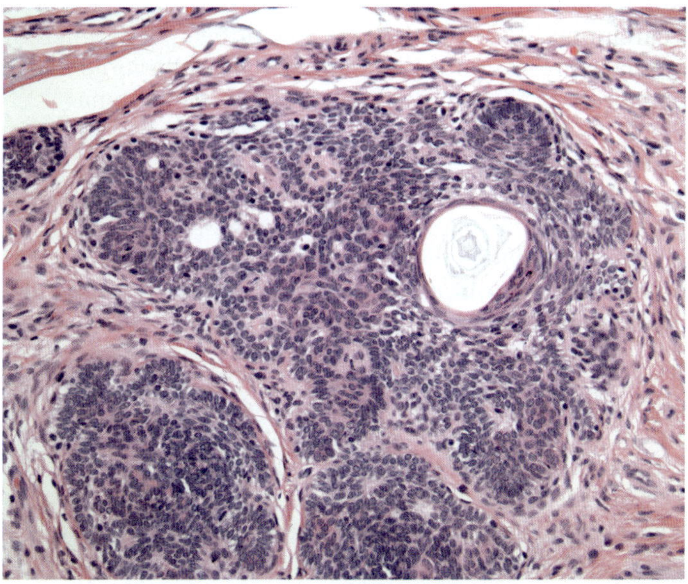

FIGURE 8.45 Keratin-containing microcysts, typically lined by cells showing infundibular differentiation with the so-called epidermal keratinization and concomitant keratohyaline granules or, less frequently, isthmic differentiation with abrupt trichilemmal keratinization, are dispersed through the lesions. Papillary mesenchymal bodies are present.

with the keratinous debris or microcalcifications (e-figs. 8.71–8.74). There is no true basaloid component in this neoplasm. At disparity with conventional trichoepithelioma, the desmoplastic form is immunoreactive for epithelial membrane antigen (EMA).

DIFFERENTIAL DIAGNOSIS. The three sclerosing adnexal neoplasms which merit consideration include the desmoplastic trichoepithelioma, the sclerosing basal cell carcinoma, and the microcystic adnexal carcinoma. The sclerosing basal cell carcinoma comprises narrow columns of atypical basaloid cells showing apoptosis and mitotic activity accompanied by rare and abortive slitlike stromal retraction (e-figs. 8.75–8.77). The stroma in turn shows a desmoplastic morphology with plump stromal cells admixed with thickened collagen bundles. The tumor is often associated with a superficial and/or nodular basal cell carcinoma from which it takes derivation and typically arises in sun-damaged stroma.[105] The absence of stromal retraction, mitotic activity, and individual cell necrosis distinguishes the desmoplastic trichoepithelioma from this tumor. The microcystic adnexal carcinoma typically seen in the midface of a middle-aged or an elderly woman shows keratinous microcysts surmounting vertically or haphazardly oriented ill-defined tubular structures comprising rather banal epithelium showing only an occasional mitotic figure. The microcystic adnexal carcinoma is widely infiltrative, frequently penetrating into subcutaneous tissue and to all margins of a given punch biopsy specimen (e-figs. 8.78–8.80). The tumor shows neurotropism that is absent in a desmoplastic trichoepithelioma. Slitlike stromal retraction is not a feature of the microcystic adnexal carcinoma. Furthermore, the desmoplastic trichoepithelioma is positive for EMA, whereas the sclerosing basal cell carcinoma does not express this antigen. The microcystic adnexal carcinoma expresses both EMA and carcinoembryonic antigen (CEA); CEA is not expressed in the desmoplastic trichoepithelioma.[155–158]

Pilomatricoma

Classically appearing as a dome-shaped nodule in the head and neck of children and infants, the pilomatricoma is also referred to as the *calcifying epithelioma of Malherbe*.[159–164] It is the prototypic lesion that produces matrical differentiation comprising shadow cells that in turn derive from a germinative epithelial layer.

HISTOPATHOLOGY. Early on its development, the pilomatricoma can show brisk mitotic activity and has cells that are proplastic with large oval nuclei and prominent nucleoli. These features may be worrisome for malignancy but in fact the tumors are well circumscribed, lacking invasion of adjacent structures or necrosis. In addition to the admixed areas of germinative and shadow cells, the pilomatricoma is associated with calcified deposits in the adjacent stroma with a foreign body giant cell reaction. Residual shadow cell sheets undergo dystrophic calcification, giving the lesion its alternate epithet (Figs. 8.46 and 8.47, e-figs. 8.81–8.85). Over time, these lesions lose their brisk mitotic activity and undergo progressive calcification.

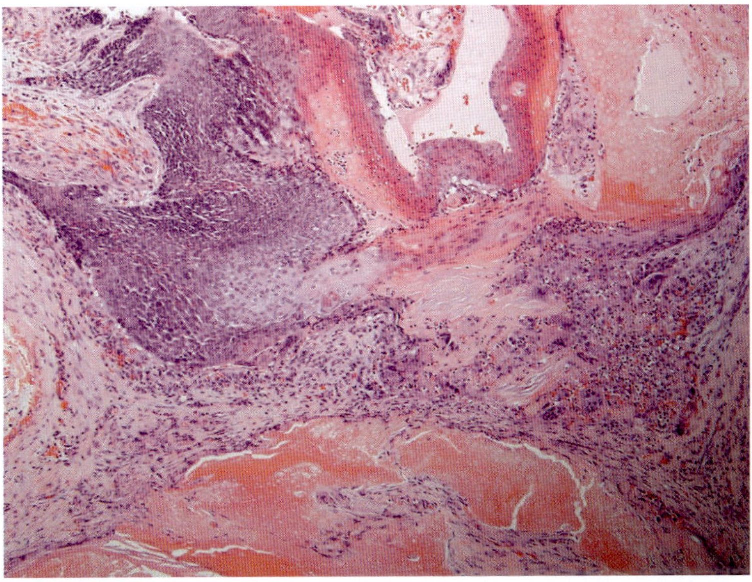

FIGURE 8.46 Early on its development, the pilomatricoma can show brisk mitotic activity and has cells which are proplastic with large oval nuclei and prominent nucleoli. This particular cell component represents the neoplastic counterpart of the anagen hair bulb and cortical epithelium.

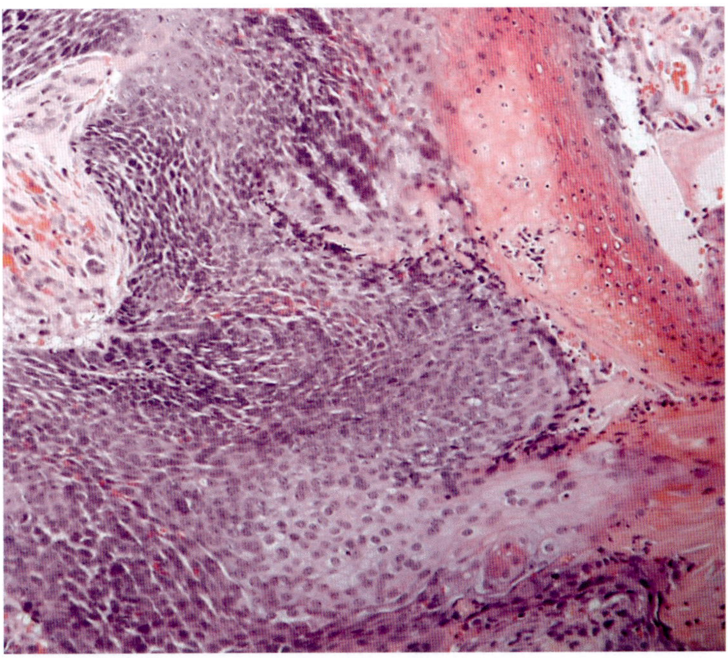

FIGURE 8.47 Like the normal hair cortex, the cortical-like cells undergo hard keratinization resulting in the formation of the so-called ghost cells.

Ultimately, the lesion eventuates as the so-called ancient pilomatricoma with a florid foreign body reaction and abundant calcification in the adjacent stroma.[163,164] Metaplastic bone formation in these lesions may ensue. A perforating variant of the pilomatricoma is uncommonly seen, whereby the necrotic material and shadow cells are extruded through the epidermis or through a hair follicle.[163,165–169]

DIFFERENTIAL DIAGNOSIS. The most important concern is with respect to the malignant pilomatricoma. The distinction is made based upon invasion of adjacent structures, an infiltrative growth pattern, and stromal desmoplasia. Metastatic tumor would of course clinch the diagnosis. There is a form of basal cell carcinoma with matrical differentiation; these are typically otherwise classical nodular basal cell carcinomas that show central matrical change within tumor cell nests.

PILOSEBACEOUS PROLIFERATIONS WITH MESENCHYMAL ELEMENTS

Basaloid Follicular Hamartoma

The basaloid follicular hamartoma occurs in two discrete clinical manifestations, a linear unilateral basal cell nevus and a generalized hair follicle hamartoma[170–174] although there is a spectrum ranging from solitary, linear or regionalized plaques or papules to generalized hamartomata. There is an association with alopecia or myasthenia gravis.[172,175] These lesions are frequently seen in excision specimens of other forms of tumor and in our experience, are infrequent findings in the territory of excised basal cell carcinomas for which the putative biologic basis of basal cell carcinoma, the basaloid follicular hamartoma, may in some instances be a precursor. These lesions are now commonly held to represent hamartomata as opposed to neoplastic proliferations and in that sense they represent a unilineal lesion which is cognate to the "hemifacial mixed appendage tumor," seen as a facial plaque in young children, that has components of basaloid follicular hamartoma admixed with eccrine and apocrine proliferations.

HISTOPATHOLOGY. The histopathology of the basaloid follicular hamartoma is that of a branching basaloid proliferation lacking cellular atypia or mitotic activity that is folliculocentric in nature and typically 1 to 2 mm in transverse diameter (e-figs. 8.86 and 8.87). As it may reflect the replacement of a pre-existing follicular bulge, there may be a central hair shaft in the native hair follicle structure from which it arises.

DIFFERENTIAL DIAGNOSIS. Stromal retraction artifact and mesenchymal mucinosis are also absent which should enable easy distinction from basal cell carcinoma.

NEOPLASMS WITH FOLLICULAR-BASED MESENCHYMAL DIFFERENTIATION

The stroma around the hair follicle is a characteristic loose mesenchyme containing plump elongated cells which is distinctive from the interfollicular dermis. Certain neoplasms and hamartomata can manifest a very similar stroma. These include the trichodiscoma, the perifollicular fibroma, the fibrofolliculoma, and the follicular myxoma.

Trichodiscoma

The trichodiscoma is thought to represent a lesion showing differentiation toward the hair disc or *haarscheibe*, a structure said to contain receptors for proprioception.[176] Held to be a neoplasm, the trichodiscoma presents as small nodules in the head and neck region in a patient in any age group[176–179]; lesions may be grouped or regional or generalized to form *trichodiscomatosis*.[177,180] Lesions are nontender.[181]

HISTOPATHOLOGY. The trichodiscoma manifests a dermal paucicellular fibrovascular stroma sometimes containing an elastic tissue visible with histochemical preparations and admixed with mesenchymal mucin and an elastic tissue that indents in a platelike fashion the peripheral wall of the follicular isthmus or infundibulum (e-figs. 8.88 and 8.89).[176,180] There is no differential diagnosis.

Perifollicular Fibroma

A recent broad review of the literature suggests that in fact the perifollicular fibroma is probably not a clue to the autosomal dominant genodermatosis Birt–Hogg–Dube syndrome (see next section). The lesions present as a few or multiple pale firm papules of the midface (e-fig. 8.90). As the name suggests, the histomorphology comprises perifollicular condensations of stroma. We view the perifollicular fibroma as a variant of angiofibroma or fibrous papule and thus to represent a form of involuting intradermal melanocytic nevus.

Fibrofolliculoma

Although clinically the perifollicular fibroma and fibrofolliculoma both can show central facial papules, the histomorphology is distinctive. In particular, in fibrofolliculoma the fibrous mantle around the pilosebaceous unit indents it and is associated with an anastomosing web of follicular epithelium (e-figs. 8.91 and 8.92). It is this lesion that is the important clue to the Birt–Hogg–Dube syndrome[182,183] and in some patients is a clue to the presence of multiple connective tissue nevi as well. With respect to the former, three Winnipeg physicians, Arthur Birt, Georgie Hogg, and Ian Dube, first recognized an association between multiple fibrofolliculomas and visceral malignancies (in particular ovary, colonic, and renal tumors); this condition is associated as well with multiple trichodiscomas and acrochordons.[184–187]

Follicular Myxoma

A rare tumor typically seen in patients under age 25, the follicular myxoma is typified by a myxoid stroma around a group of pilosebaceous structures that are often distorted and may interconnect.[99,188,189] The overlying epidermis may show reactive epithelial hyperplasia and/or papillomatosis. An identical lesion is described in the so-called NAME syndrome comprising nevi with atrial myxomas, myxoid cutaneous tumors including neurofibromas and freckles.[190]

Neurofollicular Hamartoma

These benign lesions that have an invariable location on the nose of older adults are somewhat reminiscent of sebaceous gland hyperplasia.

HISTOPATHOLOGY. These tumors have a low power architecture somewhat reminiscent of sebaceous gland hyperplasia or of trichodiscoma but with a characteristic investure of the perifollicular stroma by S100 positive spindled cells of presumptive schwannian derivation (see Fig. 8.53, e-figs. 8.93–8.95).[191–195]

Pilar Neurocristic Hamartoma

It is unclear whether the pilar neurocristic hamartoma represents a true hamartoma or a neoplastic proliferation of germinative epithelium often associated with pigment bearing dendritic cells.[193–195] The pilar neurocristic hamartoma manifests as a plaque or papule with pigmentation in the skin of the head and neck and can occur in any age group. We have seen a case arising in a 14-year-old African American on the back of her neck.[195] On occasion, these lesions give rise to a melanoma.

HISTOPATHOLOGY. The pilar neurocristic hamartoma manifests sheets of germinative cells admixed with pigmented cells with dendritic processes similar to the critical cell of the blue nevus of the dermal melanocytosis (e-figs. 8.96–8.100). Ultrastructurally, these can be shown to represent melanocytes while other cells manifest Schwann cell features. These lesions are folliculocentric, thus the designation *pilar neurocristic hamartoma*.[194]

Trichoblastoma

In 1970, Headington introduced the term trichoblastoma to describe a primitive follicular tumor of germinative epithelial derivation. While there are malignant variants, these neoplasms are essentially benign. They present clinically as nodules and can occur anywhere on the skin surface although are relatively uncommon on the distal extremities. They can be up to 2 cm in size. Unlike other follicular-based adnexal neoplasms, there is no particular association with any syndromic complex.[196–198]

HISTOPATHOLOGY. These tumors are distinctive histologically. They are relatively simple in composition comprising a monotypic populace of basaloid germinative appearing cells with a high nuclear to cytoplasmic ratio, without tumor cell necrosis or substantial atypia. The cells are characteristically arranged in cords or as small rounded islands that may exhibit a germinative bulbar organization including in the context of focal mesenchymal hair papillae body formation. Rarely, these benign cellular elements will exhibit an infiltrative pattern into perineural spaces. The stroma surrounding the trichoblastoma is a cellular fibroblast-rich one recapitulating that of normal hair papillae (e-figs. 8.101–8.105). At times, the stroma can be myxoid. Unlike trichoepithelioma, an attempt at hair shaft differentiation and other components derived from the hair germ including inner root sheath is not seen. It is a benign abortive germinative follicular epithelial neoplasm that does not differentiate beyond the hair (Figs. 8.48 and 8.49). The mesenchymal participation in lesions of trichoblastoma can be prominent. In cases where the stroma

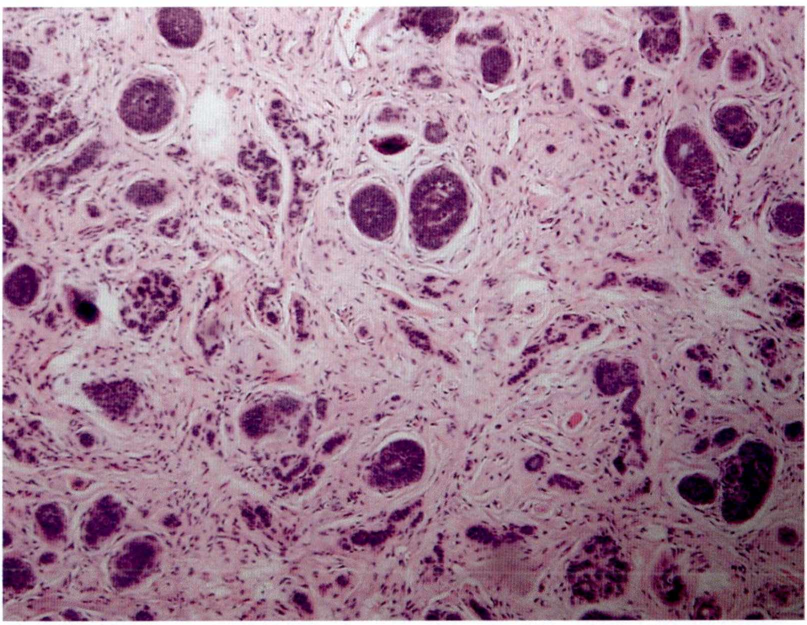

FIGURE 8.48 The cells are characteristically arranged in cords or as small rounded islands that may exhibit a germinative bulbar organization including in the context of focal mesenchymal hair papilla formation. The stroma surrounding the trichoblastoma is a cellular fibroblastic-rich one exactly recapitulating that found in the normal hair papilla. At times the stroma is myxoid.

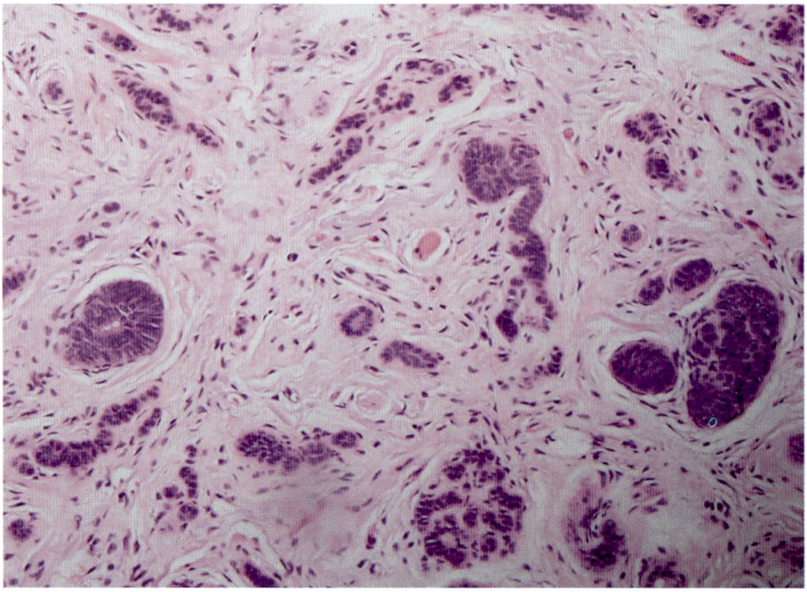

FIGURE 8.49 The cells are characteristically arranged in cords or as small rounded islands that may exhibit a germinative bulbar organization including in the context of focal mesenchymal hair papillae body formation. The stroma surrounding the trichoblastoma is a cellular fibroblastic-rich one exactly recapitulating that found in normal hair papillae. At times the stroma is myxoid.

becomes the dominant component of the tumor, the designation of trichoblastic fibroma has been used by some authors. Melanin pigment can occur and in certain cases, can be prominent. The melanin is due to pigment synthesizing melanocytes, which may be intimately admixed with germinative epithelial elements.[196–198]

Trichogerminoma

Closely related to the trichoblastoma is the trichogerminoma. There are differentiating points clinically including their predilection to involve the trunk in adult males and their progressive slowly growing course over a few years.[199,200]

HISTOPATHOLOGY. These tumors have in common with trichoblastoma their primitive germinative follicular epithelial derivation along with distinctive stromal changes identical to those encountered in the normal hair papillae (Fig. 8.50). As with the trichoblastoma, the mesenchymal component of this tumor is an important constituent of the neoplasm. Basaloid structures reminiscent of hair germ with mesenchymal body are shown in Figure 8.51. In addition to the foci of characteristic narrow cordlike arrangement seen in trichoblastoma, the tumor cells in trichogerminoma are also arranged in large lobules (Figs. 8.50–8.52).[199,200]

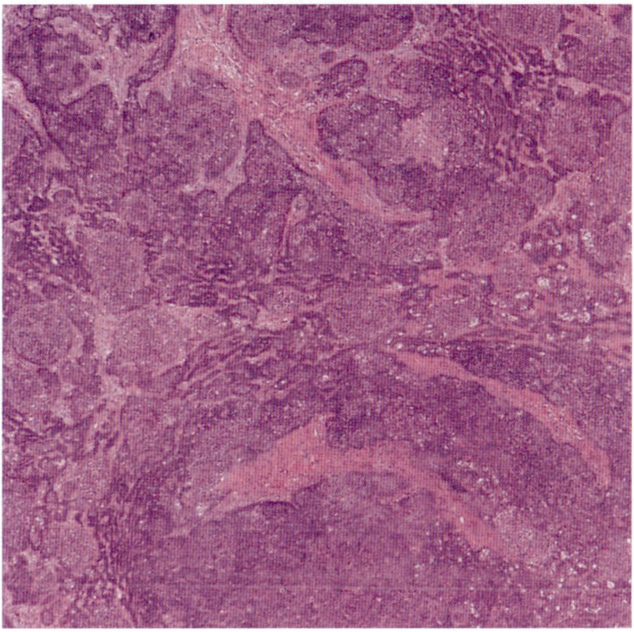

FIGURE 8.50 These tumors have in common with trichoblastoma their primitive germinative follicular epithelial derivation along with distinctive stromal changes identical to those encountered in the normal hair papillae. As with the trichoblastoma, the mesenchymal component of this tumor is an important constituent of the neoplasm. The tumor exhibits a cellular lobulated arrangement.

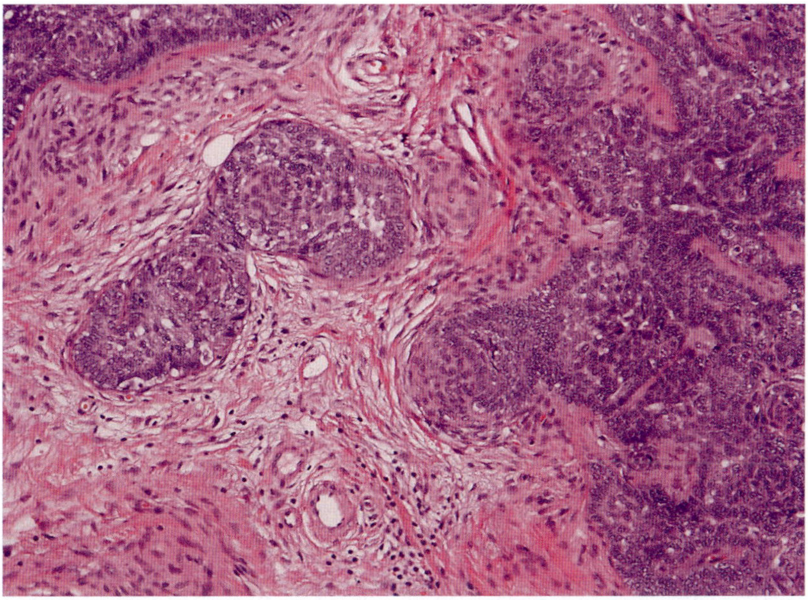

FIGURE 8.51 Basaloid structures reminiscent of hair germ with a mesenchymal body are observed.

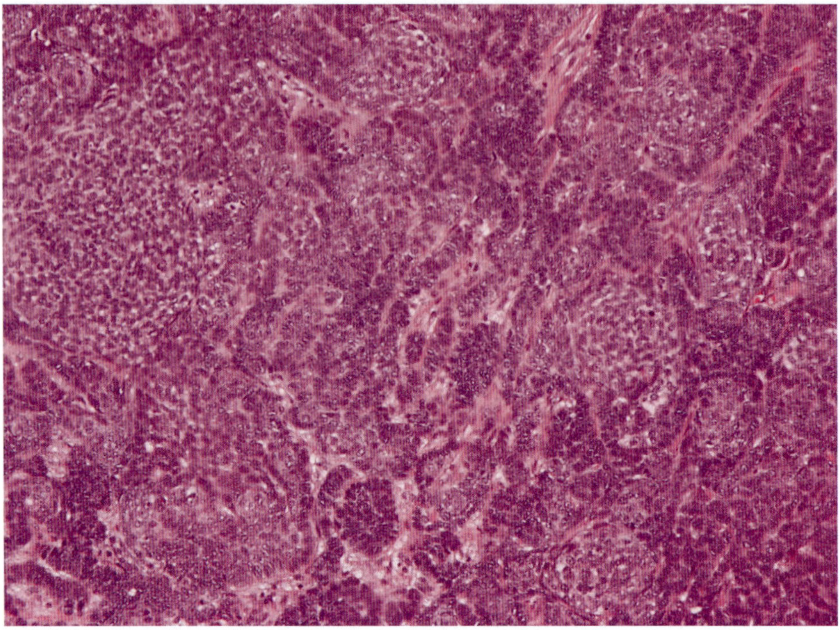

FIGURE 8.52 In addition to the foci of characteristic narrow cordlike arrangement seen in trichoblastoma, the tumor cells in trichogerminoma are also arranged in large lobules.

REFERENCES

1. Sharma HS, Meorkamal MZ, Zainol H, Dharap AS. Eccrine cylindroma of the ear canal–report of a case. *J Laryngol Otol* 1994;108:706–709.
2. Wollina U, Rulke D, Schaarschmidt H. Dermal cylindroma: Expression of intermediate filaments, epithelial and neuroectodermal antigens. *Histol Histopathol* 1992; 7:575–582.
3. Crain RC, Helwig EB. Dermal cylindroma (dermal eccrine cylindroma). *Am J Clin Pathol* 1961;35:504–515.
4. Goette DK, McConnell MA, Fowler VR. Cylindroma and eccrine spiradenoma coexistent in the same lesion. *Arch Dematol* 1982;118:273–274.
5. Cecchi R, Crudeli F, Fedi E, Giomi A. Multiple trichoepitheliomas, cylindromas, and eccrine spiradenomas observed in the same family. *G Ital Dermatol* 1985;120:149–152.
6. Tunggal L, Ravaux J, Pesch M, et al. Defective laminin 5 processing in cylindroma cells. *Am J Pathol* 2002;160:459–468.
7. Cotton DW, Slater DN, Rooney N, et al. Giant vascular eccrine spiradenomas: A report of two cases with histology, immunohistology, and electron microscopy. *Histopathology* 1986;10:1093–1099.
8. Van der Putte SC. The pathogenesis of familial multiple cylindromas, trichoepitheliomas, milia, and spiradenomas. *Am J Dermatopathol* 1995;17:271–280.
9. Lee MW, Kelly JW. Dermal cylindroma and eccrine spiradenoma. *Australas J Dermatol* 1996;37:48–49.
10. Kersting DW, Helwig EB. Eccrine spiradenoma. *Arch Dermatol* 1956;73:199–227.
11. Shelley WB, Wood MG. A zosteriform network of spiradenomas. *J Am Acad Dermatol* 1980;2:59–61.

12. Kao GF, Laskin WB, Weiss SW. Eccrine spiradenoma occurring in infancy, mimicking a mesenchymal tumor. *J Cutan Pathol* 1990;17:214–219.
13. Pruzam DL, Esterly NB, Prose NS. Eruptive syringoma. *Arch Dermatol* 1989; 125:1119–1120.
14. Isaacson D, Turner ML. Localized vulvar syringomas. *J Am Acad Dermatol* 1979; 1:352–356.
15. Henner MS, Shapiro PE, Ritter JH, et al. Solitary syringoma: A report of five cases and comparison with microcystic adnexal carcinoma. *Am J Dermatopathol* 1995; 17:465–470.
16. Lee MW, Goldberg LH, Dorsey K, Baer SC. Syringoma resembling confluent and reticulated papillomatosis of Gougerot–Carteaud. *Cutis* 1998;61:227–228.
17. Karam P, Benedetto AN. Syringomas: New approach to an old technique. *Int J Dermatol* 1996;35:219–220.
18. Hashimoto K, DiBella D, Borsuk GM. Eruptive hidradenoma and syringoma. *Arch Dermatol* 1967;96:500–519.
19. Brown SM, Freeman RG. Syringoma limited to the vulva. *Arch Dermatol* 1971; 114:331–333.
20. Yesudian P, Thambiah A. Familial syringoma. *Dermatologica* 1975;151:32–35.
21. Feibelman CE, Maize JC. Clear cell syringoma: A study by conventional and electron microscopy. *Am J Dermatopathol* 1984;6:139–150.
22. Ambrojo P, Caballero-Martinez AA, Sanchez-Yus E, Furio V. Clear cell syringoma. *Dermatologica* 1989;178:164–166.
23. Pinkus H, Rogin JR, Goldman P. Eccrine poroma. *Arch Dermatol* 1956;74:511–521.
24. Freeman RG, Knox JM, Spiller WF. Eccrine poroma. *Am J Clin Pathol* 1961; 36:444–450.
25. Hyman AB, Brownstein MH. Eccrine poroma: An analysis of 45 new cases. *Dermatologica* 1968;138:29–38.
26. Goldner R. Eccrine poromatosis. *Arch Dermatol* 1970;101:606–608.
27. Palazzo J, Stenn KS, Wolf ER. Eccrine tubular poroma. *J Cutan Pathol* 1987;14:365.
28. Pylyser K, DeWolf-Peeters C, Marien K. The histology of eccrine poroma: A study of 14 cases. *Dermatologica* 1983;167:243–249.
29. Mehregan AH, Levson DN. Hidroacanthoma simplex. *Arch Dermatol* 1969;100:303–305.
30. Hu CH, Marques AS, Winkelmann RK. Dermal duct tumor. *Arch Dermatol* 1978; 114:1659–1664.
31. Aloi FG, Pippione M. Dermal duct tumor. *Appl Pathol* 1986;4:175–178.
32. Pechere M, Roten S, Piletta P, Krischer J. Pigmented eccrine poroma. *Ann Dermatol Venereol* 1998;125:281.
33. Rahbari H. Syringoacanthoma: Acanthotic lesion of the acrosyringium. *Arch Dermatol* 1984;120:751–756.
34. Mascaro JM. Considerations on fibro-epithelial tumors. Exocrine syringofibradenoma. *Ann Dermatol Syphiligr (Paris)*. 1963;90:143–153.
35. Crowson AN, Magro CM. Desmoplastic trichilemmoma and its association with basal cell carcinoma. *Am J Dermatopathol* 1996;18:43–48.
36. Crowson AN, Magro CM, Kadin M, Stranc M. Differential expression of bcl-2 oncogene in human basal cell carcinoma. *Hum Pathol* 1996;27:355–359.
37. Weedon D, Lewis J. Acrosyringeal nevus. *J Cutan Pathol* 1977;4:166–168.
38. Takeda H, Mitsuhashi Y, Yoshikawa K, et al. Eccrine syringofibroadenoma: Report of a case and analysis of cytokeratin expression. *Dermatology* 1998;196:242–245.
39. Kanitakis J, Zambruno G, Euvrard S, et al. Eccrine syringofibroadenoma. *Am J Dermatopathol* 1987;9:37–40.

40. Civatte J, Jeanmougin M, Barrandon Y, Simenez-DeFranch A. Syringofibroadenoma eccrino de Mascaro. *Med Cutan Ibero Lat Am* 1981;9:193–196.
41. Rulon DB, Helwig EB. Papillary eccrine adenoma. *Arch Dermatol* 1977;113:596–598.
42. Cooper PH, Frierson HF. Papillary eccrine adenoma. *Arch Pathol Lab Med* 1984; 108:55–57.
43. Urmacher C, Lieberman PH. Papillary eccrine adenoma: A light microscopic and immunohistochemical study. *Am J Dermatopathol* 1987;9:243–249.
44. Urmacher C, Lieberman PH. Papillary eccrine adenoma. Light-microscopic, histochemical, and immunohistochemical studies. *Am J Dermatopathol* 1987;9(3):243–249.
45. Sexton M, Maize JC. Papillary eccrine adenoma: A light microscopic and immunohistochemical study. *J Am Acad Dermatol* 1988;18:1114–1120.
46. Biernat W, Kordek R, Wozniak L. Papillary eccrine adenoma: A case of cutaneous sweat gland tumor with secretory and ductular differentiation. *Pol J Pathol* 1994; 45:319–322.
47. Aloi F, Pich A. Papillary eccrine adenoma: A histopathological and immunohistochemical study. *Dermatologica* 1991;182:47–51.
48. Falck VG, Jordaan JH. Papillary eccrine adenoma: A tubulopapillary hidradenoma with eccrine differentiation. *Am J Dermatopathol* 1986;8:64–72.
49. Tellechea O, Reis JP, Marques C, et al. Tubular apocrine adenoma with eccrine and apocrine immunophenotypes or papillary tubular adenoma? *Am J Dermatopathol* 1995;17:499–505.
50. Johnson BL Jr, Helwig EB. Eccrine acrospiroma. *Cancer* 1969;23:641–657.
51. Hashimoto K, DiBella RJ, Lever WF. Clear cell hidradenoma. *Arch Dermatol* 1967;96:18–38.
52. Cooper PH, Frierson HF Jr, Morrison AG. Malignant transformation of eccrine spiradenoma. *Arch Dermatol* 1985;121:1445–1448.
53. Santa Cruz DJ. Sweat gland carcinoma: A comprehensive review. *Semin Diagn Pathol* 1987;4:38–74.
54. Woolworth H Jr, Dockerty MB, Wilson RB, Pratt JH. Papillary hidradenoma of the vulva. *Am J Obstet Gynecol* 1971;110:501–508.
55. Meeker JH, Neubechker RD, Helwig EB. Hidradenoma papilliferum. *Am J Clin Pathol* 1962;37:182–195.
56. Hashimoto K. Hidradenoma papilliferum: An electron microscopic study. *Acta Dermatol Venereol* 1973;53:22–30.
57. Santa Cruz DJ, Prioleau PG, Smith ME. Hidradenoma papilliferum of the eyelid. *Arch Dermatol* 1981;117:55–56.
58. Shenoy YMV. Malignant perianal papillary hidradenoma. *Arch Dermatol* 1961; 83:965–967.
59. Falck VG, Jordaan HF. Papillary eccrine adenoma. A tubulopapillary hidradenoma with eccrine differentiation. *Am J Dermatopathol* 1986;64–72.
60. Umbert P, Winkelmann RK. Tubular apocrine adenoma. *J Cutan Pathol* 1976;3:75–87.
61. Ansai S, Watanabe S, Aso K. A case of tubular apocrine adenoma with syringocystadenoma papilliferum. *J Cutan Pathol* 1989;16:230–236.
62. Fernandez RJ. Mixed tumors of the skin of the salivary gland type. *J Invest Dermatol* 1976;60:49–58.
63. Dardick I, van Nostrand AW, Phillips MJ. Histogenesis of salivary gland pleomorphic adenoma (mixed tumor) with evaluation of the role of myoepithelial cells. *Hum Pathol* 1982;13:62–75.
64. Mills SE. Mixed tumor of the skin: A model of divergent differentiation. *J Cutan Pathol* 1984;11:382–386.

65. Jaworski RC. The ultrastructure of chondroid syringoma (mixed tumor of the skin). *Ultrastruct Pathol* 1984;6:153–159.
66. Kunikane H, Ishikura H, Yamaguchi J, et al. Chondroid syringoma (mixed tumor of the skin): A clinicopathologic study of 13 cases. *Acta Pathol Jpn* 1987;37:615–625.
67. Requena L, Sanchez-Yus E, Santa Cruz DJ. Apocrine type of cutaneous mixed tumor with follicular and sebaceous differentiation. *Am J Dermatopathol* 1992;14:186–194.
68. Efskind J, Eker R. Myoepitheliomas of the skin. *Acta Dermatol Venereol* 1954; 34:279–283.
69. Bates AW, Baithun SI. Atypical mixed tumor of the skin: Histologic, immunohistochemical, and ultrastructural features in three cases and a review of the criteria for malignancy. *Am J Dermatopathol* 1998;20:35–40.
70. Troy JL, Ackerman AB. Sebaceoma: A distinctive benign neoplasm of adnexal epithelium, differentiating towards sebaceous cells. *Am J Dermatopathol* 1984;6:7–14.
71. Letizia C, Marcheggiano A, DeToma G, et al. Mixed type sweat gland adenoma: A case report. *Ann Ital Med Intern* 1993;8:248–249.
72. Czarnecki UB, Dorevitch AP. Giant senile sebaceous hyperplasia. *Arch Dermatol* 1986;122:1101–1102.
73. Kumar P, Marks R. Sebaceous gland hyperplasia and senile comedones: A prevalence study in elderly hospitalized patients. *Br J Dermatol* 1987;117:231–236.
74. Luderschmidt C, Plewig G. Circumscribed sebaceous gland hyperplasia: Autoradiographic and histoplanometric studies. *J Invest Dermatol* 1978;70:207–209.
75. Kudoh K, Hosokawa M, Miyazawa T, Tagami H. Giant solitary sebaceous gland hyperplasia clinically simulating epidermoid cyst. *J Cutan Pathol* 1988;15:396–398.
76. Bhawan J, Calhoun J. Premature sebaceous gland hyperplasia. *J Am Acad Dermatol* 1983;8:136.
77. De Villez RL, Roberts JC. Premature sebaceous gland hyperplasia. *J Am Acad Dermatol* 1982;6:933–935.
78. Dupre A, Bonafe J, Lamon R. Functional familial sebaceous hyperplasia of the face: Reverse of the Cunliffe acne-free nevus? Its inclusion among naevoid sebaceous receptor disease. *Clin Exp Dermatol* 1980;5:202–207.
79. Graham-Brown RAĊ, McGibbon DH, Sarkany I. A papular plaque-like eruption of the face due to naevoid sebaceous gland hyperplasia. *Clin Exp Dermatol* 1983;8:379–382.
80. Catalano PM, Ioannides A. Areolar sebaceous hyperplasia. *J Am Acad Dermatol* 1985;13:867–868.
81. Farina MC, Soriano ML, Escalonilla P, et al. Unilateral areolar sebaceous hyperplasia in a male. *Am J Dermatopathol* 1996;18:417–419.
82. Wick MR, Swanson PE, Barnhill RL. Sebaceous and pilar tumors. In: Barnhill R, Crowson AN, eds. *Textbook of Dermatopathology*. 2nd Ed. New York, NY: McGraw-Hill, 2004:745–784.
83. Crowson AN, Magro CM, Kadin M, Stranc M. Differential expression of bcl-2 oncogene in human basal cell carcinoma. *Hum Pathol* 1996;27:355–359.
84. Lever WF. Sebaceous adenoma: Review of the literature and report of a case. *Arch Dermatol* 1948;57:102–111.
85. Warren S, Warvi WN. Tumors of sebaceous glands. *Am J Pathol* 1943;19:441–460.
86. Prioleau PG, Santa Cruz DJ. Sebaceous gland neoplasia. *J Cutan Pathol* 1984; 11:396–414.
87. Rulon DB, Helwig EB. Cutaneous sebaceous neoplasms. *Cancer* 1974;33:82–102.
88. Brownstein MH, Shapiro L. The pilosebaceous tumors. *Int J Dermatol* 1977; 16:340–352.

89. Mehregan AH, Rahbari H. Benign epithelial tumors of the skin. II. Benign sebaceous tumors. *Cutis* 1977;19:317–320.
90. Reiffers J, Laugier P, Hunziker N. Sebaceous hyperplasias, keratoacanthomas, epitheliomas of the face, and cancer of the colon: A new entity? *Dermatologica* 1976; 153:23–33.
91. Rulon DB, Helwig EB. Multiple sebaceous neoplasms of the skin: An association with multiple visceral carcinomas, especially of the colon. *Am J Clin Pathol* 1973; 60:745–753.
92. Sciallis GF, Winkelmann RK. Multiple sebaceous adenomas and gastrointestinal carcinoma. *Arch Dermatol* 1974;110:913–916.
93. Tschang TP, Poulos E, Ho CK. Multiple sebaceous adenomas and internal malignant disease: A case report with chromosomal analysis. *Hum Pathol* 1976;7:589–594.
94. Fahmy A, Burgdorf WHC, Schosser RH, Pitha J. Muir–Torre syndrome: Reevaluation of the dermatological features and consideration of its relationship to the family cancer syndrome. *Cancer* 1973;49:1898–1903.
95. Burgdorf WHC, Pitha J, Fahmy A. Muir–Torre syndrome: Histologic spectrum of sebaceous proliferations. *Am J Dermatopathol* 1986;8:202–208.
96. Rothko F, Farmer ER, Zeligman I. Superficial epithelioma with sebaceous differentiation. *Arch Dermatol* 1980;116:329–331.
97. Friedman KJ, Boudreau S, Farmer ER. Superficial epithelioma with sebaceous differentiation. *J Cutan Pathol* 1987;14:193–197.
98. Mehregan AH, Pinkus H. Life history of organoid nevi: Special reference to nevus sebaceus of Jadassohn. *Arch Dermatol* 1965;91:574–587.
99. Morioka S. The natural history of nevus sebaceus. *J Cutan Pathol* 1985;12:200–213.
100. Lentz CL, Altman J, Mopper C. Nevus sebaceus of Jadassohn. *Arch Dermatol* 1968; 97:294–296.
101. Wilson-Jones E, Heyl T. Nevus sebaceus: A report of 140 cases with special regard to the development of secondary malignant tumors. *Br J Dermatol* 1970;82:99–105.
102. Clancy RR, Kurtz MB, Baker D, et al. Neurologic manifestations of the organoid nevus syndrome. *Arch Neurol* 1985;42:236–240.
103. Zaremba J. Jadassohn's nevus phakomatosis: A study based on a review of 37 cases. *J Ment Defic Res* 1977;22:103–122.
104. Alessi E, Wong SN, Advani HH, Ackerman AB. Nevus sebaceus is associated with unusual neoplasms: An atlas. *Am J Dermatopathol* 1988;10:116–127.
105. Crowson AN, Magro CM. Desmoplastic trichilemmoma and its association with basal cell carcinoma. *Am J Dermatopathol* 1996;18:43–48.
106. Tarkhan H, Domingo J. Metastasizing eccrine porocarcinoma developing in a nevus sebaceus of Jadassohn: Report of a case. *Arch Dermatol* 1985;121:413–415.
107. Mehregan AH, Butler JD. A tumor of the follicular infundibulum: Report of a case. *Arch Dermatol* 1961;83:924–927.
108. Mehregan AH. Tumor of follicular infundibulum. *Dermatologica* 1971;142:177–183.
109. Trunell TN, Waisman M. Tumor of the follicular infundibulum. *Cutis* 1979;23:317–318.
110. Mehregan AH. Infundibular tumors of the skin. *J Cutan Pathol* 1984;11:387–395.
111. Cribier B, Grosshans E. Tumor of the follicular infundibulum: A clinicopathologic study. *J Am Acad Dermatol* 1995;33:979–984.
112. Horn TD, Vennos EM, Bernstein BD, Cooper PH. Multiple tumors of follicular infundibulum with sweat duct differentiation. *J Cutan Pathol* 1995;22:281–287.
113. Jimenez FJ, Burchette JL Jr, Grichnik JM, Hitchcock MG. BER-EP4 immunoreactivity in normal skin and cutaneous neoplasms. *Mod Pathol* 1995;8:854–858.

114. Bhawan J. Pilar sheath acanthoma: A new benign follicular tumor. *J Cutan Pathol* 1979;6:438–440.
115. Mehregan AH, Brownstein MH. Pilar sheath acanthoma. *Arch Dermatol* 1978; 114:1495–1497.
116. Lee JYY, Hiesch G. Pilar sheath acanthoma. *Arch Dermatol* 1987;123:569–570.
117. Rahbari H, Mehregan AH, Pinkus H. Trichoadenoma of Nikolowski. *J Cutan Pathol* 1977;4:90–98.
118. Yamaguchi J, Takino C. A case of trichoadenoma arising in the buttock. *J Dermatol* 1992;19:503–506.
119. Undeutsch W, Rassner G. Das Trichoadenom (Nikolowski): Ein klinischer und histologischer Fallbericht. *Hautarzt* 1984;35:650–652.
120. Sieron J, Thein T, Pirsig W, Hemmer J. The Nikolowski trichoadenoma: A rare tumor of the ENT area. *Laryngo Rhino Otologie* 1993;72:140–142.
121. Ackerman AB, Troy JL, Rosen LB, et al. *Differential Diagnosis in Dermatopatholgy II.* Philadelphia, PA: Lea & Febiger, 1988:82–85.
122. Leonardi CL, Zhu WY, Kinsey WH, Penneys NS. Trichilemmomas are not associated with human papillomavirus DNA. *J Cutan Pathol* 1991;18:193–197.
123. Brownstein MH, Shapiro L. Trichilemmoma: Analysis of 40 new cases. *Arch Dermatol* 1973;107:866–869.
124. Hidayat AA, Font RL. Trichilemmoma of the eyelid and eyebrow: A clinicopathologic study of 31 cases. *Arch Ophthalmol* 1980;98:844–847.
125. Reifler DM, Ballitch HA II, Kessler DL, et al. Tricholemmoma of the eyelid. *Opthalmology* 1987;94:1272–1275.
126. Brownstein MH, Wolf H, Bikowski JB. Cowden's disease: A cutaneous marker of breast cancer. *Cancer* 1978;41:2393–2398.
127. Brownstein MH, Mehregan AH, Bikowski JB, et al. The dermatopathology of Cowden's syndrome. *Br J Dermatol* 1979;100:667–673.
128. Starink TM, Meijer CJLM, Brownstein MH. The cutaneous pathology of Cowden's disease: New findings. *J Cutan Pathol* 1985;12:83–93.
129. Raizis AM, Ferguson MM, George PM. Effect of nonsense mutations on PTEN mRNA stability. *Hum Genet* 2000;107:24–27.
130. Eng C. PTEN: One gene, many syndromes. *Hum Mutat* 2003;22:183–198.
131. Hunt SJ, Kilzer PB, Santa Cruz DJ. Desmoplastic trichilemmoma: Histologic variant resembling invasive carcinoma. *J Cutan Pathol* 1990;17:45–52.
132. Tellechea O, Reis JP, Baptista AP. Desmoplastic trichilemmoma. *Am J Dermatopathol* 1992;14:107–114.
133. Leppard BJ, Sanderson KV. The natural history of trichilemmal cysts. *Br J Dermatol* 1976;95:379–390.
134. Laing V, Knipe RC, Flowers FP, et al. Proliferating trichilemmal tumor: Report of a case and review of the literature. *J Dermatol Surg Oncol* 1991;17:295–298.
135. Yamaguchi J, Irimajiri T, Ohara K. Proliferating trichilemmal cyst arising in the arm of a young woman. *Dermatology* 1994;189:90–92.
136. Mann B, Salm R, Azzopardi JG. Pilar tumor: A distinctive type of trichilemmoma. *Diagn Histopathol* 1982;5:157–167.
137. Baptista AP, Silva LGE, Born MC. Proliferating trichilemmal cyst. *J Cutan Pathol* 1983;10:178–187.
138. Janitz J, Wiedersberg H. Trichilemmal pilar tumors. *Cancer* 1980;45:1594–1597.
139. Jacobson M, Ackerman AB. "Shadow" cells as clues to follicular differentiation. *Am J Dermatopathol* 1987;9:51–57.

140. Pinkus H, Sutton RL. Trichofolliculoma. *Arch Dermatol* 1965;91:46–49.
141. Gray HR, Helwig EB. Trichofolliculoma. *Arch Dermatol* 1962;86:619–625.
142. Plewig G. Sebaceous trichofolliculoma. *J Cutan Pathol* 1980;7:394–403.
143. Schulz T, Hartschuh W. Folliculosebaceous cystic hamartoma is a trichofolliculoma at its very late stage. *J Cutan Pathol* 1998;25:354–364.
144. Ramdial PK, Chrystal V, Madaree A. Folliculosebaceous hamartoma. *Pathology* 1998;30:212–214.
145. Templeton SF. Folliculosebaceous cystic hamartoma: A clinical-pathologic study. *J Am Acad Dermatol* 1996;34:77–81.
146. Aloi F, Tomasini C, Pippione M. Folliculosebaceous cystic hamartoma with perifollicular mucinosis. *Am J Dermatopathol* 1996;18:58–62.
147. Gray HR, Helwig EB. Epithelioma adenoides cysticum and solitary trichoepithelioma. *Arch Dermatol* 1963;87:102–114.
148. Zeligman I. Solitary trichoepithelioma. *Arch Dermatol* 1960;82:35–41.
149. Lever WF. Pathogenesis of benign tumors of cutaneous appendages and of basal cell epithelioma. *Arch Dermatol* Syphilol 1948;57:679–689.
150. Gaul LE. Heredity of multiple benign cystic epithelioma: "The Indiana family." *Arch Dermatol* 1953;68:517–524.
151. Pariser RJ. Multiple hereditary trichoepitheliomas and basal cell carcinomas. *J Cutan Pathol* 1986;13:111–117.
152. Rasmussen JE. A syndrome of trichoepitheliomas, milia, and cylindroma. *Arch Dermatol* 1975;111:610–614.
153. Michaelsson G, Olsson E, Westermark P. The Rombo Syndrome: A familial disorder with vermiculate atrophoderma, milia, hypotrichosis, trichoepitheliomas, basal cell carcinoma, and peripheral vasodilatation with cyanosis. *Acta Dermatol Venereol* 1981; 61:497–503.
154. Starink TM, Lane EB, Meijer CJ. Generalized trichoepitheliomas with alopecia and myasthenia gravis: Clinicopathologic and immunohistochemical study and comparison with classic and desmoplastic trichoepithelioma. *J Am Acad Dermatol* 1986;15: 1104–1112.
155. Brownstein MH, Shapiro L. Desmoplastic trichoepithelioma. *Cancer* 1977;40:2979–2986.
156. Bernstein G, Roth GJ. Sclerosing epithelial hamartoma. *J Dermatol Surg Oncol* 1978; 4:87–90.
157. MacDonald DM, Wilson-Jones E, Marks R. Sclerosing epithelial hamartoma. *Clin Exp Dermatol* 1977;2:153–160.
158. Takei Y, Fukushiro S, Ackerman AB. Criteria for histologic differentiation of desmoplastic trichoepithelioma (sclerosing epithelial hamartoma) from morphea-like basal cell carcinoma. *Am J Dermatopathol* 1985;7:207–211.
159. Forbis R, Helwig EB. Pilomatrixoma (calcifying epithelioma). *Arch Dermatol* 1961; 83:606–618.
160. Moehlenbeck FW. Pilomatrixoma (calcifying epithelioma). *Arch Dermatol* 1973; 108:532–534.
161. Taaffe A, Wyatt EH, Bury HPR. Pilomatrixoma (Malherbe). A clinical and histological survey of 78 cases. *Int J Dermatol* 1988;27:477–480.
162. Kaddu S, Soyer HP, Cerroni L, et al. Clinical and histopathological spectrum of pilomatricoma in adults. *Int J Dermatol* 1994;33:705–708.
163. Marrogi AJ, Wick MR, Dehner LP. Pilomatrical neoplasms in children and young adults. *Am J Dermatopathol* 1992;14:87–94.
164. Kaddu S, Soyer HP, Hodl S, Kerl H. Morphological stages of pilomatricoma. *Am J Dermatopathol* 1996;18:333–338.

165. Ter Poorten HJ, Sharbaugh AH. Extruding pilomatricoma: Report of a case. *Cutis* 1978;22:47–49.

166. Tsoitis G, Mandinaos C, Kanitakis JC. Perforating calcifying epithelioma of Malherbe with a rapid evolution. *Dermatologica* 1984;168:233–237.

167. Zulaica A, Peteiro C, Quintas C, et al. Perforating pilomatricoma. *J Cutan Pathol* 1988;15:409–411.

168. Alli N, Gungor E, Artuz F. Perforating pilomatricoma. *J Am Acad Dermatol* 35:116–118, 1996.

169. Shames BS, Nassif A, Bailey CS, Saltzstein SL. Secondary anetoderma involving a pilomatricoma. *Am J Dermatopathol* 1994;16:557–560.

170. Mehregan AH, Baker S. Basaloid follicular hamartoma: Report of three cases with localized and systematized unilateral lesions. *J Cutan Pathol* 1985;12:55–65.

171. Anderson TE, Best PV. Linear basal cell nevus. *Br J Dermatol* 1962;74:20–23.

172. Brown AC, Crounse RG, Winkelmann RK. Generalized hair follicle hamartoma: Associated with alopecia, aminoaciduria, and myasthenia gravis. *Arch Dermatol* 1969; 99:478–493.

173. Bleiberg J, Brodkin RH. Linear unilateral basal cell nevus with comedones. *Arch Dermatol* 1969;100:187–190.

174. Delacretaz J, Balsiger F. Hamartoma folliculaire multiple familial. *Dermatologica* 1979;159:316–324.

175. Brownstein MH. Basaloid follicular hamartoma: Solitary and multiple types. *J Am Acad Dermatol* 1992;27:237–240.

176. Pinkus H, Coskey R, Burgess GH. Trichodiscoma: A benign tumor related to Haarscheibe (hair disc). *J Invest Dermatol* 1974;63:212–218.

177. Camarasa JG, Calderon P, Moreno A. Familial multiple trichodiscomas. *Acta Dermatol Venereol* 1988;68:163–165.

178. Coskey RJ, Pinkus H. Trichodiscoma. *Int J Dermatol* 1976;15:600–601.

179. Grosshans E, Dungler T, Hanau D. Le trichodiscome de Pinkus. *Ann Dermatol Venereol* 1981;108:837–846.

180. Starink TM, Kisch LS, Meijer CJLM. Familial multiple trichodiscomas: A clinicopathologic study. *Arch Dermatol* 1985;121:888–891.

181. Moreno A, Puig LL, deMoragas JM. Multiple fibrofolliculomas and trichodiscomas. *Dermatologica* 1985;171:338–342.

182. Scully K, Bargmann H, Assaad D. Solitary fibrofolliculoma. *J Am Acad Dermatol* 1984;11:361–363.

183. Weintraub R, Pinkus H. Multiple fibrofolliculomas (Birt–Hogg–Dube) associated with a large connective tissue nevus. *J Cutan Pathol* 1977;4:289–299.

184. Junkins-Hopkins JM, Cooper PH. Multiple perifollicular fibromas: Review of a case and analysis of the literature. *J Cutan Pathol* 1994;21:467–471.

185. Schachtschabel AA, Kuster W, Happle R. Perifollicular fibroma of the skin and colonic polyps: Hornstein–Knickenberg syndrome. *Hautarzt* 1996;47:304–306.

186. Balus L, Fazio M, Sacerdoti G, et al. Fibrofolliculomes, trichodiscomes, et acrochordons: Syndrome de Birt–Hogg–Dube. *Ann Dermatol Venereol* 1983;110:601–609.

187. Birt AR, Hogg GR, Dube WJ. Hereditary multiple fibrofolliculomas with trichodiscomas and acrochordons. *Arch Dermatol* 1977;113:1674–1677.

188. Headington JT. Differentiating neoplasms of hair germ. *J Clin Pathol* 1970;23: 464–471.

189. Carney JA, Headington JT, Su WPD. Cutaneous myxomas: A major component of the complex of myxomas, spotty pigmentation, and endocrine overactivity. *Arch Dermatol* 1986;122:790–798.

190. Aterhton DJ, Pitcher DW, Wells RS, MacDonald DM. A syndrome of various cutaneous pigmented lesions, mxyoid neurofibromata, and atrial myxoma: The NAME syndrome. *Br J Dermatol* 1980;103:421–429.

191. Barr RJ, Goodman MM. Neurofollicular hamartoma: A light microscopic and immunohistochemical study. *J Cutan Pathol* 1989;16:336–341.

192. Nova MP, Zung M, Halperin A. Neurofollicular hamartoma: A clinicopathological study. *Am J Dermatopathol* 1991;13:459–462.

193. Sangueza OP, Requena L. Neurofollicular hamartoma: A new histogenetic interpretation. *Am J Dermatopathol* 1994;16:150–154.

194. Tuthill RJ, Clark WH Jr, Levene A. Pilar neurocristic hamartoma: Its relationship to blue nevus and equine melanotic disease. *Arch Dermatol* 1982;118:592–596.

195. Crowson AN, Magro CM, Clark WHC. Pilar neurocristic hamartoma (letter). *J Am Acad Dermatol* 1996;34:715.

196. Requena L, Requena I, Romero E, et al. Trichogenic trichoblastoma. An unusual neoplasm of hair germ. *Am J Dermatopathol.* 1990;12(2):175–181.

197. Aloi F, Tomasini C, Pippione M. Pigmented trichoblastoma. *Am J Dermatopathol.* 1992;14(4):345–349.

198. Wong TY, Reed JA, Suster S, et al. Benign trichogenic tumours: A report of two cases supporting a simplifiednomenclature. *Histopathology* 1993;22(6):575–580.

199. Kazakov DV, Kutzner H, Rütten A, et al. Trichogerminoma: A rare cutaneous adnexal tumor with differentiation toward the hair germ epithelium. *Dermatology* 2002; 205(4):405–408 (Review).

200. Sau P, Lupton GP, Graham JH. Trichogerminoma. Report of 14 cases. *J Cutan Pathol* 1992;19(5):357–365.

9

MALIGNANT ADNEXAL NEOPLASMS

MALIGNANT TUMORS OF THE PILOSEBACEOUS APPARATUS, THEIR MIMICS, AND PRECURSORS

Introduction

Tumors of the pilosebaceous unit can occur as proliferations of a single cell lineage or as complex proliferations showing multilineal differentiation patterns encompassing those of sweat ducts, epidermis, and stroma with its varied components. In this chapter, we focus upon the malignant adnexal proliferations, considering benign entities mainly insofar as they impact the diagnostic approach to adnexal carcinoma. We will first turn to the malignant sebaceous neoplasms, their precursors, and their mimics.

SEBACEOUS ADENOMA

Clinical Features

The sebaceous adenoma is a benign neoplasm that manifests clinically as a pale yellow papule or nodule, typically of the face, that expresses itself clinically after the age of 50 years. Tumors range in size from less than 1 cm to greater than 5 cm.[1-6] These lesions are associated with the Muir–Torre syndrome, comprising the coexpression of cutaneous neoplasms including those of sebaceous type with well-differentiated squamous epithelial neoplasms and visceral malignancies including carcinomas of breast, ovary, gastrointestinal tract, and larynx.[7-14] Occasionally, a patient may manifest a malignant lymphoma of nodal or extranodal type.[10,12,14] Sebaceous neoplasms in the setting of Muir–Torre syndrome are often difficult to classify, showing overlap features between all of the prototypic forms of sebaceous neoplasm ranging from hyperplasia to carcinoma.[13]

Histology

The prototypic sebaceous adenoma manifests 1 to 2 layers of germinative cells which mature to form central sebocytes and have an architecture comprising a sharply circumscribed sebaceous lobule surrounded by a compressed pseudocapsule of dermal stroma (Fig. 9.1A). The overlying epidermis may be attenuated but sometimes forms a collarette around

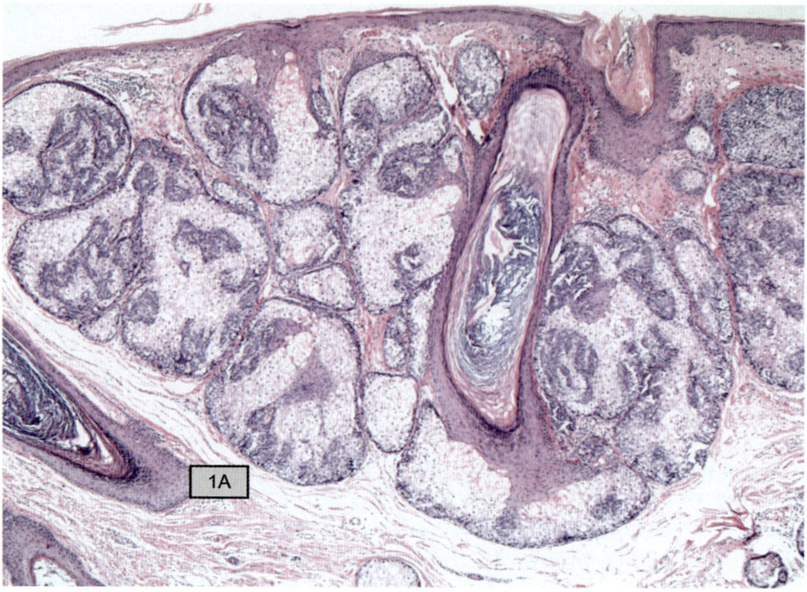

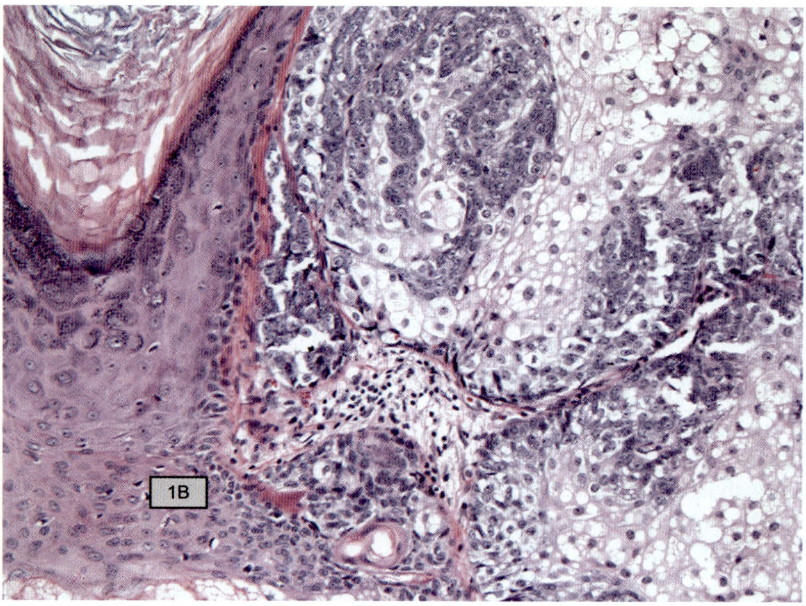

FIGURE 9.1 **Sebaceous Adenoma.** Sebaceous adenoma comprises an admixture of germinative epithelia and sebocytes in a nodular array grouped around one or more hair follicle structures **(A)**. Intermediate power microscopy shows that the germinative epithelia comprise less than 50% of the diameter of the tumor lobule but are greater than the one- to two-cell-layers thickness seen in lesions of sebaceous hyperplasia **(B)**.

the peripheral aspect of the neoplasm. Unlike sebaceous hyperplasia, occasional mitoses may be seen in the lobules of a sebaceous adenoma and, in concert with somewhat prominent nucleoli; these may provoke concern, but the pleomorphism hyperchromasia, and individual cell necrosis of the sebaceous epithelioma are not apparent (Fig. 9.1B). When seen in the context of the Muir–Torre syndrome, lesions mimicking sebaceous adenoma may open directly to the epidermal surface in a fashion that mimics nevus sebaceus.

Differential Diagnosis

The nevus sebaceus can form a confounding morphology with the sebaceous neoplasms of Muir–Torre syndrome, as can the basal cell carcinoma (BCC) with sebaceous differentiation.[15–18] The Muir–Torre syndrome is described in detail below. Another consideration in the differential diagnosis of sebaceous adenoma is the sebaceous epithelioma. Most observers equate the term sebaceous epithelioma with a BCC, typically of nodular type, showing central sebaceous differentiation. In the sebaceous epithelioma, atypical basaloid cells mimicking the germinative cells of sebaceous hyperplasia are identified in the periphery of tumor lobules but fill greater than 50% of the diameter of individual nodules and are associated with apoptosis, mitotic activity, and slitlike retraction of the tumor cell nests from the adjacent stroma accompanied by mucinotic collagen degeneration. The sebaceous adenoma, in contrast, has an increased number of germinative cell layers as opposed to sebaceous hyperplasia; typically, these constitute greater than two outside layers but less than 50% of the diameter of the tumor nodule. Individual cell necrosis, mitotic activity, and slitlike retraction of stroma are not features of sebaceous adenoma. A nevus sebaceus typically shows epidermal hyperplasia with mammillation of the surface mimicking an epidermal nevus. The sebaceous lobules in nevus sebaceus are abortive, often opening directly to the epidermal surface as opposed to through the infundibular sebaceous duct of a mature hair follicle structure. In concert with this anomaly, hairs (either polarizable terminal hairs or vellus hairs) are not seen in the folliculosebaceous anlage of the nevus sebaceus. By polarized light microscopy, one can delineate the transverse margin of a nevus sebaceus when one recognizes these mature hair shafts lateral to the lesion itself. As nevus sebaceus is a hamartoma, often with a complex mesenchymal and epithelial derivation, the stroma may appear hyperplastic and ectopic apocrine glands may be present in the dermis, sometimes with a concomitant increase in blood vessels. As nevus sebaceus can give rise to basaloid proliferations including superficial BCC and its nodular and infiltrative growth derivatives, the distinction between nevus sebaceus and sebaceous hyperplasia is an important one. Finally, the nevus sebaceus can be associated with other forms of neoplasia such as syringocystadenoma papilliferum or desmoplastic trichilemmoma.

SUPERFICIAL EPITHELIOMA WITH SEBACEOUS DIFFERENTIATION

Clinical Features

The superficial epithelioma with sebaceous differentiation manifests as a slow growing, smooth-surfaced papule or keratotic nodule on the face, trunk, or thigh.[19]

Histopathology

The lesions mimic a tumor of follicular infundibulum or superficial BCC by virtue of anastomosing cells that connect broadly to the basal layer of epidermis and have an orientation parallel to the epidermal surface. Some examples show peripheral palisading, leading some observers to suggest that this represents a form of superficial BCC with sebaceous differentiation cognate to the sebaceous epithelioma,[20,21] while other examples show squamous differentiation.

Differential Diagnosis

The presence of sebaceous differentiation distinguishes this lesion from the inverted follicular keratosis and the prototypic superficial BCC. An exceptional example of a tumor of follicular infundibulum showing sebaceous differentiation was reported in 2001,[22] but these lesions show no slitlike retraction from a mucinotic stroma.

SEBACEOMA

Introduction

The term sebaceoma was first introduced by Troy and Ackerman[23] to describe a dermal sebaceous tumor having histological overlap fcatures of sebaceous adenoma and sebaceous epithelioma.

Histopathology

These sharply circumscribed lesions have smooth borders and asymmetry and comprise aggregates of undifferentiated basaloid cells admixed with vacuolated sebocytes and sebaceous ducts (Fig. 9.2A and B). The latter may contribute, through metaplastic change, squamous epithelia to the nodules. These components are admixed in an often haphazard fashion.[24] The proportions of these components vary and have no set definition. Holocrine secretion may generate necrosis en masse, but necrosis of the tumor cells themselves is never conspicuous.[24–26] There is a verrucous or seborrheic keratosis-type lesion in which the sebaceous components connect to a hyperplastic epidermis through a proliferation of infundibular keratinocytes.[24]

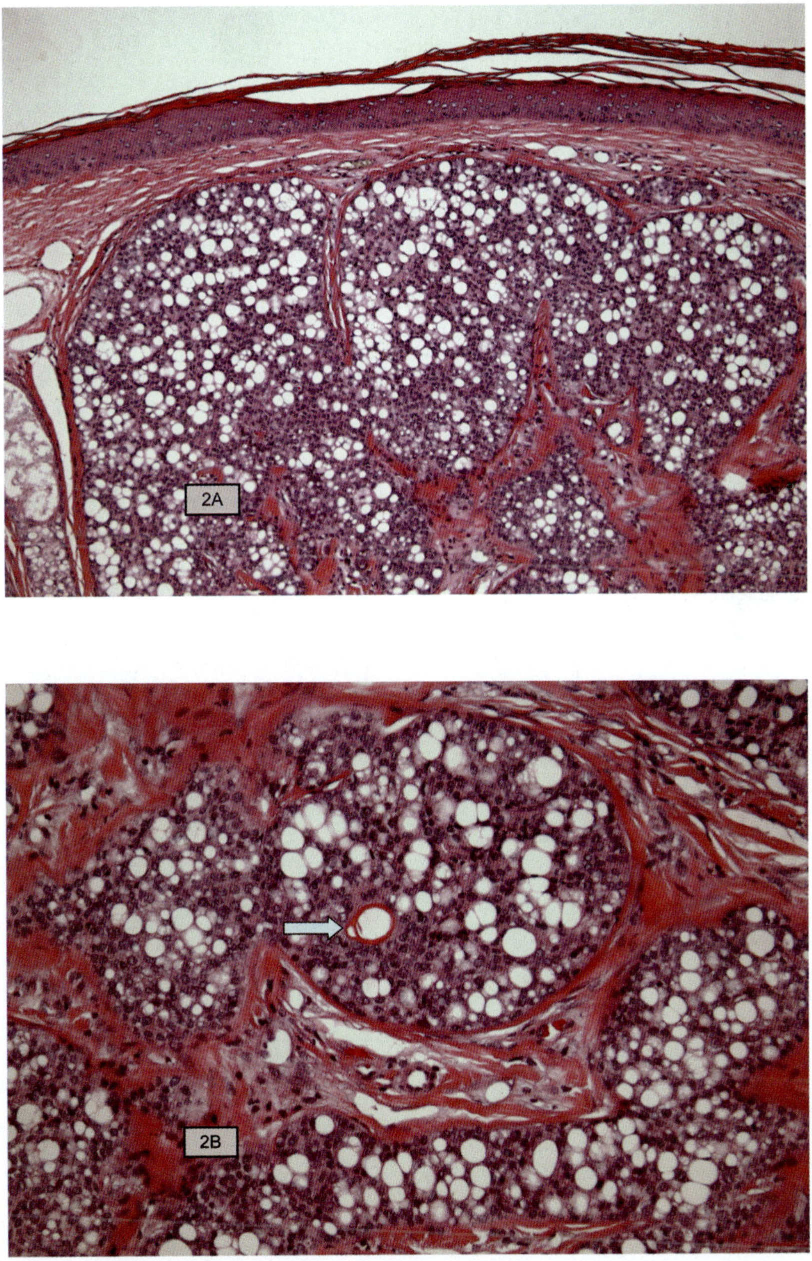

FIGURE 9.2 **Sebaceoma.** Sebaceoma is characterized by a diffuse admixture of germinative epithelia and sebocytes with no compartmentalized, organized pattern as seen in sebaceous hyperplasia and sebaceous adenoma **(A)**. Intimately admixed with these lobules of haphazardly arranged germinative cells and sebocytes are pilosebaceous ducts **(B,** *straight arrow***).** These manifest an eosinophilic lining cuticle in which keratohyalin granules are characteristically absent.

BASAL CELL CARCINOMA WITH SEBACEOUS DIFFERENTIATION (SEBACEOUS EPITHELIOMA)

Histopathology

As mentioned above, the BCC with sebaceous differentiation, a term equated by some authors and by one of us (ANC) to sebaceous epithelioma,[27] is typically a form of nodular BCC showing slitlike retraction of tumor from a mucinotic stroma with greater than 50% of the tumor lobule comprising germinative basaloid cells which demonstrate individual cell necrosis and mitotic activity (Fig. 9.3A and B).[15–18] Although the cells have a homology with the germinative cells of sebaceous adenoma, they tend to be larger with more open nuclei and more prominent nucleoli and the finding of slitlike retraction, although demonstrable in most, if not all, lesions and a principal defining feature, may be focal and difficult to identify in any particular tumor. Unlike sebaceous carcinoma, these tumors do not manifest pagetoid spread through the overlying epidermis and typically lack an infiltrative pattern of growth with a sclerosing stromal reaction. The sebaceous component in the center of the tumor lobules decorates with antibodies to epithelial membrane antigen (EMA).[27]

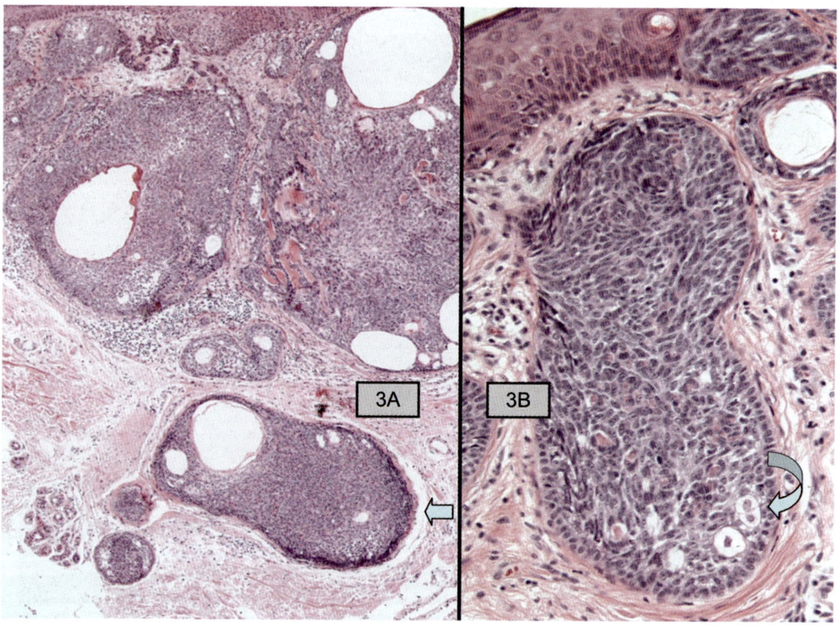

FIGURE 9.3 **Sebaceous Epithelioma.** The sebaceous epithelioma is equated by many observers with the basal cell carcinoma/epithelioma with sebaceous differentiation. The tumor comprises nodules dominated by germinative epithelia **(A)** in which slitlike stromal retraction is seen **(A**, *straight arrow***)**. In many instances, the sebocytes are difficult to identify **(B**, *curved arrow***)**. Unlike the sebaceous adenoma, the germinative epithelia in a sebaceous epithelioma comprise greater than 50% of the population in any given tumor lobule. Like other forms of basal cell carcinoma, apoptosis and mitotic activity are frequently seen within tumor lobules.

SEBACEOUS CARCINOMA

Introduction

In theory, sebaceous carcinoma can occur anywhere that sebaceous glands are located. In practice, ocular sebaceous carcinoma is far more common than its extraocular counterpart, although both are aggressive and potentially lethal malignant neoplasms.[3–5,28–39]

Clinical Features

Sebaceous carcinoma is a disorder of middle-aged and elderly individuals with a mean age of 62 to 72 years and a female preponderance.[28,40] Although ocular sebaceous carcinoma is said to have a predilection for Asians, this has not been our experience; however, this may reflect selection bias based upon our practice profiles. Patients classically develop painless nodules or papules along the eyelid margin or in palpebral conjunctiva. The upper eyelid is preferentially involved, followed by the lower lid, the caruncle, and the bulbar conjunctiva.[40] In most cases, these are solitary but on occasion, a patient develops a multicentric process. With respect to the solitary tumors, a chalazion is a frequent initial clinical misimpression. With respect to the multicentric tumors, misdiagnosis of ocular pemphigoid, actinic keratosis, and basal or squamous epithelial neoplasms is common.[30] Other locations, including elsewhere in the head and neck, the trunk, genitalia, and extremities, may be seen.[28,30,33–35,37,41] The extraocular tumors may exhibit a biological behavior that is equally aggressive to their ocular counterparts.[42] They are frequently larger, manifesting as nodular, tender or nontender, slowly or rapidly growing masses which, in some cases, ulcerate. The presence of a sebaceous carcinoma is, in some patients, a clue to internal organ malignancy in the setting of Muir–Torre syndrome.[13] Some 30% of patients with Muir–Torre syndrome manifest sebaceous carcinoma.[43,44]

Histopathology

Depending upon the degree of differentiation, the identification of sebaceous differentiation can be problematic. In low-grade tumors, multivesicular cytoplasms indent the nucleus in a fashion similar to the banal sebaceous epithelium of the sebaceous adenoma. Such tumors tend to form confluent nodular masses associated with little or no stromal desmoplasia, scattered mitoses, and mild nuclear pleomorphism with nucleolation (Figs. 9.4 and 9.5). High-grade tumors show scant cytoplasmic vacuolation with more prominent nucleoli, atypical mitoses, and abundant necrosis (Figs. 9.6–9.8). These are the tumors more likely to show pagetoid spread, although low-grade neoplasms may also do this; infiltrative patterns of growth with stromal desmoplasia and invasion of adjacent structures are features seen almost exclusively in the high-grade neoplasms (Fig. 9.6).

With respect to grading, architectural patterns rather than cytologic features are more reproducible.[29] Tumors comprising rather monomorphic rounded nodules of similar size and shape lacking a desmoplastic stroma are

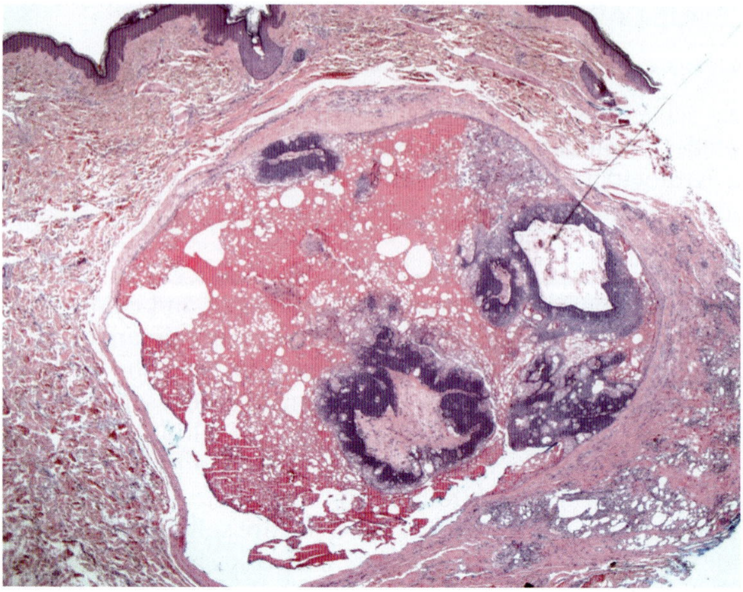

FIGURE 9.4 **Sebaceous Carcinoma, Low Grade.** The tumor illustrated is that of a 39-year-old man with a 1.8-cm diameter lesion on his right arm. A well-circumscribed nodule with a pushing contour shows the presence of atypical germinative epithelia with only scattered sebocytes and areas of necrosis.

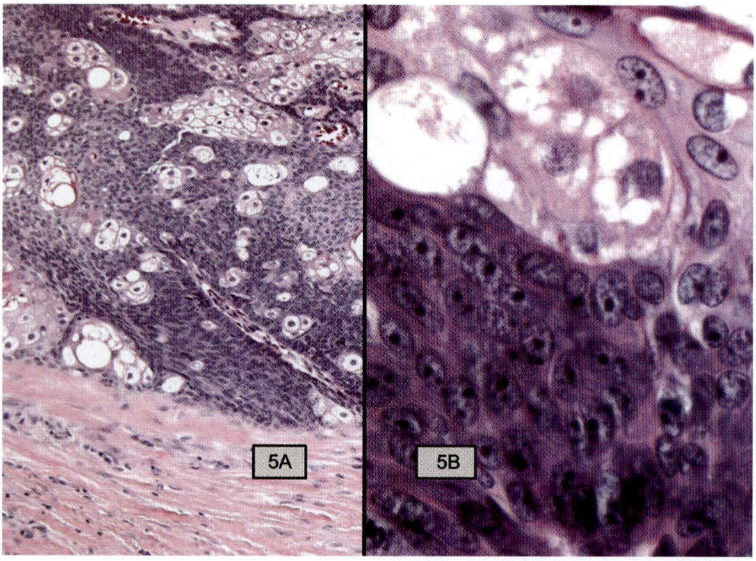

FIGURE 9.5 **Sebaceous Carcinoma, Low Grade.** High power microscopy of the same lesion illustrated in Figure 9.4 shows a dominant component of germinative epithelia within tumor lobules **(A)** that do not show slitlike retraction of stroma and are thus dissimilar from the tumor nests in a sebaceous epithelioma. Under high power microscopy **(B)**, the germinative epithelia are shown to have cytologic features of malignant neoplasia by virtue of irregularly thickened chromatinic rims and coarse, speculated chromatin patterns.

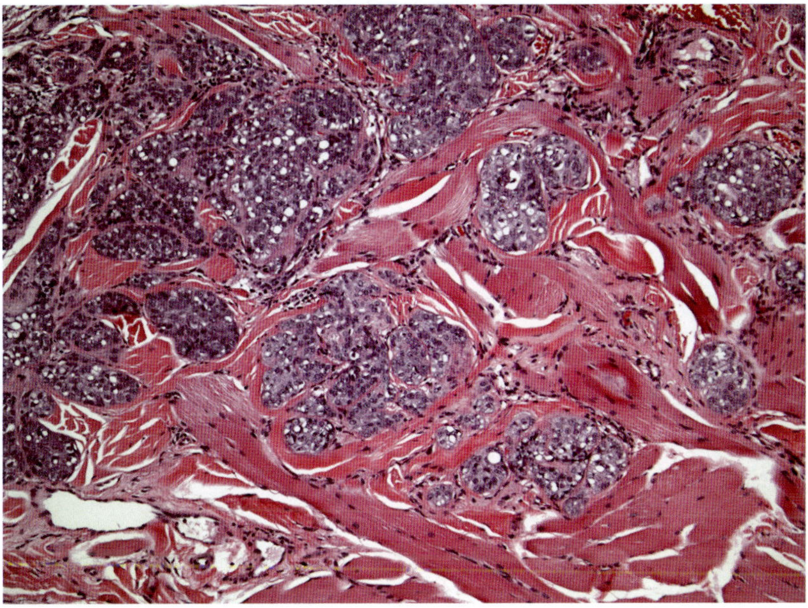

FIGURE 9.6 **Sebaceous Carcinoma, High Grade.** In this tumor from the nose of a 78-year-old man, neoplastic sebocytes show an infiltrative pattern of growth into the skeletal muscle.

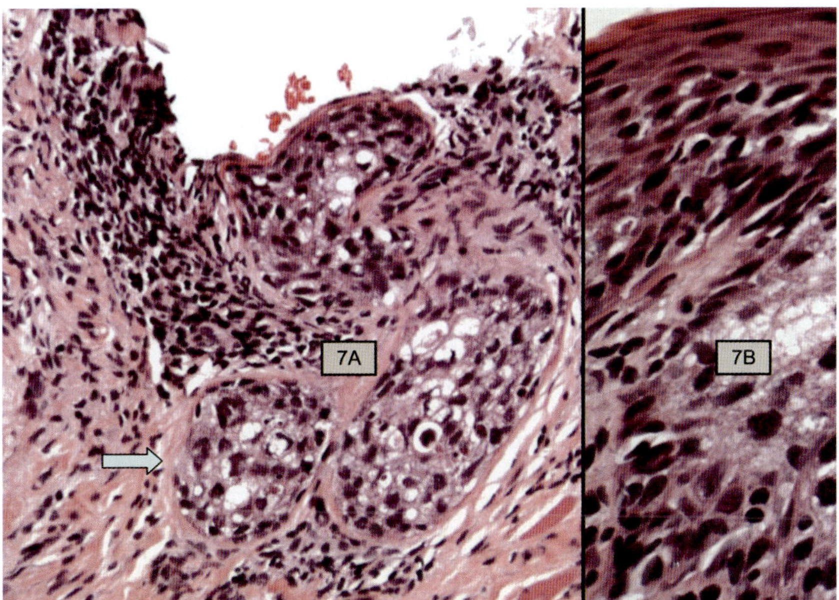

FIGURE 9.7 **Sebaceous Carcinoma, High Grade.** In addition to pagetoid spread through the epidermis of this elderly man's eyelid, the neoplastic sebocytes are shown to occupy the subepithelial sebaceous adnexal glands **(A,** *straight arrow***)**. **(B)** Fully transformed malignant nuclear change in sebocytes which show only minor and inconspicuous cytoplasmic vacuolation.

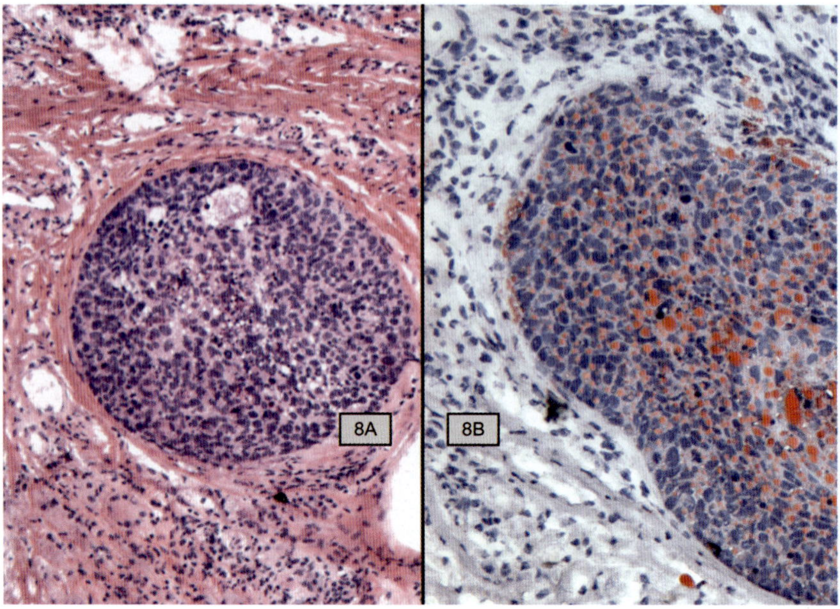

FIGURE 9.8 **Sebaceous Carcinoma.** Additional illustrations from the same lesion shown in Figure 9.7 were obtained at the time of frozen section. Neoplastic colonization of the subepithelial sebaceous adenexae is identified **(A)**. The definitive test for sebaceous differentiation is an Oil Red O histochemical preparation in frozen section material. The neutral lipid decorates with a bright red tinctorial quality **(B)**.

usually graded as I/III. Those with variably sized tumor lobules including those with jagged edges, an indistinct peripheral margin, an infiltrative pattern of growth and stromal desmoplasia, and/or a percolating growth pattern through stroma are graded as III/III. The grade II/III neoplasms show an intermediate architectural pattern with both rounded and infiltrative or jagged tumor nests. Sheetlike or syncytial growth patterns point toward grade III tumors.

As mentioned above, high-grade tumors infiltrate more aggressively, but all sebaceous carcinomas can show a pagetoid pattern of spread in the overlying epidermis. Careful attention to morphology and to immunohistochemical findings and conventional histochemistry should enable distinction (see differential diagnosis). In practical terms, when confronted with an eyelid biopsy showing a clear cell neoplasm, particularly when pagetoid epidermal involvement is identified, one must always think of sebaceous carcinoma and perform the appropriate investigative studies to include or exclude this diagnostic consideration. The Ki-67 labeling index was much higher than that of squamous cell carcinoma (SCC) in one study.[45]

Other histologic features of sebaceous carcinoma can obscure the diagnosis. In particular, those lesions showing squamous differentiation with keratin pearls, intercellular bridge formation, and cytoplasmic keratinization may strongly mimic a poorly differentiated or moderately differentiated SCC; areas of sebaceous differentiation may not be readily apparent in such tumors. There is also a sarcomatoid or spindle cell variant which mimics a spindle cell SCC.[46,47] A basaloid form comprising small cells having scant cytoplasm and showing peripheral palisading can mimic a BCC.[3,28–30,48] Apocrine differentiation is rarely described in sebaceous carcinoma.[49] Some sebaceous carcinomas manifest a trabecular or rosettelike architecture mimicking neuroendocrine neoplasia.[50] Cystic change in sebaceous neoplasms is said to be specific for Muir–Torre syndrome, where sebaceous neoplasms often prove otherwise difficult to classify precisely.[51] Associated with sebaceous neoplasms in this setting are keratoacanthomas showing sebaceous differentiation; these are seen in 20% of Muir–Torre patients and are said to be specific to the syndrome.[51]

Differential Diagnosis

One challenging differential diagnosis is that of the clear cell epithelial neoplasms, in particular, clear cell SCC and clear cell BCC. With respect to the clear cell BCCs and SCCs, the cytoplasmic vacuolation is due to glycogen; therefore, a PAS stain with and without diastase will demonstrate the abundant globules of PAS positive material. In sebaceous carcinoma, glycogen is typically less abundant but will be seen. Immunohistochemically, sebaceous carcinomas decorate strongly with EMA. In contrast, SCCs decorate weakly and BCCs are negative with this marker. Furthermore, sebaceous carcinomas decorate strongly with low-molecular weight cytokeratins (i.e., CAM 5.2), which only weakly decorate a BCC or SCC.[52] Ber-EP4 is strongly expressed in indolent growth BCC, and less so in aggressive growth variants. Extraocular sebaceous carcinomas tend to decorate with antibody CU18, which recognizes the antibreast carcinoma-associated antigen-225, anti-CA15.3 antibody, and anti-CD15 antibody.[53] Other novel markers such as the Thomsen–Friedenreich antigen, said to be expressed in sebaceous neoplasms of both benign and malignant type but not in squamous and basal cell tumors,[54] have yet to be vetted by multicenter studies. The biological basis of the visceral and sebaceous neoplasms in Muir–Torre syndrome is an aberrant mismatch repair gene (MSH2); this can be assayed immunohistochemically and is absent in the sebaceous neoplasms in this setting.[55] If one is fortunate enough to have frozen section material, an oil red O stain will demonstrate the neutral lipids present in the sebaceous carcinomas, which are absent in clear cell SCCs and BCCs. Typically, Paget disease is less challenging diagnostically. In Paget disease, the neoplastic cells, held to be of apocrine sweat gland derivation, manifest intracytoplasmic vacuoles containing epithelial mucin demonstrable with mucicarmine or Alcian blue-PAS preparations. In this disease, the cells also express carcinoembryonic antigen (CEA) and may express S100 protein, gross cystic disease fluid protein (GCDFP-15), CD15, and, in institutions which have access to these immunohistochemical markers, CA125, CA19-9,[56] CU18, CA15.3, and B6.2.[53]

Other clear cell neoplasms that can mimic sebaceous carcinoma include balloon cell melanoma, clear cell eccrine carcinoma, and metastatic clear cell carcinomas of kidney and thyroid gland. The balloon cell melanoma shows melanocyte lineage-specific markers which are expressed dominantly in the non-balloon-cell areas of the tumor. Thus, the epithelioid or sheetlike growth patterns will demonstrate Melan-A and HMB-45 positivity as well as Mit-f immunoreactivity. Melanin granules should be demonstrable in tumor cell cytoplasms but may require assiduous and time consuming high power microscopic examination. Clear cell eccrine carcinomas, like the clear cell SCCs and BCCs, are glycogen rich; they strongly express low-molecular weight cytokeratins and will be strongly EMA positive; thus, in this particular differential diagnosis, the presence of cytoplasmic glycogen in the absence of T-antigen is an important diagnostic clue. Clear cell carcinoma of thyroid gland expresses thyroid transcription factor (TTF), as will metastatic clear cell carcinoma of the lung, and in both cases, the cytoplasmic vacuolation is due to glycogen accumulation. Similarly, clear cell renal cell carcinoma is a glycogen rich tumor which, like the clear cell carcinoma of the thyroid gland, has a highly vascular stroma as would be uncharacteristic of a sebaceous carcinoma. Finally, the clear cell atypical fibroxanthoma merits consideration in the differential diagnosis of sebaceous carcinoma; the former expresses CD68 and other histiocyte lineage markers and often coexpresses EMA in the spindle cell population.[57,58] The use of procollagen I has been advocated by some authors, but there is significant overlap with spindle cell and desmoplastic melanoma and spindle cell squamous carcinoma.[59]

Distinction of sebaceous adenoma and sebaceous epithelioma from sebaceous carcinoma morphologically is discussed above. The expression of p21 in sebaceous adenoma and sebaceoma is said to have a distribution similar to that of the normal sebaceous gland, being dispersed toward the peripheral, germinative areas of the sebaceous lobule, whereas in sebaceous carcinoma, there is a loss of this topographical localization of p21 expression.[60]

The squamoid variant of sebaceous carcinoma expresses the glycoprotein BER-EP4 immunohistochemically, which SCC does not,[61] and also has, at least focally, multivesiculated sebocytes, which are absent in conventional SCC. The basaloid variant of sebaceous carcinoma is a form of poorly differentiated sebaceous carcinoma with highly atypical nuclei larger than the prototypic BCC; these tumors lack the mesenchymal mucin deposition around basaloid tumor nests that one associates with BCC. Sebocytes are rare in the basaloid sebaceous carcinoma whereas they are abundant in BCC with sebaceous differentiation and absent in conventional BCC. With respect to the differential diagnosis from sebaceous epithelioma, EMA expression is only seen in the sebaceous areas and is absent in the germinative cells, which constitute greater than 50% of the diameter of a typical tumor nodule. Both basaloid sebaceous carcinoma and BCC with sebaceous differentiation express BER-EP4.

NEVUS SEBACEUS

Introduction and Clinical Features

The nevus sebaceus may present at birth or in young life but in practical terms, patients may be unaware of these lesions until their adulthood. Thus, even patients in the fourth to sixth decades of life occasionally have a lesion biopsied to exclude a carcinoma or keratosis, which is in fact a nevus sebaceus. Typically located on the scalp, a nevus sebaceus may produce a localized area of alopecia or manifest as a tan-colored plaque with a rough surface, the latter representing the epidermal component. Prior to puberty, these lesions have no significant sebaceous component, thus the tan or a brown coloration. In and around puberty, sebaceous glands become prominent and the coloration of the plaque changes from tan-brown to yellowish and the contribution of the sebaceous component produces a verruciform surface. Rare cases are associated with systemic abnormalities such as seizures, mental retardation, or defects in visual fields.[62–67]

Histopathology

The nevus sebaceus comprises a hamartoma with contributions from epidermal and adnexal structures and mesenchymal elements, the varying proportions of which depend upon whether the patient is pre- or postpubertal. Prior to puberty, the nevus sebaceus may have no recognizable sebaceous elements and is recognizable therefore by the presence of a verruciform epidermal hyperplasia with prominence of adnexal structures, including in the context of ectopic apocrine glands. Near or after puberty, sebaceous glands become prominent. These are abortive miniaturized sebaceous glands that do not connect in the normal fashion through the sebaceous duct to the necks of the follicular bulges, but instead open directly to the epidermal surface. The lack of association with a mature pilosebaceous unit is associated in turn with a lack of polarizable terminal or vellus hairs. Thus, as mentioned above, we often use polarized light microscopy to delineate the transverse edge of the lesion; where mature hair shafts are identified, the histomorphology represents normal pilosebaceous structures of the native scalp. Like the sebaceous glands, the apocrine component is typically not conspicuous prior to puberty. A variety of additional lesions may be seen in the setting of a nevus sebaceus[68] that are, at least at inception, possibly hamartomatous in character. These include basal cell epithelioma, proliferating pilar tumor, syringocystadenoma papilliferum, trichilemmoma, apocrine adenoma, sebaceous adenoma, piloleiomyoma, and desmoplastic trichilemmoma.[69] Although these proliferations may initially be hamartomata,[70] there is no question that neoplastic transformation can occur. In a fashion cognate to that described in the transformation of superficial and nodular to infiltrative growth BCC,[71] the elaboration of cytokines by T-helper lymphocytes may immortalize basaloid epithelia. Subsequent mutagenic "hits" might then lead to an aggressive BCC. Other undisputed malignant neoplasms shown in continuity with nevi sebaceus include SCC and ductal apocrine adenocarcinoma.[72,73]

Differential Diagnosis

The nevus sebaceus is distinguished from sebaceous hyperplasia by the character of the sebaceous lobules (i.e., being miniaturized with an abortive character and opening to the epidermal surface as opposed to the pilosebaceous apparatus); nevus sebaceus lacks the prominence of germinative epithelium seen in BCC with sebaceous differentiation. Other forms of papillary epidermal hyperplasia which can mimic those of nevus sebaceus include the epidermal nevus, other hamartomas such as Becker nevus, and even old verrucae and seborrheic keratoses. Of course, verrucae and seborrheic keratoses lack the other constituents of the multilineal hamartoma which nevus sebaceus represents. Becker nevus lacks the prominence of sebaceous glands but is also a hamartoma and may show increased numbers of hair follicles and/or smooth muscle bundles.

MALIGNANT NEOPLASMS OF THE FOLLICULOSEBACEOUS APPARATUS

Malignant tumors arising in the pilosebaceous unit are rare and are often difficult to classify as they may show divergent differentiation patterns defying precise identification.

TRICHILEMMAL CARCINOMA

Clinical Features

The trichilemmal carcinoma arises in hair bearing, sun-damaged skin typically involving the face, scalp, or ears.[74–82] Either sex can be affected. Clinically, the lesion is a nodular plaque typically less than 3 cm in diameter, which may have a pale or reddish discoloration, or as an exophytic or polypoid nodule.[83] Thus, the lesion is mistaken clinically for BCC or SCC or, because of its rapid growth, keratocanthoma. Unlike trichilemmoma, the trichilemmal carcinoma is not associated with Cowden syndrome. Lesions have been said to be somewhat more indolent than conventional SCC, but aggressive local growth, recurrence, and metastasis are well-recognized risks.[84]

Histopathology

The trichilemmal carcinoma replaces the epithelium of one or more hair follicle structures generating a lobular pattern of growth and mimicking, in the affected root sheath epithelium, Bowen's disease. An infiltrative pattern of growth with stromal desmoplasia and tongues of tumor radiating

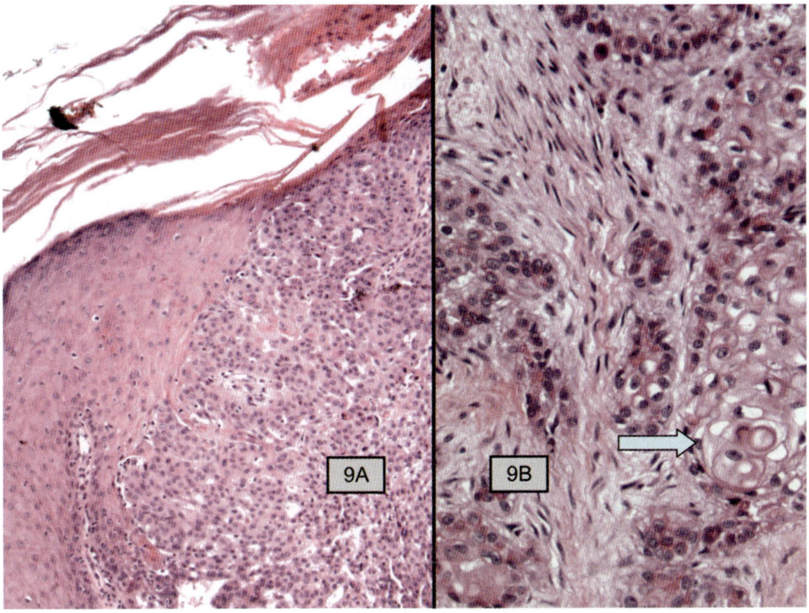

FIGURE 9.9 **Tricholemmal Carcinoma.** Tumor tongues radiate from follicular epithelia and from the intrafollicular epidermis **(A)** showing an infiltrative pattern of growth with reactive stromal desmoplasia, angioinvasion, perineural infiltration, and pagetoid spread through the intrafollicular epidermis. Note the abundant clear cell change in tumor lobules (**B**, *straight arrow*); this is due to the accumulation of intracytoplasmic glycogen as it characterizes tumors of follicular outer root sheath derivation.

from the affected follicular structures is noted (Fig. 9.9). Angioinvasion or perineural infiltration may be seen. Foci of clear cell change due to the presence of cytoplasmic glycogen are an important clue to diagnosis. In some cases, the lobules of trichilemmal carcinoma manifest peripheral palisading cognate to a trichilemmoma, but the high-grade nuclear atypia, mitoses, and individual cell necrosis enable distinction. There may be pagetoid spread of the interfollicular epidermis and of the affected follicular structures.

Differential Diagnosis

Conventional SCC arising in the interfollicular epidermis but showing clear cell differentiation, clear cell BCC, certain types of eccrine carcinoma, balloon cell melanoma, sebaceous carcinoma, and metastatic clear cell adenocarcinomas of lung, ovary, kidney, and thyroid gland all merit consideration. The diagnostic features of these differential diagnoses have been previously considered and will not be reiterated. It is noteworthy that there are certain keratins selective for the follicular epithelium, such as AE13 and AE14, that may be of assistance. One case report described CK17 and c-erb-B2 expression in a trichilemmal carcinoma, a pattern purported to confirm the outer root sheath derivation of this neoplasm.[85] The "hair differentiation" keratins are said to include CK7, CK8, CK18, and CK19; CD34 expression is also a feature that is said to support outer root sheath differentiation.[86,87]

MALIGNANT PROLIFERATING PILAR TUMOR

Introduction and Clinical Features

The rare malignant proliferating pilar tumor may arise in the background of a pre-existing pilar tumor or proliferating tricholemmal cyst. The distinction is a histopathologic one.

Histopathology

The malignant proliferating pilar tumor can be low- or high-grade in character and in either event, it manifests infiltration of the dermis and subcutaneous tissue by irregularly shaped and irregularly sized nests of malignant cells in high-grade neoplasms and lobules of proplastic atypical cells in low-grade neoplasms. The high-grade malignant proliferating pilar tumor lacks a lobular pattern and instead grows as individual cell cords or irregular nests with jagged contours associated with striking stromal desmoplasia, numerous and atypical mitotic figures, and, in some foci, a neoplastic spindle cell morphology.[88,89]

Differential Diagnosis

Early on its development, the pilomatricoma can show brisk mitotic activity and has cells which are proplastic with large oval nuclei and prominent nucleoli. These features may be worrisome for malignancy but, in fact, the tumors are well circumscribed, lacking invasion of adjacent structures and necrosis. In addition to the admixed areas of germinative and shadow cells, the pilomatricoma is associated with calcified deposits in the adjacent stroma with a foreign body giant cell reaction. Residual shadow cell sheets undergo dystrophic calcification, which gives the lesion its alternate epithet. Over time, these lesions lose their brisk mitotic activity and undergo progressive calcification. Ultimately, the lesion eventuates as a so-called ancient pilomatricoma with a florid foreign body reaction and abundant calcification in the adjacent stroma.[90,91] Metaplastic bone formation in these lesions may subsequently ensue. A perforating variant of the pilomatricoma is uncommonly seen, whereby the necrotic material and shadow cells are extruded through the epidermis or through a hair follicle.[90,92–97]

Problematic is the distinction from SCC and the ductal eccrine adenocarcinomas as well as the occasional metastatic carcinoma with squamous differentiation. The malignant proliferating pilar tumor does not connect to the overlying epidermis, shows no glandular differentiation, and is held to manifest, like the malignant trichilemmoma, a keratin immunostaining profile similar to the follicular outer root sheath. One case report described the expression of CK7 and CD34 in a carcinoma arising in a proliferating tichilemmal cyst.[87]

PILOMATRIX CARCINOMA

Clinical Features

Classically appearing as a dome-shaped nodule in the head and neck of children and infants, the pilomatricoma is also referred to as the *calcifying epithelioma of Malherbe*.[90,91,98–101] It is the prototypic lesion that produces matrical differentiation comprising shadow cells that in turn derive from a germinative epithelial layer. Its rare malignant counterpart is the pilomatrix carcinoma, a lesion with an aggressive tendency for local recurrence but little metastatic potential.[102]

Histopathology

A pilomatricoma can be mitotically active in its early phase. In contrast, pilomatrix carcinoma shows broad geographic zones of necrosis with an infiltrative margin and cytologic alterations including fully transformed malignant change.[90,91,103–115] Matrical differentiation may only be focal in these lesions. Tumors have the potential to spread to regional lymph nodes and produce fatal disseminated metastatic disease.[107,115] There is a locally invasive form of aggressive pilomatricoma that shows local occurrence but not distant metastasis. The histomorphology constitutes a point on a spectrum from the benign pilomatricoma to its malignant metastasizing counterpart. Malignant pilomatricoma shows invasion of adjacent structures, an infiltrative growth pattern, and stromal desmoplasia. Metastatic tumor would of course clinch the diagnosis.

Differential Diagnosis

The identification of matrical differentiation by virtue of ghost cells is the key step toward identifying the lineage of this neoplasm. There is a form of BCC with matrical differentiation; these are typically otherwise classical nodular BCCs that show central matrical change within tumor cell nests.

ADNEXAL CARCINOMA WITH DIVERGENT DIFFERENTIATION

On occasion, one encounters an anaplastic carcinoma with an infiltrative architecture, fully transformed cytologic criteria for malignancy, and areas suggestive of divergent differentiation toward eccrine, apocrine, sebaceous, or outer root sheath structures.[116–119]

PILAR NEUROCRISTIC HAMARTOMA

Introduction and Clinical Features

It is unclear whether the pilar neurocristic hamartoma represents a true hamartoma or a neoplastic proliferation of germinative epithelium associated with pigment bearing dendritic cells.[120–124] The pilar neurocristic hamartoma manifests as a plaque or papule with pigmentation in the skin of the head and neck and can occur in any age group. We have seen a case arising in a 14-year-old African American girl on the back of the neck.[124] On occasion, these lesions give rise to a melanoma.[125,126]

Histopathology

The pilar neurocristic hamartoma manifests sheets of germinative cells admixed with pigmented cells with dendritic processes similar to the critical cell of the blue nevus of the dermal melanocytoses. Ultrastructurally, these can be shown to represent melanocytes while other cells manifest Schwann cell features. These lesions are folliculocentric, thus the designation *pilar neurocristic hamartoma*.[123]

NEOPLASMS OF THE SWEAT GLAND APPARATUS

Introduction

Benign and malignant neoplasms may arise in the apocrine and eccrine sweat glands of humans. With respect to the latter, the acrosyrinx (the sweat duct orifice as it traverses the epidermis), the eccrine straight duct (which manifests a vertical column comprising a central cuboidal ductal cell with a peripheral myoepithelial layer as it traverses the dermis to the dermal–subcutaneous interface), and the eccrine secretory coil (a variable admixture of secretory, ductal, and myoepithelial cells at the dermal–subcutaneous interface) all can represent the source of eccrine neoplasia. The apocrine sweat ducts enter the hair follicle apparatus at the level of the follicular bulge. The apocrine apparatus typically manifests central decapitation-type secretion, manifests a coiled architecture, and is typically concentrated in the axilla and groins, i.e., the fold areas of the skin. Hamartomatous proliferations may cause apocrine ectopia with concentrations of apocrine ductal cells in, for example, the scalp of a nevus sebaceus. As the histologic expression of both eccrine and apocrine neoplasms is extremely wide, and as the tumors can be seen in combination with complex hamartomas and/or can exhibit divergent differentiation, an overwhelming and confusing lexicon of diagnostic appellations has been applied to eccrine and apocrine neoplasia. In this chapter, we describe, in some detail, the best recognized diagnostic entities for which specific nomenclature should logically be applied. When in doubt about specific subtyping, however, our practice is to identify such an adnexal neoplasm as, for example, "benign eccrine appendage neoplasm, not otherwise specified (NOS)" in the case of a benign lesion, or as a "malignant eccrine appendage tumor, NOS", for a cancerous one.

MALIGNANT SWEAT GLAND NEOPLASMS

Introduction

Malignant tumors of the sweat ducts and the secretory apparatus of sweat glands can be classified, as is the case for benign adnexal neoplasms, as those showing predominantly eccrine or predominantly apocrine differentiation.

ECCRINE CARCINOMAS

Malignant eccrine neoplasms tend to have a morphology that parallels that of malignant tumors of the ductal epithelia of the mammary glands.[127] In consequence, it is sometimes difficult to exclude metastatic disease when dealing with a primary eccrine carcinoma. In a comparison between primary sweat gland tumors and metastatic breast carcinoma to skin, Busam et al. found that the use of antibodies against epidermal growth factor receptor strongly decorated 81% of sweat gland tumors but only 17% of metastatic breast cancers ($p < 0.001$). There was no significant difference between the skin tumors and metastatic breast carcinoma when antibodies against estrogen and progesterone receptors were used.[128] In another study comparing benign and malignant primary eccrine and apocrine neoplasms to metastatic breast carcinoma, only 3.5% of these primary adnexal cancers demonstrated Her-2 positivity, whereas 10% to 23% of the breast carcinomas were positive.[129] The authors suggested that this test may be useful in distinguishing primary skin cancers from metastatic breast cancers.[129] Another study showed that primary cutaneous neoplasms stained strongly for p63 and CK5/6 with high specificity, while CK7 and CK20 were not useful.[130] When CK7 was positive in the cutaneous lesions, it exhibited focality and a specific pattern, while metastatic breast carcinoma did not express p63 or CK5/6 as strongly or as often; metastatic breast cancers diffusely expressed CK7, which was only focally positive in primary adnexal tumors. The usefulness of antibodies to CK5/6 was again shown by Plumb et al. in the differentiation of a cutaneous neoplasm from a metastatic breast carcinoma.[131] Ivan et al. presented further evidence of the usefulness of p63 in the diagnosis of adnexal cancer; in their study, none of the examples of metastatic adenocarcinoma to skin expressed p63, whereas virtually all the primary adnexal carcinomas were positive. Another study suggested using Ki-67 and p53 in atypical adnexal tumors to aid in differentiating benign from malignant lesions.[132] These studies introduce the utility of molecular methods in understanding the pathogenesis of sweat gland cancers and in attempting to differentiate them from metastatic carcinoma, especially of breast, as it affects the skin. In this chapter, we will emphasize those diagnostic features of lesions that present as primary cancers of the eccrine secretory or ductal apparatus and discuss those features that help to morphologically identify the tumors and to differentiate them from metastatic carcinomas.

ECCRINE POROCARCINOMA

Clinical Features

Eccrine porocarcinoma classically presents as a verrucous plaque or nodule of the distal extremities, particularly, the lower extremities, the head and neck, or the trunk of an elderly individual typically in the sixth to ninth decades of life.

Histopathology

The eccrine porocarcinoma is so designated as it recapitulates the morphology of the eccrine poroma with superimposed features definable as representing a neoplastic process with a potentially aggressive biological character. The latter include an infiltrative pattern of growth accompanied by a desmoplastic stromal reaction, apoptosis of tumor cells, features of high-grade cytologic atypia throughout the neoplasm, nucleolation, hypochromasia with high nucleocytoplasmic ratios indicating nuclear aneuploidy, perineural invasion, vascular invasion, and, in some observers' hands, extensive clear cell change in a population showing features of cytologic anaplasia (Figs. 9.10 and 9.11).[133–141] Some neoplasms clearly begin in the setting of a pre-existing lesion of long duration, suggesting that, for example, eccrine porocarcinoma may arise through malignant transformation of a pre-existing eccrine poroma. The presence of mutant p53 protein in both poroma and porocarcinoma lends molecular support to this hypothesis.[142] Some observers feel that an invasive pattern of growth in and of itself justifies the designation as eccrine porocarcinoma.[143] The analogy to eccrine poroma extends to an intraepidermal form of porocarcinoma in situ termed *malignant hidroacanthoma simplex*.[144–147] That, like its benign analog, shows sharply demarcated nests of tumor cells within the epidermis, the so-called Borst–Jadassohn phenomenon. The distinction

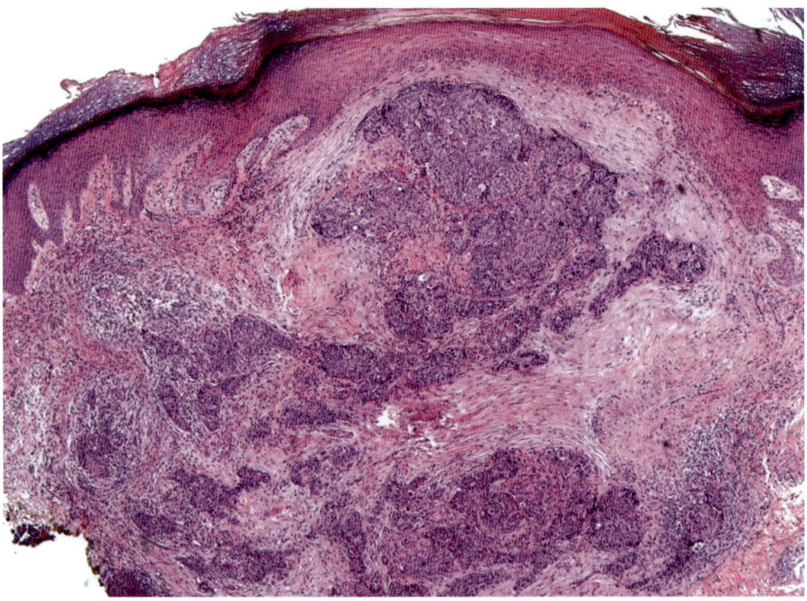

FIGURE 9.10 **Eccrine Porocarcinoma.** Eccrine porocarcinoma is characterized by infiltrative cords, lobules, and tongues of fully transformed malignant epithelia. The tumor cells have polygonal external contours and show cytoplasmic eosinophilia. There is reactive stromal desmoplasia.

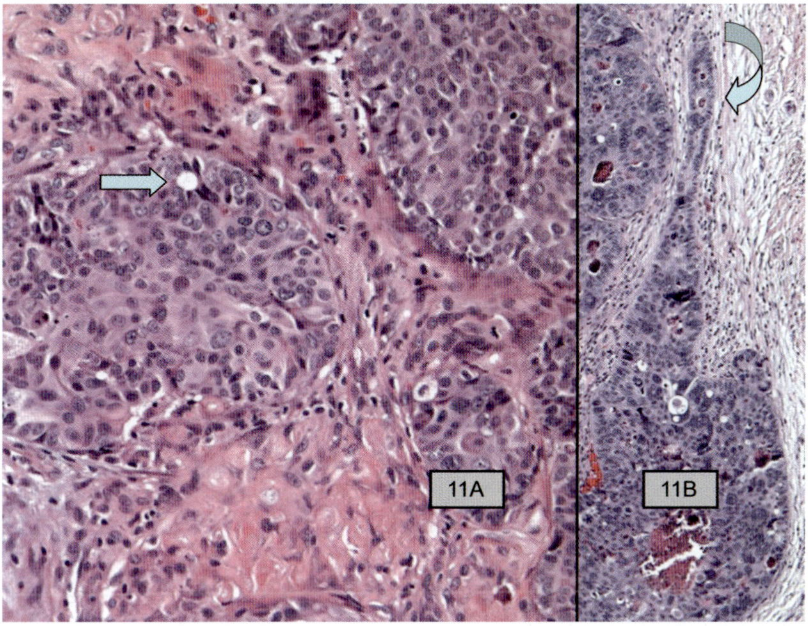

FIGURE 9.11 **Eccrine Porocarcinoma.** The same tumor illustrated in Figure 9.10 shows fully transformed malignant change with intracytoplasmic and common luminal margin formation (**A**, *straight arrow*). On occasion, one can see progressive dysplasia with neoplastic transformation of pre-existing eccrine straight ducts (**B**, *curved arrow*), a powerful clue to derivation from a pre-existing eccrine structure. In other cases of eccrine porocarcinoma, the tumor tongues and lobules radiate directly from the overlying interfollicular epidermis.

between malignant and benign hidroacanthoma simplex is based almost exclusively on the identification of cytologically malignant cells within tumor nests. An in situ component of this type may coexist with an invasive dermal-based eccrine porocarcinoma and when present, the former clearly indicates a primary neoplasm. Metastatic tumors mimicking eccrine carcinomas but showing an intraepithelial component are rare.[148]

Differential Diagnosis

With respect to the purely intraepidermal variant or those tumors showing a significant intraepithelial component, distinction from clonal seborrheic keratosis with atypia, clonal Bowen's disease, melanoma in situ, and Paget's disease is essential. The clonal seborrheic keratosis with atypia occurs in sun-damaged skin with solar elastosis being a prominent feature. Typically, therefore, lesions are on the head and neck area or on the dorsal aspects of the upper extremities. Papillomatosis with pseudohorn cyst formation should make distinction readily apparent at the light microscopic level. If not, both seborrheic keratosis and clonal Bowen disease do not strongly express cytokeratin (CK) 7, CEA, or S100 protein, which is often positive in the porocarcinoma in situ (Fig. 9.12). Melanoma in situ typically expresses S100 protein and will decorate with a Melan-A and/or HMB-45 immunohistochemical preparation; melanoma does not express CEA. The production of melanin by intraepidermal melanocytes and the delivery of melanosomes from the nurse melanocyte to the adjacent keratinocytes are phenomena which can be reduplicated in neoplastic tumors of eccrine and apocrine derivation. In consequence, melanosomes may be seen in clonal Bowen's disease, Paget's disease, and eccrine porocarcinoma in situ. The foregoing can be a cause of confusion, whereby pigmented Bowen's disease, Paget's disease, and porocarcinoma in situ can mimic melanoma. The problem is further compounded by the presence of pagetoid migration in Paget's disease or in amelanotic superficial spreading melanoma in situ; this is not, however, a feature that typifies porocarcinoma in situ.[149] Those tumors with dermal invasion must be distinguished from SCC and other forms of malignant eccrine neoplasia. The eccrine porocarcinoma, like the eccrine poroma, is composed of small cuboidal cells manifesting intercellular bridges and eosinophilic cytoplasms with sharply defined cell borders. Both the cells and their nuclei are larger than those seen in the eccrine poroma but are, nonetheless, smaller than the tumor cells of SCC. Furthermore, porocarcinoma manifests common luminal margin formation and intracytoplasmic lumina. The purely dermal-based eccrine cancers such as microcystic adnexal carcinoma and malignant eccrine

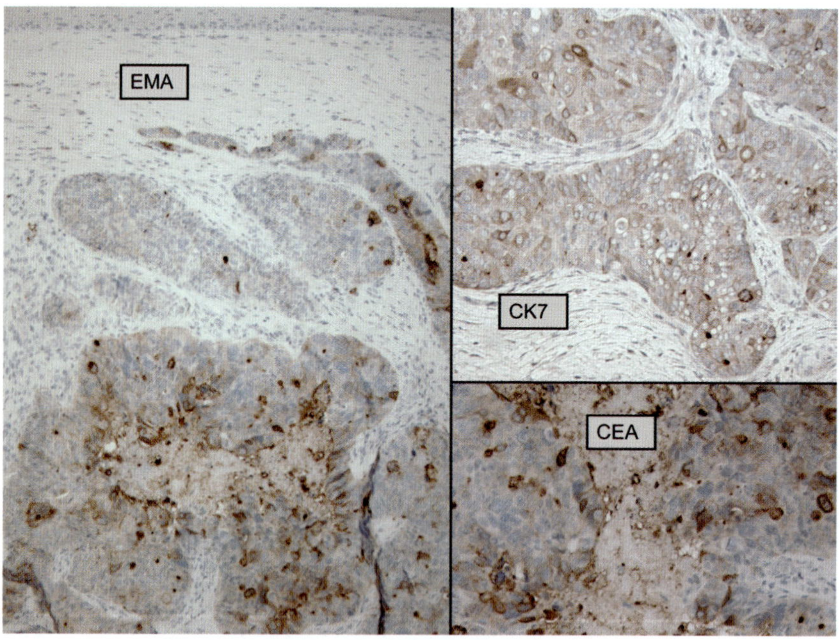

FIGURE 9.12 **Eccrine Porocarcinoma: Immunohistochemical Profile.** The neoplastic lumina in the centers of the tumor lobules frequently decorate with EMA and CEA. The tumors are floridly CK7 positive, unlike conventional SCC.

acrospiroma have no epidermal component. On occasion, metastatic disease proves impossible to distinguish from primary porocarcinoma with a dermal component.

HIDRADENOCARCINOMA

Introduction

A variety of names are applied to dominantly dermal-based malignant eccrine tumors, including hidradenocarcinoma, malignant acrospiroma, and clear cell eccrine carcinoma. This is a group associated with aggressive biological behavior and frequent distal metastases.

Clinical Features

These neoplasms present as nodules, frequently with superimposed ulceration and rapid growth, affecting the head and neck and the distal extremities of the elderly.[150–154]

Histopathology

There is a wide histomorphologic spectrum associated with malignant dermal-based eccrine proliferations. This spectrum includes both architectural and cytologic features with overlapping histologies and with more than one cytologic and/or architectural pattern often present in any given neoplasm. In general, the architectural features which characterize these tumors include polypoid neoplasms, tumors with an infiltrative peripheral margin associated with stromal desmoplasia, and variants characterized by islands of neoplastic cells showing central necrosis analogous to the comedocarcinoma of the breast. Cytologically, tumors show variable admixtures of basaloid, squamoid, and clear cells with foci of common lumenal margin formation and/or intracytoplasmic lumen production that represent evidence of eccrine ductal differentiation at the light microscopic level. From a cytologic perspective, tumors may be well differentiated (i.e., those malignant neoplasms showing an invasive peripheral margin with stromal desmoplasia and/or metastatic deposits in the absence of cytologic anaplasia) to overtly anaplastic cancers with fully transformed nuclear features of malignancy.

Differential Diagnosis

The hidradenocarcinomas call to mind a variety of differential diagnostic considerations depending upon the architectural and cytologic characteristics of the neoplasm under consideration. With respect to the clear cell hidradenocarcinomas, the differential diagnosis prominently encompasses neoplasms with clear cell differentiation and, in particular, those with malignant nuclear characteristics superimposed upon the aforementioned clear cell cytology. These include clear cell eccrine carcinoma and porocarcinoma, sebaceous carcinoma, trichilemmal carcinoma (which we consider a form of SCC with clear cell/trichilemmal differentiation), clear cell BCC, and clear cell carcinomas metastatic to the skin. With respect to the latter, the dominant diagnostic considerations are metastatic clear cell carcinoma from thyroid gland and lung. The expression of TTF seen in majority of these cases is helpful in resolving this dilemma. Some metastatic thyroid cancers also manifest expression of thyroglobulin. Metastatic clear cell carcinoma of renal primary origin manifests a prominent stromal vascularity with hemorrhage and areas of granular necrosis typically evident in biopsy material; renal cell carcinomas express the nuclear transcription factor Pax-2 (Zymed Laboratories Inc, San Francisco CA), and the cytoplasmic renal cell carcinoma marker RCC (Novocastra Laboratories Ltd, Newcastle upon Tyne, UK). Clear cell SCC of the cervix is a glycogen rich cancer with intercellular bridge formation characteristic of squamous differentiation. Unfortunately, intercellular bridges are also seen in poromas and porocarcinomas. Correlation with the clinical setting and with diagnostic imaging studies may be necessary to make these distinctions. Sebaceous carcinomas are malignant neoplasms of the sebaceous apparatus that are most frequent in the eyelids and the head and neck region but may be seen wherever sebaceous glands are identified. Sebaceous carcinomas manifest colonization of the epidermis and/or the palpebral conjunctiva in a pagetoid array. The lesions manifest an invasive pattern of growth with stromal desmoplasia and infiltration of adjacent structures. If frozen sections are available, an oil red O preparation will show intracytoplasmic fat globules in sebaceous carcinoma with variable quantities of coarse cytoplasmic glycogen (PAS positive/diastase resistant). Glycogen is more plentiful in clear cell malignant neoplasms of eccrine derivation and also those recapitulating outer root sheath derivation (i.e., trichilemmal carcinomas/SCCs with trichilemmal or clear cell differentiation). While it is generally accepted that sebaceous carcinoma is an aggressive neoplasm, clear cell BCC manifests local recurrence but typically does not metastasize. Thus, these distinctions are more than semantic in nature and accurate classification is helpful to the clinician. The immunohistochemical stains which facilitate this distinction include diffuse strong expression of EMA, low-molecular weight cytokeratin (i.e., CAM 5.2),[52] and the Thomsen–Friedenreich (T) antigen[54] in sebaceous neoplasia, versus peripheral expression of CAM 5.2 in BCC and its complete absence in SCC; EMA is expressed in neither of the two latter neoplasms.

MUCINOUS ECCRINE CARCINOMA

Introduction and Clinical Features

The mucinous eccrine carcinoma presents as a pale or violaceous nodule up to 3 cm in diameter involving the eyelids, the face, or the head and neck of elderly patients. Men and African-Americans are said to be preferentially affected.[143] This is a tumor with a propensity to local recurrence but, like its analog in the breast, mucinous carcinoma rarely metastasizes to regional lymph nodes.

Histopathology

The histopathology of mucinous eccrine carcinoma of the skin is analogous to that of its counterpart in the breast, comprising nests of variably cohesive atypical epithelia lying free in pools of mucin. The individual tumor cells manifest hyperchromatic nuclei with nucleolation and a degree of cytologic atypia which varies from low grade to frankly anaplastic (Figs. 9.13 and 9.14).[155–163] Cytoplasms are vacuolated and may show signet ring formation with peripheral displacement of the nucleus by a large intracytoplasmic vacuole. Pools of mucin dissect the stroma creating rounded and irregularly shaped aggregates of PAS positive, diastase resistant material which decorates with alcian blue or with Hale's colloidal iron.[158] Mitoses are inconspicuous as is vascular or perineural infiltration. As in the breast, colloid carcinoma of the skin may show neuroendocrine differentiation immunohistochemically by virtue of synaptophysin and/or chromogranin expression.[164] In a study of cutaneous tumors employing G-81, a monoclonal antibody reactive to dermcidin, it was suggested that eccrine carcinoma and other eccrine appendage including mixed tumors may, at times, have both eccrine and apocrine differentiation.[165]

Differential Diagnosis

Metastatic deposits from colloid carcinomas of the breast or gastrointestinal tract have an identical histomorphology. However, metastases from

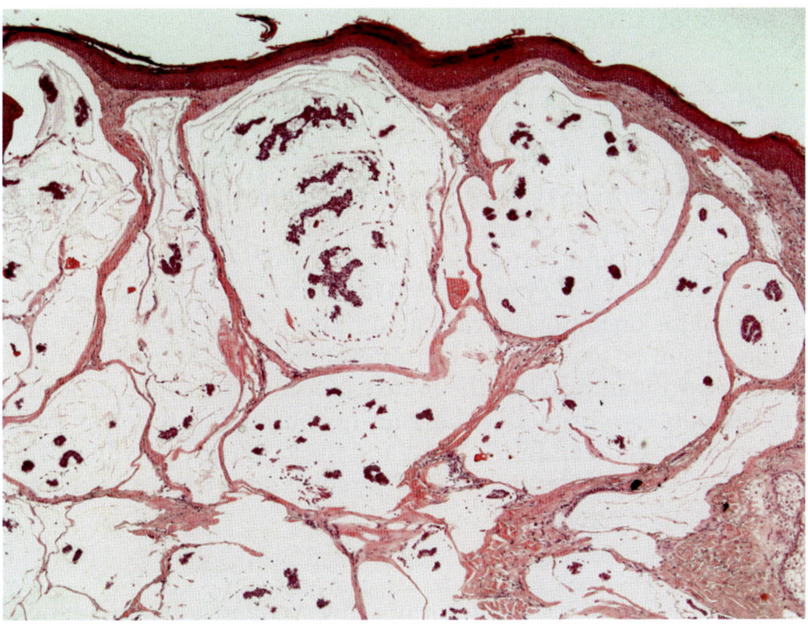

FIGURE 9.13 **Mucinous Eccrine Carcinoma.** The tumor is characterized by nests of neoplastic epithelia floating in pools of mucin.

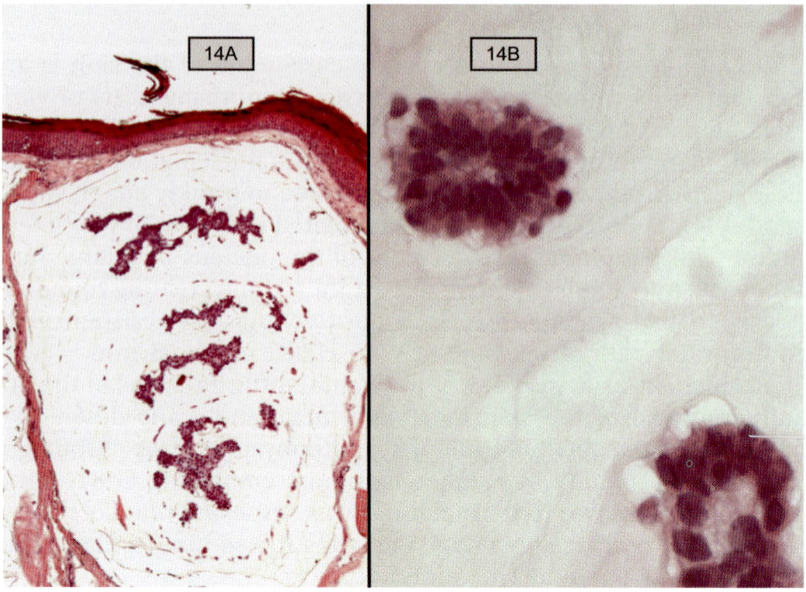

FIGURE 9.14 **Mucinous Eccrine Carcinoma.** Floating free in pools of mucin **(A)** are the neoplastic columnar epithelia often showing low-grade cytologic atypia **(B)**. Thus, the tumor has a morphology cognate to mucinous carcinomas of gastrointestinal tract and breast.

breast or gastrointestinal tract carcinomas occur late in the disease process and by that time, the clinical history and biological character of the neoplasm are almost always established.[166]

ADENOID CYSTIC CARCINOMA

Introduction and Clinical Features

Irrespective of the organ or parenchymal structure of origin, adenoid cystic carcinomas of a variety of anatomic sites show slow growth with aggressive local invasion and recurrence followed only very late in the course of disease by metastatic events.[167–170] The prototypic adenoid cystic carcinoma is a major or minor salivary gland tumor; accessory minor salivary gland-like tissue is seen in the lacrimal apparatus, the upper and lower respiratory tract, and rarely in the breast, uterine cervix, thymus gland, and prostate glands. As a primary cutaneous neoplasm, this tumor is rare, with an exceptional case seen in the head and neck, particularly the scalp, and also occasionally on the trunk. A recent report describes its appearance in the external auditory canal.[171]

Histopathology

In a fashion analogous to the tumor of salivary gland, adenoid cystic carcinoma of the skin forms tubuloalveolar structures lined by atypical basaloid epithelia and associated with the formation of myxoid matrix substance.

Globules and cylinders of brightly eosinophilic basement membrane-like material, similar to those described in the cutaneous cylindroma, complete the picture.[172–178] Mitoses are typically inconspicuous and, as mentioned above, the nuclear morphology is often deceptively bland. An important criterion in adenoid cystic carcinoma in any anatomic location is the striking propensity of these tumors to manifest perineural infiltration. In salivary gland tumors, most authorities are hesitant to make the diagnosis in the absence of this feature.[179] The same, in our view, applies to the skin.

Differential Diagnosis

Most basaloid tumors showing cylinders of eosinophilic material and/or myxoid stromal alteration with a tubuloalveolar pattern of growth are in fact BCC's showing an adenoid cystic-like pattern; these are termed "adenoid" BCCs. These tumors, however, show peripheral palisading at their exterior margin with slitlike retraction from the adjacent stroma and in most cases, as this is a form of indolent-growth neoplasm, the overall architecture is a nodular one with the absence of irregularly shaped tongues of tumor or stromal desmoplasia.[71,176] As with most indolent-growth BCCs, perineural infiltration would be most unusual in an adenoid BCC. In the center of nodular BCC including the adenoid variant, the tumors typically show apoptosis of individual cells with mitotic figures. These latter features are rare in the adenoid cystic carcinoma of the skin. Furthermore, the indolent-growth BCCs may manifest melanin production, which is absent in the adenoid cystic carcinoma, and any form of BCC may show divergent differentiation with the formation of sebaceous, pilar, or other structures. Like other forms of eccrine adnexal cancer, the adenoid cystic carcinoma typically expresses EMA, which BCC does not.

PAPILLARY DIGITAL ECCRINE ADENOCARCINOMA

This perplexing form of potentially lethal acral or near-acral adnexal cancer constitutes a significant diagnostic challenge to the unwary. In addition to high local recurrence rates, some 50% of tumors manifest distant metastases, typically to lungs and lymph nodes. As with acral melanomas, amputation at or above the nearest joint is one recommended strategy for local control.[180–182]

AGGRESSIVE DIGITAL PAPILLARY ADENOMA/ADENOCARCINOMA

Introduction

There is a peculiar group of rare neoplasms which tend to occur in adults on the acral parts, in particular, the fingers, toes, and adjacent skin of the palms and soles, as an isolated solid or solid and cystic mass. Termed *aggressive digital papillary adenoma or adenocarcinoma*, this lesion presents as a tumefactive nodule on a digit and invades the adjacent soft tissue but rarely ulcerates. Since the year 2000, the approach taken by pathologists to such neoplasms has undergone a radical change, reflecting novel publications in the peer-reviewed medical literature that in turn reflect the reported experience of national reference centers that deal with patients who develop these rare neoplasms.

Histopathology

The entity termed "aggressive digital papillary eccrine adenoma and adenocarcinoma" first appeared in the English language medical literature in 1984.[183] Papillary eccrine neoplasms in other anatomic locations were recognized prior to their identification in digits and other acral parts.[184–187] The papillary digital eccrine adenomas and adenocarcinomas typically manifest features of eccrine differentiation by virtue of showing intracytoplasmic lumina and common luminal margins (Figs. 9.15 and 9.16). The neoplasm is divergent morphologically from the typical eccrine spiradenoma or eccrine acrospiroma and other allied benign eccrine adnexal neoplasms by virtue of showing a papillary or micropapillary architecture cognate to that of in situ papillary carcinomas of ductal structures

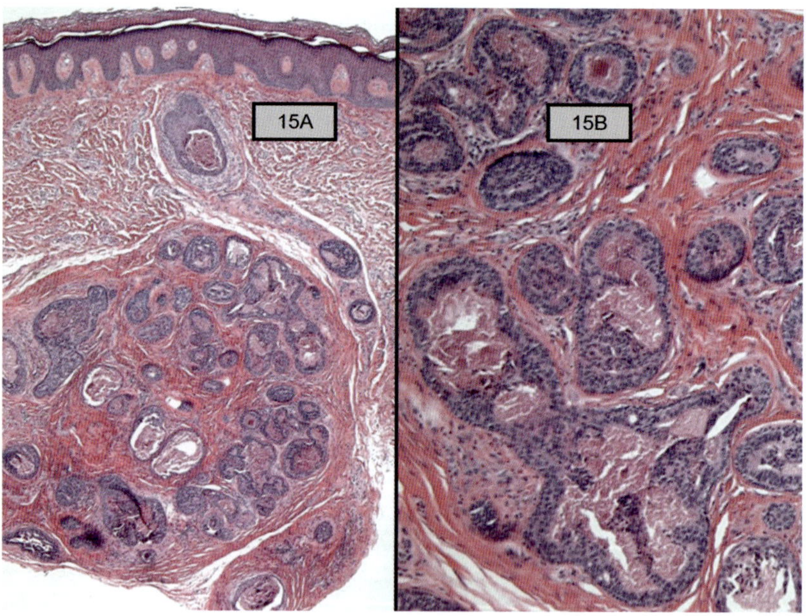

FIGURE 9.15 **Eccrine Digital Papillary Adenocarcinoma.** The low power morphology of digital papillary eccrine carcinoma **(A)** is cognate to that of ductal carcinoma in situ of the breast. Within the nests of neoplastic columnar epithelia are the areas of confluent necrosis **(B)**.

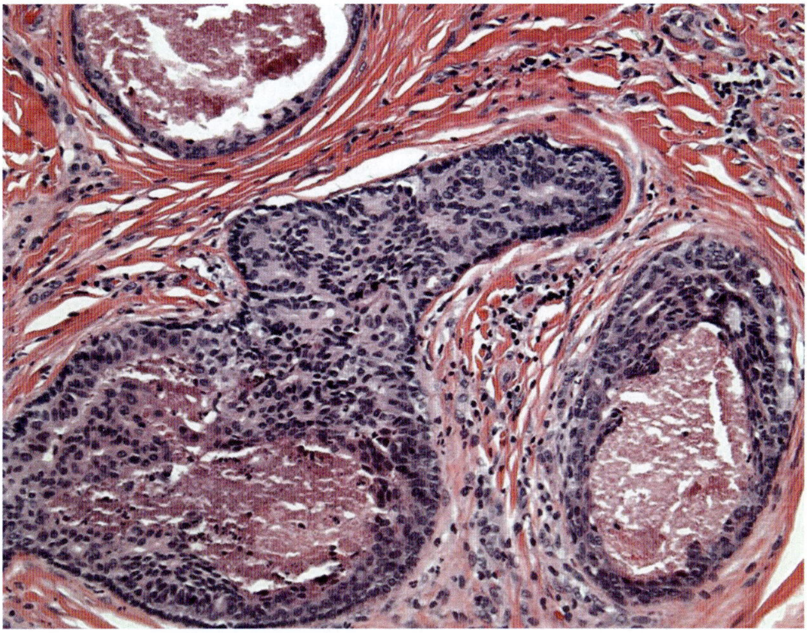

FIGURE 9.16 **Eccrine Digital Papillary Adenocarcinoma.** The neoplastic columnar epithelia form papillary tufts and buds projecting into the dilated lumina of pre-existing eccrine structures. Due to the degree of cytologic atypia, a tumor with this architectural pattern in the breast would be considered an intermediate grade cribriform/papillary carcinoma despite the abundant intraluminal necrosis.

of the human breast.[186,188–196] In particular, these neoplasms tend to manifest areas of micropapillary projections protruding into cystically dilated luminal spaces; these micropapillary structures lack fibrovascular cores. The micropapillae comprise tufts of banal or variably atypical low columnar epithelium, sometimes showing apocrine differentiation. This constellation of findings is reminiscent of the intraductal papillomas, atypical papillomas, and papillary carcinomas seen in breast ducts. Such areas may merge to form complex sheets of cells associated with stromal invasion. A subset of digital papillary eccrine neoplasms is capable of provoking distant metastatic spread with significant patient morbidity and mortality. Predicting which of these digital eccrine neoplasms belong to the subset having a metastatic potential is extremely difficult. The so-called low-grade aggressive digital papillary adenoma is distinguished from the "high-grade adenocarcinoma" by virtue of the latter showing greater pleomorphism, mitoses, and necrosis. Notwithstanding the foregoing, criteria distinguishing benign from malignant eccrine neoplasms have been elusive in the literature. Currently, all such digital eccrine papillary neoplasms are lumped together and are held to have a metastatic potential, albeit said potential is apparently greater in the more floridly atypical and mitotically active forms. Thus, the term "aggressive digital papillary adenoma" favored in an earlier era seems soon to be abandoned. Earlier textbooks in the discipline,[197] and some subspecialty textbooks of skin adnexal neoplasia,[151] distinguish papillary eccrine adenoma of acral parts from malignant papillary eccrine tumors. In earlier works, most such neoplasms were held to represent adenomas[151] lacking the capacity to generate distant metastases and/or mortality. However, even prior to 1990, it was recognized that "at least 40% of recurrent lesions (have) regional lymph node and/or pulmonary metastases."[151] The challenge of differentiating benign from malignant variants of these tumors is further clouded by the recognized capacity for histologically banal eccrine neoplasms to transform into cancers.[198] The concept of progressive transformation of benign to malignant proliferations of epithelial and other cell types has long been recognized in other tissues in humans and in animals. It is thus possible, indeed even likely, that some cases of otherwise indolent digital papillary eccrine adenoma undergo malignant transformation as well.

It is now recognized that histologic criteria did not distinguish benign (adenoma) from malignant (adenocarcinoma) in acral digital papillary eccrine adnexal neoplasms.[199] Duke's paper specifically addresses and refutes the work of Kao et al.[200] who felt that criteria existed to distinguish aggressive digital papillary adenoma from aggressive digital papillary adenocarcinoma histologically. In the hands of Kao et al., poor gland differentiation, necrosis, cytologic atypia, mitotic rates, and invasion of soft tissue, bone, or blood vessels were features that distinguished adenocarcinoma from adenoma. Despite the foregoing, the concept of papillary eccrine adenoma has persisted into the common era.[201-203]

Management

Management of the aggressive digital papillary adenoma and adenocarcinoma remains a controversial issue with some authors advising digital amputation.[180] In addition to high local recurrence, some 50% of tumors manifest distant metastases, typically to lungs and lymph nodes. As with acral melanomas, amputation at or above the nearest joint is one recommended strategy for local control.[180-182] In part because of the rarity of these tumors, modern surgical approaches such as sentinel lymphadenectomy that are commonplace for melanomas are reportable as isolated cases when applied to the digital papillary eccrine tumors.[204,205] Currently, the use of aggressive local surgical extirpation is generally advised for any digital papillary eccrine neoplasm as "originally proposed criteria for distinguishing benign (adenoma) and malignant (adenocarcinoma) do not necessarily predict biological behaviour."[205]

Differential Diagnosis

Differential diagnostic considerations include the microcystic adnexal carcinoma, hidradenoma papilliferum, syringocystadenoma papilliferum, and the nipple adenoma. Microcystic adnexal carcinoma shows thin, vertically and haphazardly oriented columns of variably atypical epithelia surmounted by keratinizing microcysts with a granular cell lining internally. It, therefore, lacks the architectural organization of the papillary eccrine and apocrine neoplasms and also does not show apocrine differentiation. Stromal desmoplasia is frequent in the microcystic adnexal carcinoma and is not seen in the digital papillary neoplasms of benign character. In contrast, the digital papillary adenocarcinomas of increasing dedifferentiation show irregularly shaped and sized nests associated with pronounced stromal fibroplasia, in concert with abundant endolumenal necrosis, overt nuclear anaplasia, and mitotic activity. These large tubulopapillary structures are thus strikingly different and simultaneously more cytologically atypical than the microcystic adnexal carcinoma and should be easily distinguished even at scanning magnification. As mentioned above, they have more in common morphologically with in situ ductal breast carcinoma than with the indolent or low-grade eccrine neoplasms. Hidradenoma papilliferum typically seen in the areas of high apocrine gland concentration such as the vulva, the perineum, and the axillae exhibits large structures with a rounded peripheral contour containing papillary proliferations of apocrine epithelium lacking cytologic atypia, necrosis, or mitotic activity. The syringocystadenoma typically opens to the epidermal surface, as seen in the setting of an underlying nevus sebaceus, and manifests banal apocrine epithelium admixed with cuboidal cells covering fibrovascular stromal cores which are rich in plasma cells. The nipple adenoma may also open to the epidermal surface to form the so-called erosive adenoma and is morphologically similar to syringocystadenoma papilliferum. Furthermore, the hidradenoma papilliferum is confined, in the majority of cases, to women. As mentioned above, the distinction of a benign eccrine papillary neoplasm from one with a metastatic potential is extremely difficult and, in the view of some authorities, impossible.

MICROCYSTIC ADNEXAL CARCINOMA

Introduction

This tumor is alluded to above. Typically a neoplasm of the mid face of young, middle-aged, or elderly woman, it has a tendency toward persistent and stubborn local recurrence but not to metastatic deposits.[182,206–209] In particular, the upper lip and the glabella are common locations; rarely, tumors appear outside the head and neck in locations such as the axilla. Local recurrence rates are approximately 50%.[210–214] Occasionally, the lesion will appear in unusual locations and settings, such as a recent case arising in the external auditory canal 15 years after radiotherapy of a nasopharyngeal carcinoma that had occurred in a 12-year-old boy.[215] Another patient showed the synchronous development of a microcystic adnexal carcinoma with a gastric carcinoma.[216]

A synonym for these tumors is *sclerosing syringomatous carcinoma* or *sclerosing sweat duct carcinoma*, which not only encompasses the neoplastic epithelia but also makes reference to the stromal desmoplasia, which is a frequent concomitant of these tumors. Currently, many microcystic adnexal carcinomas are treated with Mohs' surgery.[217]

Histopathology

The prototypic microcystic adnexal carcinoma comprises tubules of rather banal eccrine ductal epithelium, often compressed into a single column of cells, which are vertically and haphazardly oriented in the reticular dermis extending out to the peripheral margins of a punch biopsy specimen (Figs. 9.17–9.19). Surmounting the vertically oriented tubules in the papillary dermis are microcysts comprising keratinizing stratified squamous epithelia with a granular cell layer and encompassing central keratin (Fig. 9.18). The so-called sclerosing sweat duct carcinoma lacks these putative pilar microcysts[218,219] and in their absence, that designation, or in the presence of high-grade cytologic anaplasia, the terms *anaplastic syringoma* and syringoid

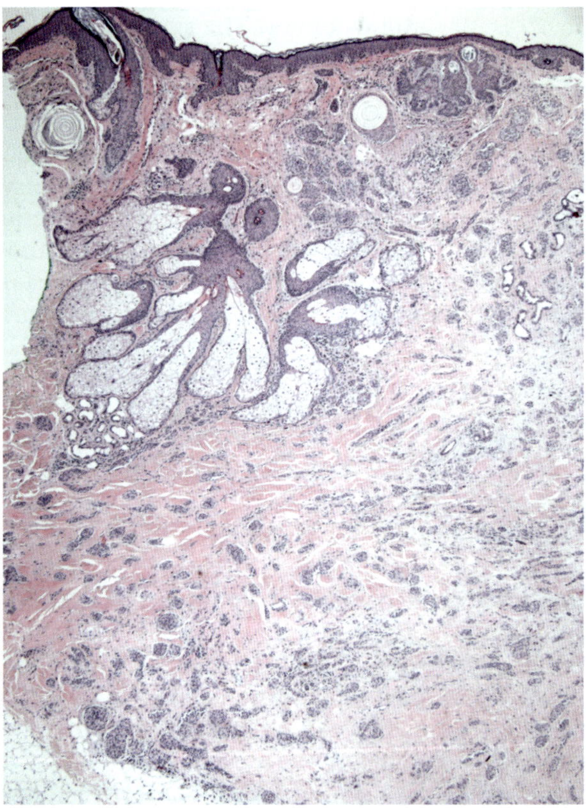

FIGURE 9.17 **Microcystic Adnexal Carcinoma.** In this low power micrograph, tumor infiltrates widely through a 4-mm punch biopsy to the deep and transverse edges of the tissue sample.

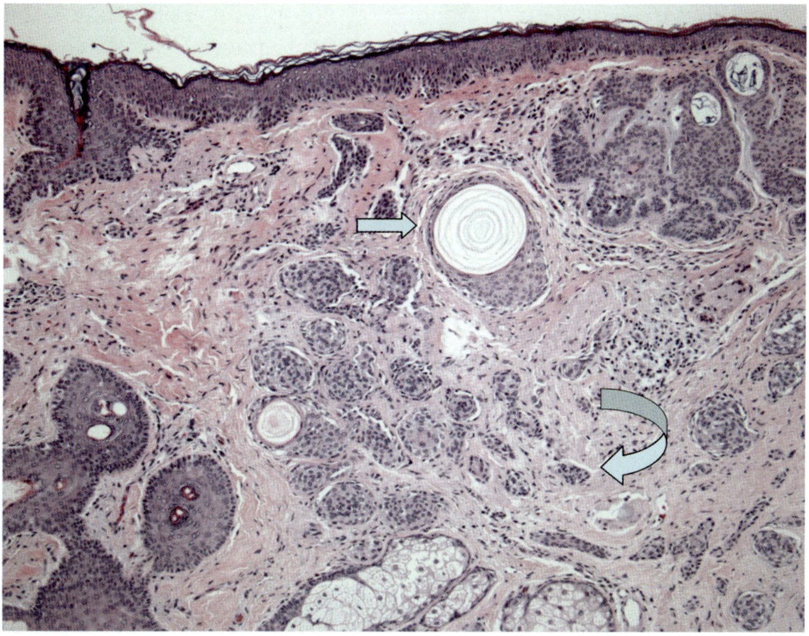

FIGURE 9.18 **Microcystic Adnexal Carcinoma.** In the superficial dermis are the microcysts of keratinous debris surrounded by squamous epithelia (*straight arrow*) showing keratohyalin granules in some foci. These keratinous microcysts surmount neoplastic tubules (*curved arrow*) which grow in a haphazard fashion through a desmoplastic stroma.

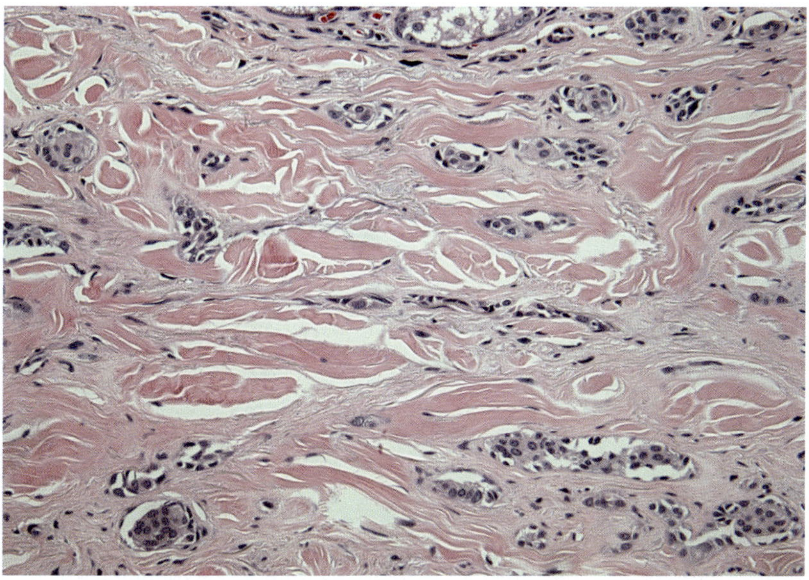

FIGURE 9.19 **Microcystic Adnexal Carcinoma.** The tumor tongues form narrow columns that grow through a desmoplastic stroma.

carcinoma have also been applied.[220,221] Neoplastic cells may infiltrate blood vessels, skeletal muscle, and perineural spaces.[222–228,153] Concentric whorls of tumor cells and clear cell change are described.[229] Inspissated secretory material and an internal lining cuticle expressing CEA (Fig. 9.20) give evidence for eccrine differentiation in these neoplasms.[218] Expression of mutant p53, c-erbB-2, bcl2, and Ki-67 is typically not observed.[230]

Differential Diagnosis

The differential diagnosis of microcystic adnexal carcinoma is that of the sclerosing adnexal neoplasms of the head and neck. These are commonly held to include the desmoplastic trichoepithelioma, the sclerosing or morpheaform BCC, the syringoma, and those rare forms of basosquamous or poorly differentiated SCC of the skin that show intracytoplasmic vacuolation suggesting gland formation, i.e., the so-called adenosquamous carcinoma of the skin. Some authors rank trichoadenoma in the differential diagnosis list for microcystic adnexal carcinoma, but in our view, this is a distinction which can be made at the light microscopic level with comparative ease. The desmoplastic trichoepithelioma typically presents as a small mid facial papule or as multiple small firm papules as distinct from the ill-defined plaque of microcystic adnexal carcinoma.[218,231,232] This clinical morphology has a histologic analog; in particular, the microcystic adnexal carcinoma is widely invasive to the edges of a 5-mm punch biopsy specimen whereas the desmoplastic trichoepithelioma might well be completely encompassed by

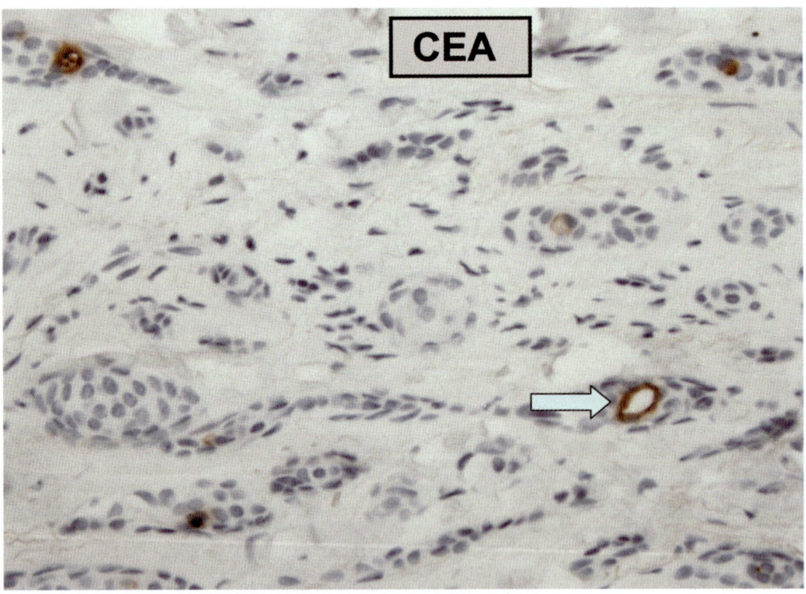

FIGURE 9.20 **Microcystic Adnexal Carcinoma: CEA immunohistochemistry.** The intracytoplasmic lumina decorate strongly with CEA (*arrow*) in this example of a microcystic adnexal carcinoma.

a biopsy of this size. Put another way, the desmoplastic trichoepithelioma is a shallow tumor whereas the microcystic adnexal carcinoma invades deeply. Like conventional trichoepithelioma, the desmoplastic form has its own modified specialized stroma and if the peripheral contour of the lesion and its interface with adjacent native dermis is identified, it has a circumscribed morphology as opposed to the ill-defined and poorly circumscribed margin of a microcystic adnexal carcinoma. Desmoplastic trichoepithelioma is often associated with horn cysts, several of which may have ruptured into the adjacent stroma with cholesterol clefts and their associated foreign body granulomatous inflammatory response. Like conventional trichoepithelioma, mitoses and individual cell necrosis should be absent. The desmoplastic trichoepithelioma may show slitlike retraction of the tumor plus the adjacent peritumoral mesenchyma from nearby stromal cells. This is distinctive from the morpheaform BCC and from the microcystic adnexal carcinoma, which characteristically does not show stromal retraction change. Trichoepithelioma is characteristically banal cytologically but this feature does not permit a distinction from the often low-grade nuclear atypia seen in microcystic adnexal carcinoma. In contrast to the foregoing, the sclerosing or morpheaform BCC shows slitlike retraction of tumor cells from the immediately adjacent stroma. Mesenchymal mucosubstances are often present in these slitlike areas of stromal retraction.[233] Mitoses are identified in morpheaform BCC but may be hard to find as the tumor volume relative to stroma is often low. Individual cell necrosis should be apparent, however. Morpheaform BCC often forms a part of an infiltrative growth tumor with larger, jagged and irregular nests and is associated with stromal desmoplasia, the fibroblasts in the mesenchymal component being plump and proplastic. Finally, there may be a component of coexistent nodular or superficial BCC which clinches the diagnosis. With respect to syringoma, these lesions show multiple layers of ductal epithelia, comma-shaped tales, and central inspissated mucosubstances. The tubular character of the syringoma and its multilayered ductal elements should enable distinction. Like the desmoplastic trichoepithelioma, it is more shallow and broad in character than is the microcystic adnexal carcinoma. Shave biopsies from this group of lesions which do not sample the tissue edges and the deep lesional margin can create diagnostic difficulties, particularly when a clinical history is not provided with the specimen.[143] One type of syringoma, namely, which is observed as a manifestation of multiple heritable syringomas, can extend deeply and can be confused with a microcystic adnexal carcinoma. In the heritable variant, there is always a well-defined pattern of cellularity with cells forming multiple layers around the ductal elements. Also, there is a definite stroma that accompanies the cellular proliferative areas as in the common syringoma. Furthemore, there is no evidence of neurotropism.[234,235] A lesion termed *syringomatous adenoma of the nipple*,[236] seen in both sexes, is held to be a form of microcystic adnexal carcinoma occurring outside the head and neck region.[143] The so-called primary adenosquamous carcinoma of skin connects to the overlying epidermis from which radiate the cytologically malignant epithelia forming intercellular bridges in concert with a glandular component comprising common lumenal margins and/or intracytoplasmic lumens. Mitoses and individual cell necrosis are a frequent finding, the latter often forming confluent zones of geographic necrosis. The tumor extends from the epidermis across a broad front and may show both perineural and vascular invasion.[237–240]

MUCOEPIDERMOID CARCINOMA OF THE SKIN

Introduction and Clinical Features

In a fashion analogous to the adenoid cystic carcinomas primary in the skin, the mucoepidermoid carcinoma is a neoplasm which recapitulates that seen in major and minor salivary glands in diverse anatomic locations.[241–243] Like adenoid cystic carcinoma in salivary gland tissue, the mucoepidermoid carcinomas in that tissue anlage tend to show multiple local recurrences and only uncommonly distant metastases; in such a scenario, the clinical history provides definitive proof.[244–247] Mucoepidermoid carcinoma has been reported to arise in a nevus sebaceus of Jadassohn.[248] As is the case with many of the adnexal carcinomas, Mohs microsurgery has been advocated in the treatment of mucoepidermoid carcinoma of the skin.[249]

Histopathology

Like their counterparts in salivary gland tissue, the primary mucoepidermoid carcinomas of the skin show an admixture of squamous epithelial elements which may be deceptively bland, associated with areas of glandular differentiation comprising low columnar mucin-containing cells often associated with mucin-containing microcysts.[241–243] Clear cell change may be seen,[247] Unlike the adenoid cystic carcinoma, perineural infiltration is rare.[143] Cytologic atypia is inconspicuous, with round to oval nuclei in the 10 to 15 μ size range showing little, if any, apoptosis and typically no mitoses.[250] These banal cytologic characteristics exclude forms of metaplasia occurring in typical SCC.[250]

Differential Diagnosis

The main diagnostic consideration would be a metastasis from a mucoepidermoid carcinoma. Prototypically, this would occur in the head and neck area. Criteria for distinguishing these two events would then become important. The presence of inflammation is said to favor a primary mucoepidermoid carcinoma as is a solitary lesion and a uninodular lesion as opposed to multifocal pattern of growth.[143] By direct extension from minor salivary gland tissue in the oral cavity and its analogs in nasopharynx or the lacrimal apparatus, mucoepidermoid carcinoma involving the skin would grow from the subcutaneous tissue and/or skeletal muscle vertically toward the skin surface, typically sparing the upper reticular and papillary dermis as well as the epidermis. In contrast, a primary mucoepidermoid carcinoma of the skin taking origin from the sweat apparatus would dominantly be centered in reticular dermis or at the dermal–subcutaneous interface. The problem of squamous syringometaplasia is less significant as the degree of atypia is typically less in this scenario; there should be evidence either of a surgical insult or of individual cell necrosis of the eccrine apparatus due to chemotherapy and/or neutrophilic hidradenitis.[251] Furthermore, a clinical history of previous cancer with appropriate chemotherapy should be available if the appropriate questions are asked. At times, mucoepidermoid carcinoma may be confused with adenosquamous carcinoma. Differentiation can be made on the basis of the presence of pancytokeratin, CK7, CEA, and EMA positivity and CK20 and GCDFP negativity. These findings indicate that this carcinoma is of adnexal origin as opposed to epidermal cell origin.[252]

CARCINOMA ARISING IN PRE-EXISTING CYLINDROMA OR ECCRINE SPIRADENOMA

Introduction and Clinical Features

Malignant degeneration of pre-existing benign eccrine adnexal tumors is a well-described phenomenon[198,253–269] and is heralded by a sudden change in tumor size or the acquisition of symptomatology such as pain or ulceration.

Histopathology

To be considered a bona fide finding, the pre-existing benign neoplasm must be identifiable. The malignant degeneration is typically characterized by sheets of undifferentiated carcinoma cells showing loose cohesion, whereby the tumor cells have high-grade nuclear atypia. The tumor may form sheets of polygonal cells with abundant eosinophilic cytoplasm, spindled areas, or admixtures of the foregoing. Mitoses and individual cell necrosis are a common finding and there may be zones of geographic necrosis as well.[143,254,257] In consequence of the foregoing, the tumor may have pure squamous, adenosquamous, glandular, or sacromatoid features. These changes do not necessarily herald imminent metastatic behavior.[259,262,263] A hybrid tumor exhibiting features of a malignant cylindroma and of a malignant spiradenoma has been described in two patients; the authors held that elevated p53 expression and increased nuclear staining with Ki-67 can be useful in distinguishing benign from malignant appendage tumors.[132]

ECCRINE DUCTAL ADENOCARCINOMA

Introduction and Clinical Features

Eccrine ductal adenocarcinoma is so named because it histologically mimics the ductal carcinomas of the breast.[127,220,270] Clinical history then becomes essential to proper interpretation.[143] This primary skin tumor is typically a slow-growing lesion up to 5 cm in diameter present for months or years prior to presentation. It is therefore quite distinctive from secondary deposits of breast cancer in the skin, which typically occur either in the skin of the ipsolateral anterior chest wall or axilla or occur as multiple disseminated metastatic seeds in a widespread disposition.[270,271] Like primary breast cancers and like the aggressive digital papillary adenoma/low-grade papillary adenocarcinoma of the digits, primary ductal eccrine adenocarcinoma is an aggressive tumor that has a high risk of disseminated metastatic seeding.

Histopathology

The eccrine ductal adenocarcinoma is characterized by solid sheets and cords of cells forming true common lumenal margins with tubuloalveolar formations, papillary components, and areas of obvious infiltration of a desmoplastic stroma.[169,272–276] In the primary location, carcinoma in situ of the eccrine straight ducts and of the secretory coil may be demonstrated in a fashion analogous to high-grade in situ ductal carcinoma of the breast.[272] A further analogy with breast cancer is the presence of a parallel immunohistochemical profile including in the context of estrogen and progesterone hormone receptors.[277,278] The foregoing necessitates correlation to a comprehensive and accurate clinical history. Areas of squamous differentiation may be seen in the eccrine ductal adenocarcinoma. Some forms show a fibromyxoid stroma, which has caused some authorities to label such lesions *malignant chondroid syringoma*,[189,272] whereas others use the term *eccrine adenocarcinoma with fibromyxoid stroma*.[189,272] These lesions may connect to the epidermal surface and so mimic forms of basal cell or SCC with myxoid stroma but invariably express EMA enabling distinction.[189,278] These tumors may collide with other forms of primary eccrine cancer.

Differential Diagnosis

As implied by the histomorphology, the differential diagnosis of the eccrine ductal adenocarcinoma is in fact a metastatic deposit of ductal carcinoma of the breast which can be distinguished by clinical history in most cases.

CLEAR CELL ECCRINE CARCINOMA

Introduction

On occasion, a malignant neoplasm with obvious eccrine features will show an overwhelming or universal clear cell cytoplasmic morphology. The designation "clear cell eccrine carcinoma" is then applied.[279,280] The clinical behavior and nosology are similar to that of the malignant acrospiroma or hidradenocarcinoma[281–287,272]; the abundant clear cell change gives the tumor a distinctive histomorphology and differential diagnosis.

Clinical Features

The tumors present typically as a solid nodular growth in the head and neck region up to 5 cm in greatest diameter.

Histopathology

Skin biopsies show a multinodular dermal proliferation with no connection to the overlying epidermis. The critical cells have abundant clear cytoplasms and neoplastic nuclei that may either be of low grade with round to oval nuclei manifesting smooth contours or may have more atypical features with irregular clearing of chromatin and irregular thickening of the chromatinic rim. The tumor masses form broad sheets separated by a fibrovascular stroma. The mitotic count is variable with no defined threshold for diagnosis. Similarly, necrosis may be absent or may manifest as individual cell necrosis and occasionally as confluent or geographic necrosis. Some cases show perineural or vascular invasion.[279,280].

Differential Diagnosis

The differential diagnosis of malignant clear cell neoplasms in the skin includes metastases from clear cell tumors of thyroid and kidney, and rarely from lung.[270,288] The metastatic renal cell tumors often have granular debris in their stroma and a finely arborizing vascular pattern; as well, they express relatively specific markers including Pax-2 and RCC. In the modern era, the use of antibodies to TTF enables easy distinction of pulmonary primary large cell carcinomata, in which TTF is almost uniformly expressed, from those primary clear cell carcinomas in the skin, in which TTF studies are negative. A proportion of clear cell neoplasms of ovary, kidney, and endometrium may have a hobnail pattern which is absent in the primary cutaneous clear cell carcinoma.[270,288–290] As with other eccrine cancers, the clear cell variant expresses CEA which is uniformly negative in renal cell cancer and is also typically not expressed in the neoplasms of ovary and endometrium.[278]

CARCINOSARCOMA

Introduction

Although occasional cases of fully transformed malignant neoplasms arising in cutaneous mixed tumors are reported,[291] the term *malignant mixed tumor* is reserved for neoplasms showing divergent differentiation with both epithelial and mesenchymal cell lines demonstrated.[143,292–302] Carcinosarcoma has been reported to arise in a patient with multiple cylindromas.[303]

Clinical Features

In the typical setting of a pre-existing indolent nodule, a patient reports rapid change with growth, ulceration, and sometimes tenderness. Despite a histopathology suggesting an aggressive neoplasm, most behave in a biologically indolent fashion.

Histopathology

The typical malignant mixed tumor comprises a neoplasm in which areas of recognizable eccrine differentiation are admixed with neoplastic mesenchymal elements, be they of chondrosarcoma, rhabdomyosarcoma, leiomyosarcoma, osteosarcoma, or fibrosarcoma types or undifferentiated sarcomatous proliferations.[292–302] In a case of carcinosarcoma arising in a cylindroma, there were both clearly malignant adnexal epithelia as well as a sarcomatous area with malignant spindle cells.[303]

Differential Diagnosis

True carcinosarcomas of breast, lung, and other sites can involve the skin by direct extension or by metastatic seeding.[304] These neoplasms prove difficult to differentiate from primary cutaneous malignant mixed tumors. With respect to pulmonary disease, application of TTF immunohistochemistry has not yet been reported in the literature to our knowledge but this seems a logical course.

BASALOID ECCRINE CARCINOMA

Introduction

A tumor of historical note, basaloid eccrine carcinoma was first reported in 1968[220,305] in a series of cutaneous neoplasms, some of which likely represent, in hind sight, Merkel cell carcinoma.[306] More recently, a small cell or basaloid variant of eccrine cancer has been described[307] which appears to represent a bona fide entity.[307]

Clinical Features

In the experience of Wick et al.,[143] these tumors are invariably long-standing acral neoplasms which, at least in some, have been proven capable of producing metastatic deposits in lymph nodes and, in at least one case, fatal dissemination to viscera.

Histopathology

Nests and cords of monotonous small basaloid cells with hyperchromatic nuclei showing frequent and atypical mitoses, individual cell and confluent necrosis, and sparse cytoplasms mimicking neuroendocrine carcinoma typify this tumor. Areas of confluent necrosis lead to microcyst formation. The stroma may be desmoplastic in nature.

Differential Diagnosis

The differential diagnosis of the basaloid eccrine carcinoma includes the "small round blue cell tumors" including the Merkel cell carcinoma, Ewing's sarcoma, mesenchymal chondrosarcoma, lymphoma, and small cell melanoma[308] or basaloid SCC. With respect to these differential diagnostic considerations, Merkel cell carcinomas express chromogranin and synaptophysin, Ewing's sarcoma expresses CD99 and contains abundant cytoplasmic glycogen, lymphomas typically express common leukocyte antigen (CD45), and small cell melanoma, in most cases, is S100 positive but may also decorate for melanocyte lineage-specific markers such as Melan-A and HMB-45. SCCs, as described above, typically do not express CEA.

PAGET'S DISEASE

Introduction

In the past, Paget's disease of the breast, and in particular of the nipple, so-called mammary Paget's disease, was held to derive from neoplastic transformation of the breast ductal system with secondary extension to the skin. In contrast, extramammary Paget's disease was thought to represent a neoplasm arising in the germinative cells of the basal layer of the epidermis.[309,310] Both processes were held to manifest apocrine differentiation, but both were held to have different paths of lesional development. However, there are cases of mammary Paget's disease lacking underlying ductal carcinoma of the breast,[311,312] and further we have seen lesions of extramammary Paget's disease with underlying sweat gland carcinoma (personal observation). An alternative cell of origin, the clear cell of Toker, represents the termination of mammary and mammary-like ducts in nipple and vulva and has been postulated as a potential alternative progenitor cell.[313]

Clinical Features

Irrespective of anatomic location, tumors present as erythematous plaques with a scaling or exudative surface. Paget's disease of the breast involves women who most often have an underlying ductal carcinoma and, as one might expect, presentations are typically greater than 40 years of age. Extramammary Paget's disease occurs with an almost equal sex distribution and appears to be concentrated in anatomic sites where apocrine glands manifest greatest density, i.e., the vulva, scrotum, perineum, axillae, perineal region, eyelids, and the ear canals. Lesions of extramammary Paget's disease have been reported in association with condyloma accuminatum.[314]

Histopathologic Features

In Paget's disease, the epidermis manifests a proliferation of single and clustered neoplastic cells showing evidence of glandular differentiation. The nuclei are round to oval with prominent nucleoli and dispersed chromatin; typically, the nuclear diameters are up to double of those adjacent keratinocyte nuclei. The glandular differentiation takes the form of intracytoplasmic lumina manifesting a basophilic cytoplasmic hue, sometimes with a sharply demarcated intracytoplasmic cuticle. The glandular epithelia may also cluster together to form common luminal margins (Fig. 9.21).

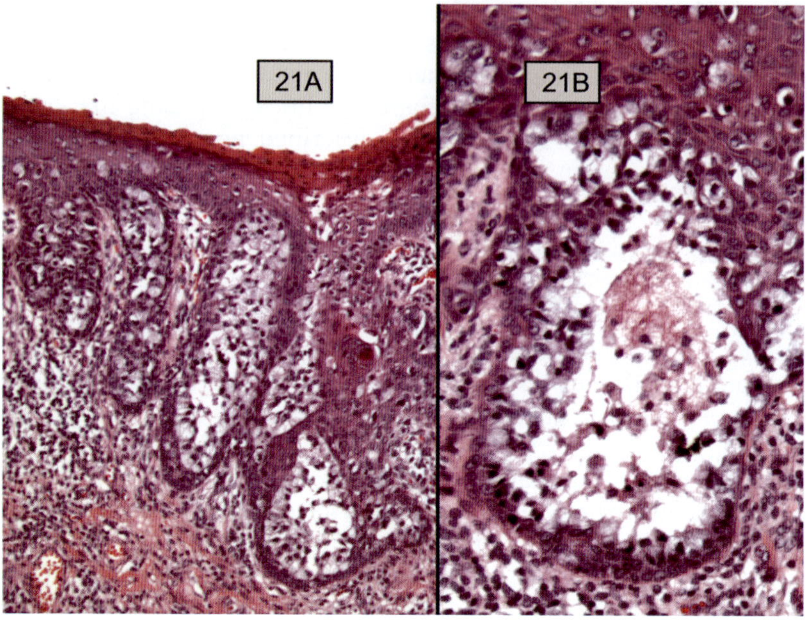

FIGURE 9.21 **Extramammary Paget's Disease.** In extramammary Paget's disease, the squamous epithelium is replaced by loosely cohesive groups of neoplastic glandular epithelia **(A)**. The neoplastic glandular epithelia appear to compress the basal layer of squamous epithelium from above **(B)**.

On occasion, the cytoplasm shows fine vacuolation.[315-320] For reasons not understood, the neoplastic glandular cells in Paget's disease often spare the basal layer of the epidermis and appear to compress it from above. As the neoplastic cells have less well-defined intercellular bridges than keratinocytes, they form loosely cohesive groups in a fashion that may mimic an acantholytic process. A rare example of Paget's disease shows marked variation of nuclear size and shape with less conspicuous glandular differentiation; this has been termed *anaplastic Paget's disease*.[321] The neoplastic cells in any event contain cytoplasmic epithelial mucins that decorate with alcian blue-PAS, PAS-diastase, and mucicarmine preparations. Histochemically, the tumors express GCDFP-15 as would be anticipated in light of their apocrine lineage,[322] in concert with CK7 and CEA.[323-326] Androgen receptors and Her2/neu are commonly expressed in both extramammary and mammary Paget's disease, while estrogen and progesterone receptors are not[327]; Her2/neu overexpression[328] implicates a potential therapeutic role for the Her2/neu receptor blocker trastuzumab.[329]

Differential Diagnosis

Neoplasms that show pagetoid migration of malignant epithelia include clonal Bowen's disease, sebaceous carcinoma, and melanomas, particularly of superficial spreading type. With respect to superficial spreading melanoma, the presence of melanin granules in the cytoplasms of the neoplastic cells is an important clue to diagnosis, but we have seen cases of pigmented Paget's disease and pigmented Bowen's disease containing melanin granules provided by nurse melanocytes to the neoplastic cells. Thus, one must fall back upon immunohistochemical methods to delineate these lesions. Melanomas express melanocyte lineage-specific markers such as HMB-45 and Melan-A, versus the expression of GCDFP-15, CK7, and CEA in Paget's disease.[323–326] Bowen's disease, in contrast, will express high-molecular weight cytokeratin but not CK7 and should not express any of the aforementioned melanocyte or apocrine lineage differentiation markers. In addition to positivity for CK20, glandular neoplasms of the genitourinary or gastrointestinal tract (i.e., endocervix, urachus, or colorectum) may cause diagnostic confusion.[330–333] Extramammary Paget's disease does not express estrogen or progesterone receptor antigenicity but has been shown to express androgen receptor proteins as discussed above.[334,335] Differential expression of claudins, proteins involved in tight junction assembly in epithelial and endothelial cells, may differentiate the cells of Paget's disease from adjacent squamous epithelia but not from breast carcinoma cells.[336] Another form of pagetoid intraepidermal carcinoma with vacuolated cells is sebaceous carcinoma, but in this entity, the cells appear vacuolated with a clear cytoplasmic morphology as opposed to basophilic mucin. It has been shown that CD 5 will strongly decorate both Paget's and extramammary Paget's disease but will not react with the cells of Bowen's disease, melanoma in situ, or sebaceous carcinoma.[337] Other immunochemical markers such as the T-antigen expressed in sebaceous carcinoma are discussed in the section on tumors of the pilosebaceous apparatus.

REFERENCES

1. Lever WF. Sebaceous adenoma. Review of the literature and report of a case. *Arch Dermatol* 1948;57:102–111.
2. Warren S, Warvi WN. Tumors of sebaceous glands. *Am J Pathol* 1943;19:441–460.
3. Prioleau PG, Santa Cruz DJ. Sebaceous gland neoplasia. *J Cutan Pathol* 1984;11:396–414.
4. Rulon DB, Helwig EB. Cutaneous sebaceous neoplasms. *Cancer* 1974;33:82–102.
5. Brownstein MH, Shapiro L.The pilosebaceous tumors. *Int J Dermatol* 1977;16:340–352.
6. Mehregan AH, Rahbari H. Benign epithelial tumors of the skin. II. Benign sebaceous tumors. *Cutis* 1977;19:317–320.
7. Reiffers J, Laugier P, Hunziker N. Sebaceous hyperplasias, keratoacanthomas, epitheliomas of the face, and cancer of the colon: A new entity? *Dermatologica* 1976;153:23–33.
8. Rulon DB, Helwig EB. Multiple sebaceous neoplasms of the skin: An association with multiple visceral carcinomas, especially of the colon. *Am J Clin Pathol* 1973;60:745–753.
9. Sciallis GF, Winkelmann RK. Multiple sebaceous adenomas and gastrointestinal carcinoma. *Arch Dermatol* 1974;110:913–916.
10. Housholder MS, Zeligman. Sebaceous neoplasms associated with visceral carcinomas. *Arch Dermatol* 1980;116:61–64.

11. Tschang TP, Poulos E, Ho CK. Multiple sebaceouss adenomas and internal malignant disease: A case report with chromosomal analysis. *Hum Pathol* 1976;7:589–594.
12. Fahmy A, Burgdorf WHC, Schosser RH, Pitha J. Muir–Torre syndrome. Reevaluation of the dermatological features and consideration of its relationship to the family cancer syndrome. *Cancer* 1973;49:1898–1903.
13. Burgdorf WHC, Pitha J, Fahmy A. Muir–Torre syndrome. Histologic spectrum of sebaceous proliferations. *Am J Dermatopathol* 1986;8:202–208.
14. Davis DA, Cohen PR. Genitourinary tumors in men with the Muir–Torre syndrome. *J Am Acad Dermatol* 1995;33:909–912.
15. Lasser A, Carter DM. Multiple basal cell epitheliomas with sebaceous differentiation. *Arch Dermatol* 1973;107:91–93.
16. McMullan FH. Sebaceous epithelioma. *Arch Dermatol* 1955;71:725–727.
17. Zackheim HS. The sebaceous epithelioma. *Arch Dermatol* 1964;89:711–724.
18. Okuda C, Ito M, Fujiwara H, Takenouchi T. Sebaceous epithelioma with sweat gland differentiation. *Am J Dermatopathol* 1995;17:523–528.
19. Rothko F, Farmer ER, Zeligman I. Superficial epithelioma with sebaceous differentiation. *Arch Dermatol* 1980;116:329–331.
20. Friedman KJ, Boudreau S, Farmer ER. Superficial epithelioma with sebaceous differentiation. *J Cutan Pathol* 1987;14:193–197.
21. Lee MJ, Kim YC, Lew W. A case of superficial epithelioma with sebaceous differentiation. *Yonsei Med J* 2003;30:347–350.
22. Mahalingam M, Bhawan J, Finn R, Stefanato CM. Tumor of the follicular infundibulum with sebaceous differentiation. *J Cutan Pathol* 2001;28:314–317.
23. Troy JL, Ackerman AB. Sebaceoma: A distinctive benign neoplasm of adnexal epithelium differentiating toward sebaceous cells. *Am J Dermatopathol* 1984;6:7–13.
24. Misago N, Mihara I, Ansai S-I, Narisawa Y. Sebaceoma and related neoplasms with sebaceous differentiation. *Am J Dermatopathol* 2002;24:294–304.
25. Zaim MT. Sebocrine adenoma: An adnexal adenoma with sebaceous and apocrine poroma-like differentiation. *Am J Dermatopathol* 1988;10:311–318.
26. Grosshans E, Hanau D. L'adenome infundibulaire: Un porome folliculaire a' differenciation sebacee et apocrine. *Ann Dermatol Venereol* 1981;108:59–66.
27. Misago N, Suse T, Uemura T, Narisawa Y. Basal cell carcinoma with sebaceous differentiation. *Am J Dermatopathol* 2004;26:298–303.
28. Wick MR, Goellner JR, Wolfe JT III, Su WPD. Adnexal carcinomas of the skin. II. Extraocular sebaceous carcinomas. *Cancer* 1985;56:1163–1172.
29. Wolfe JT III, Wick MR, Campbell RJ. Sebaceous carcinomas of the oculocutaneous adnexa and extraocular skin. In: Wick MR, ed. *Pathology of Unusual Malignant Cutaneous Tumors*. New York: Marcel Dekker, 1985:77–106.
30. Wolfe JT III, Campbell RJ, Yeatts RP. Sebaceous carcinoma of the eyelid: Errors in clinical and pathologic diagnosis. *Am J Surg Pathol* 1984;8:597–606.
31. Rao NA, Hidayat AA, McLean IW, Zimmerman LE. Sebaceous carcinoma of the ocular adnexa: A clinicopathologic study of 104 cases, with five-year followup data. *Hum Pathol* 1982;13:113–122.
32. Ni C, Kuo PK. Meibomian gland carcinoma: A clinicopathological study of 156 cases with long-period followup of 100 cases. *Jpn J Ophthalmol* 1979;23:388–401.
33. Graham RM, McKee PH, McGibbon D. Sebaceous carcinoma. *Clin Exp Dermatol* 1984;9:466–471.
34. Doxanas MT, Green WR. Sebaceous gland carcinoma: Review of 40 cases. *Arch Ophthalmol* 1984;102:245–249.
35. Ausidio RA, Lodeville O, Quaglivolo V, Clemente C. Sebaceous carcinoma arising from the eyelid and from extraocular sites. *Tumori* 1987;73:531–535.

36. Nguyen GK, Mielke BW. Extraocular sebaceous carcinoma with intraepidermal (pagetoid) spread. *Am J Dermatopathol* 1987;9:304–305.
37. Nelson BR, Hamlet KR, Gillard M, et al. Sebaceous carcinoma. *J Am Acad Dermatol* 1995;33:1–15.
38. Harvey PA, Parsons MA, Rennie IG. Primary sebaceous carcinoma of lacrimal gland: A previously unreported primary neoplasm. *Eye* 1994;8:592–595.
39. Ansai S, Hashimoto H, Aoki T, et al. A histochemical and immunohistochemical study of extraocular sebaceous carcinoma. *Histopathology* 1993;22:127–133.
40. Shields JA, Demirci H, Marr BP, et al. Sebaceous carcinoma of the eyelids: Personal experience with 60 cases. *Ophthalmology* 2004;111:2151–2157.
41. Oppenheim AR. Sebaceous carcinoma of the penis. *Arch Dermatol* 1981;117:306–307.
42. Bassetto F, Baraziol R, Sottosanti MV, et al. Biological behaviour of the sebaceous carcinoma of the head. *Dermatol Surg* 2004;30:472–476.
43. Cohen PR, Kohn SR. Association of sebaceous gland tumors and internal malignancy: The Muir-Torre syndrome. *Am J Med* 1991;90:606–613.
44. Moreno C, Jacyk WK, Judd MJ, Requena L. Highly aggressive extraocular sebaceous carcinoma. *Am J Dermatopathol* 2001;23:450–455.
45. Ohara M, Sotozono C, Tsuchihashi Y, Kinoshita S. Ki-67 labeling index as a marker of malignancy in ocular surface neoplasms. *Jpn J Ophthalmol* 2004;48:524–529.
46. Luderschmidt C, Plewig G. Circumscribed sebaceous gland hyperplasia: Autoradiographic and histoplanometric studies. *J Invest Dermatol* 1978;70:207–209.
47. Kudoh K, Hosokawa M, Miyazawa T, Tagami H. Giant solitary sebaceous gland hyperplasia clinically simulating epidermoid cyst. *J Cutan Pathol* 1988;15:396–398.
48. Nakamura SI, Nakayama K, Nishihara K, Imai T. Sebaceous carcinoma, with special reference to the histopathologic differential diagnosis. *J Dermatol* 1988;15:55–59.
49. Misago N, Narisawa Y. Sebaceous carcinoma with apocrine differentiation. *Am J Dermatopathol* 2001;23:50–57.
50. Kazakov DV, Kutzner H, Rutten A, et al. Carcinoid-like pattern in sebaceous neoplasms: Another distinctive, previously unrecognized pattern in extraocular sebaceous carcinoma and sebaceoma. *Am J Dermatopathol* 2005;27:195–203.
51. Abbott JJ, Hernandez-Rios P, Amirkhan RH, et al. Cystic sebaceous neoplasms in Muir-Torre syndrome. *Arch Pathol Lab Med* 2003;127:614–617.
52. Sinard JH. Immunohistochemical distinction of ocular sebaceous carcinoma from basal cell and squamous carcinoma. *Arch Ophthalmol* 1999;117:776–783.
53. Ansai S, Mitsuhashi Y, Kondo S, Manabe M. Immunohistochemical differentiation of extra-ocular sebaceous carcinoma from other skin cancers. *J Dermatol* 2004;31:998–1008.
54. Hassanein AM. Sebaceous carcinoma and the T-antigen. *Semin Cutan Med Surg* 2004; 23:62–72.
55. Rishi K, Font RL. Sebaceous gland tumors of the eyelids and the conjunctiva in the Muir-Torres syndrome: A clinicopathological study of five cases and literature review. *Ophthal Plast Reconstr Surg* 2004;20:31–36.
56. Swanson PE, Wick MR. Immunohistochemistry of cutaneous tumors. In: Leong ASY, ed. *Applied Immunohistochemistry for the Surgical Pathologist.* London: Edward Arnold, 1993:269–308.
57. Crowson AN, MacInnes C, Carlson-Sweet K, et al. Clear cell atypical fibroxanthoma: A clinicopathological study. *J Cutan Pathol* 2002;29:374–381.
58. Crowson AN, Taylor JR, Magro CM. Clear cell vs 'conventional' atypical fibroxanthoma: A clinicopathologic study of 10 cases. *Lab Invest* 2003;90A.
59. Jensen K, Wilkinson B, Wines N, Koosard S. Procollagen 1 expression in atypical fibroxanthoma and other tumors. *J Cutan Pathol* 2004;31:57–61.

60. McBride SR, Leonard N, Reynolds NJ. Loss of p21 (WAF1) compartmentalisation in sebaceous carcinoma compared with sebaceous hyerplasia and sebaceous adenoma. *J Cutan Pathol* 2002;55:763–766.
61. Jimenez FJ, Burchette JL Jr, Grichnik JM, Hitchcock MG. BER–EP4 immunoreactivity in normal skin and cutaneous neoplasms. *Mod Pathol* 1995;8:854–858.
62. Mehregan AH, Pinkus H. Life history of organoid nevi: Special reference to nevus sebaceus of Jadassohn. *Arch Dermatol* 1965;91:574–587.
63. Morioka S. The natural history of nevus sebaceus. *J Cutan Pathol* 1985;12:200–213.
64. Lentz CL, Altman J, Mopper C. Nevus sebaceus of Jadassohn. *Arch Dermatol* 1968;97: 294–296.
65. Wilson-Jones E, Heyl T. Nevus sebaceus: A report of 140 cases with special regard to the development of secondary malignant tumors. *Br J Dermatol* 1970;82:99–105.
66. Clancy RR, Kurtz MB, Baker D, et al. Neurologic manifestations of the organoid nevus syndrome. *Arch Neurol* 1985;42:236–240.
67. Zaremba J. Jadassohn's nevus phakomatosis: A study based on a review of 37 cases. *J Ment Defic Res* 1977;22:103–122.
68. Alessi E, Wong SN, Advani HH, Ackermon AB. Nevus sebaceus is associated with unusual neoplasms: An atlas. *Am J Dermatopathol* 1988;10:116–127.
69. Crowson AN, Magro CM. Desmoplastic trichilemmoma and its association with basal cell carcinoma. *Am J Dermatopathol* 1996;18:43–48.
70. Ng WK. Nevus sebaceus with apocrine and sebaceous differentiation. *Am J Dermatopathol* 1996;18:420–423.
71. Crowson AN, Magro CM, Kadin M, et al. Differential expression of bcl-2 oncogene in human basal cell carcinoma. *Hum Pathol* 1996;27:355–359.
72. Domingo J, Helwig EB. Malignant neoplasms associated with nevus sebaceus of Jadassohn. *J Am Acad Dermatol* 1979;1:545–556.
73. Tarkhan H, Domingo J. Metastasizing eccrine porocarcinoma developing in a nevus sebaceus of Jadassohn: Report of a case. *Arch Dermatol* 1985;121:413–415.
74. Headington JT. Tumors of the hair follicle: A review. *Am J Pathol* 1976;85:480–505.
75. Ten Seldam REJ. Tricholemmocarcinoma. *Australas J Dermatol* 1977;18:62–72.
76. Krumrey KW. The tricholemmal carcinoma: Report of a case with review of the literature. *Aktuel Dermatol* 1984;10:70–72.
77. Schell H, Haneke E. Tricholemmal carcinoma: Report of 11 cases. *Hautarzt* 1986;37: 384–387.
78. Grouls V. Tricholemmale Keratose und tricholemmales Karzinom. *Hautarzt* 1987;38: 335–341.
79. Boscaino A, Terracciano LM, Donofrio V, et al. Trichilemmal carcinoma: A study of seven cases. *J Cutan Pathol* 1992;19:94–99.
80. Swanson PE, Marrogi AJ, Williams DJ, et al. Trichilemmal carcinoma. *J Cutan Pathol* 1992;19:100–109.
81. Reis JP, Tellechea O, Cunha MF, Baptista AP. Trichilemmal carcinoma: Review of eight cases. *J Cutan Pathol* 1993;20:44–49.
82. Wong TY, Suster S. Trichilemmal carcinoma: A clinicopathologic study of 13 cases. *Am J Dermatopathol* 1994;16:463–473.
83. Garrett AB, Azmi FH, Ogburia KS. Trichilemmal carcinoma: A rare cutaneous malignancy: A report of two cases. *Dermatol Surg* 2004;30:113–115.
84. Lai TF, Huilgol SC, James CL, Celva D. Trichilemmal carcinoma of the upper eyelid. *Acta Ophthalmol Scand* 2003;81:536–538.
85. Allee JE, Cotsarelis G, Solky B, Cook JL. Multiple recurrent trichilemmal carcinoma with perineural invasion and cytokeratin 17 positivity. *Dermatol Surg* 2003;29:886–889.

86. Ohnishi T, Watanabe S. Immunohistochemical analysis of cytokeratin expression in various trichogenic tumors. *Am J Dermatopathol* 1999;21:337–343.

87. Haas N, Audring H, Sterry W. Carcinoma arising in a proliferating trichilemmal cyst expresses fetal and trichilemmal hair phenotype. *Am J Dermatopathol* 2002;24:340–344.

88. Mori O, Hachisuka H, Sasai Y. Proliferating trichilemmal cyst with spindle cell carcinoma. *Am J Dermatopathol* 1990;12:479–484.

89. Alvarez-Quinones M, Garijo MF, Fernandez F, et al. Malignant aneuploid spindle cell transformation in a proliferatiing trichilemmal tumor. *Acta Dermatol Venereol* 1993;73:444–446.

90. Marrogi AJ, Wick MR, Dehner LP. Pilomatrical neoplasms in children and young adults. *Am J Dermatopathol* 1992;14:87–94.

91. Kaddu S, Soyer HP, Hodl S, et al. Morphological stages of pilomatricoma. *Am J Dermatopathol* 1996;18:333–338.

92. Ter Poorten HJ, Sharbaugh AH. Extruding pilomatricoma: Report of a case. *Cutis* 1978;22:47–49.

93. Tsoitis G, Mandinaos C, Kanitakis JC. Perforating calcifying epithelioma of Malherbe with a rapid evolution. *Dermatologica* 1984;168:233–237.

94. Zulaica A, Peteiro C, Quintas C, et al. Perforating pilomatricoma. *J Cutan Pathol* 1988; 15:409–411.

95. Alli N, Gungor E, Artuz F. Perforating pilomatricoma. *J Am Acad Dermatol* 1996;35: 116–118.

96. Lee WS, Yoo MS, Ahn SK. Anetodermic cutaneous changes overlying pilomatricoma. *Int J Dermatol* 1995;34:144–145.

97. Shames BS, Nassif A, Bailey CS, Saltzstein SL. Secondary anetoderma involving a pilomatricoma. *Am J Dermatopathol* 1994;16:557–560.

98. Forbis R, Helwig EB. Pilomatrixoma (calcifying epithelioma). *Arch Dermatol* 1961;83: 606–618.

99. Moehlenbeck FW. Pilomatrixoma (calcifying epithelioma). *Arch Dermatol* 1973;108: 532–534.

100. Taaffe A, Wyatt EH, Bury HPR. Pilomatrixoma (Malherbe). A clinical and histological survey of 78 cases. *Int J Dermatol* 1988;27:477–480.

101. Kaddu S, Soyer HP, Cerroni L, et al. Clinical and histopathological spectrum of pilomatricoma in adults. *Int J Dermatol* 1994;33:705–708.

102. Bassarova A, Nesland JM, Sebloev T, et al. Pilomatrix carcinoma with lymph node metastases. *J Cutan Pathol* 2004;31:330–335.

103. Inglefield CJ, Muir IF, Gray ES. Aggressive pilomatricoma in childhood. *Ann Plast Surg* 1994;33:656–658.

104. Lopansri S, Mihm MC. Pilomatrix carcinoma or calcifying epitheliocarcinoma of Malherbe: A case report and review of the literature. *Cancer* 1980;45:2368–2373.

105. Gray M, Parhizgar B, Beerman H. Malignant pilomatrixoma. *Arch Dermatol* 1984;120: 770–773.

106. Manivel JC, Wick MR, Mukai K. Pilomatrix carcinoma: An immunohistochemical comparison with benign pilomatrixoma and other benign lesions of pilar origin. *J Cutan Pathol* 1986;13:22–29.

107. Gould E, Kurzon R, Kowalczyk AP, Saldana M. Pilomatrix carcinoma with pulmonary metastases: A report of a case. *Cancer* 1984;54:370–372.

108. Van der Walt JD, Rohlova B. Carcinomatous transformation in a pilomatrixoma. *Am J Dermatopathol* 1984;6:63–69.

109. Weedon D, Bell J, Maize J. Matrical carcinoma of the skin. *J Cutan Pathol* 1980;7:39–42.

110. Reed RJ, Lamar LM. Invasive hair matrix tumors of the scalp: Invasive pilomatrixoma. *Arch Dermatol* 1966;94:310–316.

111. Martelli G, Giardini R. Pilomatrix carcinoma: A case report and review of the literature. *Eur J Surg Oncol* 1994;20:703–704.

112. Panico L, Manivel JC, Pettinato G, et al. Pilomatrix carcinoma. *Tumori* 1994;80:309–314.

113. Sau P, Lupton GP, Graham JH. Pilomatrix carcinoma. *Cancer* 1993;71:2491–2498.

114. Zagarella SS, Kneale KL, Stern HS. Pilomatrix carcinoma of the scalp. *Aust J Dermatol* 1992;33:39–42.

115. Niedermeyer HP, Peris K, Hofler H. Pilomatrix carcinoma with multiple visceral metastases: Report of a case. *Cancer* 1996;77:1311–1314.

116. Rahbari H, Mehregan AH. Pilary complex carcinoma: An adnexal carcinoma of the skin with differentiation towards the components of the pilary complex. *J Dermatol* 1993;20:630–637.

117. Sanchez-Yus E, Requena L, Simon P, Sanchez M. Complex adnexal tumor of the primary epithelial germ with distinct patterns of superficial epithelioma with sebaceous differentiation, immature trichoepithelioma, and apocrine adenocarcinoma. *Am J Dermatopathol* 1992;14:245–252.

118. Wick MR, Swanson PE, LeBoit PE, Cooper PH. Lymphoepithelioma-like carcinomas of the skin with adnexal differentiation. *J Cutan Pathol* 1991;18:93–102.

119. Requena L, Sanchez-Yus E, Jimenez E, Roo E. Lymphoepithelioma-like carcinoma of the skin: A light microscopic and immunohistochemical study. *J Cutan Pathol* 1994;21: 541–548.

120. Barr RJ, Goodman MM: Neurofollicular hamartoma. A light microscopic and immunohistochemical study. *J Cutan Pathol* 1989;16:336–341.

121. Nova MP, Zung M, Halperin A: Neurofollicular hamartoma. A clinicopathological study. *Am J Dermatopathol* 1991;13:459–462.

122. Sangueza OP, Requena L: Neurofollicular hamartoma. A new histogenetic interpretation. *Am J Dermatopathol* 1994;16:150–154.

123. Tuthill RJ, Clark WH Jr, Levene A. Pilar neurocristic hamartoma: Its relationship to blue nevus and equine melanotic disease. *Arch Dermatol* 1982;118:592–596.

124. Crowson AN, Magro CM, Clark WHC. Pilar neurocristic hamartoma (letter). *J Am Acad Dermatol* 1996;34:715.

125. Pathy AL, Helm TN, Elston D, et al. Malignant melanoma arising in a blue nevus with features of pilar neurocristic hamartoma. *J Cutan Pathol* 1993;20:459–464.

126. Pearson JP, Weiss SW, Headington JT. Cutaneous malignant melanotic neurocristic tumors arising in neurocristic hamartomas: A melanocytic tumor morphologically and biologically distinct from common melanoma. *Am J Surg Pathol* 1996;20:665–677.

127. Page DL, Anderson TJ, Sakamoto G. Infiltrating carcinoma: Major histological types. In: Page DL, Anderson TJ, eds. *Diagnostic Histopathology of the Breast*. New York: Churchill-Livingstone, 1987:193–295.

128. Busam KJ, Tan LK, Granter SR, et al. Epidermal growth factor, estrogen, and progesterone receptor expression in primary sweat gland carcinomas and primary and metastatic mammary carcinomas. *Mod Pathol* 1999;12:786–793.

129. Hiatt KM, Pilow JL, Smoller BR. Her-2 expression in cutaneous eccrine and apocrine neoplasms. *Mod Pathol* 2004:17:28–32.

130. Qureshi HS, Ormsby AH, Lee MW, et al. The diagnostic utility of p63, CK5/6, CK 7, and CK 20 in distinguishing primary cutaneous adnexal neoplasms from metastatic carcinomas. *Cutan Pathol* 2004;31:145–152.

131. Plumb SJ, Argenyi ZB, Stone MS, De Young BR. Cytokeratin 5/6 immunostaining in cutaneous adnexal neoplasms and metastatic adenocarcinoma. *Am J Dermatopathol* 2004;26:447–451.

132. Carlsten JR, Lewis MD, Saddler K et al. Spiradenocylindrocarcinoma: A malignant hybrid tumor. *J Cutan Pathol* 2005;32:166–171.
133. Goedde TA, Bumpers H, Fiscella J, et al. Eccrine porocarcinoma. *J Surg Oncol* 1994;55: 261–264.
134. Poiares-Baptista A, Tellechea O, Reis JP, et al. Eccrine porocarcinoma: A review of 24 cases. *Ann Dermatol Venereol* 1993;120:107–115.
135. Snow SN, Reizner GT. Eccrine porocarcinoma of the face. *J Am Acad Dermatol* 1992;27:306–311.
136. Yamamoto O, Haratake J, Yokoyama S, et al. A histopathological and ultrastructural study of eccrine porocarcinoma with special reference to its subtypes. *Virchows Arch A Pathol Anat Histopathol* 1992;420:395–401.
137. Turner JJ, Maxwell L, Bursle GA. Eccrine porocarcinoma. *Pathology* 1982;14:469–475.
138. Shaw M, McKee PH, Lowe D, Black MM. Malignant eccrine poroma: A study of twenty seven cases. *Br J Dermatol* 1982;107:675–680.
139. Bottles K, Sagebiel RW, McNutt NS, et al. Malignant eccrine poroma. *Cancer* 1984; 53:1579–1585.
140. Ryan JF, Darley CR, Pollock DJ. Malignant eccrine poroma: Report of three cases. *J Clin Pathol* 1986;39:1099–1104.
141. Mehregan AH, Hashimoto K, Rahbari H. Eccrine adenocarcinoma: A clinicopathologic study of 35 cases. *Arch Dermatol* 1983;119:104–114.
142. Akalin T, Sen S, Yuceturk A, Kandiloglu G. p53 protein expression in eccrine poroma and porocarcinoma. *Am J Dermatopathol* 2001;23:402–406.
143. Wick MR, Swanson PE, Barnhill RL. Sweat gland tumors. In: Barnhill RL, Crowson AN, eds. *Textbook of Dermatopathology*. 2nd Ed. New York: McGraw-Hill Co., 2004: 745–784.
144. Miyashita M, Suzuki H. In situ porocarcinoma: A case with malignant expression in clear tumor cells. *Int J Dermatol* 1993;32:749–750.
145. Bardach H. Hidroacanthoma simplex with in situ porocarcinoma. *J Cutan Pathol* 1978;5:236–248.
146. Isikawa K. Malignant hidroacanthoma simplex. *Arch Dermatol* 1972;104:529–532.
147. Moreno R, Salvatella N, Guix M, et al. Malignant hidroacanthoma simplex. *Dermatologica* 1984;169:318–322.
148. Manteaux A, Cohen PR, Rapini RP. Zosteriform and epidermotropic metastasis: Report of two cases. *J Dermatol Surg Oncol* 1992;18:97–100.
149. Hara K, Kamiya S. Pigmented eccrine porocarcinoma: A mimic of malignant melanoma. *Histopathology* 1995;27:86–88.
150. Wick MR, Swanson PE. *Cutaneous Adnexal Tumors: A Guide to Pathologic Diagnosis*. Chicago, IL: ASCP Press, 1991.
151. Hashimoto K, Mehregen AH, Kumakiri M. *Tumors of Skin Appendages*. Boston, MA: Butterworths, 1987:48–51.
152. Van der Putte SC. The pathogenesis of familial multiple cylindromas, trichoepitheliomas, milia, and spiradenomas. *Am J Dermatopathol* 1995;17:271–280.
153. Cooper PH. Carcinomas of sweat glands. *Pathol Annu* 1987;22(Pt 1):83–124.
154. Ohta M, Hiramoto M, Fujii M, Togo T. Nodular hidradenocarcinoma on the scalp of a young woman: Case report and review of literature. *Dermatol Surg* 2004;30: 1265–1268.
155. Fukamizu H, Tomita K, Inoue K, Takigawa M. Primary mucinous carcinoma of the skin. *J Dermatol Surg Oncol* 1993;19:625–628.
156. Ghamande SA, Kasznick J, Griffiths CT, et al. Mucinous adenocarcinomas of the vulva. *Gynecol Oncol* 1995;57:117–120.

157. Katoh N, Hirano S, Hosokawa Y, et al. Mucinous carcinoma of the skin: Report of a case with DNA cytofluorometric study. *J Dermatol* 1994;21:117–121.
158. Mendoza S, Helwig EB. Mucinous (adenocystic) carcinoma of the skin. *Arch Dermatol* 1971;103:68–78.
159. Rodriguez MM, Lubowitz RM, Shannon GM. Mucinous (adenocystic) carcinoma of the eyelid. *Arch Ophthalmol* 1973;89:493–494.
160. Grossman JR, Izuno GT. Primary mucinous (adenocystic) carcinoma of the skin. *Arch Dermatol* 1974;110:274–276.
161. Santa Cruz DJ, Meyers JH, Gnepp DR, Perez BM. Primary mucinous carcinoma of the skin. *Br J Dermatol* 1978;68:645–653.
162. Yeung KY, Stinson JC. Mucinous (adenocystic) carcinoma of sweat glands with widespread metastasis. *Cancer* 1977;39:2556–2562.
163. Pilgram JP, Kloss SG, Wolfish PS, Heng MCY. Primary mucinous carcinoma of the skin with metastases to the lymph nodes. *Am J Dermatopathol* 1985;7:461–469.
164. Rahilly MA, Beattie GJ, Lessells AM. Mucinous eccrine carcinoma of the vulva with neuroendocrine differentiation. *Histopathology* 1995;27:82–86.
165. Minami Y, Uede K, Sagawa K, et al. Immunohistochemical staining of cutaneous tumours with G-81, a monoclonal antibody to dermcidin. *Br J Dermatol* 2004;141: 165–169.
166. Rosen T. Cutaneous metastases. *Med Clin North Am* 1980;64:885–900.
167. Koh BK, Choi JM, Yi JY, et al. Recurrent primary cutaneous adenoid cystic carcinoma of the scrotum. *Int J Dermatol* 2001;40:724–725.
168. Chu SS, Chang YL, Lou PJ. Primary cutaneous adenoid cystic carcinoma with regional lymph node metastasis. *J Laryngol Otol* 2001;115:673–675.
169. Urso C, Bondi R, Paglierani M, et al. Carcinomas of sweat glands: Report of 60 cases. *Arch Pathol Lab Med* 2001;125:498–505.
170. Chang SE, Ahn SJ, Choi JH, et al. Primary adenoid cystic carcinoma of skin with lung metastasis. *J Am Acad Dermatol* 1999;40:640–642.
171. DeLucia A, Gambardella T, Carra P, Motta. A case of highly aggressive adenoid cystic carcinoma of the external auditory canal. *Acta Otorhinolaryngol Ital* 2004;24:354–356.
172. Wassef M, Thomas V, Deffrennes D, Saint-Guily JL. Primary adenoid cystic carcinoma of the skin: Histologic and ultrastructural study of two cases localized in the external auditory canal. *Ann Pathol* 1995;15:150–155.
173. Eckert F, Pfau A, Landthaler M. Adenoid cystic sweat gland carcinoma: A clinicopathologic and immunohistochemical study. *Hautarzt* 1994;45:318–323.
174. Matsumura T, Kumakiri M, Ohkaware A, Yoshida T. Adenoid cystic carcinoma of the skin: An immunohistochemical and ultrastructural study. *J Dermatol* 1993;20:164–170.
175. Cooper PH, Adelson GL, Holthaus WH. Primary cutaneous adenoid cystic carcinoma. *Arch Dermatol* 1984;120:774–777.
176. Wick MR, Swanson PE. Primary adenoid cystic carcinoma of the skin. *Am J Dermatopathol* 1986;8:2–13.
177. Seab JA, Graham JH. Primary cutaneous adenoid cystic carcinoma. *J Am Acad Dermatol* 1987;17:113–118.
178. Van der Kwast TH, Vuzevski VD, Ramaekers F. Primary cutaneous adenoid cystic carcinoma. *Br J Dermatol* 1988;118:567–576.
179. Dardick I, van Nostrand AW, Phillips MJ. Histogenesis of salivary gland pleomorphic adenoma (mixed tumor) with evaluation of the role of myoepithelial cells. *Hum Pathol* 1982;13:62–75.
180. Inaloz HS, Patel GK, Knight AG. An aggressive treatment for aggressive digital papillary adenocarcinoma. *Cutis* 2002;69:179–182;quiz 210.

181. Smith KJ, Skelton HG, Holland TT. Recent advances and controversies concerning adnexal neoplasms. *Dermatol Clin* 1992;10(1):117–160.

182. Goldstein DJ, Barr RJ, Santa Cruz DJ. Microcystic adnexal carcinoma: A distinct clinicopathologic entity. *Cancer* 1982;50:566–572.

183. Kao GF, Graham JH, Helwig EB. Aggressive digital papillary adenoma and adenocarcinoma [Abstract]. *Arch Dermatol* 1984;120:1612.

184. Rulon DB, Helwig EB. Papillary eccrine adenoma. *Arch Dermatol* 1977;113:596–598.

185. Elpern DJ, Farmer ER. Papillary eccrine adenoma. *Arch Dermatol* 1978;114(8):1241.

186. Cooper PH, Frierson HF. Papillary eccrine adenoma. *Arch Pathol Lab Med* 1984;108:55–57.

187. Urmacher C, Lieberman PH. Papillary eccrine adenoma: A light microscopic and immunohistochemical study. *Am J Dermatopathol* 1987;9:243–249.

188. Falck VG, Jordaan HF. Papillary eccrine adenoma. A tubulopapillary hidradenoma with eccrine differentiation. *Am J Dermatopathol* 1986;8:64–72.

189. Swanson PE, Cherwitz DL, Neumann MP, Wick MR. Eccrine sweat gland carcinoma: A histologic and immunohistochemical study of 32 cases. *J Cutan Pathol* 1987;14(2):65–86.

190. Sexton M, Maize JC. Papillary eccrine adenoma: A light microscopic and immunohistochemical study. *J Am Acad Dermatol* 1988;18:1114–1120.

191. Kanitakis J, Hermier C, Thivolet J. Papillary eccrine adenoma. *Am J Dermatopathol* 1988;10(2):180–182.

192. Jerasutus S, Suvanprakorn P, Wongchinchai M. Papillary eccrine adenoma: An electron microscopic study. *J Am Acad Dermatol* 1989;20(6):1111–1114.

193. Hashimoto K, Kato I, Taniguchi Y, et al. Papillary eccrine adenoma. Immunohistochemical and ultrastructural analyses. *J Dermatol Sci* 1990;1:65–71.

194. Requena L, Pena M, Sanchez M, Sanchez Yus E. Papillary eccrine adenoma–a light-microscopic and immunohistochemical study. *Clin Exp Dermatol* 1990;15(6):425–428.

195. Aloi F, Pich A. Papillary eccrine adenoma: A histopathological and immunohistochemical study. *Dermatologica* 1991;182:47–51.

196. Fox SB, Cotton DW. Tubular apocrine adenoma and papillary eccrine adenoma. Entities or unity? *Am J Dermatopathol* 1992;14(2):149–154.

197. Lever WF, Schaumberg-Lever, G. *Histopathology of the Skin*. 7th Ed. Philadelphia, PA: JB Lippincott & Co., 1989:638–639.

198. Galadari E, Mehregan AH, Lee KC. Malignant transformation of eccrine tumors. *J Cutan Pathol* 1987;14:15–22.

199. Duke WH, Sherrod TT, Lupton GP. Aggressive digital papillary adenocarcinoma (aggressive digital papillary adenoma and adenocarcinoma revisited). *Am J Surg Pathol* 2000;24(6):775–784.

200. Kao GF, Helwig EG, Graham JH. Aggressive digital papillary adenoma and adenocarcinoma. A clinicopathological study of 57 patients, with histochemical, immunopathological, and ultrastructural observations. *J Cutan Pathol* 1987;14(3):129–146.

201. Guccion JG, Patterson RH, Nayar R, Saini NB. Papillary eccrine adenoma: An ultrastructural and immunohistochemical study. *Ultrastructural Pathol* 1998;22:263–269.

202. Ichikawa E, Okabe S, Umebayashi Y, et al. Papillary eccrine adenoma: Immunohistochemical studies of keratin expression. *J Cutan Pathol* 1997;24:564–570.

203. Elder DE, Elenitsas R, Ragsdale B. Tumors of the epidermal appendages. In: Elder DE, Johnson BE, Jaworsky C, et al. eds. *Lever's Histopathology of the Skin*. 8th Ed. Philadelphia, PA: JB Lippincott Co., 1997:747–803.

204. Malafa MP, McKesey P, Stone S, et al. Sentinel node biopsy for aggressive digital papillary adenocarcinoma. *Dermatol Surg* 2000;26(6):580–583.

205. Daigeler A, Fansa H, Tammer M, Schneider W. Aggressive digital papillary adenocarcinoma–a case report. *Handchir Mikrochir Plast Chir* 2002;34(2):137–139.

206. Wick MR, Cooper PH, Swanson PE, et al. Microcystic adnexal carcinoma: An immunohistochemical comparison with other cutaneous appendage tumors. *Arch Dermatol* 1990;126:189–194.

207. Nickoloff BJ, Fleischmann HE, Carmel J. Microcystic adnexal carcinoma: Immunohistologic observations suggesting dual (pilar and eccrine) differentiation. *Arch Dermatol* 1986;122:290–294.

208. Callahan EF, Vidimos AT, Bergfeld WF. Microcystic adnexal carcinoma (MAC) of the scalp with extensive pilar differentiation. *Dermatol Surg* 2002;28:536–539.

209. Ongenae KC, Verhaegh ME, Vermeulen AH, Naeyaert JM. Microcystic adnexal carcinoma: An uncommon tumor with debatable origin. *Dermatol Surg* 2001;27:979–984.

210. Ohtsuka H, Nagamatsu S. Microcystic adnexal carcinoma: Review of 51 Japanese patients. *Dermatology* 2002;204:190–193.

211. Snow S, Madjar DD, Hardy S, et al. Microcystic adnexal carcinoma: Report of 13 cases and review of the literature. *Dermatol Surg* 2001;27:401–408.

212. Chiller K, Passaro D, Scheuller M, et al. Microcystic adnexal carcinoma: Forty-eight cases, their treatment, and their outcome. *Arch Dermatol* 2000;136:1355–1359.

213. Carroll P, Goldstein GD, Brown CW Jr. Metastatic microcystic adnexal carcinoma in an immunocompromised patient. *Dermatol Surg* 2000;26:531–534.

214. Friedman PM, Friedman RH, Jiang SB, et al. Microcystic adnexal carcinoma: Collaborative series review and update. *J Am Acad Dermatol* 1999;41: 225–231.

215. Beer KT, Buhler SS, Mullis P, et al. A Microcystic adnexal Carcinoma in the auditory canal 15 years after radiotherapy of a 12-year-old boy with nasopharynx carcinoma. *Strahlender Onkol* 2005;181:405–410.

216. Ohtsuka H, Nozawa R, Kushida Y. Synchronous microcystic adnexal carcinoma and gastric cancer with review of the literature. *J Dermatol* 2005;32:43–47.

217. Kachemoune A, Olbricht SM, Johnson DS. Microcytstic adnexal carcinoma: Report of four cases treated with Mohs' micrographic surgical technique. *Int J Dermatol.* 2005;44:507–512.

218. Cooper PH, Mills SE, Leonard DD, et al. Sclerosing sweat duct (syringomatous) carcinoma. *Am J Surg Pathol* 1985;9:422–433.

219. Cooper PH. Sclerosing carcinomas of sweat ducts (microcystic adnexal carcinoma). *Arch Dermatol* 1986;122:261–264.

220. Berg JW, McDivitt RW. Pathology of sweat gland carcinomas. *Pathol Annu* 1968; 3:123–144.

221. Lipper S, Peiper SC. Sweat gland carcinoma with syringomatous features. *Cancer* 1979;44:157–163.

222. Cooper PH, Mills SE. Microcystic adnexal carcinoma. *J Am Acad Dermatol* 1984; 10:908–914.

223. McAlvany JP, Stonecipher MR, Leshin B, et al. Sclerosing sweat duct carcinoma in an 11 year old boy. *J Dermatol Surg Oncol* 1994;20:767–768.

224. Batsakis JG, El-Naggar AK, Weber RS. Two perplexing skin tumors: Microcystic adnexal carcinoma and keratoacanthoma. *Ann Otol Rhinol Laryngol* 1994;103:829–832.

225. LeBoit PE, Sexton M. Microcystic adnexal carcinoma of the skin. A reappraisal of the differentiation and differential diagnosis of an underrecognized neoplasm. *J Am Acad Dermatol* 1993;29:609–618.

226. Hesse RJ, Scharfenberg JC, Ratz JL, Griener E. Eyelid microcystic adnexal carcinoma. *Arch Ophthalmol* 1995;113:494–496.

227. Verdier-Sevrain S, Thomine E, Lauret P, Hemet J. Syringomatous carcinoma: Apropos of three cases with a review of the literature. *Ann Pathol* 1995;15:280–284.

228. Schlipper JH, Holecek BU, Sievers KW. A tumor derived from Ebner's glands: Microcystic adnexal carcinoma of the tongue. *J Laryngol Otol* 1995;109:1211–1214.

229. Yus ES, Caballero LR, Salazar IG, Menchero SC. Clear cell syringoid eccrine carcinoma. *Am J Dermatopathol* 1987;9:225–231.

230. Smith KJ, Williams J, Corbett D, Skelton H. Microcystic adnexal carcinoma: An immunohistochemical study including markers of proliferation and apoptosis. *Am J Surg Pathol* 2001;25:464–471.

231. Pruzam DL, Esterly NB, Prose NS. Eruptive syringoma. *Arch Dermatol* 1989;125: 1119–1120.

232. Brownstein MH, Shapiro L. Desmoplastic trichoepithelioma. *Cancer* 1977;40:2979–2986.

233. Salasche SJ, Amonette RA. Morpheaform basal cell epitheliomas. *J Dermatol Surg Oncol* 1981;7:387–394.

234. Smith KJ, Skelton HG. Familial syringomas: An example of gonadal mosaicism. *Cutis* 2001;68:293–295.

235. Draznin M. Hereditary syringomas: A case report. *Dermatol Online J* 2004;115:19.

236. Biernat W, Jablkowski W. Syringomatous adenoma of the nipple. *Pol J Pathol* 2000;51: 201–202.

237. Banks ER, Cooper PH. Adenosquamous carcinoma of the skin: A report of 10 cases. *J Cutan Pathol* 1991;18:227–234.

238. Weidner N, Foucar E. Adenosquamous carcinoma of the skin: An aggressive mucin- and gland-forming squamous carcinoma. *Arch Dermatol* 1985;121:775–779.

239. Sakamoto F, Ito M, Oguro K, et al. Adenosquamous carcinoma of the skin: Ultrastructural and immunohistochemical studies. *Jpn J Dermatol* 1990;100:1183–1190.

240. Azorin D, Lopez-Rios F, Ballestin C, et al. Primary cutaneous adenosquamous carcinoma: A case report and review of the literature. *J Cutan Pathol* 2001;28: 542–545.

241. Landman G, Farmer ER. Primary cutaneous mucoepidermoid carcinoma: Report of a case. *J Cutan Pathol* 1991;18:56–59.

242. Wenig BL, Sciubba JJ, Goodman RS, Platt N. Primary cutaneous mucoepidermoid carcinoma of the anterior neck. *Laryngoscope* 1983;93:464–467.

243. Friedman KJ. Low-grade primary cutaneous adenosquamous (mucoepidermoid) carcinoma. *Am J Dermatopathol* 1989;11:43–50.

244. Smoller BR, Narurkar V. Mucoepidermoid carcinoma metastatic to the skin: An histologic mimic of a primary sweat gland carcinoma. *J Dermatol Surg Oncol* 1992; 18:365–368.

245. Metcalf JS, Maize JC, Shaw EB. Bronchial mucoepidermoid carcinoma metastatic to skin: Report of a case and review of the literature. *Cancer* 1986;58:2556–2559.

246. Barsky SH, Martin SE, Matthews M, et al. "Low grade" mucoepidermoid carcinoma of the bronchus with "high grade" biological behavior. *Cancer* 1983;51:1505–1509.

247. Revercomb CH, Reitmeyer WJ, Pulitzer DR. Clear cell variant of mucoepidermoid carcinoma of the skin. *J Am Acad Dermatol* 1993;29:642–644.

248. Diwan AH, Smith KJ, Brown R, Skelton HG. Mucoepidermoid carcinoma arising within nevus sebaceus of Jadassohn. *J Cutan Pathol* 2003;30:652–655.

249. Wildemore JK, Lee JB, Humphreys TR. Mohs surgery for malignant eccrine neoplasms. *Dermatol Surg* 2004;30:1574–1579.

250. Fernandez-Figueras MT, Fuente MJ, Bielsa I, et al. Low-grade mucoepidermoid carcinoma on the vermilion border of the lip. *Am J Dermatopathol* 1997;19:197–201.

251. Harris TJ, Jine JD, Berman RS, et al. Neutrophilic eccrine hidradenitis. A distinctive type of neutrophilic dermatosis associated with myelogenous leukemia and chemotherapy. *Arch Dermatol* 1982;118:263–266.

252. Riedlinger WF, Hurley MY, Dehner LP, Lind AC. Mucoepidermoid carcinoma of the skin: A distinct entity from adenosquamous carcinoma: A case study with a review of the literature. *Am J Surg Pathol* 2005;29:131–135.

253. Bondeson L. Malignant dermal eccrine cylindroma. *Acta Dermatol Venereol* 1979;59: 92–94.

254. Boulond A, Clerens A, Signard H. Cylindrome malin. *Dermatologica* 1979;158:203–207.

255. Urbanski SJ, From L, Abramowicz A. Metamorphosis of dermal cylindroma: Possible relation to malignant transformation. *J Am Acad Dermatol* 1985;12:188–195.

256. Rockerbie N, Solomon AR, Woo TY, et al. Malignant dermal cylindroma in a patient with multiple dermal cylindromas, trichoepitheliomas, and bilateral dermal analogue tumors of the parotid gland. *Am J Dermatopathol* 1989;11:353–359.

257. Lyon JB, Rouillard LM. Malignant degeneration of turban tumor of the scalp. *Trans St John's Hosp Dermatol Soc* 1961;46:74–77.

258. Grouls V, Iwaszkiewicz J, Berndt R. Malignant dermal cylindroma. *Pathologe* 1991;12: 157–160.

259. Dabska M. Malignant transformation of eccrine spiradenoma. *Pol Med J* 1972;11: 388–396.

260. Evans HL, Su WPD, Smith JL, Winkelmann RK. Carcinoma arising in eccrine spiradenoma. *Cancer* 1979;43:1881–1884.

261. Cooper PH, Frierson HF Jr, Morrison AG. Malignant transformation of eccrine spiradenoma. *Arch Dermatol* 1985;121:1445–1448.

262. Wick MR, Kaye VN, Swanson PE, Pittelkow MR. Sweat gland carcinoma ex eccrine spiradenoma. *Am J Dermatopathol* 1987;9:90–98.

263. Argenyi AZ, Nguyen AV, Balogh K, et al. Malignant eccrine spiradenoma: A clinicopathologic study. *Am J Dermatopathol* 1990;12:335–343.

264. Varsa EW, Jordan SW. Fine needle aspiration cytology of malignant spiradenoma arising in congenital eccrine spiradenoma. *Acta Cytol* 1990;34:275–277.

265. Zamboni AC, Zamboni WA, Ross DS. Malignant eccrine spiradenoma of the hand. *J Surg Oncol* 1990;43:131–133.

266. Yaremchuk MJ, Elias LS, Graham RR, Wilgis EF. Sweat gland carcinoma of the hand: Two cases of malignant eccrine spiradenoma. *J Hand Surg* 1984;9:910–914.

267. McKee PH, Fletcher CD, Rasbridge SA. The enigmatic eccrine epithelioma (eccrine syringomatous carcinoma). *Am J Dermatopathol* 1990;12:552–561.

268. Pizinger K, Michal M. Malignant cylindroma in Brooke–Spiegler syndrome. *Dermatology* 2000;201:255–257.

269. Jamshidi M, Nowak MA, Chiu YT, et al. Giant malignant eccrine spiradenoma of the scalp. *Dermatol Surg* 1999;25: 45–48.

270. Brownstein MH, Helwig EB. Metastatic tumors of the skin. *Cancer* 1972;29: 1298–1307.

271. Brownstein MH, Helwig EB. Patterns of cutaneous metastasis. *Arch Dermatol* 1972;105: 862–868.

272. Wick MR, Goellner JR, Wolfe JT III, Su WPD. Adnexal carcinomas of the skin: I. Eccrine carcinomas. *Cancer* 1985;56:1147–1162.

273. El-Domeiri AA, Brasfield RD, Huvos AG, et al. Sweat gland carcinoma: A clinicopathologic study of 83 patients. *Ann Surg* 1971;173:270–274.

274. Kay S, Hall WEB. Sweat gland carcinoma with proved metastases. *Cancer* 1954;7: 373–376.

275. Okada N, Ota J, Sato K, Kitano Y. Metastasizing sweat gland carcinoma. *Arch Dermatol* 1984;120:768–769.

276. Miller WL. Sweat gland carcinoma: A clinicopathologic problem. *Am J Clin Pathol* 1967;47:767–780.
277. Swanson PE, Mazoujian G, Mills SE, et al. Immunoreactivity for estrogen receptor protein in sweat gland tumors. *Am J Surg Pathol* 1991;15:835–841.
278. Swanson PE, Wick MR. Immunohistochemistry of cutaneous tumors. In: Leong ASY, ed. *Applied Immunohistochemistry for the Surgical Pathologist*. London: Edward Arnold, 1993:269–308.
279. Wong TY, Suster S, Nogita T, et al. Clear cell eccrine carcinomas of the skin: A clinicopathologic study of nine patients. *Cancer* 1994;73:1631–1643.
280. Suster S. Clear cell tumors of the skin. *Semin Diagn Pathol* 1996;13:40–59.
281. Headington JT, Niederhuber JE, Beals TF. Malignant clear cell acrospiroma. *Cancer* 1978;41:641–647.
282. Kersting DW. Clear cell hidradenoma and hidradenocarcinoma. *Arch Dermatol* 1963;87:323–333.
283. Keasbey LE, Hadley GG. Clear cell hidradenoma: Report of three cases with widespread metastases. *Cancer* 1954;7:934–952.
284. McKenzie DH. A clear-cell hidradenocarcinoma with metastases. *Cancer* 1957;10: 1021–1023.
285. Chung CK, Hefferman AH. Clear cell hidradenoma with metastasis. *Plast Reconstr Surg* 1971;48:177–179.
286. Czarnecki DB, Aarous I, Dowling JP. Malignant clear cell hidradenoma: A case report. *Acata Dermatol Venereol* 1982;62:173–176.
287. Hernandez-Perez E, Cestoni-Parducci R. Nodular hidradenoma and hidradenocarcinoma: A 10 year review. *J Am Acad Dermatol* 1985;12:15–20.
288. Kwon TJ, Ro JY, Mackay B. Clear-cell carcinoma: An ultrastructural study of 57 tumors from various sites. *Ultrastruct Pathol* 1996;20:519–527.
289. Tolia BM, Whitmore WF. Solitary metastasis from renal cell carcinoma. *J Urol* 1975;114: 836–838.
290. Connor DH, Taylor HB, Helwig EB. Cutaneous metastases of renal cell carcinoma. *Arch Pathol* 1963;76:339–346.
291. Sharvill DE. Mixed salivary-type tumor of the skin with malignant recurrence. *Br J Dermatol* 1962;74:103–104.
292. Rosborough D. Malignant mixed tumors of the skin. *Br J Surg* 1963;50:697–699.
293. Matz LR, McCully DJ, Stokes BAR. Metastasizing chondroid syringoma: A case report. *Pathology* 1961;1:77–81.
294. Hilton JMN, Blackwell JB. Metastasizing chondroid syringoma. *J Pathol* 1972;167–170.
295. Webb JN, Stott WG. Malignant chondroid syringoma of the thigh. *J Pathol* 1975;116: 43–46.
296. Botha JBC, Kahn LB. Aggressive chondroid syringoma. *Arch Dermatol* 1978;114:954–955.
297. Ishimura E, Iwamoto H, Kobashi Y, et al. Malignant chondroid syringoma. Report of a case with widespread metastasis and review of pertinent literature. *Cancer* 1983;52:1966–1973.
298. Scott A, Metcalf S. Cutaneous malignant mixed tumor. *Am J Dermatopathol* 1988;10: 335–342.
299. Shvili D, Rothem A. Fulminant metastasizing chondroid syringoma of the skin. *Am J Dermatopathol* 1986;8:321–325.
300. Harrist TJ, Aretz TH, Mihm MC Jr, et al. Cutaneous malignant mixed tumor. *Arch Dermatol* 1981;117:719–724.
301. Pinto de Moraes H, Herrera GA, Mendonca AM, et al. Metastatic malignant mixed tumor of the skin: Ultrastructural and immunohistochemical characterization, histogenetic

considerations, and comparison with benign mixed tumors of skin and salivary glands. *Appl Pathol* 1986;4:199–208.

302. Redono C, Rocamora A, Villoria F, et al. Malignant mixed tumor of the skin: Malignant chondroid syringoma. *Cancer* 1982;49:1690–1696.
303. De Francesco V, Frattasio A, Pillon B, et al. Carcinosarcoma arising in a patient with multiple cylindromas. *Am J Dermatopathol* 2005;27:21–26
304. Wick MR, Swanson PE. "Carcinosarcomas"–current perspectives and a historical review of nosological concepts. *Semin Diagn Pathol* 1993;10:118–127.
305. Wick MR, Coffin CM. Sweat glands and pilar carcinomas. In: Wick MR, ed. *Pathology of Unusual Malignant Cutaneous Tumors*. New York: Marcel Dekker, 1985:1–76.
306. Toker C. Trabecular carcinoma of the skin. *Arch Dermatol* 1972;105:107–110.
307. Busam DJ, Gellis S, Shimamura A, et al. Small cell sweat gland carcinoma in childhood. *Am J Surg Pathol* 1998;22: 215–220.
308. Crowson AN, Magro CM, Mihm MC Jr. *The Melanocytic Proliferations: A Comprehensive Textbook of Pigmented Lesions*. New York: John Wiley and Sons, 2001.
309. Jones, RE, Ackerman AB. Extramammary Paget's disease: A critical reappraisal. *Am J Dermatopathol* 1979;1:101–132.
310. Kuan, SF, Montag AG, Hart J, et al. Differential expression of mucin genes in mammary and extramammary Paget's disease. *Am J Surg Pathol* 2001;25:1469–1477.
311. Jones RE. Mammary Paget's disease without underlying carcinoma. *Am J Dermatopathol* 1985;7:361–365.
312. Mori, O. Hachisuka H, Nakano S, et al. A case of mammary Paget's disease without an underlying carcinoma: Microscopic analysis of the DNA content in Paget cells. *J Dermatol* 1994;21:160–165.
313. Willman JH, Golitz LE, Fitzpatrick JE. Vulvar clear cells of Toker. precursors of extramammary Paget's disease. *Am J Dermatopathol* 2005;27:185–188.
314. Honda Y, Egawa K. Extramammary Paget's disease not only mimicking but also accompanying condyloma accuminatum. *Dermatology* 2005;210:315–318.
315. Lee SC, Roth LM, Ehrlich C, et al. Extramammary Paget's disease of the vulva: A clinicopathologic study of 13 cases. *Cancer* 1977;39:2540–2549.
316. Boehm F, Morris JML. Paget's disease and apocrine gland carcinoma of the vulva. *Obster Gynecol* 1971;38:185–192.
317. Hart WR, Millman JB. Progression of intraepithelial Paget's disease of the vulva to invasive carcinoma. *Cancer* 1977;40:2333–2337.
318. Mitsudo S, Nakanishi I, Koss LG. Paget's disease of the penis and adjacent skin: Its association with fatal sweat gland carcinoma. *Arch Pathol Lab Med* 1981;105:518–520.
319. Knauer WJ Jr, Whorton CM. Extramammary Paget's disease originating in Mill's glands of the eyelid. *Trans Am Acad Ophthalmol Otolaryngol* 1963;67:829–833.
320. Nadji M, Morales AR, Girtanner RE, et al. Paget's disease of the skin: A unifying concept of histogenesis. *Cancer* 1982;50:2203–2206.
321. Rayne SC, Santa Cruz DJ. Anaplastic Paget's disease. *Am J Surg Pathol* 1992;16: 1085–1091.
322. Mazoujian G, Pinkus GS, Haagensen DE. Extramammary Paget's disease: Evidence for an apocrine origin. *Am J Surg Pathol* 1984;8:43–50.
323. Satoh F, Umemura S, Osamura RY. Immunohistochemical analysis of GCDFP-15 and GCDFP-24 in mammary and non-mammary tissue. *Breast Cancer* 2000;7:49–55.
324. Kariniemi AL, Ramaekers F, Lehto VP, Virtanen I. Paget cells express cytokeratins typical of glandular epithelia. *Br J Dermatol* 1985;112:179–183.
325. Hitchcock A, Topham S, Bell J, et al. Routine diagnosis of mammary Paget's disease. *Am J Surg Pathol* 1992;16:58–61.

326. Helm KF, Goellner JR, Peters MS. Immunohistochemical stains in extramammary Paget's disease. *Am J Dermatopathol* 1992;14:402–407.

327. Liegl B, Horn LC, Moinfar F. Androgen receptors are frequently expressed in mammary and extramammary Paget's disease. *Mod Pathol* 2005;18:1283–1288.

328. Reich O, Liegl B, Tamussino K, Regauer S. P185HER2 overexpression and HER2 oncogene amplification in recurrent vulvar Paget's disease. *Mod Pathol* 2005;18:354–357.

329. Brummer O, Stegner HE, Bohmer G, et al. HER-2/neu expression in Paget's disease of the vulva and female breast. *Gynecol Oncol* 2004;95:336–340.

330. Takeshita K, Kzumoi S, Ebuchi M, et al. A case of rectal carcinoma concomitant with pagetoid lesion in the perianal region. *Gastroenterol Jpn* 1978;13:85–95.

331. McKee PH, Hertogs KT. Endocervical adenocarcinoma and vulvar Paget's disease: A significant association. *Br J Dermatol* 1980;103:443–448.

332. Degefu S, O'Quinn AG, Dhurandhar HN. Paget's disease of the vulva and urogenital malignancies. *Gynecol Oncol* 1986;25:347–354.

333. Ojeda VJ, Heenen PJ, Watson SH. Paget's disease of the groin associated with adenocarcinoma of the urinary bladder. *J Cutan Pathol* 1987;14:227–231.

334. Fujimoto A, Takata M, Hatta N, Takehara K. Expression of structurally unaltered androgen receptor in extramammary Paget's disease. *Lab Invest* 2000;80:1465–1471.

335. Diaz-de-Leon E, Carcangiu ML, Prieto VG, et al. Extramammary Paget disease is characterized by the consistent lack of estrogen and progesterone receptors but frequently expresses androgen receptor. *Am J Clin Pathol* 2000;113:572–575.

336. Soini Y. Claudins 2,3,4 and 5 in Paget's disease and breast carcinoma. *Hum Pathol* 2004;35:1531–1536.

337. Bogner PN, Su LD, Fullen DR. Cluster designation 5 staining of normal and nonlymphoid neoplastic skin. *J Cutan Pathol* 2005;32:50–54.

10

SOFT TISSUE NEOPLASMS OF THE SKIN AND SUPERFICIAL SUBCUTIS

A complete description of every entity that shows fibrous, vascular, adipose, muscle, cartilage, bone, or neural differentiation is beyond the scope of this book. The reader is referred to excellent reviews of this subject already in print.[1-3] This chapter focuses on entities that are commonly seen in biopsies of the skin, with particular emphasis on those that pose diagnostic challenges, or where diagnostic errors have significant consequences.

TUMORS OF FIBROUS TISSUE

Hypertrophic Scar and Keloid

Both hypertrophic scars and keloids begin as granulation tissue. With time, collagen gradually increases, myofibroblasts mature, and inflammation dissipates, leading to a decline in cellularity. Keloids are easily distinguished from scars clinically by their tendency to extend from the site of initial injury. Histologically, mature keloids have characteristic bands of hyalinized collagen (e-fig. 10.1). In practice, it is not uncommon to see cicatrices which are clinically diagnosed as hypertrophic, but in which small foci of keloidal collagen are nevertheless present. It is not clear whether this represents the earliest stage of keloid formation, but it is the authors' practice to defer to the clinical impression when only a small amount of keloidal collagen is involved.

Otherwise, the differential diagnosis may include dermatofibroma, which is usually more cellular, has a storiform pattern, and is also characterized by epidermal changes, including acanthosis and hyperpigmentation. It may not always be possible to distinguish a paucicellular dermatofibroma from a scar, and some authors indeed consider dermatofibromas to be reactive entities, related to cicatrices. A minority of dermatofibromata are clonal, and for the most part, these are lesions dominated by epithelioid cells, perhaps best classified as "benign fibrous histiocytomata." Fibromatoses are usually far more cellular than scars, and occur in deeper soft tissues at characteristic sites (palms, soles, and penis).

Angiofibroma

Angiofibromas are proliferations of thin-walled blood vessels in fibrous tissue which may occur sporadically or in one of three specific clinical settings:

- Fibrous papule: A solitary lesion on the central face of adults (characteristically on the nose). Some authors classify these separately from angiofibromas.
- Adenoma sebaceum: A lesion characteristic of tuberous sclerosis, typically occurring as multiple lesions of the face with a preference for the nasolabial fold.
- Pearly penile papule: A small, clinically distinctive lesion occurring in groups or rows on the coronal margin and sulcus of an uncircumcised penis that may sometimes clinically resemble a condyloma.

The histologic features are similar, regardless of the clinical context. Lesions are usually rounded, but may be pedunculated, with a flattened epidermis and an underlying network of coarse collagen fibers, often showing arrangements around follicles and, sometimes, blood vessels. Fibroblasts are often plump and stellate to spindled. Blood vessels are increased in numbers and often ectatic.

Acquired digital fibrokeratoma, formerly known as Koenen's tumor, acral fibrokeratoma, acquired periungual fibrokeratoma, garlic clove fibroma, subungual fibroma, or periungual fibroma, may also be seen in tuberous sclerosis, although most cases are sporadic. It characteristically occurs on the digits and, in particular, the proximal nail fold. Its histology is related to that of the angiofibroma, but the epidermis is more hyperplastic, sometimes with an arborizing retiform pattern, and the stroma shows an increase in telangiectatic vessels admixed with thick collagen bundles oriented in a vertical or haphazard pattern, and spindled to stellate fibroblasts (e-fig. 10.2). In some cases, vessels are not prominent, and on this basis, these lesions are often reported as fibromas rather than angiofibromas.

Circumscribed Storiform Collagenoma

Circumscribed storiform collagenoma (sometimes referred to as hypocellular fibroma or sclerotic fibroma) is a hypocellular lesion with a characteristic storiform and whorled pattern (e-fig. 10.3) which typically occurs as an isolated sporadic lesion, where we postulate that it relates to the dermatofibroma. The presence of multiple lesions may be a marker of Cowden's syndrome.

Fibroma of Tendon Sheath

Fibroma of tendon sheath typically arises as a small, painless nodule on the hands or feet of young adults, particularly men. Although attachments to the tendon or tendon sheath can be demonstrated at the time of surgery, these tumors of soft tissue nevertheless frequently present in skin biopsies. Histologically, the tumors are well circumscribed and are composed of uniform, spindled fibroblasts and myofibroblasts arranged in short fascicles (Fig. 10.1). Collagen bands are present and may be arranged in characteristic concentric whorls. Vascular channels are often slitlike and appear compressed. More cellular examples may sometimes show an occasional giant cell; the differential diagnosis with giant cell tumor of tendon sheath may be exceptionally difficult in some cases, suggesting a morphologic spectrum. Some cases show a strong resemblance to nodular fasciitis (NF), although this should have a "tissue-culture" appearance and an inflammatory background. Some cellular cases may show similarities to fibromatosis; however, the clinical presentation and site are different.

DERMATOMYOFIBROMA. Dermatomyofibroma typically occurs as a plaque on the upper trunk or back of young female patients, with a particular emphasis on the limb girdles (shoulders, axillae, and upper arms). Microscopically, it consists of an ill-defined proliferation of bland, spindle-cell-shaped myofibroblasts. It is easily confused with dermatofibroma, but may be distinguished by its horizontal parallel fascicles, which show sparing of the skin adnexae (e-fig. 10.4A).

Although the absence of nuclear pleomorphism and hyperchromasia should reassure the pathologist and prevent the diagnosis of a higher grade sarcoma, a large, cellular example of a dermatomyofibroma (which

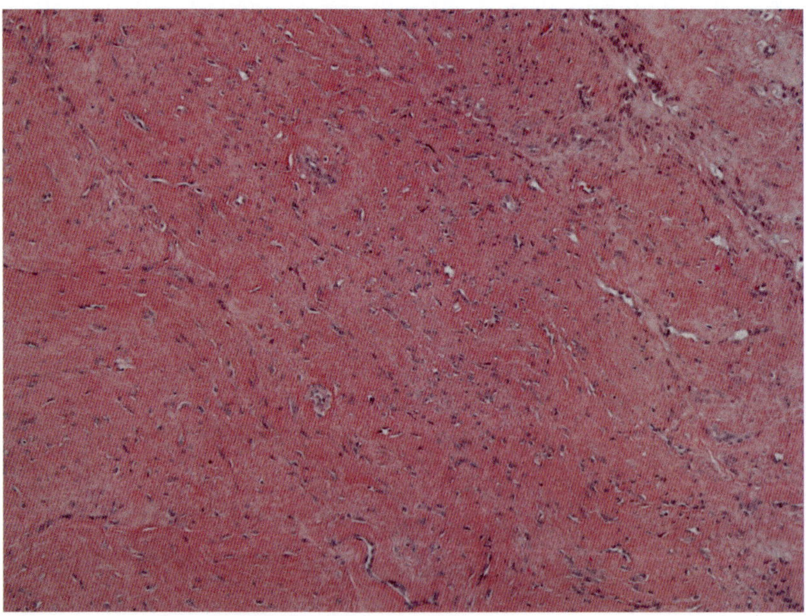

FIGURE 10.1 **Fibroma of Tendon Sheath.** Nodules of paucicellular fibrous tissue are surrounded by narrow cleftlike spaces.

may extend to all biopsy margins) may resemble dermatofibrosarcoma protuberans (DFSP). However, dermatomyofibroma should show at most focal infiltration into the subcutis or skeletal muscle.

Nodular Fasciitis

NF is a mass-forming fibrous proliferation, which often occurs in the subcutaneous tissue, although intradermal cases have been reported. It is of interest because of its tendency to be confused with sarcoma, particularly in a superficial biopsy. NF typically occurs on the upper extremity, trunk, or head and neck and sometimes shows origin from fascia, when completely excised. A related entity, intravascular fasciitis, shows origin in small- to medium-sized vessels. NF characteristically grows rapidly with a short preoperative duration and symptoms of soreness or tenderness. It is almost always less than 5 cm in greatest dimension. Histologically, the lesion appears infiltrative or circumscribed and is often very cellular, being composed of plump spindle-shaped fibroblasts or myofibroblasts. Although mitotic activity may be high, there are no atypical mitotic figures and the nuclei are also highly regular, lacking nuclear hyperchromasia and pleomorphism (e-fig. 10.4). It generally has myxoid foci (sometimes described as feathery or "tissue-culture-like"). Being fibroblastic, NF occasionally has a collagenous background. In cellular areas, the myofibroblasts may grow in curved fascicles, and there is sometimes a storiform pattern mimicking dermatofibroma (or DFSP). NF, however, is characterized by a background chronic inflammatory infiltrate which frequently shows multinucleated giant cells. Extravasated erythrocytes are also often identified, although there is not the heavy hemosiderin deposition seen in aneurysmal fibrous histiocytoma, a lesion of much longer duration. There may also be a proliferation of small vessels, mimicking granulation tissue.

The most important feature in distinguishing NF from a malignancy of soft tissue is that, despite its high mitotic rate and occasionally infiltrative border, it lacks cytologic atypia. Low grade myxofibrosarcoma, in particular, may be distinguished by the presence of occasional hyperchromatic cells, as well as characteristic curvilinear vessels and lipoblastlike cells with vacuolated cytoplasm. Fibromatosis may be distinguished both by its characteristic clinical presentation, as well as its uniform high degree of cellularity (lacking the characteristic myxoid areas of NF).

NF is a benign entity which rarely recurs following excision, and may regress spontaneously following a biopsy. Cases of recurrent NF should be regarded with suspicion.

Fibromatosis

Superficial fibromatoses characteristically arise in fascia at three sites:

- Penile fibromatosis (Peyronie's disease).
- Palmar fibromatosis (Dupuytren's contracture).
- Plantar fibromatosis (Ledderhose's disease).

The lesions show a variety of histologic appearances, beginning as highly cellular proliferations of plump myofibroblasts and proceeding to paucicellular, mitotically inactive masses composed primarily of hyalinized stromal collagen. At any stage, tumor cells are uniform, spindle-shaped, may have wavy nuclei with discrete nucleoli, and are characteristically arranged in interlacing fasicles with a wavy collagenous stroma (e-fig. 10.5). While benign, these lesions have a tendency to recur and sometimes show destructive growth.

Dermatofibroma (Fibrous Histiocytoma)

Dermatofibroma is a very common dermal tumor which shows a wide range of histologic appearances. These characteristically occur on the limbs and trunk with only rare cases on the face.

The lesions are characterized by a variably cellular proliferation of spindle-shaped to round cells, resembling fibroblasts or histiocytes, centered in the reticular dermis with an occasional lesion showing extension into the superficial subcutis (e-fig. 10.6). It has ill-defined margins with trapping of bundles of dermal collagen at the lateral edges. In addition to these fibrohistiocytic spindled cells, there may be siderophages, lipophages, and multinucleated cells (typically of Touton type). Often the dermatofibroma reflects a response to trauma, and has an epicenter in the midreticular dermis; the lipid presumably reflects extravasated platelets and the hemosiderin a breakdown product of extravasated red blood cells. A perivascular mononuclear cell infiltrate is noted at the periphery. The overlying epidermis generally shows acanthosis, and occasionally shows induction of hair follicles, resembling a superficial basal cell carcinoma. When all these features are present, this lesion rarely causes diagnostic difficulty; however, a small biopsy from the center of a dermatofibroma may resemble dermatofibrosarcoma protuberans, as the overall circumscription and the lateral entrapment of collagen bundles will not be appreciated. Polarized light microscopy may be helpful as dermatofibroma entraps and ultimately produces polarizable dermal collagen, whereas the fibrous tissue laid down by DFSP is only weakly birefringent. In difficult cases, an immunohistochemical panel is usually diagnostic: CD34 may be focally weakly positive in dermatofibroma, but should be strongly diffusely positive in DFSP. Smooth muscle actin is positive in a majority of cases of dermatofibroma, as is factor XIIIa.

Histologic variants of dermatofibroma may cause greater diagnostic difficulty. The most commonly occurring variant is cellular fibrous histiocytoma (cellular dermatofibroma), a lesion which shares the histologic and immunohistochemical features of dermatofibroma, but which is more cellular and has a greater tendency for nondestructive recurrence. Extremely rare but well-publicized instances of metastasizing cellular fibrous histiocytoma have been reported, and the WHO has recommended complete excision on the basis of these case reports[4]; although it is not clear that wide excision would always be in the patient's best interest. Cellular fibrous histiocytoma will sometimes mimic leiomyosarcoma or leiomyoma. However, these smooth muscle tumors show fascicular, as opposed to a storiform, growth pattern; have ovoid to cigar-shaped nuclei (with blunt rather than tapered ends); and strongly express smooth muscle actin as well as desmin and h-caldesmon, whereas fibrous histiocytomas express smooth-muscle actin weakly, if at all, and rarely express the other smooth-muscle markers.

Aneurysmal fibrous histiocytoma may be clinically concerning because of its similarity to melanoma or Kaposi sarcoma (KS). Histologically, it is characterized by pseudovascular spaces with extravasation of erythrocytes and hemosiderin accumulation (e-fig. 10.7). Distinction from a melanocytic proliferation may be made with a simple iron stain that will reveal that the pigment is indeed hemosiderin; distinction from KS may be made with the aid of clinical information, or an immunohistochemical stain for human herpes virus 8 (HHV-8). In addition, as these are pseudovascular spaces, they will be negative for vascular markers such as CD31 and CD34.

Epithelioid cell histiocytoma is the rarest of the subtypes mentioned here, and is characterized histopathologically by sheets of angulated epithelioid cells with abundant eosinophilic cytoplasm and a round to ovoid, centrally located nucleus, often mimicking a Spitz nevus both histopathologically and clinically. Melanocytic markers, however, are reliably negative, and factor XIIIa is expressed in 50% to 70% of cases.

Atypical Fibroxanthoma

Atypical fibroxanthoma (AFX) is a controversial entity considered by many as a benign tumor with little, if any, potential for metastasis. These almost always occur on the sun-damaged skin of older adults, in particular, the forehead, bald scalp, superior ears, and forearms. Histologically, they show an anaplastic proliferation within the superficial dermis, which is commonly polypoid with erosion of the overlying epidermis and an epidermal collarette below. The tumor itself must be completely excised to permit a confident diagnosis, as AFX should have a well-rounded, deep margin without infiltration of the subcutis. The overlying epidermis shows no evidence of a melanocytic or keratinocytic precursor lesion.

The cells themselves are highly pleomorphic, with frequent bizarre forms. Some cases show a lesser degree of cytologic atypia and are characterized by a proliferation of spindled cells. Mitotic activity is generally high, and atypical mitotic figures are present (Fig. 10.2). However, necrosis and vascular invasion should not be present.

The differential diagnosis may include leiomyosarcoma in cases that show prominent fasciculation and spindle cell features. However, AFX, while occasionally positive for actin, is reliably negative for desmin.

AFX is a diagnosis of exclusion, and requires immunohistochemistry to rule out spindle cell squamous cell carcinoma and malignant melanoma. In particular, the authors employ multiple broad-spectrum keratins stains, with an emphasis on high molecular weight cytokeratins. S-100 must also be negative. Nevertheless, it should be noted that in the absence

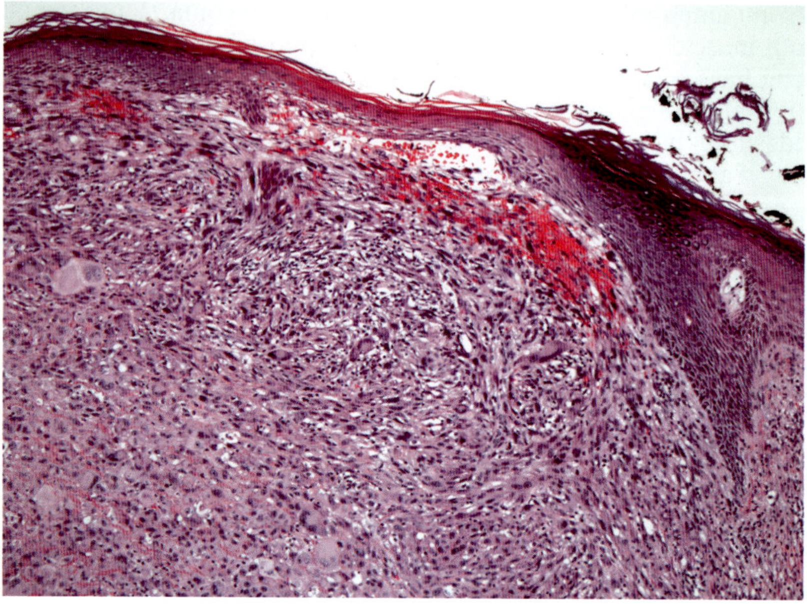

FIGURE 10.2 **Atypical Fibroxanthoma.** A diffuse dermal proliferation of pleomorphic and hyperchromatic spindled cells, epithelioid cells, xanthomatous cells, and multinucleated giant cells with elevated mitotic activity.

of positivity for a variety of keratins, as well as S-100, a benign diagnosis cannot be confidently rendered unless the lesion has been completely excised to ensure the absence of necrosis, vascular invasion, and deep infiltration of the subcutis. Many of the reported cases of so-called metastatic AFX either had infiltration of the subcutis, or were not fully examined pathologically.[5–7]

Giant Cell Tumor of Tendon Sheath

This neoplasm, which arises from tendons, typically occurs as a painless swelling on the hands and feet of young adults. It is closely related to diffuse-type giant cell tumor, an entity which occurs in the deep soft tissues and joints, and is therefore not seen on skin biopsies. A variant involving soft tissue (giant cell tumor of soft tissue) may also be seen on skin biopsy. Although these tumors may histologically resemble a fibroma of tendon sheath (see above), they are much more likely to cause diagnostic confusion with sarcomas.

Giant cell tumors of tendon sheath are lobulated, well-circumscribed tumors that are usually at least partially encapsulated, and made up of a variable mixture of mononuclear cells, multinucleated giant cells, hemosiderin-laden macrophages, and hyalinized stroma (Fig. 10.3). Although the tumor takes its name from the giant cells, the mononuclear cells are just as characteristic, having an ovoid, round, or reniform, eccentric, often grooved nucleus and abundant, palely eosinophilic cytoplasm (the so-called

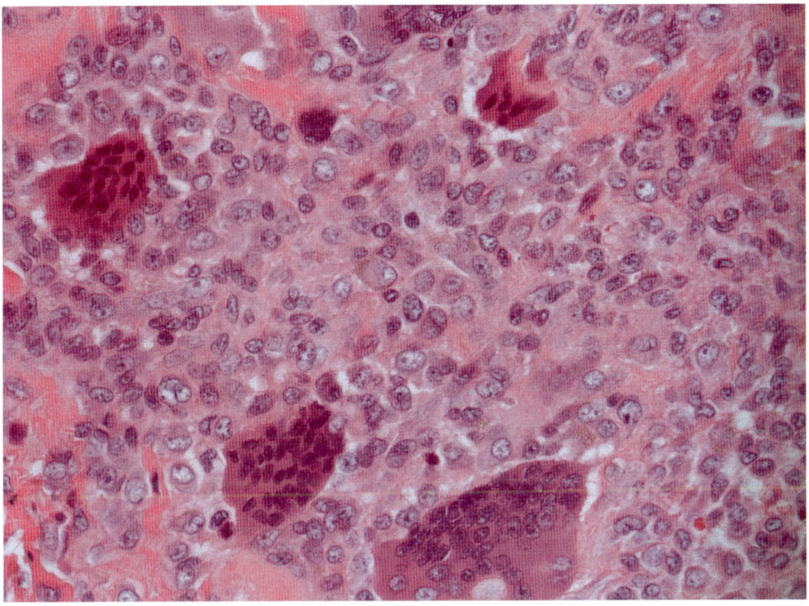

FIGURE 10.3 **Giant Cell Tumor of Tendon Sheath.** Multinucleated giant cells may be conspicuous and have numerous nuclei, and pigment deposition is also common; but the so-called ladybird cell (center) is the most reliable histologic finding.

lady bird cell). Mitotic activity may be brisk (rarely, up to 20/10 hpf) but necrosis is very rare.

Malignant forms of giant cell tumor of tendon sheath are extremely rare, but the presence of cytologic atypia or necrosis should prompt an immunohistochemical evaluation to rule out epithelioid sarcoma. Giant cell tumor of tendon sheath is characteristically positive for CD68, but unlike epithelioid sarcoma should be negative for all keratins as well as epithelial membrane antigen (EMA).

Infantile Digital Fibromatosis

Infantile digital fibromatosis is a clinically distinctive lesion, also known as inclusion body fibromatosis. It occurs on the fingers and toes of young children, infants, and neonates, and consists of interlacing bundles of fibroblasts and myofibroblasts. This entity rarely poses a diagnostic challenge once its characteristic paranuclear eosinophilic intracytoplasmic inclusions are appreciated (see e-fig. 10.4B). Ultrastructurally, these inclusions are composed of actin, and in the event of any diagnostic uncertainty, they may be identified with Masson's trichrome stain, phosphotungstic acid-hematoxylin (PTAH), or immunohistochemistry for actin.

Myofibroma/Myofibromatosis

This tumor typically presents in one of two clinical contexts. In infants and young children, it often occurs in the context of systemic disease–so-called myofibromatosis, which often involves the bones, lungs, and gastrointestinal tract as well as the skin. However, in adults, the tumor is almost always localized to a single location, in which setting it is called "solitary myofibroma" for clarity.

Diagnosis on a biopsy specimen can be quite challenging as recognition requires the presence of two distinct patterns, often in alternating zones which may not be adequately represented in a small specimen. The first pattern is composed of whorls or broad fascicles of bland myofibroblasts with a hyaline or pseudochondroid stroma; in adults, this is generally the predominant pattern (e-fig. 10.8). The second, frequently seen at the center of the lesion, is usually cellular, composed of primitive, round to spindled cells with scant cytoplasm and often staghorn vessels. The mitotic rate may be high in these areas (e-fig. 10.9).

If only the primitive zone is sampled (a rare occurrence in adults) a false concern for malignancy may be raised due to the presence of mitotic activity, necrosis, and even apparent foci of vascular invasion. By contrast, the outer, mature zone may give a nonspecific impression of a benign or low-grade myofibroblastic lesion or leiomyoma. It is only following complete excision that a correct diagnosis will be made. The immunophenotype is unrevealing, with both zones being positive only for vimentin and actins.[8]

Cutaneous Myxoma/Angiomyxoma

These benign tumors are most often located at acral sites, on the head, neck, and genital regions; depending on their histologic features, a diagnosis of myxoma, cellular myxoma, or angiomyxoma may be appropriate. In all cases, there is a poorly circumscribed, paucicellular, myxoid mass composed primarily of extracellular matrix, with a few bland stellate to spindled nuclei (Fig. 10.4). Nuclear atypia must not be present: the presence of bizarre cells, in particular, should raise the possibility of acral myxoinflammatory fibroblastic sarcoma. An epithelial component may occasionally be present in angiomyxomas. Although small vessels may be abundant in angiomyxoma, the presence of thick-walled, curvilinear vessels should prompt concern for myxofibrosarcoma. Although most myxomas are sporadic, rarely, cutaneous myxomas may be the initial presentation of Carney complex.

Dermatofibrosarcoma Protuberans (Giant Cell Fibroblastoma)

Although traditionally categorized separately, DFSP and giant cell fibroblastoma are now seen by many as histologic variants of a single entity. The basis for combining the two is their shared prognosis, cytogenetic abnormalities, and immunohistochemical profile, and their tendency to show overlapping histologic features—both on initial presentation and at recurrence. DFSP is characterized by monomorphic spindle cells which widely infiltrate subcutaneous adipose tissue and dermis (Fig. 10.5) (although usually sparing the superficial dermis). The tumor is often quite cellular. By contrast, giant cell fibroblastoma typically occurs in much younger patients and features pseudovascular spaces lined by floretlike giant cells,

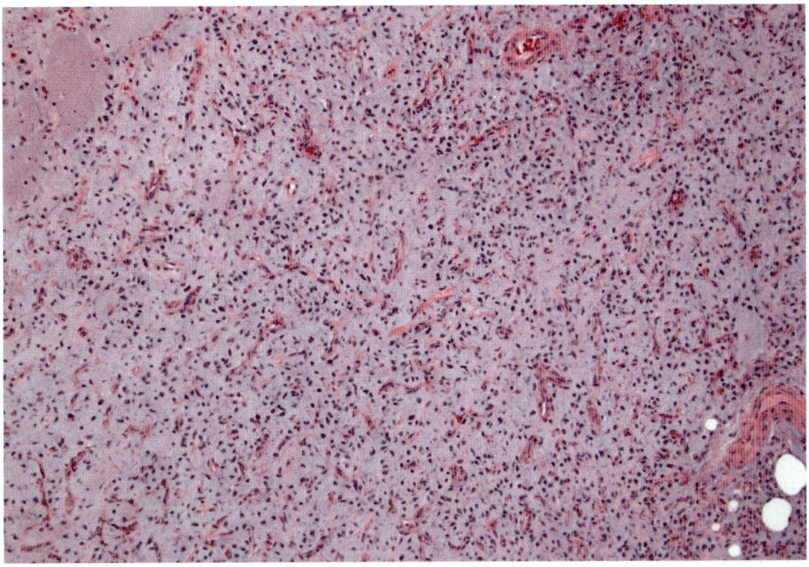

FIGURE 10.4 **Cellular Myxoma.** When examining a myxoid tumor, thin-walled "chicken wire" vessels such as these should reassure the pathologist that the tumor is a myxoma, not a myxofibrosarcoma.

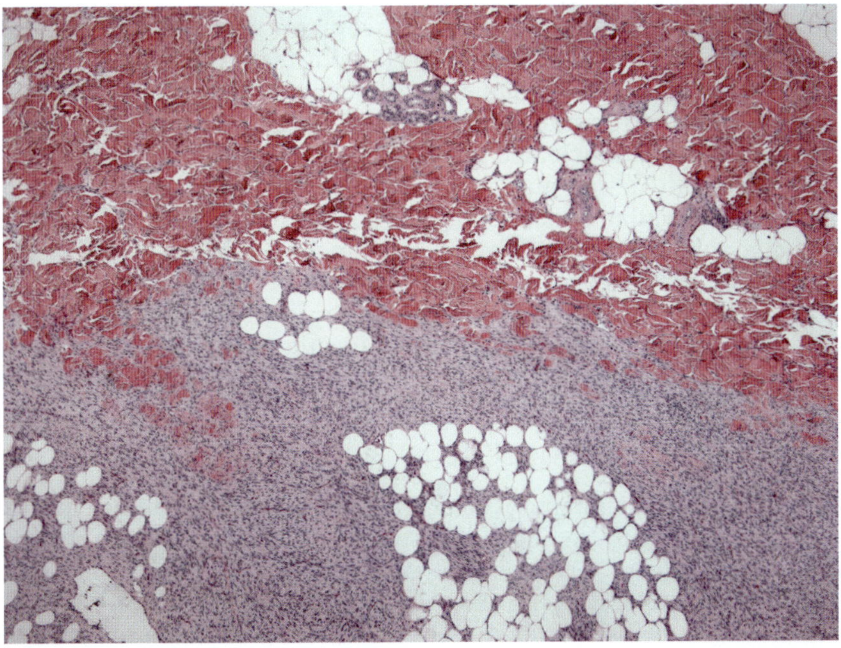

FIGURE 10.5 **Dermatofibrosarcoma Protuberans.** Extension into the subcutis along septa is characteristic Dermatofibrosarcoma Protuberans.

with a characteristic myxoid matrix in at least some areas. Because of its similarity to vascular tumors, it is important that CD31, as well as CD34, be used to exclude vascular neoplasms.

Although they are rarely seen on a biopsy specimen, it is important to search for areas of fibrosarcomalike histology, with long fascicles of monomorphic but hyperchromatic spindle cells with increased mitotic activity resembling low-grade fibrosarcoma. These areas of fibrosarcomatous change are believed to herald an increased likelihood of metastasis which is otherwise rare in this tumor.

The differential diagnosis with dermatofibroma has been discussed above. A small percentage of tumors, the so-called Bednar tumors, may show pigment deposition in admixed slender dendritic cells cognate to those of the blue nevus; negativity for S-100 in the critical cells will rule out a melanocytic lesion. Immunohistochemical stains must be interpreted with caution, however, as dendritic nevomelanocytes are frequently present: these cells may stain positively with S-100 and other melanocytic markers. Myxoid cases of DFSP may resemble myxofibrosarcoma: the diagnosis of DFSP depends on a truly monomorphous population of cells, while the presence of nuclear pleomorphism, together with characteristic curvilinear vessels, should raise concern for myxofibrosarcoma.

Plexiform Fibrohistiocytic Tumor

This tumor characteristically occurs in the upper extremities of boys and young men. Although spontaneous regression has been reported,[9] the tumor is considered to be a low-grade neoplasm because of the potential for persistent recurrence as well as even metastasis. It is characterized by a complex arrangement of nodules and fascicles of fibroblastic cells which interdigitate and entrap subcutaneous adipose tissue. Nodules of histiocytes associated with multinucleated giant cells are seen in the background, and for this reason, the lesion may be mistaken for a granulomatous inflammatory process. Vascular invasion may be present, but the mitotic rate is low, and atypia and necrosis are absent. Recognition of the fascicles of fibroblastic cells is essential for a correct diagnosis. When necrosis is present within the histiocytic nodules, an infectious process or epithelioid sarcoma should be considered. Plexiform fibrohistiocytic tumor may also resemble cellular neurothekeoma, but it is negative for NKI/C3 and microopthalmia transcription factor.

Angiomatoid Fibrous Histiocytoma

Once considered a subtype of malignant fibrous histiocytoma, this low-grade tumor typically involves the subcutis but may arise in the deep dermis. It is frequently pseudoencapsulated and consists of large blood-filled cystic spaces and areas of hemorrhage in addition to solid nests of fibroblastlike and histiocytelike cells. A chronic inflammatory infiltrate may be present, and often includes hemosiderin-laden macrophages and giant cells. It characteristically presents in adolescents and young adults.

The differential diagnosis typically includes vascular neoplasms, but angiomatoid fibrous histiocytoma is negative for all vascular markers. Desmin and EMA are occasionally positive.

Fibrosarcoma

Once considered the most common sarcoma, adult fibrosarcoma has all but disappeared from the medical literature, following the introduction of immunohistochemistry and molecular techniques. Some equate it with fibrosarcomatous change in DFSP (see above) but this simplification risks confusing this narrowly defined histologic change with the older, now vanishing entity.

Myxofibrosarcoma

Myxofibrosarcoma (formerly "myxoid malignant fibrous histiocytoma"), is a tumor commonly seen on the arms and legs of older adults. It shows a spectrum of differentiation, and, unlike most sarcomas, its histologic grade correlates clearly with behavior. At the well-differentiated end of this spectrum, the tumor may be hypocellular, comprising scattered hyperchromatic cells in a mucinous background. Keys to recognizing low-grade myxofibrosarcoma are a multilobular pattern of growth, true nuclear atypia, and thick-walled, arcuate (or curvilinear) vessels with surrounding stromal condensation. At the other end of the spectrum, a poorly differentiated myxofibrosarcoma may resemble other poorly differentiated sarcomas, with focal myxoid areas resembling a lower-grade myxofibrosarcoma. Although a cutoff has been proposed, this distinction may be of little clinical relevance, as high-grade myxofibrosarcoma apparently has the same prognosis as so-called malignant fibrous histiocytoma (pleomorphic sarcoma).

Occasionally, tumor cells in myxofibrosarcoma may have vacuolated cytoplasms and indented nuclei, mimicking lipoblasts. However, the cytoplasm will stain positively for mesenchymal mucin with Alcian blue. In addition, myxoid liposarcoma shows a distinctive "chicken-wire" vasculature, distinct from the characteristic arcuate vessels of myxofibrosarcoma.[10]

Low-Grade Fibromyxoid Sarcoma

Typically a tumor of deep soft tissue, low grade fibromyxoid sarcoma would only rarely be seen on skin biopsy. It is nevertheless important because its appearance may mimic a benign entity. It is recognized by its characteristic arcades of small blood vessels, perivascular sclerosis and alternating zones of heavily collagenized, hypocellular zones with more cellular myxoid nodules. The collagenized areas show short, whorling fascicles. One characteristic subtype shows giant collagen rosettes.

Epithelioid Sarcoma

An uncommon malignancy of unknown lineage that most frequently presents in the skin and superficial soft tissues of the limbs of young adults, epithelioid sarcoma is important to pathologists because of its tendency to mimic a necrobiotic granuloma. When fully excised, it shows a characteristic nodular growth pattern showing areas of necrosis surrounded by eosinophilic, epithelioid, and spindle cells showing slight nuclear atypia, vesicular nuclei, and small nucleoli. Superficial shave biopsy may show only these cellular areas; fortunately, even if the characteristic histologic appearance is lacking, this tumor will show immunoreactivity for a variety of cytokeratins as well as EMA, unlike histiocytic lesions.

A "proximal type" epithelioid sarcoma has also been described; these resemble a poorly differentiated carcinoma and frequently show rhabdoid features. They are typically confined to the deep soft tissues of the pelvis, perineum, and genitals.[11]

TUMORS OF FAT, MUSCLE, CARTILAGE, AND BONE

Lipoma

These typically arise as solitary, subcutaneous masses between the age of 40 and 60 years, although in approximately 5% of patients, multiple lipomata may be present.[3] Lipomas are composed of mature white adipocytes with a thin fibrous capsule, although this capsule may not be seen in a biopsy specimen.

At one extreme, lipomata may be indistinguishable from normal subcutaneous tissue, if the capsule is not visible. However, a variety of concerning features may also occur. Fat necrosis may raise concern for malignancy, although careful examination of the nuclear features shows neither the hyperchromasia nor the scalloping that characterize a lipoblast. The presence of variation in adipocyte size should raise concern for a malignant lesion; however, many such lesions, upon careful examination, show no other features of malignancy and are appropriately categorized as lipomas. In our experience, the presence of fibrous septa with stromal hyperchromatic cells is the most useful feature in distinguishing atypical lipomatous tumor from simple lipoma and a firm diagnosis of atypical lipomatous tumor may be made on this finding alone. Other findings which should raise concern for atypical lipomatous tumor include a size greater than 5 cm, or presence in a lower limb. Lipoblasts are characteristic of liposarcomas, but may sometimes be seen in lipomas.

Angiolipomas show the same histologic features as lipomas, but with an increase in small vessels, which characteristically show fibrin microthrombi. As a practical matter, this distinction is unimportant except that angiolipomata are more often painful or tender.

Spindle Cell Lipoma/Pleomorphic Lipoma

Although widely considered a variant of lipoma, this tumor may show little or no adipocytic differentiation. It commonly occurs in the subcutis of the head, neck, and back of older men. Its most reliable histologic features are refractile,

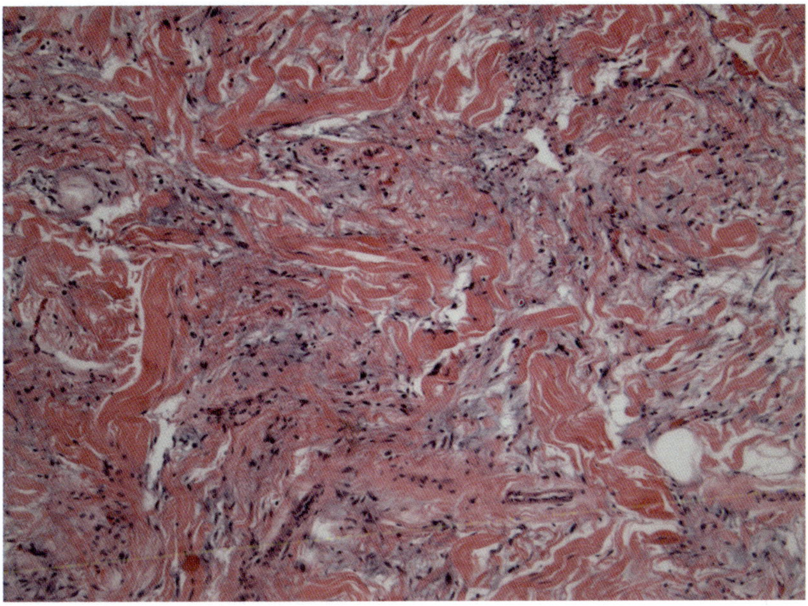

FIGURE 10.6 **Spindle Cell Lipoma.** Bundles of ropelike collagen associated with bland spindled cells; adipocytes are usually present.

"ropey" collagen, and uniform spindle cells in a myxoid matrix (Fig. 10.6). The cells have slender, bipolar processes, but unlike perineurioma, the cells are immunohistochemically positive for CD34 rather than EMA. Foci of bony or cartilaginous metaplasia may occur; in the presence of nuclear pleomorphism, however, this should prompt consideration of pleomorphic lipoma. In difficult cases, immunohistochemistry for MDM2 and CDK4 may be useful in ruling out an atypical lipomatous tumor. Other worrisome features include size greater than 4 cm, and mitotic activity.[12,13]

Pleomorphic lipomas may have similar features to those seen above, but have small, spindle to rounded, hyperchromatic cells, with multinucleated cells often showing a characteristic "floretlike" pattern (resembling the petals of a flower).

Hibernoma

A tumor of brown fat which typically occurs on the upper back or axillae of young to middle-aged adults; diagnosis of hibernoma is usually straightforward and even its large size (up to 24 cm) should not prompt concern so long as nuclei are regular (lacking the hyperchromasia and scalloping of true lipoblasts), uniform, and lack mitotic activity(e-fig. 10.10).[14]

Atypical Lipomatous Tumor

Atypical lipomatous tumor (also known as well-differentiated liposarcoma, or atypical lipoma), although rare, is the most common malignant

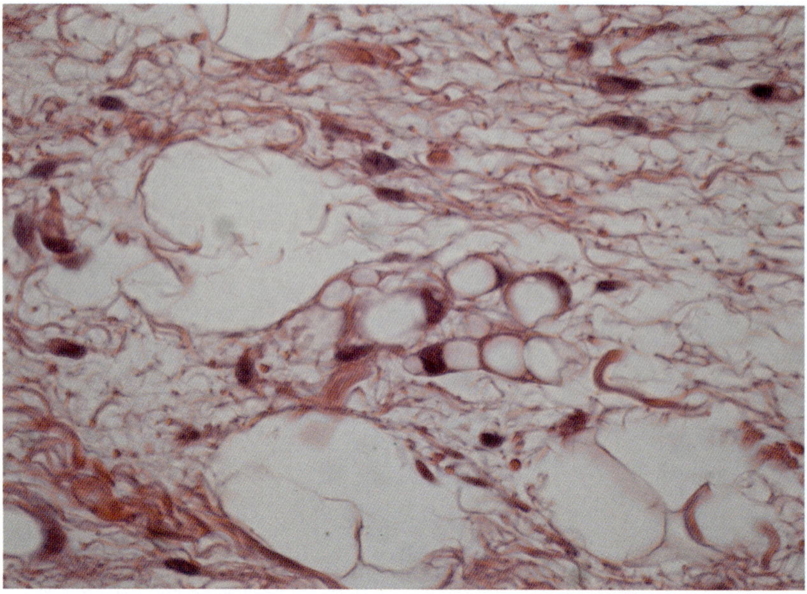

FIGURE 10.7 **Atypical Lipomatous Tumor.** Careful examination usually reveals lipoblasts; but the presence of hyperchromatic spindled cells alone is highly worrisome.

tumor of adipocytes in the subcutis. It may even occur within the dermis, although it should be emphasized that the large majority of superficial adipocytic lesions are benign lipomata. As their name implies, atypical lipomatous tumors may strongly resemble lipomas. Important differences include variation in adipocyte size, and the presence of fibrous septa with hyperchromatic stromal cells (Fig. 10.7). The older literature has emphasized the importance of lipoblasts, manifesting multiple cytoplasmic vacuoles scalloping a hyperchromatic nucleus. While rare, true lipoblasts may be present in an atypical lipomatous tumor; they are not required for a diagnosis. Most authorities require multiple vacuoles for a cell to qualify as a lipoblast. In principle, univacuolar (signet-ring cell) lipoblasts exist, but these may be indistinguishable from small vessels on routinely stained sections; for this reason, most authors consider them to be insufficient evidence for the diagnosis.

In cases where the diagnosis is in doubt, immunohistochemistry for MDM2 and CDK4 has recently become available and may be useful as these markers are positive in greater than 90% of atypical lipomatous tumors and less than 10% of lipomas.[15–17]

Myxoid Liposarcoma/Round Cell Liposarcoma

While these entities are usually included in reviews of adipocytic lesions, myxoid liposarcoma, and round cell liposarcoma occur almost exclusively in the deep soft tissues of the proximal lower extremity. The dermatopathologist should be highly wary of making such a diagnosis when no such deep-seated mass is present. Moreover, when encountering a highly cellular malignant lesion with foci of apparent liposarcomatous differentiation, the dermatopathologist should be aware that atypical lipomatous tumors may dedifferentiate into pleomorphic sarcomas indistinguishable from so-called malignant fibrous histiocytoma (pleomorphic sarcoma). In such cases, the original, well-differentiated, tumor is often seen only in small areas discovered at final resection, if at all.

SMOOTH MUSCLE TUMORS

Smooth muscle tumors of the skin fall into three categories: smooth muscle hamartomas, benign smooth muscle neoplasms, and leiomyosarcomata.

Smooth Muscle Hamartomas

These lesions occur mainly on the trunk in children, and are composed of disordered bundles of smooth muscle. They are in many cases, although not always, associated with other components of a Becker's nevus, namely, mammilated epidermal hyperplasia and, in some cases, basal layer pigmentation.

Leiomyoma/Angioleiomyoma

Leiomyomata are generally solitary, but often multiple, benign smooth muscle lesions of the dermis or subcutis. They are typically circumscribed, but not sharply so, and are not encapsulated. By definition, mitotic activity and atypia should be minimal (<1 mitotic figure per fifty 40× hpf). Small amounts of fibrous stroma are typically present between smooth muscle bundles, but a large fibrous component should prompt consideration of smooth muscle hamartoma as a diagnosis. If necessary, smooth muscle differentiation can be confirmed using immunohistochemistry for actin, desmin, and h-caldesmon.

Although they may resemble leiomyomas, angioleiomyomas are clinically distinctive, usually being a solitary, painful, or tender lesion on the lower extremity of a woman. Histologically, angioleiomyoma forms a spectrum with leiomyoma, although numerous vascular spaces are present intrinsic to the mass; these spaces are typically compressed and slitlike but may be cavernous. In either case, the smooth muscle of the vascular wall merges imperceptibly with the surrounding tumor.[1]

Leiomyosarcoma

Leiomyosarcomas may arise in either the subcutis or the dermis, and are typically solitary lesions of adults. They usually have obvious mitotic activity and nuclear pleomorphism (Fig. 10.8); necrosis is another sign of

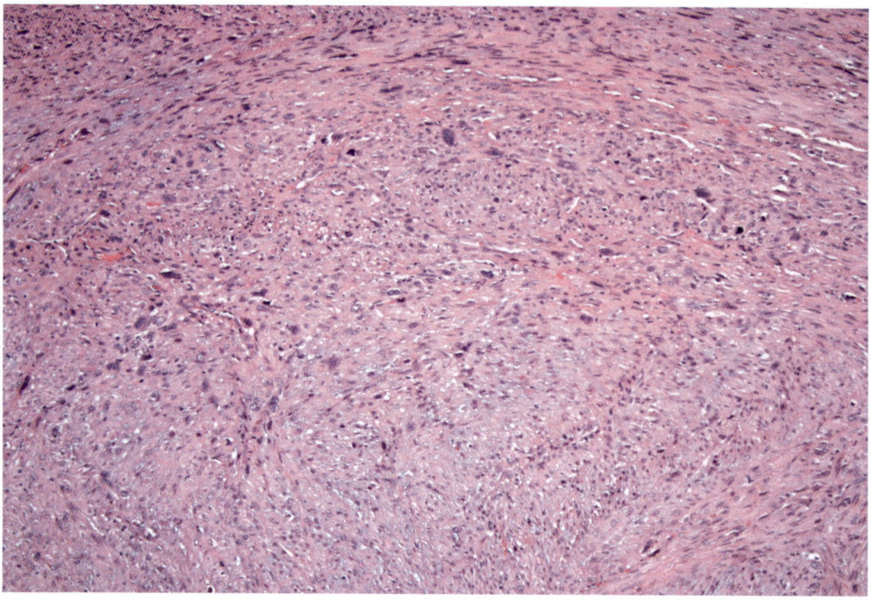

FIGURE 10.8 **Characteristic Case of Leiomyosarcoma (Atypical Leiomyomatous Tumor).** Disordered fascicles of spindle cells in the dermis. Nuclei have blunted ends; hyperchromasia and nuclear pleomorphism are prominent; and there is abundant eosinophilic cytoplasm.

malignancy. However, well-differentiated lesions may be difficult to distinguish from leiomyoma (Fig. 10.9); in such cases, it may be helpful to examine the edges of the tumor, if they have been sampled, as leiomyosarcoma is less circumscribed than leiomyoma. When the edges of the tumor are not visible, or the nuclear features are equivocal, it may be best to defer the final diagnosis to the excision specimen. Mitotic activity greater than 1/50 hpf may also be a useful criterion, although the precise threshold of mitotic activity required for a diagnosis of malignancy is not universally agreed upon.

When the tumor is confined to the dermis, the distinction between leiomyoma and leiomyosarcoma may be of little importance as smooth muscle tumors of the skin rarely, if ever, metastasize; for this reason, some authorities prefer the term "atypical leiomyomatous tumor" for such lesions. When the tumor arises from the subcutis, however, it should be referred to and treated as a sarcoma, as such lesions metastasize in up to 50% of cases. One should consider uterine or other potentially metastasizing smooth muscle tumors in the appropriate clinical circumstances.[18]

TUMORS OF SKELETAL MUSCLE

Malignant skeletal muscle tumors are exceptionally rare in skin, except as metastases, or as part of an underlying soft-tissue mass.

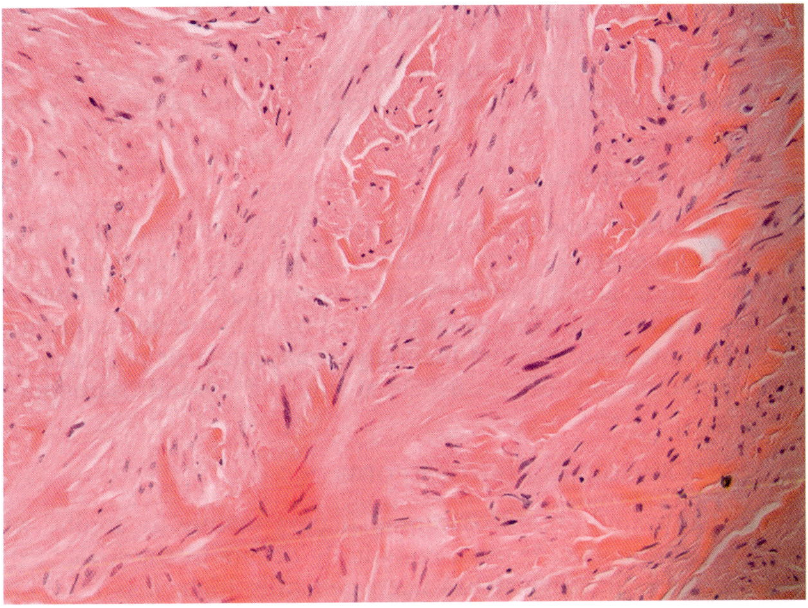

FIGURE 10.9 **Leiomyosarcoma.** An occasional atypical nucleus is present, along with mitotic activity, in a tumor consisting of disordered fascicles of smooth muscle. Despite the milder findings, such cases do qualify as leiomyosarcoma (atypical leiomyomatous tumor).

Rhabdomyomatous Mesenchymal Hamartoma

Rhabdomyomatous mesenchymal hamartoma typically occurs near the midline of the head and neck in infants and young children; it may also be congenital. Microscopically, it consists of bundles of mature (not fetal), vertically oriented skeletal muscle fibers surrounded by mature fibrous and adipose tissue. Peripheral nerves may be present in variable numbers.

Rhabdomyoma

In contrast to rhabdomyomatous mesenchymal hamartomas, rhabdomyomas should consist almost exclusively of skeletal muscle. These are of two kinds:

- Adult-type rhabdomyomas occur predominantly in the head and neck of adults, usually men. They consist of large, round to polygonal cells with abundant, brightly eosinophilic cytoplasm. Cross striations are present.
- Fetal-type rhabdomyomas typically present in infants or children under the age of 5, and may be congenital. They occur as solitary lesions of the face and neck, and cluster, in particular, around the eyes and ears. They consist of disordered fetal skeletal muscle, often with areas of maturation. Mitotic activity, necrosis, and pleomorphism are absent.[19,20]

In cases where it is necessary to confirm skeletal muscle differentiation, immunohistochemistry for myogenin, myoglobin, desmin, and actin HHF-35 will generally be positive, although smooth muscle actin and h-caldesmon are usually negative.

TUMORS OF CARTILAGE AND BONE

Setting aside osteoma cutis, true neoplasms of bone and cartilage do not occur as primary skin tumors, although lesions of the subcutis may be seen in a skin biopsy.

Extraskeletal Chondroma

Extraskeletal chondroma is a benign lesion that typically occurs as a solitary, well-circumscribed tumor of the hands and feet of adults, usually no more than 2 cm in greatest dimension. It is composed of a variably cellular, mature cartilage which may show focal ossification and even marked nuclear pleomorphism. Myxoid foci may occur, but their presence should prompt consideration of extraskeletal myxoid chondrosarcoma (see below).[21,22]

Extraskeletal Myxoid Chondrosarcoma

Extraskeletal myxoid chondrosarcoma occurs mainly in adults, with a 2:1 male predominance. It most commonly occurs in the lower extremity. Although 5-year survival has been generally high, it is now known that most patients eventually die of disease, but often only after 10 to 20 years.[23,24] Microscopically, the tumor is lobulated and has a mucoid or myxoid stroma. Within the stroma, there are interlacing cords and strands of ovoid to spindle-shaped cells which may show no obvious chondroblastic differentiation. Mitoses are often scarce, and the cytology may be deceptively bland, with no necrosis.

Although both tumors may show a mixture of cartilaginous and myxoid features, skeletal myxoid chondrosarcoma can be distinguished from extraskeletal chondroma by virtue of its multilobular architecture and the tendency of its cells to form nests and strands. If necessary, a reciprocal (9;22) translocation can be demonstrated in most cases of extraskeletal myxoid chondrosarcoma. Other entities that may enter into the differential diagnosis include mixed tumor of skin, which has an epithelial component; myxoma, which is less cellular; and neurothekeoma, which is both myxoid and multilobulated, but characteristically occurs in the dermis, whereas extraskeletal myxoid chondrosarcoma is a tumor of subcutaneous soft tissues.

Myositis Ossificans/Fibroosseous Pseudotumor of Digits

Myositis ossificans is a reactive lesion, related to nodular fasciitis, which usually occurs in muscle, but may also occur in the dermis or subcutis where it is sometimes referred to as panniculitis ossificans or fasciitis ossificans. It frequently arises in physically active young men and may be related to trauma in up to 50% of cases. Initial growth may be rapid, but the tumor is ultimately self-limiting.[3]

In early lesions, the tumor resembles NF, with numerous proliferating fibroblasts oriented randomly or in short fascicles. Mitoses may be

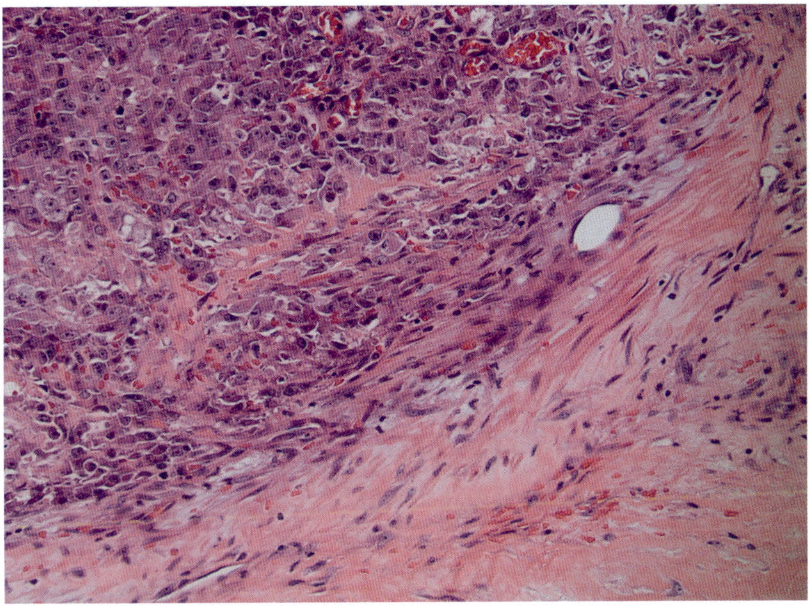

FIGURE 10.10 **Metastatic Osteosarcoma** This example of metastatic osteosarcoma in skin shows malignant cells with a trace of osteoid formation.

numerous, but nuclear pleomorphism and hyperchromasia are absent. With time, trabecular bone develops around the periphery, rimmed by active osteoblasts and osteoclasts. Eventually, in mature lesions, the center becomes less cellular and more collagenized, whereas the bony periphery gradually matures, and may eventually develop hematopoietic marrow. This phenomenon of zoning–with bone at the periphery and cellular, fibroblastic areas at the center–helps to distinguish this lesion from extraskeletal osteosarcoma, which it may otherwise resemble, but in which the pattern of zonation is reversed.

Extraskeletal Osteosarcoma

Extraskeletal osteosarcoma is a rare lesion of older adults that typically arises in the soft tissue of the legs, and may be associated with a history of irradiation to the affected site.

Histologically, the tumor is characterized by atypical cells which, by definition, must be at least focally associated with an osteoid or a chondroid matrix. Atypia is usually present and may be pronounced, with atypical mitotic figures, and often an infiltrative border. Zonation, when present, is generally the opposite of myositis ossificans, with osteoid at the center and cellular areas at the periphery; newly formed "malignant" osteoid (Fig. 10.10) laid down by neoplastic osteoblasts, and not just mature bone, is required for the diagnosis.

NEURAL AND NEUROENDOCRINE TUMORS

Traumatic Neuroma

Traumatic neuromas are usually solitary, skin-colored lesions which occur at sites of prior trauma, commonly on the extremities. They are often painful and, in the special case of neuromas occurring at the site of an amputation, cause lancinating pain. The supernumerary digit, which occurs congenitally on the lateral-volar aspect of the hand, is a polypoid lesion that shares the histologic features of a traumatic neuroma. Some authors have speculated that it results from in utero amputation of a true digit.[25] They do not contain cartilage or bone.

Although they result in a mass, traumatic neuromas are not true neoplasms, but disorganized reactive proliferations of axons, Schwann cells, and perineural cells in a dense fibroblastic stroma. As such, the constituent cells stain positively with S-100, and neurofilament protein highlights axons. EMA is positive in perineural cells.

Palisaded Encapsulated Neuroma (Palisaded Neuroma)

Palisaded neuroma is a small, solitary, dome-shaped lesion which characteristically occurs on the face of adults, although 10% of cases occur elsewhere. It is known by a variety of names–true neuroma, solitary circumscribed neuroma, spontaneous neuroma–reflecting the fact that encapsulation is typically not complete. Microscopically, the lesion is a generally well-circumscribed dermal nodule composed of tightly woven fascicles of spindled cells separated by artefactual, cleftlike spaces. Rudimentary Verocay bodies are often present. A thin capsule, if present, may be highlighted with immunohistochemistry for EMA. Rarely, a connection with the originating nerve may be discovered. Immunohistochemistry for S-100 is positive, and some[26] but not all authors[27] have found axons within the lesion. The distinction between palisaded neuroma and schwannoma (neurilemmoma) is of limited importance as both lesions are benign, although palisaded encapsulated neuroma is a feature of multiple endocrine neoplasia 2b (MEN2b). The schwannoma typically has a thick capsule and shows a peripheral nerve branch from which it takes origin. In general, palisaded neuroma is a dermal tumor, whereas schwannoma is a tumor of the subcutaneous soft tissue. Unlike neurofibroma, the palisaded neuroma compresses adjacent structures; the constituent cells of a neurofibroma percolate around, but do not displace, adnexae.

Neurofibroma

Neurofibromas most commonly occur as sporadic, frequently painless, skin-colored, pink or brown, dome-shaped to pedunculated lesions which may occur anywhere on the body. Multiple neurofibromas are not uncommon, particularly in older adults; but when present in combination with findings such as café au lait macules, Lisch nodules, axillary freckling, and a variety of visceral abnormalities, they are the primary finding of classic

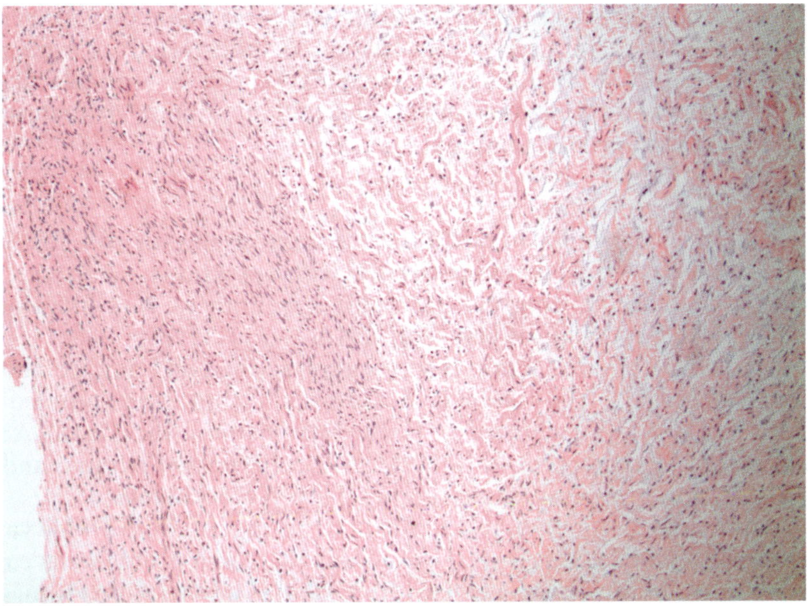

FIGURE 10.11 **Neurofibroma.** In rare cases, the nerve of origin can be identified (left).

von Recklinghausen's neurofibromatosis (NF1). In such cases, the neurofibromata tend to arise in adolescence. Rarely, the pathologist may see a biopsy specimen of a deep, plexiform neurofibroma, once thought to occur only in NF1.

Microscopically, the lesions are circumscribed but unencapsulated lesions composed of spindled cells with indistinct cell borders and wavy nuclei with tapered ends ("seagull-shaped") (Fig. 10.11). The stroma can be variably fibrous, myxoid, areolar, or vascular. Mast cells are typically scattered throughout the lesion. The originating nerve twig is rarely observed, and neurofilaments are immunohistochemically present. Mitotic activity is usually nonexistent, and, although the cells are often uniformly hyperchromatic, nuclear pleomorphism should prompt careful scrutiny for mitotic activity, in the presence of which, a diagnosis of malignant peripheral nerve sheath tumor (neurofibrosarcoma, malignant schwannoma) must be considered (see below). Neurofibromas that have atypia in the absence of mitotic activity are called "Atypical neurofibromas" and have a benign prognosis.

Neurofibromas are S-100 positive, and the differential diagnosis with a fully neurotized nevus is difficult, if not impossible, except in patients with known NF1.[28]

Malignant Peripheral Nerve Sheath Tumor

Although a well-established entity in soft tissues, this diagnosis should be approached with extreme caution in the skin, as it is generally indistinguishable from sarcomatoid melanoma, a far more common entity. Except in cases where a diagnosis of NF1 has already been made or a progenitor nerve or neurofibroma can be convincingly demonstrated, or which are negative for S-100 and other melanoma markers, it is probably best to favor a diagnosis of malignant melanoma (either primary or metastatic) even when no epidermal component is present.

Perineurioma

Perineurioma is a benign tumor almost always arising in soft tissues or peripheral nerves which is not associated with any known syndrome, and displays a bewildering range of histologic appearances, but, like normal perineurial cells, stains positively with EMA.

Microscopically, the lesion is well circumscribed and may be nodular or dumbbell-shaped. The tumor cells are usually short and spindled and arranged in a storiform, whorled, or fasciculated pattern (Fig. 10.12). A sclerosing variant is characterized by a densely collagenized stroma, and the tumor cells may show epithelioid or granular cell morphology.

In practice, the tumor may be difficult to distinguish from a wide variety of low-grade spindle cell lesions. Dermatofibrosarcoma protuberans can be excluded using immunohistochemistry for CD34, as perineurioma is, at, most focally CD34 positive; and, unlike true neural lesions, is S-100 negative.[29]

Neurothekeoma

A benign tumor presenting typically on the arms or face of middle-aged adults (mean age 48.4 years),[1] the neurothekeoma is an unencapsulated,

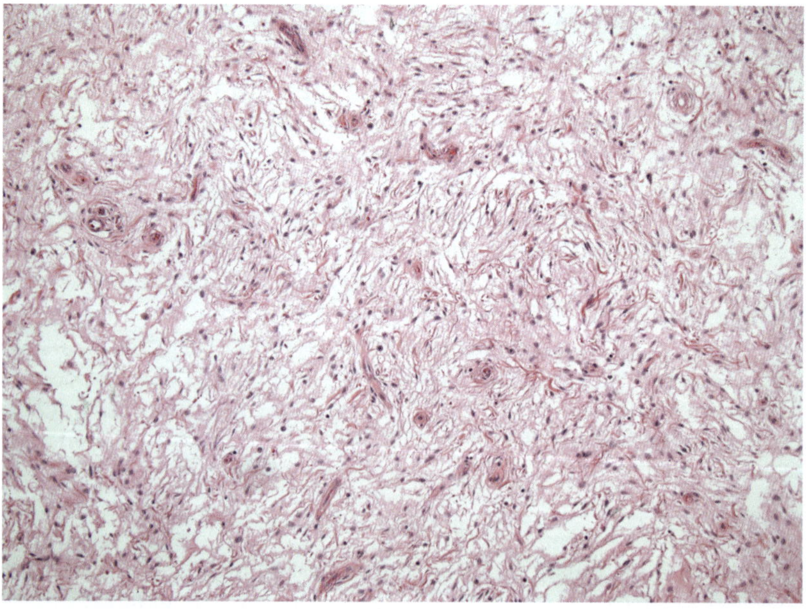

FIGURE 10.12 **Perineurioma.** In this area with marked edema, the slender, bipolar cytoplasmic processes can be seen easily.

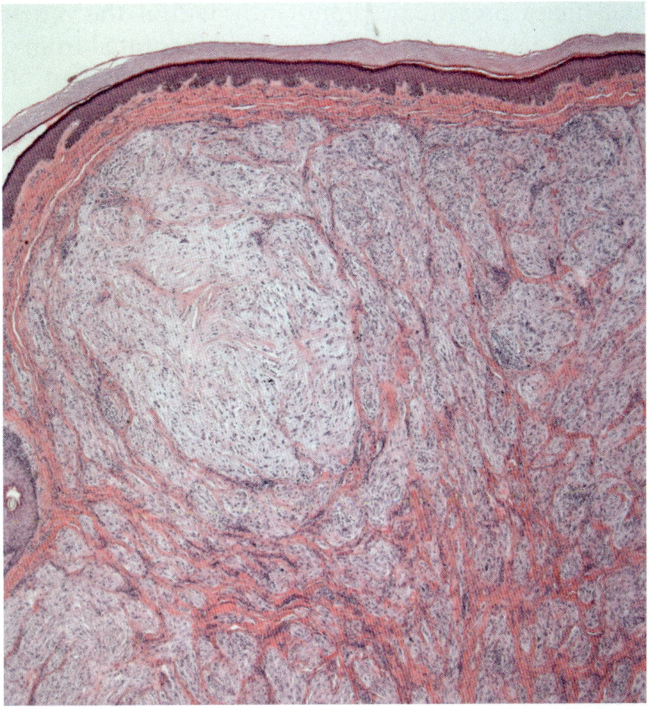

FIGURE 10.13 **Neurothekeoma.** In some examples, mucin is inconspicuous.

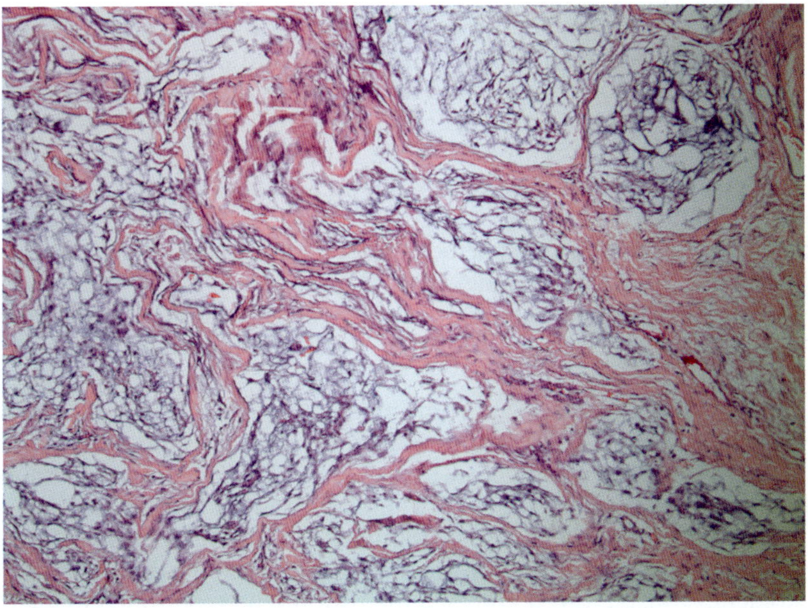

FIGURE 10.14 A more typical case showing multilobular proliferation of bland, spindle-shaped cells arranged in a mucinous stroma and separated by fibrous septa.

multilobulated mass present predominantly within the reticular dermis. The tumor lobules are of variable size, and are separated from one another by thin fibrovascular septa (Fig 10.13). There is abundant, myxomatous stroma (Fig. 10.14) with sparsely distributed spindled, stellate, and polygonal cells with minimal nuclear pleomorphism. Mitotic activity is rare or absent. Immunohistochemistry for neural markers S-100, CD57, and neuron-specific enolase (NSE) is positive.[30]

Cellular Neurothekeoma

Although traditionally considered a variant of neurothekeoma, cellular neurothekeoma is categorized separately here because of its lack of convincing immunohistochemical similarity to neurothekeoma. Cellular neurothekeoma is benign, like neurothekeoma, and tends to occur on the head, neck, and arms, although in a somewhat younger age group (average, 24 years old).[31] Microscopically, it shows a diffuse, ill-defined pattern of growth in the dermis and subcutis. The cells are epithelioid, with vesicular nuclei and abundant, eosinophilic cytoplasm, and are arranged in nests and fascicles (e-fig. 10.11). Occasional giant cells may be present. Cytologic atypia is not uncommon, and typical mitotic figures are often present. Myxoid change, however, is rare.

As mentioned above, cellular neurothekeoma is consistently negative for S-100, but is generally positive with micro-opthalmia transcription factor, NSE and NKI-C3.

Granular Cell Tumor

Granular cell tumor is generally a solitary lesion of adults, with a 3:1 female predominance. 10% are multifocal, predominantly in African Americans. While the skin is often involved, the most common site is the tongue.[32] The tumor is histologically distinctive, consisting of fascicles or sheets of polygonal cells with abundant, granular, eosinophilic cytoplasm and small, often hyperchromatic, centrally placed nuclei (Fig. 10.15). The granules are PAS positive and diastase resistant, and ultrastructurally correlate with lysosomes; characteristically, the granules are fine, but occasional giant granules may be seen. Interspersed between tumor cells, there may be histiocytic cells with coarse, triangular granules known as "angulate bodies." The overlying epidermis characteristically shows marked pseudoepitheliomatous hyperplasia, often mimicking well-differentiated squamous cell carcinoma or a verruca.

Although it does not arise from any recognized neural structure, granular cell tumor shows immunohistochemical evidence of neural differentiation (staining positively with S-100 and NSE) but is also positive for histiocytic markers CD68 and α_1-antitrypsin (but not lysozyme).

Approximately 2% to 3% of granular cell tumors behave in a malignant fashion, and, unfortunately, such behavior is usually difficult to predict histologically. Suspicious features, which should be mentioned in a pathology report, include mitotic activity greater than 2/10 hpf; marked cytologic

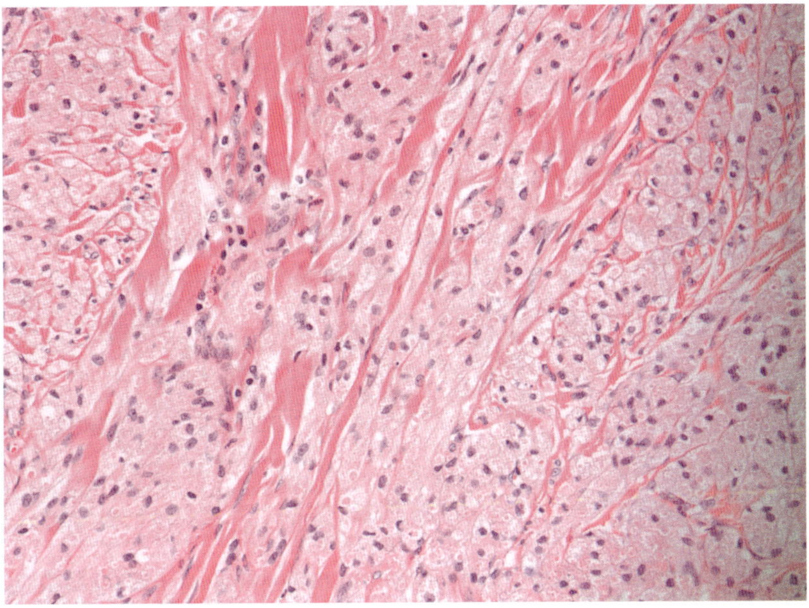

FIGURE 10.15 **Granular Cell Tumor.** Cuboidal cells with regular, round to ovoid nuclei and granular, eosinophilic cytoplasm.

atypia, with prominent nucleoli or spindling; lymphovascular invasion; and necrosis. Perineural spread (e-fig. 10.12) and low levels of mitotic activity are both common features, and do not discriminate between lesions that pursue a benign and those that pursue a malignant course.[3]

Merkel Cell Carcinoma (Primary Neuroendocrine Carcinoma of Skin)

Merkel cell carcinoma typically occurs on the sun-exposed skin of older adults, where it arises as a solitary pink to violaceous nodule. It is highly malignant and frequently recurs locally in spite of wide excision. Hematogenous and lymphatic spread are common, and usually fatal.

Merkel cell carcinoma usually grows at sheets, nests, or trabeculae within the dermis and, usually, subcutis (hence the former designation, trabecular carcinoma of the skin). The cells resemble high-grade neuroendocrine carcinoma of other sites, with a high nucleocytoplasmic ratio, finely dispersed chromatin with a distinctive steel-gray color and indistinct nucleoli, sharp nuclear borders, nuclear molding and abundant mitotic and apoptotic activity (Fig. 10.16). Foci of squamous differentiation may be present, and a pagetoid component is, infrequently, present in the epidermis. Bowen's disease co-exists in up to 10% of cases.

Immunohistochemistry is vital in the differential diagnosis of Merkel cell carcinoma. Metastatic small cell carcinoma of the lung is nearly indistinguishable from Merkel cell carcinoma on routine sections.

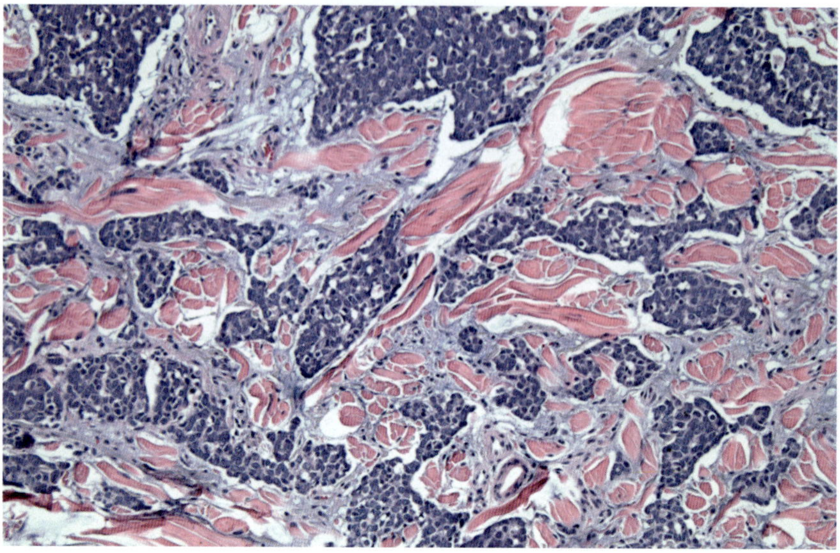

FIGURE 10.16 **Merkel Cell Carcinoma.** A dermal proliferation of neuroendocrine cells with a high N:C ratio, sharp nuclear membranes, finely dispersed chromatin, and abundant mitotic and apoptotic activity. Without immunohistochemistry, it is indistinguishable from metastatic small cell carcinoma.

Immunohistochemically, whereas small cell carcinoma of the lung is characteristically positive with TTF-1 and negative with CK20, Merkel cell carcinoma is generally negative with TTF-1, and shows a characteristic paranuclear dotlike positivity with CK20 (although more diffuse staining is acceptable). Absence of S-100 protein expression rules out melanoma which might be considered in that minority of cases which contain an intraepidermal component. Where squamous cell carcinoma is considered because of foci of squamous differentiation, the characteristic expression pattern of CK20, as well as supportive expression with chromogranin, synaptophysin, and CD56 may be necessary. Squamous cell carcinoma should be negative with CK20 and positive with p63 and high molecular weight cytokeratins such as 34β E2.

Cutaneous Meningioma

Cutaneous meningiomas may occur in one of three clinical presentations: In type I, tumors are composed of arachnoidal cells that are misplaced during embryogenesis. Type II cutaneous meningiomas develop along the course of the cranial nerves, and are therefore primarily located on the head and neck. Type III cutaneous meningiomas result from direct extension or metastasis of meningeal meningiomas. Histologically, cutaneous meningioma is generally composed of ovoid to spindled meningoendothelial cells within the deep dermis or subcutis, often with an infiltrative growth pattern, and forming pseudovascular spaces. In the most common form, the cells have a concentric, whorled architecture. The tumor may resemble a vascular neoplasm, but is negative for CD31 and CD34, and positive with EMA.[33]

Glial Heterotopia

Glial heterotopias are rare developmental anomalies that are, in principle, always congenital, although rarely they will be first noticed in adulthood. They typically present as a firm, subcutaneous mass adjacent to the bridge of the nose, often with associated hypertelorism; such cases are often known as nasal gliomas. An intranasal lesion may also be present, which may manifest with respiratory obstruction. Other rarer sites include the lip, oral cavity, scalp, and midline of the back. Although the lesion is benign, preoperative radiologic evaluation is mandatory to exclude the presence of communication with the frontal lobes.

Histologically, nasal gliomas are composed of well-circumscribed nodules of well-differentiated astrocytes in a loose, neurofibrillar stroma arising in the dermis to subcutaneous tissue. Oligodendrocytes and neurons may also be present. Nasal gliomas form a histologic spectrum with, and may be indistinguishable from, encephaloceles. Diagnosis can be confirmed with immunohistochemistry for glial fibrillary acidic protein (GFAP).[34]

Vascular Lesions

The subclassification of benign vascular lesions has traditionally been a frustrating field, with high interobserver variability plaguing attempts to distinguish lymphatic vessels from blood vessels, venous forms from arterial or capillary, and neoplasms from malformations. Our own approach in this chapter has been to follow the WHO[1] as closely as possible with particular emphasis on entities with malignant potential and benign entities with difficult differential diagnoses or implications for systemic disease.

Telangiectasias

Telangiectasias are pre-existing blood vessels which have become abnormally dilated, rather than a proliferation of new vessels. They are a characteristic finding in a number of genodermatoses: Louis Bar's syndrome (ataxia-telangiectasia), unilateral nevoid telangiectasia, hereditary benign telangiectasia, generalized essential telangiectasia, hereditary hemorrhagic telangiectasia (Osler–Weber–Rendu's disease), Cockayne's syndrome, Bloom's syndrome, and Rothmund Thompson's syndrome. These entities have been described in greater detail elsewhere.[35] Acquired telangiectasias most commonly result from chronic sun exposure, but may also be drug induced; idiopathic acquired telangiectasias make up the so-called costal fringe, a clinically distinctive pattern of telangiectasias on the anterior thorax of elderly men.

Spider angioma (nevus araneus) is, despite its Latin name, an acquired lesion consisting of numerous telangiectasias in the papillary dermis radiating from a central, thick-walled arteriole. They are associated with pregnancy and chronic liver disease, but are also common as a solitary, sporadic lesion, being present in 10% to 15% of normal adults.[36]

Venous Lake

Venous lake is an acquired venous ectasia characteristically occurring on the head and neck of older adults. Clinically, it may resemble a pigmented lesion, or it may suddenly change or become symptomatic owing to thrombosis. Histologically, it consists of a single dilated vein. It may be histologically indistinguishable from the so-called capillary aneurysm.

Nevus Flammeus

Known clinically as "salmon patch" or "port wine stain," nevus flammeus is a congenital proliferation of dilated, thin-walled venules occurring either in the superficial dermis, or scattered throughout the dermis. It is unilateral, and typically occurs on the head and neck. As such, it is generally clinically distinctive. The pathologist, however, should be aware that it is associated with various syndromes (Table 10.1).

Angioma Serpiginosum

Angioma serpiginosum is clinically distinctive vascular proliferation consisting of multiple red-violaceous puncta, which may form groups but characteristically have a gyrate or serpiginous configuration. They most often occur on the legs, but may arise anywhere on the skin (except the palms and soles). They characteristically occur before puberty, and are more common in girls than boys. Histologically, they consist of dilated capillaries in the upper half of the dermis.[37]

TABLE 10.1 Nevus Flammeus: Associated Syndromes

Cobb's syndrome	Nevus flammeus, often in a dermatomal distribution, overlying a vascular malformation in the spinal cord
Sturge–Weber's syndrome (encephalotrigeminal angiomatosis)	Unilateral nevus flammeus in the distribution of the trigeminal nerve, associated with ipsilateral vascular malformations, underlying tram-track calcifications of the temporal and occipital cortex, progressive skeletal and soft tissue hypertrophy of the affected area, and ipsilateral glaucoma
Klippel–Trenaunay's syndrome (angiosteohypertrophy syndrome)	Unilateral nevus flammeus with edema and skeletal and soft tissue hypertrophy of the underlying limb and underlying vascular malformations

Hemangioma of Infancy

A common tumor, occurring in approximately 10% of infants,[38] it typically presents congenitally or in the perinatal period, with a 3:1 female predominance. It may proliferate rapidly in the first year but typically regresses slowly afterward. Rarely, large facial hemangiomas may be associated with the PHACES syndrome.[35]

Microscopically, the lesion is a multilobular proliferation of plump endothelial cells with tiny, slitlike lumina surrounded by multilaminated basement membranes. Mitotic figures may be numerous. Mast cells are abundant. The lesions characteristically involve the dermis, but may extend into the subcutis. Perineural extension can occur. Involuting lesions show larger lumina, flattened endothelial cells and pericytes, and a more conspicuous, loose connective tissue stroma.

Unusually for a vascular tumor, hemangiomas of infancy show strong immunohistochemical expression of GLUT1.

Cherry Hemangioma

Also known as Campbell de Morgan spots or senile hemangiomas, cherry hemangiomas are common skin lesions. They are rare before puberty, begin to appear in early adulthood, and are almost universally present in late life. Clinical diagnosis is rarely challenging. Microscopically, they manifest clusters of rounded capillaries with thickened basement membranes and variably inflamed stroma.

Sinusoidal Hemangioma

An acquired vascular proliferation of adults, formerly known as "cavernous hemangioma," it typically occurs in the subcutis or deep dermis as a well-circumscribed nodule of back-to-back dilated vascular channels. Diagnosis is rarely challenging when the lesion is completely excised; however, Masson change may occur as a result of thrombosis, simulating angiosarcoma. Angiosarcoma, however, is distinct even in a small biopsy, and can be recognized (see below) by its diffuse infiltration, mitotic activity, cytologic atypia of endothelial cells, and often, multilayering.

Hobnail Hemangioma

Hobnail hemangioma, also known as targetoid hemosiderotic hemangioma, is a benign lesion of adults important mainly in that it must be distinguished from KS. Microscopically, hobnail hemangioma consists of a wedge-shaped vascular proliferation of dilated, thin-walled vascular spaces lined by hyperchromatic, flat to hobnailed endothelial cells. Hemorrhage and perilesional hemosiderin deposition are often present, and may correspond to a clinically targetoid appearance. If the base of the lesion is included, vessels can be seen to dissect collagen bundles and surround dermal appendages in the deep dermis to subcutis, mimicking patch stage KS. However, immunohistochemistry for HHV-8 is uniformly negative.

Glomeruloid Hemangioma

Glomeruloid hemangioma is a rare, distinctive, acquired benign vascular proliferation which is of significance because it is believed to occur only in patients with POEMS syndrome (Crow–Fukase's syndrome) (Table 10.2).

In approximately one third of cases of POEMS syndrome, multiple cutaneous vascular lesions will be present, of which only a minority are glomeruloid hemangiomas. Clinically, glomeruloid hemangiomas appear to be small, firm, red to violaceous papules of the trunk and proximal extremities.[39] Microscopically, they are characterized by multiple tufts of proliferating, coiled capillaries expanding within ectatic, thin-walled vessels in the dermis to form structures cognate to renal glomeruli (Fig. 10.17). The current view is that these lesions are a reactive vascular proliferation,

TABLE 10.2 **POEMS Syndrome**

P	Polyneuropathy
O	Organomegaly
E	Endocrinopathy
M	Monoclonal antibody
S	Skin changes

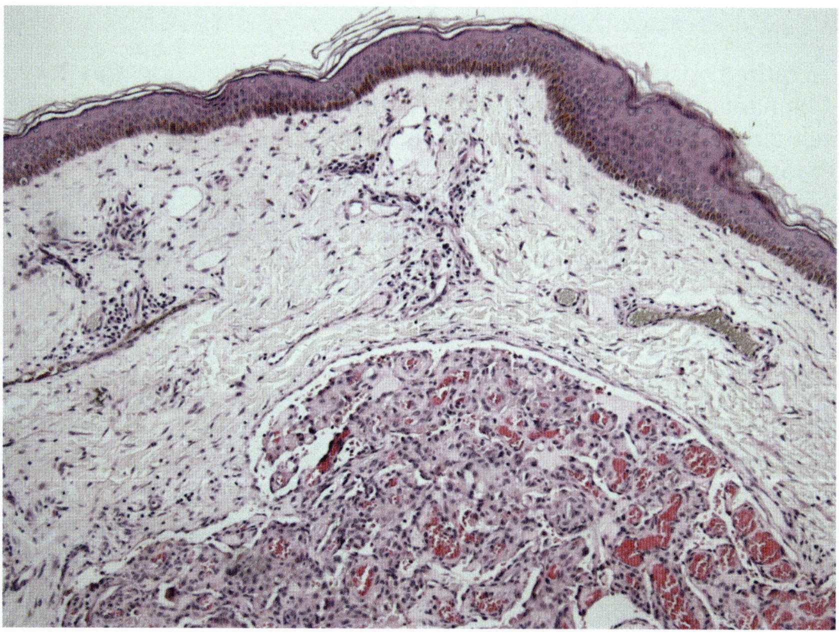

FIGURE 10.17 **Glomeruloid Hemangioma.** A proliferation of vascular spaces surrounded by a crescentic, cleftlike vascular space.

akin to reactive angioendotheliomatosis (RAE), possibly occurring in response to the circulating paraproteinemia.[40]

Microvenular Hemangioma

Microvenular hemangioma is an acquired hemangioma of adults that is significant because its poorly circumscribed appearance at low power may simulate an invasive neoplasm such as KS. Its clinical appearance is that of a solitary angioma, that may occur anywhere on the body, although the forearms are the most common site.

Microscopically, it consists of a poorly circumscribed proliferation of small, thin-walled vessels with largely collapsed lumina (Fig. 10.18). The surrounding dermis often shows some sclerosis, and in cases where the deep dermis has been sampled, tufted vascular proliferations, resembling glomeruloid hemangioma, may be seen. (It is possible that, in patients with POEMS syndrome, a spectrum may exist.) Background inflammation is usually minimal, unlike KS, and immunohistochemistry for HHV-8 is negative.

Angiolymphoid Hyperplasia with Eosinophilia

Angiolymphoid hyperplasia with eosinophilia (ALHE) is a benign, possibly reactive vascular proliferation that has been known in the past by a wide array of names: epithelioid hemangioma, cutaneous histiocytoid angioma, atypical pyogenic granuloma, intravenous atypical vascular

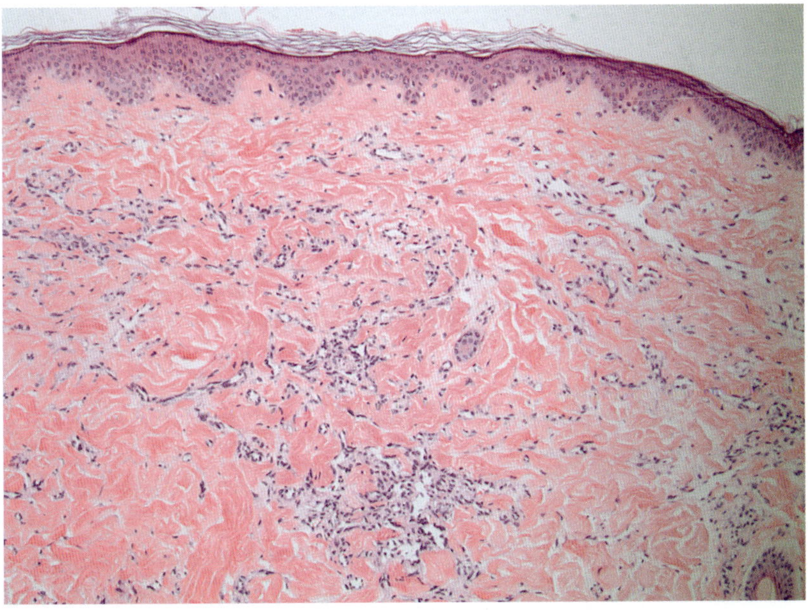

FIGURE 10.18 **Microvenular Hemangioma.** Uniform, collapsed-looking vascular spaces with plump, but not atypical, endothelial cells.

proliferation, and nodular angioblastic hyperplasia with eosinophilia and lymphofolliculosis. It characteristically occurs on the head and neck, may be quite large (up to 10 cm), and may be pulsatile. Multiple lesions may occur, being either grouped or following the lines of Blaschko. Although ALHE was once categorized with Kimura's disease, it is now considered a distinct entity as lymphadenopathy, eosinophilia, temporal arteritis, proteinuria, and elevated serum IgE are not present.[41]

Histologically, ALHE is a mixed inflammatory and vascular proliferation in the dermis and sometimes subcutis. Endothelial cells have a characteristic epithelioid appearance, with abundant eosinophilic cytoplasms, are often protuberant, and may form projections into vascular lumina with distinct vacuoles (Fig. 10.19) or even solid sheets resembling epithelioid hemangioendothelioma (EHE) (e-fig. 10.13). The inflammatory milieu, however, is characteristic, with eosinophils, multinucleated giant cells, plasma cells, mast cells, and lymphocytes which may even form follicles.[42]

Although considered benign, this entity may repeatedly recur if incompletely excised.

Spindle Cell Hemangioma

Once called "spindle cell hemangioendothelioma" and considered to be an entity of uncertain malignant potential, spindle cell hemangioma is now believed to be benign. Its importance flows mainly from the fact that it may be mistaken for KS. It may also form a part of Maffucci's syndrome

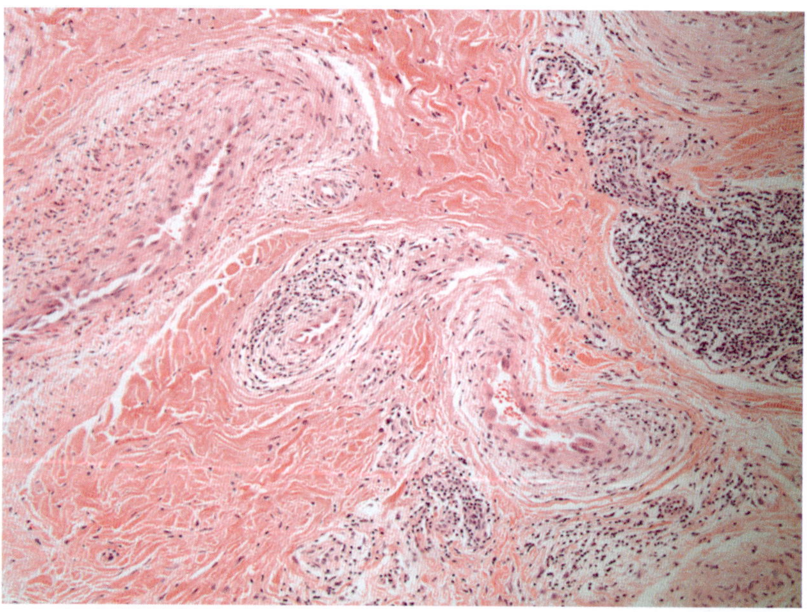

FIGURE 10.19 **ALHE.** The epithelioid change in the endothelial cells is striking. Note the lymphoid follicle at right.

(in association with multiple enchondromas) or Klippel–Trenaunay's syndrome. It presents as a purplish nodule ranging in size from a few millimeters up to 10 cm or more. Microscopically, it may occur either in the dermis or deeper soft tissues. It is circumscribed but unencapsulated, and consists of zones of cavernous endothelial-lined spaces, interwoven with solid areas consisting of short fascicles of spindle cells interspersed with slitlike vascular spaces (Fig. 10.20). In some cases, the lesion appears to be at least partly intravascular. Despite occasional intracytoplasmic lumina, the spindle cells are unexpectedly negative for vascular markers CD31 and CD34, as well as HHV-8.

Although now considered benign, spindle cell hemangioma may exhibit multiple recurrences, apparently related to its histologic extension into pre-existing vessels.

(Acquired) Tufted Angioma

Tufted angioma is a rare, acquired, benign lesion of children and young adults occurring mainly on the upper chest, neck, and back that is important because, despite its benign status and indolent growth, it may grow to cover large areas of the body.

Microscopically, the lesions consist of multiple lobules within the dermis and subcutis. Some lobules bulge the walls of thin-walled vessels at their periphery, imparting a distinctive semilunar appearance. The lobules themselves consist of solid whorls of pericytic cells

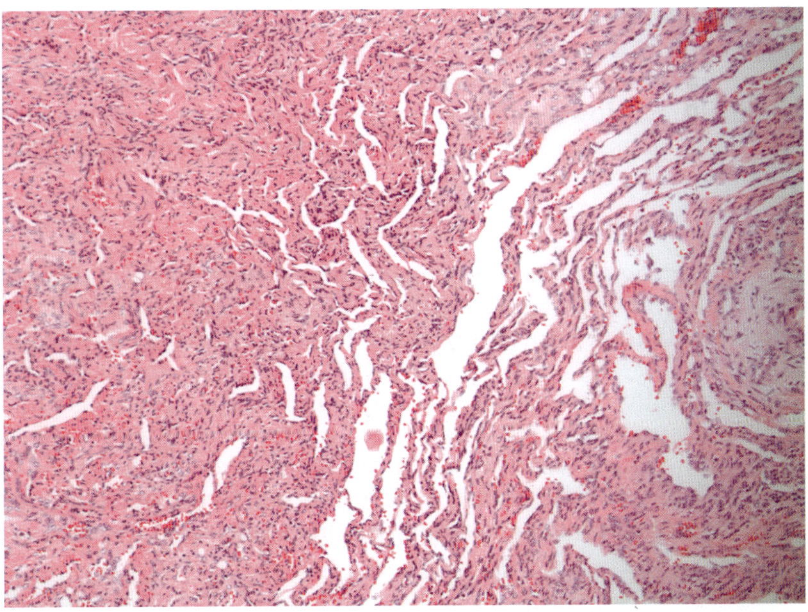

FIGURE 10.20 **Spindle Cell Hemangioma.** A mixture of cavernous spaces, slitlike vascular spaces resembling Kaposi sarcoma, and more cellular areas with inconspicuous vascular channels.

arranged around identifiable, apparently pre-existing vessels. The tumor stains positively with vascular markers CD31 and CD34; the pericytic cells may be identified with immunohistochemistry for smooth muscle actin (SMA).[43]

Bacillary Angiomatosis

Although quite rare today, bacillary angiomatosis remains important because it may histologically simulate pyogenic granuloma and because it is a treatable condition that is closely associated with HIV disease. Microscopically, the lesion closely resembles pyogenic granuloma, showing a lobular proliferation of small vessels with variable reactive changes in the overlying epidermis. Careful examination, however, reveals multiple aggregates of amorphous, slightly basophilic material. A Warthin–Starry or Giemsa stain will stain the causative coccobacillary organisms, which are usually either *Bartonella henselae* or *B. quintana*.

Reactive Angioendotheliomatosis

RAE is an uncommon reactive condition associated with a wide variety of chronic systemic illnesses, including sarcoidosis, cardiac valvular disease, rheumatoid arthritis, alcoholic cirrhosis, polymyalgia rheumatica, antiphospholipid syndrome, cryoglobulinemia, and renal disease. In many cases, the patients are immunosuppressed as a result of solid organ transplantation.[44]

Histologically, there are clusters of tightly packed capillaries extending from the dermis to the superficial subcutis, some of which appear to proliferate within existing vessels. Endothelia often appear reactive, and there is often extravasation of erythrocytes, suggesting a degree of vascular incompetence. However, a distinct layer of pericytes is always present. Irregular vascular spaces, as in KS, are not present, and the lesion lacks the solid, cellular areas of tufted angioma.

Verrucous Hemangioma

Verrucous hemangioma is a rare, clinically distinctive hemangioma of neonates and young children, which is clinically verrucous and, unlike hemangioma of infancy, rarely regresses. It is large and typically occurs on the leg.

Histologically, it is characteristically composed of cavernously dilated, thin-walled vessels in the superficial dermis, showing a gradual transition to smaller, thin-walled vessels extending deep into the subcutis (Fig. 10.21). The superficial vessels are usually closely apposed to the overlying epidermis in an angiokeratomalike fashion, with acanthosis and hyperkeratosis.

Pyogenic Granuloma

Pyogenic granulomata (PG) are clinically distinctive, exophytic, rapidly growing lesions which are apparently reactive, and often arise at sites of recent trauma or in response to pregnancy, endocrine alterations, or

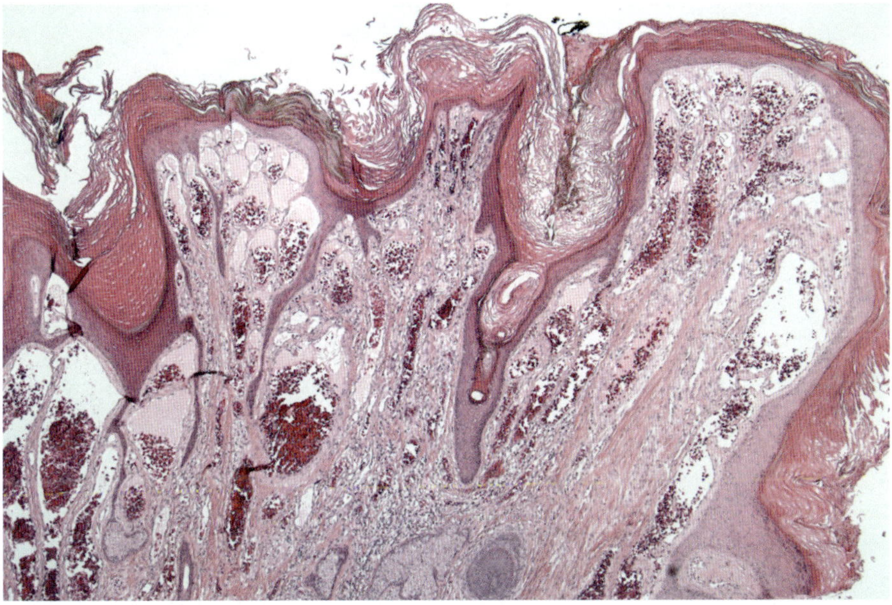

FIGURE 10.21 **Verruciform Hemangioma.** The superficial component resembles an angiokeratoma, but the vascular component extends deeply into the subcutis.

medications. These lesions may occur anywhere, but are typically seen on the fingers, face, and oral or nasal mucosa of children and young adults.

Histologically, they show a variety of features depending on lesional age. Initially, they are indistinguishable from granulation tissue (by definition, since they arise at sites of superficial trauma). As it progresses, a PG becomes increasingly polypoid, and the vascular proliferation becomes gradually more organized as proliferating capillaries arranged in lobules. Mitoses are often present, and the surrounding stroma is typically inflamed; however, the vascular proliferation is typically circumscribed and confined to the superficial dermis. In such typical, fully formed lesions, the overlying epidermis is eroded (Fig. 10.22), although with time this re-epithelializes, leaving a lesion histologically indistinguishable from a mature hemangioma. At this stage, the lesions are often referred to as "lobular capillary hemangiomas."

Although completely benign, PGs frequently recur when treated with electrodessication and curettage.

Cavernous Malformation

Also known as "cavernous hemangioma," these lesions are now thought of as malformations rather than true neoplasms. They may be associated with Maffucci's syndrome, and are characteristic of the blue rubber bleb nevus syndrome. Histologically, they are characterized by gaping, venous, endothelial-lined spaces in a fibrous stroma, reminiscent of the corpus cavernosum. Smooth muscle is often present, and, as vascular malformations, heterogeneity rather than homogeneity (as in hemangiomas) is their true

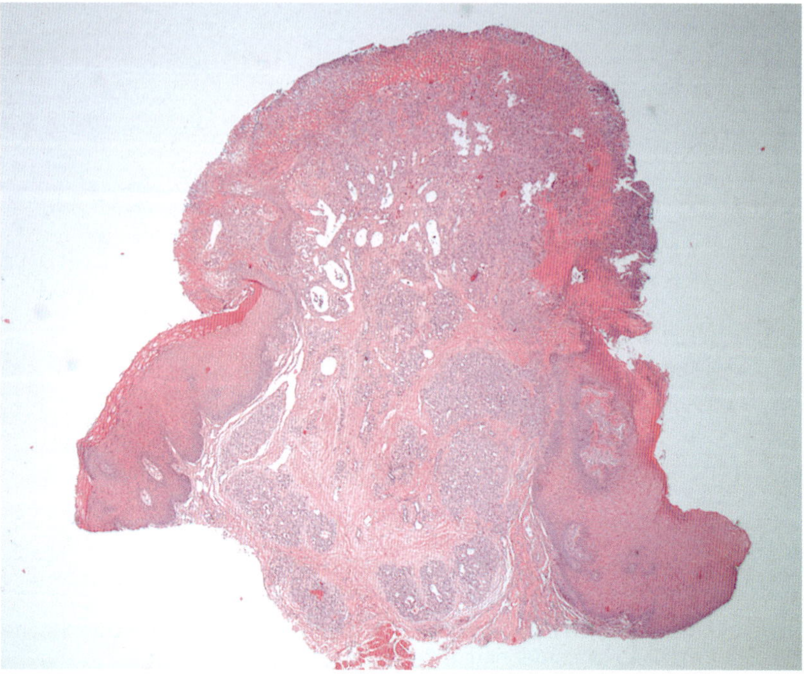

FIGURE 10.22 **Pyogenic Granuloma.** A polypoid example with a lobular proliferation of capillary spaces and ulceration of the overlying epidermis.

hallmark (Fig. 10.23). As such, in addition to the classic cavernous spaces described above, many examples will have capillary, arterial, or apparent lymphatic spaces. Examples which are devoid of blood, and are filled entirely with lymph, are referred to as cavernous lymphatic malformations. Glomangiomas (see below) may be architecturally indistinguishable from cavernous malformations, but have polygonal, SMA-positive glomus cells in their walls.

Angiokeratomas

Angiokeratomas are benign vascular proliferations of the superficial dermis that induce epidermal changes and, when multiple, may be associated with Fabry's disease (angiokeratoma corporis diffusum) (Table 10.3).

Histologically, the lesion shows ectatic, thin-walled vascular spaces in the superficial dermis that are so closely apposed to the dermoepidermal junction that some appear to be present within the epidermis; indeed, in many cases, hemorrhage is present even into the stratum corneum (e-fig 10.14). There is associated acanthosis and hyperkeratosis. In Fabry's disease, there may be subtle vacuolization of the endothelium and vascular and arrector pili smooth muscle; these vacuoles may be highlighted with a PAS stain or lipid stain, and correspond to the characteristic ultrastructural finding: electron-dense lamellar inclusion bodies.

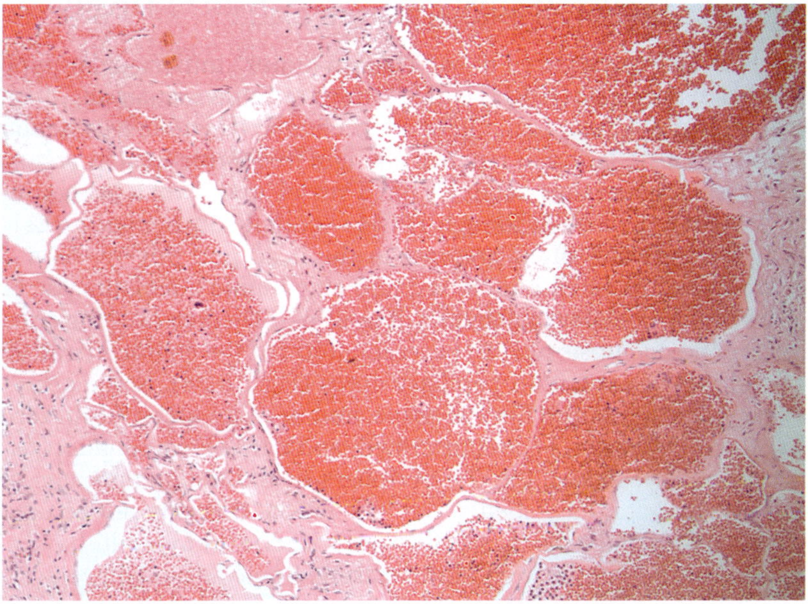

FIGURE 10.23 Cavernous Malformation. Widely dilated vascular spaces, filled with blood, with a flattened endothelial lining.

TABLE 10.3 Clinical Types of Angiokeratoma

Type	Description
Mibelli type	Lesions on dorsal fingers and toes
Fordyce type	Lesions on scrotum or vulva
Angiokeratoma corporis diffusum	Lesions covering the entire body, associated with Fabry's disease, β-galactosidase deficiency, or fucosidosis
Angiokeratoma circumscriptum	Multiple lesions in groups or bands on an extremity
Solitary angiokeratoma	Solitary lesion occurring anywhere on the body

(Acral) Arteriovenous Hemangioma

Formerly known as cirsoid aneurysm, and variously thought of as a hamartoma, a proliferation originating in the Sucquet–Hoyer canal, or a simple sporadic hemangioma, arteriovenous hemangioma is similar to other hemangiomas in that it is a well-circumscribed proliferation of mature blood vessels. It is distinctive only in that it is composed of thick-walled arterial and venous structures (e-fig. 10.15) and tends to occur on the face.

Intravascular Papillary Endothelial Hyperplasia

Although sometimes referred to as "Masson tumor," intravascular papillary endothelial hyperplasia (IPEH) is also known as intravascular angiomatosis or vegetant intravascular hemangioendothelioma. It is not a true neoplasm, but simply a constellation of reactive changes frequently seen in organizing thrombi which, when they occur within a vessel, may form a mass and may mimic angiosarcoma, even though IPEH is completely benign. IPEH may occur at any age, and often presents in the head and fingers. As a deep, dermal nodule, it is often blue to red and may mimic a melanocytic lesion if solitary and a vascular malignancy if multiple. The key histologic feature for making the diagnosis of IPEH is recognition of the characteristic glassy, eosinophilic material within papillary cores (Fig. 10.24). Some areas may show transition to mature fibrous tissue, and in other areas, fibrin thrombi may be seen. The lesion is circumscribed, and careful examination usually discloses a thin vessel wall at the periphery of the lesion, although, if the submitting physician has "shelled out" the lesion, this may not be present.

The endothelial cells themselves are variable, but should have a low mitotic rate and do not exhibit multilayering. Some authors have accepted severe cytologic atypia in lesions of IPEH,[45] but such cases are quite rare. In any event, the presence of severe cytologic atypia should prompt careful consideration of the possibility of angiosarcoma.[46]

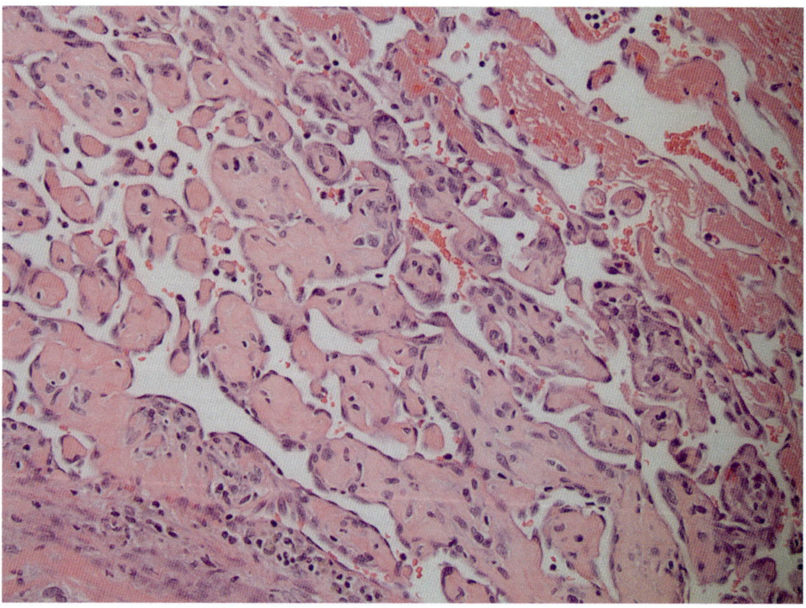

FIGURE 10.24 **Intravascular Papillary Endothelial Hyperplasia.** Papillary fronds with hyalinized cores, a fibrin thrombus, and hemosiderin deposition can all be seen in this example.

Glomus Tumor

The term "glomus tumor" includes at least two distinct benign entities, both of which are characterized by the presence of glomus cells: polygonal, epithelioid cells with round, regular, centrally located nuclei with a moderate amount of pale eosinophilic cytoplasm. They often have a well-defined cell membrane which may be highlighted by PAS or toluidine blue stains. Glomus cells are normally present in the Sucquet–Hoyer canal (arteriovenous anastomosis). While glomus tumors may appear epithelioid, their immunohistochemical profile suggests kinship to pericytes: actins, calponin, and h-caldesmon are typically positive; desmin is variable; and vascular markers CD34 and CD31 are occasionally positive with a higher frequency of positivity for factor XIIIa. Keratins are negative. Two main categories of glomus tumor exist: the solid type (or glomus tumor proper) and glomangioma. Solid type glomus tumors are generally painful or tender dermal nodules occurring on the fingers and toes of adults. They are often subungual. Glomangiomas are also typically solitary, although multiple lesions may occur. They clinically resemble hemangiomas and may occur anywhere on the trunk or extremities. They are usually not tender. Histologically, glomangiomas resemble cavernous malformations (see above) with variably dilated vessels; however, unlike a cavernous malformation, a glomangioma has a variably thick layer of glomus cells in its walls (Fig. 10.25, e-fig. 10.16). Solid type

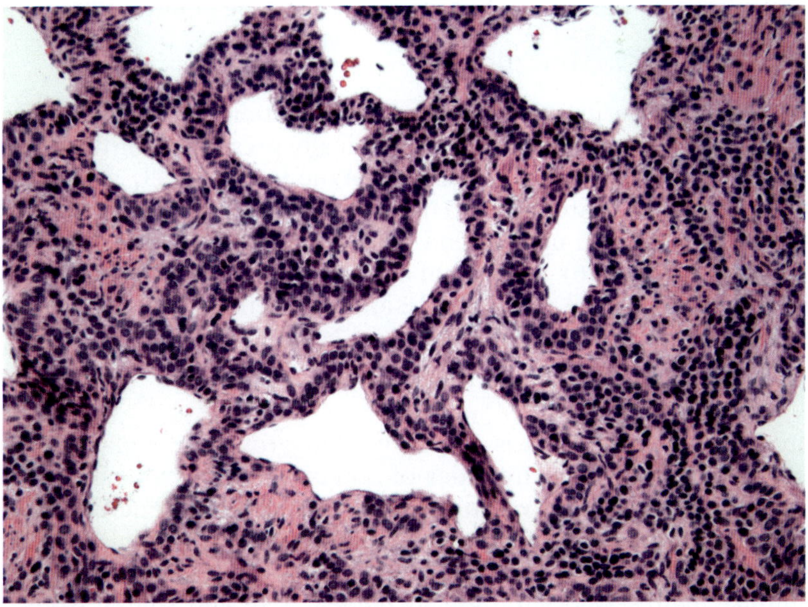

FIGURE 10.25 **Glomangioma.** A proliferation of banal glomus cells interrupted by numerous cavernous vascular spaces.

TABLE 10.4 Criteria for Malignancy in Glomus Tumor
1. Size >2 cm and subfascial or visceral location;
2. Atypical mitotic figures; or
3. Marked nuclear atypia together with any level of mitotic activity

glomus tumors, by contrast, consist of nests of glomus cells surrounding capillary-sized vessels and set in a variably hyalin to myxoid stroma (e-fig. 10.17). Glomus cells typically extend along vessel walls beyond the main tumor mass.

In cases where the glomus tumors show a transition to smooth muscle cells, the term "glomangiomyoma" may be used; similarly, a glomus tumor with prominent staghorn vessels is sometimes referred to as a "glomangiopericytoma."

MALIGNANT GLOMUS TUMORS OR GLOMANGIOSARCOMAS

Malignant glomus tumors (glomangiosarcomas) exist, but are rare. The WHO has recently elaborated the following criteria for malignancy (Table 10.4).[47]

Tumors with marked nuclear atypia, but devoid of mitotic activity, are considered benign and are known as symplastic glomus tumors.

Lymphangioma Circumscriptum

Lymphangioma circumscriptum is a proliferation of lymphatic vessels occurring in the superficial dermis. It typically presents at birth or in early childhood, and most frequently occurs on the tongue, neck, axillae, shoulders, and proximal extremities. Histologically it consists of dilated lymphatic channels which may extend from the superficial dermis deep into the subcutis (Fig. 10.26). Epidermal hyperplasia, analogous to that seen in angiokeratoma, may be seen. The lesions are benign, although, owing to their deep extension, they not uncommonly recur.

Progressive Lymphangioma

Progressive lymphangioma is a benign, slow-growing neoplasm typically occurring on the lower extremities of adults. Histologically, it consists of thin-walled, often dilated vascular spaces which tend to decrease in size as they extend deeper. The nuclei are often hyperchromatic but lack the characteristic features of angiosarcoma, namely, multilayering of endothelia, mitotic figures, and variation in nuclear size and shape. Excision is usually curative.

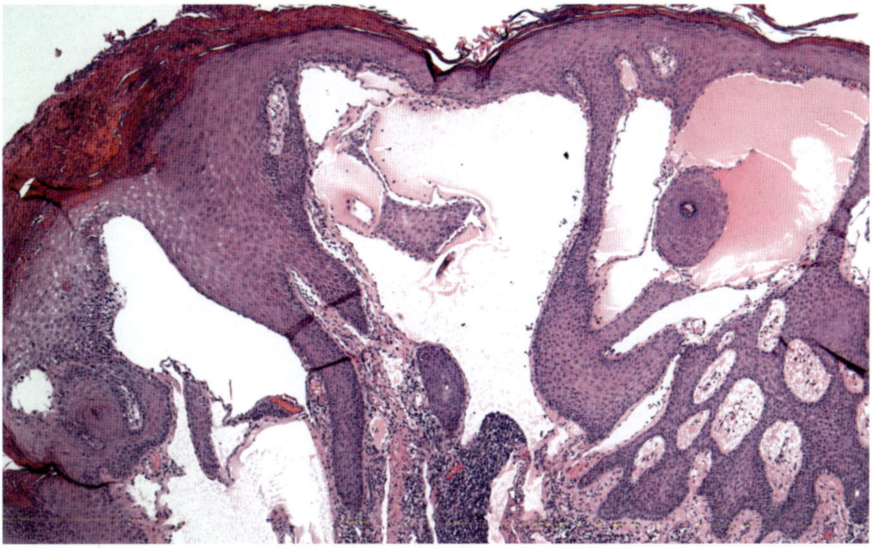

FIGURE 10.26 **Lymphangioma Circumscriptum.** Lymph-filled vascular spaces in the superficial dermis with overlying verrucous change in the epidermis, cognate to angiokeratoma.

VASCULAR TUMORS OF INTERMEDIATE MALIGNANT POTENTIAL

Epithelioid Hemangioendothelioma

EHE is a rare endothelial tumor with metastatic potential that typically occurs in viscera or deep soft tissue but which may rarely present in the skin, especially in the extremities. Histologically, it consists of nests and cords of plump, epithelioid to spindled cells in a fibromyxoid stroma. These rarely form well-defined vascular channels, but often contain endocytoplasmic vacuoles. Vascular markers are typically positive although keratins may also be positive, raising the differential diagnosis of epithelioid angiosarcoma, however, epithelioid angiosarcoma usually has necrosis and a greater degree of cytologic atypia.

Papillary Intralymphatic Angioendothelioma

Also known as Dabska tumor, papillary intralymphatic angioendothelioma (PILA) is a very rare tumor of infants and children that usually presents as a slow-growing plaque or nodule on the extremities. Microscopically, the tumor is composed of thin-walled, dilated vascular spaces from which blood is often absent. Endothelial cells are often hobnailed and hyperchromatic, but the diagnosis requires prominent intraluminal tufts studded by endothelial cells, and with hyalinized cores. Mitotic figures are rare, and cytologic atypia is not striking. The differential diagnosis is generally with hobnail hemangioma, and the correct diagnosis depends on recognition

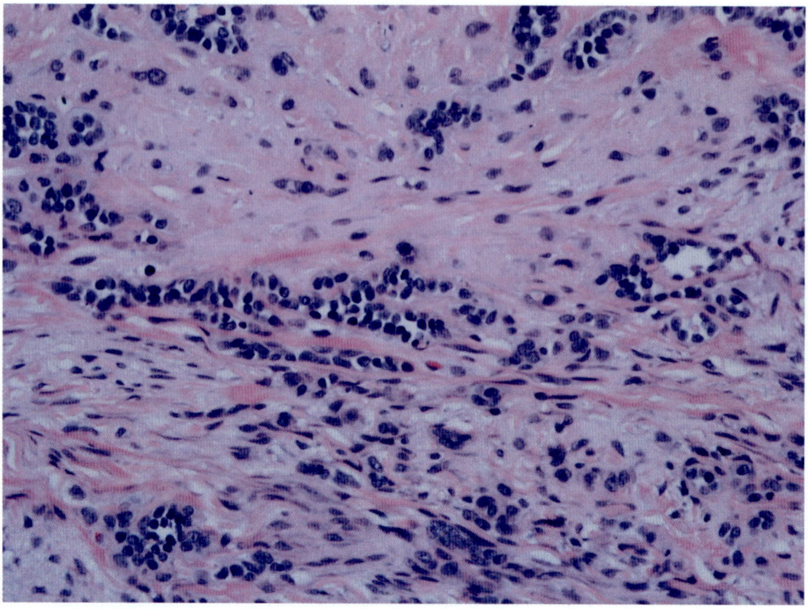

FIGURE 10.27 **Retiform Hemangioendothelioma.** Vascular channels lined by uniform hobnail endothelial cells, architecturally resembling the rete testis. Lymphocytic inflammation may be prominent; however, if intraluminal papillary structures are seen, intravascular papillary endothelial hyperplasia (Dabska tumor) should be considered.

of the papillary intravascular fronds. Occasionally, the distinction from retiform hemangioendothelioma (Fig. 10.27) cannot be reliably made. Although the metastatic potential of the tumor is now disputed, the original series[48] considered the tumor malignant; for this reason, wide local excision remains the treatment of choice.

KAPOSI SARCOMA

KS is a tumor frequently associated with HHV-8 infection of endothelial cells which tends to occur either in elderly males, typically of Mediterranean, eastern European, or Saudi descent (classic KS) or in immunocompromised patients, mostly either advanced HIV disease (HIV-associated KS) patients or solid organ transplant recipients (iatrogenic KS). An endemic form is found in equatorial Africa but will not be discussed further here. Although traditionally referred to as a sarcoma, KS is rarely lethal in an immunocompetent host; however, spread to lymph nodes, gastrointestinal tract, and lungs may occur.

Classic KS typically presents as multiple nodules on the extremities which may be reddish-blue, purplish, or brown. HIV-associated KS, by contrast, often involves the face, oral mucosa, or genitals as well as the lower extremities.

Regardless of clinical context, the histologic appearance of KS progresses through a series of appearances corresponding to the clinical presence of patches, plaques, or nodules. Patch-stage KS may be extremely subtle, resembling a hemangioma; however, in its recognizable form, it consists of irregular, thin-walled vascular channels dissecting collagen fibers in the upper reticular dermis, often surrounding pre-existing vessels and adnexae, sometimes leading to the so-called promontory sign, a pre-existing vessel protruding into the lumen of a neoplastic vascular space. The surrounding stroma often has lymphocytes, plasma cells, extravasated erythrocytes, and hemosiderin deposition. Plaque-stage KS is made up of similar components, but is much more obvious histologically. Hyalin globules are also often found, and areas of spindle cells may occur. Nodules of KS are composed of fascicles of mitotically active uniform atypical spindled endothelial cells which are often vertically oriented (Fig. 10.28). Between these are apparently vascular, slitlike spaces, in which red blood cells can be found. Hyalin globules are more common, both within the cytoplasm of the spindled cells and in the extracellular space, and, toward the edges of the lesion, the characteristic irregular vascular spaces of plaque-stage KS can be found.

HHV-8 is now generally accepted as the etiologic agent in all stages of KS. Immunohistochemistry for HHV-8 is positive in the majority of cases; roughly 20% of KS cases do not express HHV-8, however, and the diagnosis should not be dismissed in its absence.[49–51]

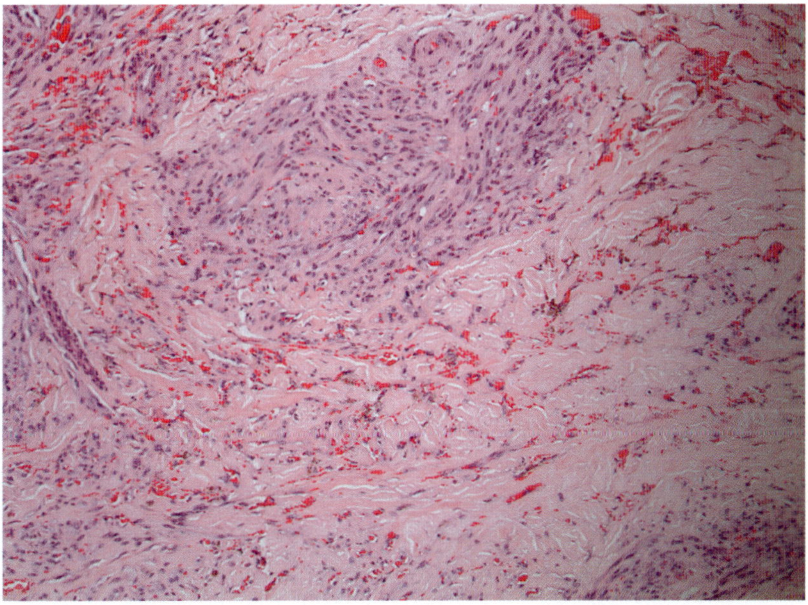

FIGURE 10.28 **Nodular Stage Kaposi Sarcoma.** In nodular stage, characteristic cellular areas coexist with areas more typical of patch stage KS.

MALIGNANT VASCULAR LESIONS

Angiosarcoma

Angiosarcoma (or lymphangiosarcoma) is a malignancy of endothelial cells. It characteristically occurs in the head and neck of elderly patients, especially men, but may also occur at a site of radiation exposure or in a setting of chronic lymphedema. Stuart–Treves's syndrome, or angiosarcoma occurring in a lymphedematous arm following ipsilateral mastectomy with axillary dissection, is nowadays rare. In any of these settings, angiosarcoma usually presents as a poorly defined erythematous to bluish plaque, resembling a bruise but with no tendency to regress.

Microscopically, the lesions consist of small, jagged, thin-walled vessels that infiltrate between collagen bundles in the reticular dermis (Fig. 10.29). Endothelial cells are often atypical, mitotically active, and show crowding or multilayering; papillary projections may also occur. These well-differentiated lesions are generally poorly marginated, and margin status may be unclear even in large resection specimens. More poorly-differentiated examples also occur which may stain with only one of a panel of endothelial markers; an epithelioid variant also exists which may stain positively with some keratins. In these situations, the histologic differential diagnosis will often be with pleomorphic sarcoma (so-called malignant fibrous histiocytoma) or poorly differentiated carcinoma, respectively. Without immunohistochemical

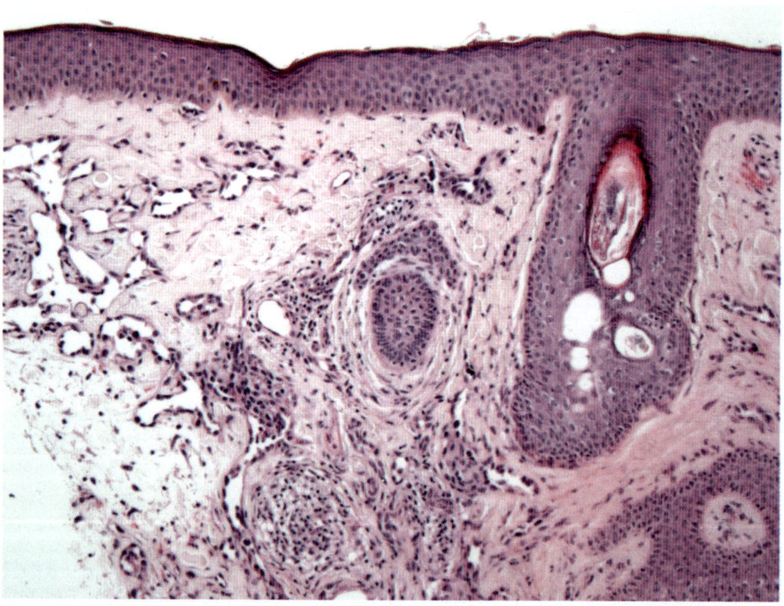

FIGURE 10.29 **Angiosarcoma.** Jagged vascular spaces lined by atypical endothelial cells dissect dermal collagen bundles. In well-differentiated examples such as this, distinction from KS may be difficult.

or ultrastructural evidence of endothelial differentiation, a diagnosis of angiosarcoma may, indeed, be impossible to make.

Regardless of the degree of histologic differentiation, the prognosis is poor with frequent distant metastasis.

REFERENCES

1. LeBoit PE, Burg G, Weedon D, et al. eds. *World Health Organization Classification of Tumors Pathology and Genetics, Skin Tumors*. Lyon, France: IARCPRESS, 2006.
2. Fletcher CD, Unni KK, Mertens F, eds. *World Health Organization Classification of Tumors, Pathology and Genetics, Tumors of Soft Tissue and Bone*. Lyon, France: IARCPRESS, 2002.
3. Weiss SW, Goldblum JR. *Enzinger and Weiss' Soft Tissue Tumors with CD ROM*. 5th Ed. Philadelphia, PA: Mosby, 2008.
4. LeBoit PE, Burg G, Weedon D, Sarasin A, eds. *World Health Organization Classification of Tumors Pathology and Genetics, Skin Tumors*. Lyon, France: IARCPRESS, 2006:262.
5. Fretzin DF, Helwig EB. Atypical fibroxanthoma of the skin: A clinical pathologic study of 140 cases. *Cancer* 1973;31:1541–1552.
6. Dahl I. Atypical fibroxanthoma of the skin: A clinical pathologic study of 57 cases. *Acta path Microbiol Scand Sect A* 1976,84:183–197.
7. Kuwano H, Hashimoto H, Enjoji M. Atypical fibroxanthoma distinguishable from spindle cell carcinoma in sarcoma-like skin lesions. *Cancer* 1985;55:172–180.
8. Beham A, Badve S, Suster S, Fletcher CDM. Solitary fibroma in adults: Clinicopathological analysis of a series. *Histopathology* 1993;22:335–341.
9. Hollowood K, Holley MP, Fletcher CD. Plexiform fibrohistiocytic tumor: Clinical pathological, immunohistochemical and ultrastructural analysis in favor of a myofibroblastic lesion. *Histopathology* 1992;19:503–513.
10. Mentzel T, Calonje E, Wadden C, Fletcher CD. Myxofibrosarcoma: Clinical pathologic analysis of seventy-five cases with emphasis on the low grade variant. *Am J Surg Pathol* 1996;20:391–405.
11. Chase DR, Enzinger FM. Epithelioid sarcoma: Diagnosis, prognostic indicators, and treatment. *Am J Surg Pathol* 1985;9:241–263.
12. Enzinger FM, Harvey DA. Spindle cell lipoma. *Cancer* 1975;36:1852–1859.
13. Fletcher CDM, Martin-Bates E. Spindle cell lipoma: A clinical pathologic study with some original observations. *Histopathology* 1987;11:803–817.
14. Furlong MA, Fanburg-Smith JC, Miettinen M. The morphologic spectrum of hibernoma: A clinical pathologic study of 70 cases. *Am J Surg Pathol* 2001;25(6):809–814.
15. Binh MBN, Sastre-Garau X, Guillou L, et al. MDM2 and CDK4 immunostainings are useful adjuncts in diagnosing well-differentiated and dedifferentiated liposarcoma subtypes: A comparative analysis of 559 soft tissue neoplasms with genetic data. *Am J Surg Pathol* 2005;29:1340–1347.
16. Enzinger FM, Winslow DJ. Liposarcoma. A study of 103 cases. *Virchows Arch A* 1962; 335:367–388.
17. Evans HL. Liposarcomas and atypical lipomatous tumors: A study of 66 cases followed for a minimum of 10 years. *Surg Pathol* 1988;1:41–54.
18. Jensen ML, Jensen OM, Michalski W, et al. Intradermal and subcutaneous leiomyosarcoma: A clinical pathologic and immunohistochemical study of 41 cases. *J Cutan Pathol* 1996;23:458–463.
19. Kapadia SB, Meis JM, Frisman DM, et al. Adult rhabdomyoma of the head and neck: A clinical pathologic and immunophenotypic study. *Human Pathol* 1993;28:608–617.

20. Kapadia SB, Meis JM, Frisman DM, et al. Fetal rhabdomyoma of the head and neck: A clinical pathologic and immunophenotypic study of 24 cases. *Human Pathol* 1993;24:754–765.
21. Chung EB, Enzinger FM. Chondroma of soft parts. *Cancer* 1978;41:1414–1424.
22. Humphrey S, Pambakian H, McKee PH, Kindblom LG. Soft tissue chondroma: A study of 15 tumours. *Histopathology* 1986;10:147–159.
23. Meis-Kindblom JM, Bergh P, Gunterberg B, Kindblom LG. Extraskeletal myxoid chondrosarcoma: a reappraisal of its morphologic spectrum and prognostic factors based on 117 cases. *Am J Surg Pathol* 1999;23:636–650.
24. Saleh G, Evans HL, Ro JY, Ayala AG. Extraskeletal myxoid chondrosarcoma. *Cancer.* 1992;70:2827–2830.
25. Barnhill RA, Crowson AN, eds. *Textbook of Dermatopathology*. 2nd Ed. New York, NY: McGraw-Hill, 2004:893–914.
26. Argenyi ZB. Immunohistochemical characterization of palisading, encapsulated euroma. *J Cut Pathol* 1989;16:293.
27. Kossard S, Kumar A, Wilkinson B. Neural spectrum: palisaded encapsulated neuroma and verocay body poor dermal schwannoma. *J Cut Pathol* 1999;26:31–36.
28. Van Paesschen MA, Goovaerts G, Buyssens N. A study of the so-called neurotization of nevi. *Am J Dermatopathol* 1990;12:242–248.
29. McKee PH, Calonje E, Granter S. *Pathology of the Skin*. 3rd ed. Philadelphia, PA: Mosby, 2005:1586–1788.
30. Laskin WB, Fetsch JF, Miettinen M. The “neurothekeoma”: immunohistochemical analysis distinguishes the true nerve sheath myxoma from its mimics. *Human Pathol* 2000;31:1230–1241.
31. Barnhill RL, Mihm MC. Cellular neurothekeoma: a distinctive variant of neurothekeoma mimicking nevomelanocytic tumors. *Am J Surg Pathol* 1990;14:113–120.
32. Neville BW, Damm DD, Allen CM, Bouquot JE. *Oral and Maxillofacial Pathology*. 3rd Ed. Philadelphia, PA: W.B. Saunders; 2002:465–466.
33. Lopez DA, Silver DN, Helwig EB. Cutaneous meningiomas: A clinical pathologic study. *Cancer* 1974;34:728–744.
34. Theaker JM, Fletcher CDM. Heterotopic glial nodules: A light microscopy and immunohistochemical study. *Histopathology* 1991;8:255–260.
35. Spitz JL, Ed. *Genodermatoses: A Full Color Guide to Genetic Skin Disorders*. 2nd Ed. Philadelphia, PA: Lippincott, Williams & Wilkins, 2005.
36. Bean WB. Notes on the natural history of vascular spiders in healthy persons. *Arch Intern Med* 1960;106:35–38.
37. Stephenson J, Lincoln C. Angioma serpiginosum. *Arch Dermatol* 1967;95:16–22.
38. Holmdahl K. Cutaneous hemangiomas in premature infants. *Acta Paediatr Scand* 1955;44:370–379.
39. Odom, RB. *Andrews' Diseases of the Skin: Clinical Dermatology*. 9th Ed. Philadelphia, PA: WB Saunders, 2000:752.
40. LeBoit PE, Burg G, Weedon D, Sarasin A, eds. *World Health Organization Classification of Tumors Pathology and Genetics, Skin Tumors*. Lyon, France: IARCPRESS, 2006: 235–237.
41. Kuo T-T, Shih L, Chan H-L. Kimura's disease. Involvement of regional lymph nodes and distinction from angiolymphoid hyperplasia with eosinophilia. *Am J Surg Pathol* 1988;12:843–854.
42. Zeitouni NC, Hanna S, Loree TR, et al. Angiolymphoid hyperplasia with eosinophilia: A classic clinical presentation with histologic features of angiosarcoma. *Dermatol Surg* 2002;28:772–775.
43. Hunt SJ, Santa Cruz DJ, Barnhill R. In: Barnhill, RL, Crowson AN, eds. *Textbook of Dermatopathology*. 2nd Ed. New York, NY: McGraw-Hill, 2004:833.

44. McMenamin ME, Fletcher CDM. Reactive angioendotheliomatosis: a study of fifteen cases demonstrating a wide clinicopathologic spectrum. *Am J Surg Pathol* 2002;26:685–697.
45. Renshaw A, Rosai J. Benign atypical vascular lesions of the lip. A study of twelve cases. *Am J Surg Pathol* 1993;17:557–565.
46. Kuo T, Sayers C, Rosai J. Masson's "vegetant intravascular hemangioendothelioma:" A lesion often mistaken for angiosarcoma: Study of seventeen cases located in the skin and soft tissues. *Cancer* 1976;38:1227–1236.
47. Fletcher CD, Krishnan Unni K, Mertens F, eds. *World Health Organization Classification of Tumors, Pathology and Genetics, Tumors of Soft Tissue and Bone*. Lyon, France: IARCPRESS, 2002:136–137.
48. Dabska M. Malignant endovascular papillary angioendothelioma of the skin in childhood. Clinical pathologic study of six cases. *Cancer* 1969;24:503–510.
49. Chang Y, Cesarman E, Pessin MS, et al. Identification of herpes virus-like DNA sequences in AIDS-associated Kaposi sarcoma. *Science* 1994;266:1865–1869.
50. Patel RM, Goldblum JR, Hsi ED. Immunohistochemical detection of human herpes virus-8 latent nuclear antigen-1 is useful in the diagnosis of Kaposi sarcoma. *Mod Pathol* 2004;17:456–460.
51. Antman K, Chang Y. Kaposi's sarcoma. *New Eng J Med* 2000;342:1027–1038.

11

MEDICOLEGAL ASPECTS OF NEOPLASTIC DERMATOLOGY

INTRODUCTION

Medical malpractice litigation is rising at an explosive rate in the United States and, to a lesser extent, in Canada. The impact of medical malpractice litigation on health care costs and the cost of insurance is dramatic. Certain specialist categories are becoming uninsurable in some parts of the United States, while in others, clinicians are retiring early, restricting or changing practice, or changing states of residence in consequence of medical malpractice claims and of the cost and availability of insurance. This, in turn, has had the real effect of denying care to patients in some communities in the United States. Dermatology and dermatopathology are impacted by this trend. In particular, the misdiagnosis of melanoma is alleged to account for 13% of all malpractice claims in the period from 1995 to 2001.[2] One study suggested that melanoma was the second most common cause of malpractice litigation in the United States.[3] A survey of 1,807 physicians in 1999 showed that 58% had experienced a medical malpractice claim at some point in their careers.[4] Although historically pathologists have been at a much lower risk of malpractice litigation than other specialists, lawsuits against pathologists are increasing geometrically as the public becomes more informed about the role of the pathologist in medical care.[5] Dermatology, by contrast, has a much higher profile and a greater risk of litigation, as the patient is far more familiar with his clinician than with the pathologist who was formerly deemed to be in the background of patient care. Those clinicians who practice cosmetic dermatology are at even greater risk. However, the greatest malpractice awards in dermatology have been melanoma claims.[6] The attendant morbidity and mortality which flow from the mistaken underdiagnosis or nonrecognition of melanoma is the explanation for the latter; the two main causes for melanoma malpractice awards are delay in diagnosis and mistaken diagnosis, which most typically represents an error by the histopathologist.[7]

Certain steps can be taken by pathology laboratories to reduce, but never completely eliminate, the risk of medical malpractice claims. In this review, attention is paid to the source of medical malpractice claims and an abbreviated approach to specific strategies for risk management is presented.

Malpractice, Negligence, and the Burden of Proof

The four standards which must be justified to establish the validity of a medical malpractice claim are *duty, breach* (i.e., negligence), *proximal cause* (i.e., causation of injury), and *damage*.[1,5,8,9] The concept of duty relates to the responsibility of a physician to a patient and flows from the relationship between the patient and his or her physician. A pathologist who picks up a slide for interpretation and then issues a report at once establishes the relationship between himself and the patient. The duty incumbent upon the pathologist is the accurate, specific, and timely reportage of a biopsy or resection specimen. Errors in interpretation or delays in reporting can be directly attributable to the pathologist. They may also flow from other events only indirectly under the control of the pathologist, such as typographical errors in the stenographic pool, specimen labeling errors, or substandard or erroneous technical performance at any step in the preparation of the tissue for histological interpretation. The responsibility for the erroneous actions of one or more of his employees who are directly under the control of the pathologist may constitute *vicarious liability*.[9] In the event that the pathologist recognizes that poor technical quality may impact his interpretation in a given case and fails to correct the technical deficiency, he may be considered to have exercised *negligent supervision*. The demonstration of negligence, also termed *breach*, is the failure to execute the accepted standard of care. Unfortunately, the definitions of breach and of what constitutes an accepted standard of care are so open to interpretation, particularly in jury trials in the United States, that the standard may be in constant flux and thus unobtainable. Formerly, breach was defined as a failure to treat within the standard of care[1] and did not necessarily imply error. Rather, the onus was on the practicing physician to exert a standard of care similar to that which a reasonable, qualified physician in his area would, at that time, have exercised. This local standard is apposite in some states, such as Tennessee. In other jurisdictions, a national standard of care is applied. Expert testimony is typically utilized to define the standard of care in any given malpractice case[8,10]; therefore, the opinions or modes and methods of practice of one's peers in the region where one practices may be diluted by said expert testimony. In consequence, the attorneys for both plaintiff and defendant will typically obtain depositions from nationally and/or internationally recognized authorities in a given subspecialty of pathologic practice and, in consequence, disputes arise as to what constitutes the real "standard of care" in any particular malpractice proceeding. Members of the lay public, and even specialist and subspecialist physicians serving on juries at such trials, may find it impossible to assess said testimony appropriately.

The issue of causation of injury by a particular medical error is termed *proximal cause*. In essence, it must be established that the failed standard of care has somehow resulted in a patient injury which would not have been sustained had the purported appropriate care been rendered. The final issue is *damage*, that is, the injury sustained by the patient as a direct result of the error generated by the physician's inability to meet the standard of care. In general terms, all four of the aforementioned issues must be established to be operative by the plaintiff's attorneys or the plaintiff's case will fail. If no injury has been sustained, no intelligent jury will generate an award and no competent attorney will seek a remedy. If an injury has been sustained but cannot be linked to the action of a given physician, the case will be dismissed. The burden of proof upon the plaintiff's attorneys is to show that there is a breach (i.e., negligence), that the negligence was causative of specific damage, and that an injury was sustained. These issues are not absolute and the onus on the plaintiff's attorneys is thus to establish that a preponderance of the evidence implicates the physician as he relates to the patient and that his actions as a professional and the damage sustained in consequence by the patient are linked. In attempting to establish these relationships, the plaintiff's attorneys will produce *relevant evidence*, that is, information intended to prove negligence, causation, and injury. The plaintiff's attorneys cannot present information concerning the record of the defendant, including in the context of previous medicolegal action against him. By contrast, the records of the expert witnesses may be evidentiary.

Only about 1 in 30 calls from patients to legal firms eventuate in a lawsuit,[8] and most of these lawsuits do not generate indemnity payments.[1,11,12] Tort reform, when the result of effective and well-designed legislation, has a tendency to reduce malpractice damage awards and consequently, to reduce the cost of medical malpractice insurance. In particular, those states which have imposed hard caps on noneconomic damages (i.e., pain and suffering of patients and their families) experience a reduction in insurance premiums and also in the number of medical malpractice claims. It has been suggested that attorneys in such states find the financial rewards of malpractice litigation less satisfying and in consequence, are less apt to encourage their clients to litigate.[11,13]

In Canada, a national organization, the Canadian Medical Protective Association (CMPA) insures virtually all physicians in the country, has a strong financial reserve, and repeatedly uses the same limited number of malpractice attorneys in each major center. In consequence, the expertise of defense attorneys is high compared to that of attorneys representing the plaintiff in a typical malpractice lawsuit. The number of medical malpractice claims *per capita* in Canada, along with the size of the indemnity awards, is vastly lower than is seen in the United States. However, owing to the more litigious climate in the United States, CMPA may refuse to insure a Canadian physician involved in a malpractice claim resulting from services rendered to an American citizen.

Nature of Error in Dermatopathologic Practice

In the laboratory, errors can occur in any of the preanalytical, the analytical, or the postanalytical phases. This applies to anatomical as well as to clinical laboratory practice. With respect to anatomical pathology, preanalytical errors include the quality of the biopsy sample (i.e., inadequate size, crush artifact, or choice of a biopsy site that does not adequately represent the lesion), mishandling or mislabeling of a specimen in the gross dissection room, poor technical quality, or loss of the tissue element, prior to its receipt on the desk of the pathologist who will interpret the case. Analytical errors are typically errors of interpretation: The pathologist fails to recognize clues to diagnosis, missing important findings which impact classification or prognosis, or misinterprets specific findings needed to arrive at a correct case construction. Reports which are unequivocal on suboptimal biopsies or which imply certainty where uncertainty exists, and therefore lack caveats concerning the limits of interpretation of the case, are another source of concern. The key question is whether the resulting report generates or, in the hands of a clinician exercising an adequate standard of care, ought to generate appropriate therapy for the patient. Postanalytic errors include, among others, stenographic errors in the report such as key typographical errors, misidentification of site or patient, and the failure to transmit the report to the clinician.

Several different types of neoplastic skin lesions have been the source of medicolegal action. Of these, as mentioned above, melanocytic neoplasms are by far the most common. Glusac describes 'four principles' that underlie this fact.[1] First, melanocytic neoplasms are said to be perhaps the most common neoplasms in human beings. Second, melanoma is, by size, arguably the most lethal human neoplasm. That is, at a similar size of a few millimeters, a cancer of thyroid, breast, or colon is unlikely to even be discovered or, if discovered, is often eminently curable by simple excision. A melanoma a few millimeters in diameter, if in vertical growth phase, may kill.[14] Third, the distinction between melanoma and nevus can be challenging at the light microscopic, and even at the molecular level[15,16] just as it is at the clinical level.[17,18] Various studies have shown that even expert melanocytic lesion pathologists are unable to obtain a concordant view on one-quarter to two-third of studied lesions.[19,20] These figures vary with the subset of melanocytic lesions under discussion, with the particularly treacherous Spitzoid melanomas and atypical Spitz's tumors, generating the least consensus.[21] With respect to the latter, Barnhill et al. demonstrated a lack of consensus among members of an expert panel for 17 of 30 cases; 13 of 21 lesions held to be Spitz tumors metastasized.[21] Another group showed sentinel lymph node parenchymal metastases in 5 of 10 patients with Spitzoid lesions.[22] In our hands and in the experience of others, predicting a malignant phenotype in melanocytic proliferations in childhood is particularly challenging.[23] The fourth consideration is that melanoma, as it is a disease of young as well as old patients, has the potential to cause great loss of life with attendant social and economic disruption for the family members of the deceased, as it results in more lost years of life per case fatality than any other neoplastic disorder, except perhaps leukemia.[1,24]

Underdiagnosis

With respect to the underdiagnosis of melanoma, several factors can increase the risk of such events. First of all, as mentioned above, partial samples of melanocytic tumors may fail to represent the most aggressive morphology in any given lesion.[25] Crush artifact can obscure the morphology and, in the case of heavily inflamed melanocytic proliferations, the inflammatory reaction itself can obscure the cytology of the neoplastic melanocytes. The clinician may choose the wrong area to biopsy; in particular, a pre-existing dysplastic or banal common acquired nevus in the territory of a superimposed melanoma may be the only portion of the lesion sampled. By contrast, areas of whitish discoloration representing regression may be sampled without the accompanying neoplastic melanocytes necessary to establish the histologic diagnosis. Crush and cautery artifact also obscure morphological details.

The second problem in underdiagnosis of melanoma is represented by those melanocytic proliferations which mimic benign nevi. In particular, nevoid melanoma,[26–33] minimal deviation melanoma,[26,34–39] desmoplastic melanoma,[33,40–45] and the atypical spitzoid melanocytic proliferations [21,33] represent special problems in melanocytic tumor pathology.

With respect to the aforementioned specific scenarios, some of them have a repeating theme. The first is that of the nodular melanoma misdiagnosed as a nevus. The clinician will often report a "changing nevus" which by itself may have none of the specific atypical "ABCD" features—that is, asymmetry, irregular border, peculiar or irregular coloration, or large diameter (i.e., greater than 6 mm). In particular, nevoid melanoma and the so-called minimal deviation melanoma both manifest as changing lesions in the setting of pre-existing, often longstanding, melanocytic nevi. We have also seen several cases in childhood of combined nevi or longstanding Spitz tumors undergoing malignant degeneration, including in the context of metastases in sentinel and nonsentinel lymph nodes. As malignant change may be local and focal within a particular neoplasm, step sections are often a useful adjunct in the setting of a changing melanocytic nevus. It is essential, however, that the clinician provides this history with submission of the biopsy. Clinicians are counseled equally to be aware of discordance between their clinical impression and the pathology report.[2] Communication between clinician and pathologist is an essential aspect of patient care and also an important line of defense for them and their patients. Most of us have had the personal experience of a telephone call from an experienced clinician requesting step levels to exclude a melanoma in a pre-existing dysplastic nevus, only to find that, in fact, deeper levels through the block showed a fully developed cancer which was not apparent at the time the report was generated. Of all melanoma claims, it is suggested that over 80% involve shave, punch, or incisional biopsies, while fewer than 20% involve complete excisions.[2] The ideal melanocytic tumor biopsy is one which encompasses the entire lesion plus a 2 to 3 mm margin of adjacent normal skin. If a melanoma is detected and the depth is sufficient to merit sentinel lymph node biopsy, the procedure can still be performed as the lymphatic bed of the neoplasm has not been so perturbed as to produce a disordered pattern of lymphatic drainage. A proper diagnosis facilitated by not only a complete excisional biopsy, but also prognostic microstaging, as described elsewhere in this book, is far more likely to be accurate in a fully excised lesion.

Another frequent medicolegal case scenario is that of a melanoma diagnosed as a dysplastic nevus with positive margins. This is an area which is in flux. Formerly, we did not recommend complete excision of partially excised dysplastic nevi if only mild cytologic and architectural atypia was present.[33] However, most of us have had the experience of a subsequent late recurrence of an incompletely excised, mildly dysplastic nevus and/or progression to melanoma at that location. If a clinician opts not to re-excise a dysplastic nevus with positive margins, the patient must be counseled to promptly report any recurrent or residual pigmented lesion at that location. Clinical follow-up is thus of paramount importance.

The fourth case scenario is that of melanoma misdiagnosed as a Spitz's nevus. Spitz nevi are aneuploid in roughly 25% of cases.[33] Nevi which are aneuploid, and thus biologically unstable, cannot be determined by light microscopy alone. Our practice, therefore, is to advise complete excision of all Spitz's nevi with only rare exceptions. Such exceptions would include those which would require mutilating surgery or functional compromise of anatomical structures, especially in young children. Some dermatologists would dispute this recommendation as being excessive, but most would not argue that any Spitzoid neoplasm in an adult should not be completely excised.

The fifth case scenario is that of the desmoplastic melanoma, misinterpreted clinically and pathologically as a scar or dermatofibroma.

The sixth case scenario is that of a patient who presents with metastatic melanoma of unknown primary site only to recall the removal and discard or destruction of a skin lesion in the past. Any and all pigmented skin lesions removed from a patient should be submitted for histopathological analysis. One could make the argument that pedunculated skin taglike lesions with no suggestion of pigmentation should also be submitted for histology, in light of the danger of missing a verrucous nevoid melanoma.

Owing to the time delay between the underdiagnosis of melanoma and the subsequent recurrence and/or metastatic events and their subsequent evaluation, diagnosis, therapy and outcome, litigation in cases of underdiagnosed melanoma typically takes 3 to 10 years to mature.

Overdiagnosis

The opposite problem is overdiagnosis with excessive therapy; this can include mutilating surgical procedures and/or adjuvant therapy. The latter includes interferon alpha therapy which has potential toxic side effects. The advent of the sentinel lymph node biopsy, which causes little in the way of functional impairment, including in the context of lymphedema, has lessened the impact of unnecessary lymph node dissection in overdiagnosed melanocytic lesions. In consequence, the sentinel lymph node biopsy is held by some observers to have a role in establishing the metastatic potential of any given "borderline" or prognostically indeterminate melanocytic proliferation.[33]

Certain types of lesions are particularly prone to be the source of an overdiagnosis of melanoma. The effect of ultraviolet irradiation on promoting melanocyte activation, and the impact or psoralens and plant products such as in the setting of phytophotodermatitis or psoralen with ultraviolet light (PUVA) therapy are two such pitfalls.[46,47] Another is the histologic appearance of nevi of peculiar anatomic sites (i.e., milk line, flexural, auricular, genital, or acral nevi).[33,48,49] All may generate a histomorphology suspicious for melanoma.[50] Other potential pitfalls for overdiagnosis include the pigmented spindle cell nevus and the combined nevus, including in the context of the deep penetrating nevus. With respect to the deep penetrating/inverted type A nevus and its combined nevus variant, our policy, based upon sobering experience, is to recommend complete excision of such lesions. As overdiagnosis is only detected through peer case review, such events often go unappreciated by the clinician and the patient.

From the standpoint of nonmelanocytic neoplasms which represent a potential medicolegal pitfall, the misclassification of basal cell carcinoma and a failure to recognize infiltrative neoplasms such as microcystic adnexal carcinoma, squamous cell carcinoma (particularly in the case of neurotropism), and atypical intraepithelial proliferations, such as clonal Bowen's disease and porocarcinoma in situ are all potential pitfalls. In addition to the foregoing, inaccurate interpretation of margins has been a source of medicolegal action.

Strategies for the Avoidance of Potentially Litigious Diagnostic Errors

Several caveats flow from the aforementioned considerations. First and foremost, proper and full communication between pathologist and clinician is essential. The pathology requisition must be adequately and accurately documented in terms of the patient's name, age, sex, the site of the biopsy, and the clinical concerns. The "chain of control" of the biopsy from the clinician's office through the courier system to the pathology gross laboratory must be intact and must utilize a verifiable regimen for specimen tracking. The gross laboratory prosector, either the pathologist or the pathologist's assistant, should be fully acquainted with the proper methods of handling and description of specimens. The histopathology laboratory requires equipment which is well maintained to ensure adequate tissue processing. Histotechnologists of experience and capability are necessary to provide good sections. With respect to specimen embedding and paraffin blocks, the pieces of tissue must be close enough together to facilitate good sectioning and also to help ensure that the pathologist does not fail to examine a tissue element.[1] Secondly, if too many tissue elements are incorporated into the tissue cassette prior to paraffin embedding, orientation of the tissue elements by the histotechnologist is compromised and microscopic interpretation becomes more difficult. Similarly, the orientation of the tissue elements to the block face by an experienced histotechnologist will help avoid tangential sections which may compromise interpretation and also make accurate Breslow thickness measurements difficult or impossible. Incomplete sections are problematic not only for margin assessment, but also for evaluation of features essential for the diagnosis of melanoma. Small punch or shave biopsies (i.e., 3 mm in transverse diameter) when embedded as single tissue elements and then sectioned, may not adequately represent a pigmented lesion which presumably is roughly central in the biopsy. Correlation with the clinical impression is, therefore, essential to ensure that if a dysplastic nevus was suspected, appropriate step levels were cut through the block to identify the territory of interest. Curettage biopsies of melanocytic neoplasms are not recommended due to fragmentation and misorientation of the tissue elements.[1] Most of us are familiar with examples of misdiagnosis in curetted melanocytic proliferations.

Even when all of the aforementioned steps are taken correctly and the quality of histotechnology is high, certain cases will prove problematic, even to the most experienced, compulsive, astute, and talented histopathologist. The question arises as to what one ought to do when confronted with a biopsy, which defies precise classification and represents a prognostically indeterminate nevomelanocytic proliferation. Our strategy for the reporting of such prognostically indeterminate nevomelanocytic proliferations has been described elsewhere in some detail.[33] Simply put, our intention is to express our uncertainty about the prognostic attributes of a neoplasm in the pathology report. We believe that the patient is best served when a prognostically indeterminate nevomelanocytic proliferation is treated as though it were melanoma, including in the context of sentinel lymph node biopsy. The latter is a nonmutilating procedure with limited associated morbidity[51] which has been traditionally reserved for melanomas in the 1 to 4 mm depth range, or those tumors less than 1 mm in thickness that show either a vertical growth phase component or substantial regression at the primary site. Unfortunately, no significantly beneficial adjuvant therapy has been demonstrated for melanomas greater than 4 mm in depth or those with distant metastases. The largest series available suggests that completion lymphadenectomy for patients with positive sentinel lymph node deposits produces a statistically significant survival benefit, as opposed to those patients in whom there was a delay for completion lymphadenectomy following a positive sentinel lymph node while clinicians waited for clinically evident lymph node metastases. Our diagnostic strategy, therefore, is to proceed to completion lymphadenectomy when prognostically significant sentinel lymph node deposits are identified in the sentinel lymphadenectomy specimen (see Chapter 5).

Our second strategy is to liberally obtain additional opinions. Obtaining one or more additional opinions of experienced and skilled melanocytic tumor pathologists is a critical component of due diligence. It also shows to the referring clinician and to the patient and his or her family, that an effort has been made in good faith to arrive at the best possible diagnosis. For the most challenging melanocytic proliferations, and in particular, for those in children, we invariably put two or more signatures to the pathology report and frequently seek expert outside consultative opinion.

The more frequent scenario in litigation following underdiagnosis of melanoma is that a lesion with a metastatic potential has been considered to be benign without any equivocation or caveats applied in the pathology report. To prevent such events without a 100% review policy would be impossible. Thus, at Regional Medical Laboratory in Tulsa, Oklahoma, 100% of all anatomic pathology reports with the complete slides from the case are reviewed by a second pathologist and tracked in a complex computerized database. While the turnaround time standard for the primary report ranges from 24 to 48 h, depending upon the nature of the specimen, the turnaround time standard for the review system is currently 72 h. Thus, within a maximum of five business days after receipt of the specimen, two pathologists will have reviewed the case and their opinions will have been recorded in an electronic database. The intent of review is to avoid the complication of underdiagnosis, namely metastatic disease in an unsuspecting patient. Rapid correction of errors with immediate verbal communication to the clinician and the subsequent generation of a revised report documenting both the error and the time and date of the direct notification of the clinician ensue. This form of 100% review is laborious, expensive, and time consuming.[52] Detection of clinically significant diagnostic errors by systems such as this is reported to be in the range of 0.26 to 1.7%.[52–55]

A representative sample of data from a laboratory utilizing a 100% review system is provided in Table 11.1. The data presented covers a period of 54 months from May, 2000 to October, 2004. Of 35,756 reports generated at that facility, significant errors were identified in 25 reports (0.070% of cases). A *significant error* is defined as one which, if left uncorrected, has the potential to generate an adverse patient outcome. *Insignificant errors* constitute those mistakes, such as, for example, typographical miscues that do not alter the substance of the report and which, if corrected, would not alter patient care. The *insignificant error* rate was approximately 2.4 times the *significant error* rate. Not shown in these data and

TABLE 11.1 **Results of Surgical Pathology Review**

	No. of Surgical Reports	No. of Significant Errors	No. of Insignificant Errors
May 2000–Oct 2000	4227	3	9
Nov 2000–April 2001	3965	2	9
May 2001–Oct 2001	4237	3	15
Nov 2001–April 2002	3972	2	–
May 2002–Oct 2002	3969	4	3
Nov 2002–April 2003	3634	2	2
May 2003–Oct 2003	3819	0	0
Nov 2003–April 2004	4068	3	–
May 2004–Oct 2004	3865	6	9
Total	35756	25	47
Significant Error Rate	0.070%		

–Not Recorded.

undefinable in such systems, are those errors which were made in the original surgical pathology report and not detected in the review process.

CONCLUSION

Medical malpractice litigation is a significant factor impacting health care costs, insurance rates, affordability and availability of care in the United States and Canada. Various factors–historic, legal, and financial–make this problem far more serious in the United States. Tort reform has the capacity and potential to alleviate the burden of medicolegal cost to the system and to practitioners, but it is no panacea. A free and honest communication flow between clinician and pathologist, rigorous control of the tissue trail from the clinician's office to the laboratory, comprehensive quality assurance mechanisms in the gross and histopathology laboratories, careful pathological interpretations that recognize the limitations of the art and science which we apply to our discipline, and a comprehensive review system which is open and transparent to clinical practitioners are the best lines of defense in a litigious environment.

ACKNOWLEGMENTS

I am indebted to Dr C.T. Dolan of Regional Medical Laboratory in Tulsa, OK, and Mr R.L. Sewell of Short, Wiggins, Margo and Adler in Oklahoma City for their kindness in reviewing this material.

REFERENCES

1. Glusac EJ. Under the microscope: Doctors, lawyers, and melanocytic neoplasms. *J Cutan Pathol* 2003;30:287–293.
2. Sullivan M. How to protect yourself from melanoma claims. *Skin and Allergy News* 2005;April:24–25.
3. Troxel DB, Sabella JD. Problem areas in pathology practice. Uncovered by a review of malpractice claims. *Am J Surg Pathol* 1994;18:821–831.
4. Forster J, ed. Malpractice survey snapshot: Who's been sued–and who won. *Med Econ* 1999;76:58–60, 65, 69.
5. Epstein JI. Pathologists and the judicial process: How to avoid it. *Am J Surg Pathol* 2001;25:527–537.
6. Altman J. The National Association of Insurance Commissioners (NAIC) medical malpractice closed claim study 1975–1978. *J Am Acad Dermatol* 1981;5:721–725.
7. Jackson R. Malignant melanoma: A review of 75 malpractice cases. *Int J Dermatol* 1997;36:497–498.
8. Gittler GJ, Goldstein EJC. Medicolegal case reviews. *Clin Infect Dis* 1996;23:1152–1155.
9. Martello J. Basic medical legal principles. *Clin Plast Surg* 1999;26:9–14.
10. Petrek FR Jr, Slovis MR, Esq. The defendant in a medical malpractice suit: An integral part of the defense team. *Pediatr Radiol* 1998;28:905–912.
11. Ellington DP, Rosenthal RS. The defense perspective. *Med Malpractice* 1997;94:323–327.
12. Moran T. So you've been sued. Tips for enduring and avoiding the malpractice roller coaster ride. *Tex Med* 1995;91:24–31.
13. Zuckerman S, Bovbjerg RR, Sloan F. Effects of tort reforms and other factors on medical malpractice insurance premiums. *Inquiry* 1990;27:167–182.
14. Clark WH Jr, Elder DE, Van Horn M. The biologic forms of malignant melanoma. *Hum Pathol* 1986;17:443–450.
15. Piepkorn M, Odland PB. Quality of care in the diagnosis of melanoma and related melanocytic lesions. *Arch Dermatol* 1997;133:1393–1396.
16. Smith KJ, Barrett TL, Skelton HG. Spindle cell and epithelioid cell nevi with atypia and metastasis (malignant Spitz nevus). *Am J Surg Pathol* 1989;13:931–939.
17. Grant-Kels JM, Bason ET, Grin CM. The misdiagnosis of malignant melanoma. *J Am Acad Dermatol* 1999;40:539–548.
18. Andersen WK, Silvers DN. 'Melanoma? It can't be melanoma!' A subset of melanomas that defies clinical recognition. *JAMA* 1991;266:3463–3465.
19. Farmer ER, Gonin R, Hanna MP. Discordance in the histopathologic diagnosis of melanoma and melanocytic neoplasms between expert pathologists. *Hum Pathol* 1996; 27:528–531.
20. Corona R, Mele A, Amini M, et al. Interobserver variability on the histopathologic diagnosis of cutaneous melanoma and other pigmented skin lesions. *J Clin Oncol* 1996;14:1218–1223.
21. Barnhill RL, Argenyi ZB, From L, et al. Atypical Spitz Nevi/tumors; lack of consensus for diagnosis, discrimination from melanoma, and prediction of outcome. *Hum Pathol* 1999;30:513–520.
22. Lohmann CM, Coit DG, Brady MS, et al. Sentinel lymph node biopsy in patients with diagnostically controversial spitzoid melanocytic tumors. *Am J Surg Pathol* 2002;26:47–55.
23. Wechsler J, Bastuji-Garin S, Spatz A, et al. Reliability of the histopathologic diagnosis of malignant melanoma in childhood. *Arch Dermatol* 2002;138:625–628.
24. Albert VA, Koh HK, Geller AC, et al. Years of potential life lost: Another indicator of the impact of cutaneous malignant melanoma on society. *J Am Acad Dermatol* 1990; 23:308–310.

25. Troxel DB. Diagnostic errors in surgical pathology uncovered by a review of malpractice claims. Part IV. Melanoma. *Int J Surg Pathol* 2001;9(1):61–63.
26. Philips ME, Margolis RJ, Merot Y, et al. The spectrum of minimal deviation melanoma: A clinicopathologic study of 21 cases. *Hum Pathol* 1986;17:796–806.
27. Suster S, Ronnen M, Bubis JJ. Verrucous pseudonevoid melanoma. *J Surg Oncol* 1987; 36:134–137.
28. Wong TY, Duncan LM, Mihm MC Jr. Melanoma mimicking dermal and Spitz's nevus ("nevoid melanoma"). *Semin Surg Oncol* 1993;9:188–193.
29. McNutt NS, Urmacher C, Hakimian J, et al. Nevoid malignant melanoma: Morphologic patterns an immunohistochemical reactivity. *J Cutan Pathol* 1995;22:502–517.
30. Wong TY, Suster S, Duncan LM, Mihm MC Jr. Nevoid melanoma: A clinicopathological study of seven cases of malignant melanoma mimicking spindle and epithelioid cell nevus and verrucous dermal nevus. *Hum Pathol* 1995;26:171–179.
31. Kossard S, Wilkinson B. Small cell (naevoid) melanoma: A clinicopathologic study of 131 cases. *Australas J Dermatol* 1997;38(Suppl. 1): S54–S58.
32. Blessing K, Grant JJ, Sanders DS, et al. Small cell malignant melanoma: A variant of naevoid melanoma. Clinicopathological features and histological differential diagnosis. *J Clin Pathol* 2000; 53:591–595.
33. Crowson AN, Magro CM, Mihm MC Jr. The melanocytic proliferations: A comprehensive textbook of pigmented lesions. New York: John Wiley and Sons; 2001:281–397.
34. Muhlbauer J, Margolis R, Mihm MC, Reed R. Minimal deviation melanoma: A histologic variant of cutaneous malignant melanoma in vertical growth phase. *J Invest Dermatol* 1983;80:63s–65s.
35. Philips ME, Margolis RJ, Merot Y, et al. Common and uncommon melanocytic nevi and borderline melanomas. *Semin Oncol* 1975;2:119–147.
36. Reed RJ. Minimal deviation melanoma. *Hum Pathol* 1990;21:1206–1211.
37. Reed RJ, Martin P. Variants of melanoma. *Semin Cutan Med Surg* 1997;16:137–158.
38. Reed RJ. Minimal deviation melanoma. Borderline and intermediate melanocytic neoplasia. *Clin Lab Med* 2000;20:745–758.
39. Podnos YD, Jimenez JC, Zainabadi K, et al. Minimal deviation melanoma. *Cancer Treat Rep* 2002;28:219–221.
40. Conley J, Lattes R, Orr W. Desmoplastic malignant melanoma (a rare variant of spindle cell melanoma). *Cancer* 1971;28:914–936.
41. Bruijn JA, Mihm MC Jr, Barnhill RL. Desmoplastic melanoma. *Histopathology* 1992; 20:197–205.
42. Skelton HG, Smith KJ, Laskin WB, et al. Desmoplastic malignant melanoma. *J Am Acad Dermatol* 1995;32:717–725.
43. Carlson JA, Dickersin GR, Sober AJ, Barnhill RL. Desmoplastic neurotropic melanoma. A clinicopathologic analysis of 28 cases. *Cancer* 1995;75:478–494.
44. Egbert B, Kempson R, Sagebiel. Desmoplastic malignant melanoma. A clinicopathologic study of 25 cases. *Cancer* 1988;62:2033–2041.
45. LeBoit PE, Ming ME. Litigious melanocytic proliferations and how to avoid them. *Pathol Case Rev* 1999;4:77–86.
46. Tronnier M, Wolff HH. UV-irradiated melanocytic nevi simulating melanoma in situ. *Am J Dermatopathol* 1995; 17:1–6.
47. Somach SC, Taira JW, Patha JV, et al. Pigmented lesions in actinically damaged skin. Histopathologic comparison of biopsy and excisional specimens. *Arch Dermatol* 1996; 132:1297–1302.
48. LeBoit PE. A diagnosis for maniacs. *Am J Dermatopathol* 2000;22:556–558.

49. Rongioletti F, Ball RA, Marcus R, Barnhill RL. Histopathological features of flexural melanocytic nevi: A study of 40 cases. *J Cutan Pathol* 2000; 27:215–217.

50. Kerl H. Pseudomelanomas: Pitfalls in the diagnosis of malignant melanoma. *Am J Dermatopathol* 1992; 14:75.

51. Morton DL, Cochran AL, Thompson JF, et al. Sentinel node biopsy for early-stage melanoma. *Ann Surg* 2005;242:302–313.

52. Safrin R, Bark C. Surgical Pathology Signout. Routing review of every case by a second pathologist. *Am J Surg Pathol* 1994;17:1190–1192.

53. Lind A, Bewtra C, Healy JC, et al. Prospective peer review in surgical pathology. *Am J Clin Pathol* 1995;104:560–566.

54. Abt A, Abt L. The effect of interinstitutional anatomic pathology consultation on patient care. *Arch Pathol Lab Med* 1995;119:514–517.

55. Wakely S, Baxendine-Jones J, Gallagher PJ, et al. Aberrant diagnoses by individual surgical pathologists. *Am J Surg Pathol* 1998;22:77–82.

INDEX

Page numbers in *italics* denote figures; those followed by a "t" denote tables.

N